CONTENTS

ADDITIONAL SUMMARIES AND EVALUATIONS OF EVIDENCE FOR CARCINOGENICITY IN EXPERIMENTAL ANIMALS, AND SUMMARIES OF OTHER RELEVANT DATA, FOR SELECTED AGENTS FOR WHICH THERE ARE NO DATA ON CARCINOGENICITY IN HUMANS

NOTE TO THE READER

The term 'carcinogenic risk' in the *IARC Monographs* series is taken to mean the probability that exposure to an agent will lead to cancer in humans.

Inclusion of an agent in the *Monographs* does not imply that it is a carcinogen, only that the published data have been examined. Equally, the fact that an agent has not yet been evaluated in a monograph does not mean that it is not carcinogenic.

The evaluations of carcinogenic risk are made by international working groups of independent scientists and are qualitative in nature. No recommendation is given for regulation or legislation.

Anyone who is aware of published data that may alter the evaluation of the carcinogenic risk of an agent to humans is encouraged to make this information available to the Unit of Carcinogen Identification and Evaluation, International Agency for Research on Cancer, 150 cours Albert Thomas, 69372 Lyon Cedex 08, France, in order that the agent may be considered for re-evaluation by a future Working Group.

Although every effort is made to prepare the monographs as accurately as possible, mistakes may occur. Readers are requested to communicate any errors to the Unit of Carcinogen Identification and Evaluation, so that corrections can be reported in future volumes.

IARC WORKING GROUP ON THE EVALUATION OF CARCINOGENIC RISKS TO HUMANS: OVERALL EVALUATIONS OF CARCINOGENICITY: AN UPDATING OF *IARC MONOGRAPHS* VOLUMES 1-42

Lyon, 10-18 March 1987

LIST OF PARTICIPANTS

Members[1]

O. Axelson, Department of Occupational Medicine and Industrial Ergonomics, University Hospital, 581 85 Linköping, Sweden

P. Bannasch, Abteilung für Cytopathologie, Deutches Krebsforschungszentrum, Postfach, 6900 Heidelberg 1, Federal Republic of Germany

P.A. Bertazzi, Institute of Occupational Health, Clinica del Lavoro 'Luigi Devoto', University of Milan, via S. Barnaba 8, 20122 Milan, Italy

A. Blair, Environmental Epidemiology Branch, National Cancer Institute, Room 4C-16, Landow Building, Bethesda, MD 20892, USA

A.L. Brown, Medical School, University of Wisconsin-Madison, 1205 Medical Sciences Center, 1300 University Avenue, Madison, WI 53706, USA (*Chairman*)

A.I. Bykorez, Institute for Oncology Problems, Vasilkovskaya str. 45, 252 127 Kiev, USSR

I.N. Chernozemsky, Cancer Cell and Molecular Biology Group, Darvenitza, Sofia 1156, Bulgaria

G. Della Porta, Division of Experimental Oncology A, Istituto Nazionale per lo Studio e la Cura dei Tumori, via Venezian 1, 20133 Milan, Italy

H.J. Evans, MRC Clinical and Population Cytogenetics Unit, Western General Hospital, Crewe Road, Edinburgh EH4 2XU, UK

---

[1]Unable to attend: B.K. Armstrong, NH & MRC Research Unit in Epidemiology and Preventive Medicine, University Department of Medicine, The Queen Elizabeth II Medical Centre, Nedlands, Western Australia 6009, Australia

R.A. Griesemer, Biology Division, Oak Ridge National Laboratory, PO Box Y, Oak Ridge, TN 37830, USA

J.M. Harrington, Institute of Occupational Health, University of Birmingham, PO Box 363, Birmingham B15 2TT, UK

K. Hemminki, Institute of Occupational Health, Topeliuksenkatu 41 a A, 00250 Helsinki, Finland

S. Hernberg, Institute of Occupational Health, Topeliuksenkatu 41 a A, 00250 Helsinki, Finland

K. Hooper, Hazard Evaluation System and Information Services (HESIS), Department of Health Services/Department of Industrial Relations, 2151 Berkeley Way, Berkeley, CA 94704, USA

N. Ito, First Department of Pathology, Nagoya City University Medical School, 1 Kawasumi, Mizuho-cho, Mizuho-ku, Nagoya 467, Japan

D.G. Kaufman, Department of Pathology, School of Medicine, University of North Carolina, Chapel Hill, NC 27514, USA

R. Kroes, National Institute of Public Health and Environment, PO Box 1, 3720 BA Bilthoven, The Netherlands

T.M. Mack, Department of Preventive Medicine, University of Southern California, 2025 Zonal Avenue, Los Angeles, CA 90033, USA

E.E. McConnell, Toxicology Research and Testing Program, National Institute of Environmental Health Sciences, PO Box 12233, Research Triangle Park, NC 27709, USA

A.B. Miller, Department of Preventive Medicine and Biostatistics, Faculty of Medicine, McMurrich Building, University of Toronto, Toronto, Ontario M5S 1A8, Canada (*Vice-Chairman*)

M.C. Pike, Imperial Cancer Research Fund, Radcliffe Infirmary, Oxford OX2 6HE, UK

A. Pinter, Department of Morphology, National Institute of Hygiene, Gyali ut 2-6, 1966 Budapest, Hungary

D.B. Thomas, Program in Epidemiology, Fred Hutchinson Cancer Research Center, 1124 Columbia Street, Seattle, WA 98104, USA

I.B. Weinstein, College of Physicians and Surgeons, Columbia University Cancer Center, Institute of Cancer Research, 701 West 168th Street, New York, NY 10032, USA

G.M. Williams, Division of Pathology and Toxicology, American Health Foundation and New York Medical College, 1 Dana Road, Valhalla, NY 10595, USA

Representatives and observers

Representative of the National Cancer Institute
S.M. Sieber, Division of Cancer Etiology, National Cancer Institute, Building 31, Room 11A03, Bethesda, MD 20892, USA

Representatives of the Commission of the European Communities

A. Berlin, Commission of the European Communities, Health and Safety Directorate, Bâtiment Jean Monnet, Plateau du Kirchberg, BP 1907, 2920 Luxembourg, Grand Duchy of Luxembourg (14-18 March)

M. Repetto, Istituto Nacional de Toxicologia, Carretera San Geronimo, Apartado Postal 863, Seville 41080, Spain

M.-Th. van der Venne, Commission of the European Communities, Health and Safety Directorate, Bâtiment Jean Monnet, Plateau du Kirchberg, BP 1907, 2920 Luxembourg, Grand Duchy of Luxembourg (10-13 March)

Representative of the International Programme on Chemical Safety, World Health Organization

G.C. Becking, World Health Organization, Interregional Research Unit, MD A206, PO Box 12233, Research Triangle Park, NC 27709, USA

Representative of the Institute of Medical Science, University of Tokyo, Japan

T. Matsushima, Department of Molecular Oncology, Institute of Medical Science, University of Tokyo, 4-6-1 Shirokonedai, Minato-ku, Tokyo 108, Japan

Representative of the National Institute for Occupational Safety and Health

T.J. Meinhardt, Division of Standard Development and Technology Transfer, National Institute for Occupational Safety and Health, 4676 Columbia Parkway, Cincinnati, OH 45226, USA

Representative of the American Petroleum Institute

R.A. Scala, Exxon Biomedical Sciences, Inc., Mettlers Road, PO Box 235, East Millstone, NJ 08873, USA

Representative of the Chemical Manufacturers' Association

R.J. Mollenaar, Dow Chemical Company, 1803 Building, Midland, MI 48640, USA

Representative of the European Chemical Industry Ecology and Toxicology Centre

M. Sharratt, BP Group Occupational Health Centre, 10 Occam Road, Surrey Research Park, Guildford, Surrey GU2 5YQ, UK

Secretariat

A. Aitio, Unit of Carcinogen Identification and Evaluation
H. Bartsch, Unit of Environmental Carcinogens and Host Factors
J.R.P. Cabral, Unit of Mechanisms of Carcinogenesis
E. Cardis, Unit of Biostatistics Research and Informatics
M. Friesen, Unit of Environmental Carcinogens and Host Factors
M.-J. Ghess, Unit of Carcinogen Identification and Evaluation

L. Haroun[1], Unit of Carcinogen Identification and Evaluation (*Co-Secretary*)

E. Heseltine, Lajarthe, 24290 Montignac, France

J. Estève, Unit of Biostatistics Research and Informatics

J. Kaldor, Unit of Biostatistics Research and Informatics

D. Mietton, Unit of Carcinogen Identification and Evaluation

R. Montesano, Unit of Mechanisms of Carcinogenesis

I. O'Neill, Unit of Environmental Carcinogens and Host Factors

C. Partensky, Unit of Carcinogen Identification and Evaluation

I. Peterschmitt, Unit of Carcinogen Identification and Evaluation, Geneva, Switzerland

R. Saracci, Unit of Analytical Epidemiology

L. Shuker, Unit of Carcinogen Identification and Evaluation (*Co-Secretary*)

L. Simonato, Unit of Analytical Epidemiology

L. Tomatis, Director

A. Tossavainen[2], Unit of Carcinogen Identification and Evaluation

V. Turusov, Office of the Director

H. Vainio[2], Unit of Carcinogen Identification and Evaluation (*Head of the programme*)

J.D. Wilbourn, Unit of Carcinogen Identification and Evaluation

H. Yamasaki, Unit of Mechanisms of Carcinogenesis

Secretarial assistance

J. Cazeaux

M. Lézère

S. Reynaud

---

[1]Present address: 29 South Sixth Avenue, La Grange, IL 60525, USA

[2]Present address: Institute of Occupational Health, Topeliuksenkatu 41 a A, 00250 Helsinki, Finland

IARC MONOGRAPHS PROGRAMME ON THE EVALUATION OF CARCINOGENIC RISKS TO HUMANS[1]

PREAMBLE

1. BACKGROUND

In 1969, the International Agency for Research on Cancer (IARC) initiated a programme to evaluate the carcinogenic risk of chemicals to humans and to produce monographs on individual chemicals. The *Monographs* programme has since been expanded to include consideration of exposures to complex mixtures of chemicals (which occur, for example, in some occupations and as a result of human habits) and of exposures to other agents, such as radiation and viruses. With Supplement 6, the title of the series was modified from *IARC Monographs on the Evaluation of the Carcinogenic Risk of Chemicals to Humans* to *IARC Monographs on the Evaluation of Carcinogenic Risks to Humans*, in order to reflect the widened scope of the programme.

The criteria established in 1971 to evaluate carcinogenic risk to humans were adopted by the working groups whose deliberations resulted in the first 16 volumes of the *IARC Monographs* series. Those criteria were subsequently re-evaluated by working groups which met in 1977(1), 1978(2), 1979(3), 1982(4) and 1983(5). The present preamble was prepared by a Working Group which met in September 1986.

2. OBJECTIVE AND SCOPE

The objective of the programme is to prepare, with the help of international working groups of experts, and to publish in the form of monographs, critical reviews and evaluations of evidence on the carcinogenicity of a wide range of agents to which humans are or may be exposed. The *Monographs* may also indicate where additional research efforts are needed.

[1]This project is supported by PHS Grant No. 5 UO1 CA33193-05 awarded by the US National Cancer Institute, Department of Health and Human Services, and with a subcontract to Tracor Jitco, Inc. and Technical Resources, Inc. Since 1986, this programme has also been supported by the Commission of the European Communities.

The *Monographs* represent the first step in carcinogenic risk assessment, which involves examination of all relevant information in order to assess the strength of the available evidence that, under certain conditions of exposure, an agent could alter the incidence of cancer in humans. The second step is quantitative risk estimation, which is not usually attempted in the *Monographs*. Detailed, quantitative evaluations of epidemiological data may be made in the *Monographs*, but without extrapolation beyond the range of the data available. Quantitative extrapolation from experimental data to the human situation is not undertaken.

These monographs may assist national and international authorities in making risk assessments and in formulating decisions concerning any necessary preventive measures. **No recommendation is given for regulation or legislation, since such decisions are made by individual governments and/or other international agencies.** The *IARC Monographs* are recognized as an authoritative source of information on the carcinogenicity of chemicals and complex exposures. A users' survey, made in 1984, indicated that the *Monographs* are consulted by various agencies in 45 countries. Each volume is printed in 4000 copies for distribution to governments, regulatory bodies and interested scientists. The *Monographs* are also available *via* the Distribution and Sales Service of the World Health Organization.

3. SELECTION OF TOPICS FOR MONOGRAPHS

Topics are selected on the basis of two main criteria: (a) that they concern agents for which there is evidence of human exposure, and (b) there is some evidence or suspicion of carcinogenicity. The term agent is used to include individual chemical compounds, groups of chemical compounds, physical agents (such as radiation), biological factors (such as viruses) and mixtures of agents such as occur in occupational exposures and as a result of personal and cultural habits (like smoking and dietary practices). Chemical analogues and compounds with biological or physical characteristics similar to those of suspected carcinogens may also be considered, even in the absence of data on carcinogenicity.

The scientific literature is surveyed for published data relevant to an assessment of carcinogenicity; the IARC surveys of chemicals being tested for carcinogenicity[6] and directories of on-going research in cancer epidemiology[7] often indicate those agents that may be scheduled for future meetings. An ad-hoc working group convened by IARC in 1984 gave recommendations as to which chemicals and exposures to complex mixtures should be evaluated in the *IARC Monographs* series[8].

As significant new data on subjects on which monographs have already been prepared become available, re-evaluations are made at subsequent meetings, and revised monographs are published.

4. DATA FOR MONOGRAPHS

The *Monographs* do not necessarily cite all of the literature on a particular agent. Only those data considered by the Working Group to be relevant to making an evaluation are included.

With regard to biological and epidemiological data, only reports that have been published or accepted for publication in the openly available scientific literature are reviewed by the working groups. In certain instances, government agency reports that have undergone peer review and are widely available are considered. Exceptions may be made on an ad-hoc basis to include unpublished reports that are in their final form and publicly available, if their inclusion is considered pertinent to making a final evaluation (see p. 29 *et seq.*). In the sections on chemical and physical properties and on production, use, occurrence and analysis, unpublished sources of information may be used.

5. THE WORKING GROUP

Reviews and evaluations are formulated by a working group of experts. The tasks of this group are five-fold: (i) to ascertain that all appropriate data have been collected; (ii) to select the data relevant for the evaluation on the basis of scientific merit; (iii) to prepare accurate summaries of the data to enable the reader to follow the reasoning of the Working Group; (iv) to evaluate the results of experimental and epidemiological studies; and (v) to make an overall evaluation of the carcinogenicity of the agent to humans.

Working Group participants who contributed to the consideration and evaluation of the agents within a particular volume are listed, with their addresses, at the beginning of each publication. Each participant who is a member of a working group serves as an individual scientist and not as a representative of any organization, government or industry. In addition, representatives from national and international agencies and industrial associations are invited as observers.

6. WORKING PROCEDURES

Approximately one year in advance of a meeting of a working group, the agents to be evaluated are announced and participants are selected by IARC staff in consultation with other experts. Subsequently, relevant biological and epidemiological data are collected by IARC from recognized sources of information on carcinogenesis, including data storage and retrieval systems such as CANCERLINE, MEDLINE and TOXLINE. Bibliographical sources for data on genetic and related effects and on teratogenicity are the Environmental Mutagen Information Center and the Environmental Teratology Information Center, both located at the Oak Ridge National Laboratory, USA.

The major collection of data and the preparation of first drafts of the sections on chemical and physical properties, on production and use, on occurrence, and on analysis are carried out under a separate contract funded by the US National Cancer Institute. Efforts are made to supplement this information with data from other national and international sources. Representatives from industrial associations may assist in the preparation of sections on production and use.

Production and trade data are obtained from governmental and trade publications and, in some cases, by direct contact with industries. Separate production data on some agents may not be available because their publication could disclose confidential information.

Information on uses is usually obtained from published sources but is often complemented by direct contact with manufacturers.

Six months before the meeting, reference material is sent to experts, or is used by IARC staff, to prepare sections for the first drafts of monographs. The complete first drafts are compiled by IARC staff and sent, prior to the meeting, to all participants of the Working Group for review.

The Working Group meets in Lyon for seven to eight days to discuss and finalize the texts of the monographs and to formulate the evaluations. After the meeting, the master copy of each monograph is verified by consulting the original literature, edited and prepared for publication. The aim is to publish monographs within nine months of the Working Group meeting.

7. EXPOSURE DATA

Sections that indicate the extent of past and present human exposure, the sources of exposure, the persons most likely to be exposed and the factors that contribute to exposure to the agent under study are included at the beginning of each monograph.

Most monographs on individual chemicals or complex mixtures include sections on chemical and physical data, and production, use, occurrence and analysis. In other monographs, for example on physical agents, biological factors, occupational exposures and cultural habits, other sections may be included, such as: historical perspectives, description of an industry or habit, exposures in the workplace or chemistry of the complex mixture.

The Chemical Abstracts Services Registry Number, the latest Chemical Abstracts Primary Name and the IUPAC Systematic Name are recorded. Other synonyms and trade names are given, but the list is not necessarily comprehensive. Some of the trade names may be those of mixtures in which the agent being evaluated is only one of the ingredients.

Information on chemical and physical properties and, in particular, data relevant to identification, occurrence and biological activity are included. A separate description of technical products gives relevant specifications and includes available information on composition and impurities.

The dates of first synthesis and of first commercial production of an agent are provided; for agents which do not occur naturally, this information may allow a reasonable estimate to be made of the date before which no human exposure to the agent could have occurred. The dates of first reported occurrence of an exposure are also provided. In addition, methods of synthesis used in past and present commercial production and different methods of production which may give rise to different impurities are described.

Data on production, foreign trade and uses are obtained for representative regions, which usually include Europe, Japan and the USA. It should not, however, be inferred that those areas or nations are necessarily the sole or major sources or users of the agent being evaluated.

Some identified uses may not be current or major applications, and the coverage is not necessarily comprehensive. In the case of drugs, mention of their therapeutic uses does not necessarily represent current practice nor does it imply judgement as to their clinical efficacy.

Information on the occurrence of an agent in the environment is obtained from data derived from the monitoring and surveillance of levels in occupational environments, air, water, soil, foods and animal and human tissues. When available, data on the generation, persistence and bioaccumulation of the agent are also included.

Statements concerning regulations and guidelines (e.g., pesticide registrations, maximal levels permitted in foods, occupational exposure limits) are included for some countries as indications of potential exposures, but they may not reflect the most recent situation, since such limits are continuously reviewed and modified. The absence of information on regulatory status for a country should not be taken to imply that that country does not have regulations with regard to the agent.

The purpose of the section on analysis is to give the reader an overview of current methods cited in the literature, with emphasis on those widely used for regulatory purposes. No critical evaluation or recommendation of any of the methods is meant or implied. Methods for monitoring human exposure are also given, when available. The IARC publishes a series of volumes, *Environmental Carcinogens: Selected Methods of Analysis*(9), that describe validated methods for analysing a wide variety of agents.

8. BIOLOGICAL DATA RELEVANT TO THE EVALUATION OF CARCINOGENICITY TO HUMANS

The term 'carcinogen' is used in these monographs to denote an agent that is capable of increasing the incidence of malignant neoplasms; the induction of benign neoplasms may in some circumstances (see p. 23) contribute to the judgement that an agent is carcinogenic. The terms 'neoplasm' and 'tumour' are used interchangeably.

Some epidemiological and experimental studies indicate that different agents may act at different stages in the carcinogenic process, probably by fundamentally different mechanisms. In the present state of knowledge, the aim of the *Monographs* is to evaluate evidence of carcinogenicity at any stage in the carcinogenic process independently of the underlying mechanism involved. There is as yet insufficient information to implement a classification of agents according to their mechanism of action(5).

Definitive evidence of carcinogenicity in humans is provided by epidemiological studies. Evidence relevant to human carcinogenicity may also be provided by experimental studies of carcinogenicity in animals and by other biological data, particularly those relating to humans.

The available studies are summarized by the working groups, with particular regard to the qualitative aspects discussed below. In general, numerical findings are indicated as they appear in the original report; units are converted when necessary for easier comparison. The Working Group may conduct additional analyses of the published data and use them in their assessment of the evidence and may include them in their summary of a study; the results of such supplementary analyses are given in square brackets. Any comments are also made in square brackets; however, these are kept to a minimum, being restricted to those instances in which it is felt that an important aspect of a study, directly impinging on its interpretation, should be brought to the attention of the reader.

9. EVIDENCE FOR CARCINOGENICITY IN EXPERIMENTAL ANIMALS

For several agents (e.g., 4-aminobiphenyl, bis(chloromethyl)ether, diethylstilboestrol, melphalan, 8-methoxypsoralen(methoxsalen) plus UVR, mustard gas and vinyl chloride), evidence of carcinogenicity in experimental animals preceded evidence obtained from epidemiological studies or case reports. Information compiled from the first 41 volumes of the *IARC Monographs*(10) shows that, of the 44 agents for which there is *sufficient* or *limited evidence* of carcinogenicity to humans (see p. 30), all 37 that have been tested adequately experimentally produce cancer in at least one animal species. Although this association cannot establish that all agents that cause cancer in experimental animals also cause cancer in humans, nevertheless, **in the absence of adequate data on humans, it is biologically plausible and prudent to regard agents for which there is** *sufficient evidence* **(see p. 30) of carcinogenicity in experimental animals as if they presented a carcinogenic risk to humans**.

The monographs are not intended to summarize all published studies. Those that are inadequate (e.g., too short a duration, too few animals, poor survival; see below) or are judged irrelevant to the evaluation are generally omitted. They may be mentioned briefly, particularly when the information is considered to be a useful supplement to that of other reports or when they provide the only data available. Their inclusion does not, however, imply acceptance of the adequacy of the experimental design or of the analysis and interpretation of their results. Guidelines for adequate long-term carcinogenicity experiments have been outlined(e.g., 11).

The nature and extent of impurities or contaminants present in the agent being evaluated are given when available. Mention is made of all routes of exposure by which the agent has been adequately studied and of all species in which relevant experiments have been performed. Animal strain, sex, numbers per group, age at start of treatment and survival are reported.

Experiments in which the agent was administered in conjunction with known carcinogens or factors that modify carcinogenic effects are also reported. Experiments on the carcinogenicity of known metabolites and derivatives may be included.

(a) Qualitative aspects

The overall assessment of the carcinogenicity of an agent involves several considerations of qualitative importance, including (i) the experimental conditions under which the test was performed, including route and schedule of exposure, species, strain, sex, age, duration of follow-up; (ii) the consistency with which the agent has been shown to be carcinogenic, e.g., in how many species and at which target organs(s); (iii) the spectrum of neoplastic response, from benign tumours to malignant neoplasms; and (iv) the possible role of modifying factors.

Considerations of importance to the Working Group in the interpretation and evaluation of a particular study include: (i) how clearly the agent was defined; (ii) whether the dose was adequately monitored, particularly in inhalation experiments; (iii) whether the doses used were appropriate and whether the survival of treated animals was similar to that of controls; (iv) whether there were adequate numbers of animals per group; (v) whether animals of both sexes were used; (vi) whether animals were allocated randomly to groups; (vii) whether the duration of observation was adequate; and (viii) whether the data were adequately reported. If available, recent data on the incidence of specific tumours in historical controls, as well as in concurrent controls, should be taken into account in the evaluation of tumour response.

When benign tumours occur together with and originate from the same cell type in an organ or tissue as malignant tumours in a particular study and appear to represent a stage in the progression to malignancy, it may be valid to combine them in assessing tumour incidence. The occurrence of lesions presumed to be preneoplastic may in certain instances aid in assessing the biological plausibility of any neoplastic response observed.

Among the many agents that have been studied extensively, there are few instances in which the only neoplasms induced were benign. Benign tumours in experimental animals frequently represent a stage in the evolution of a malignant neoplasm, but they may be 'endpoints' that do not readily undergo transition to malignancy. However, if an agent is found to induce only benign neoplasms, it should be suspected of being a carcinogen and it requires further investigation.

(b) Quantitative aspects

The probability that tumours will occur may depend on the species and strain, the dose of the carcinogen and the route and period of exposure. Evidence of an increased incidence of neoplasms with increased exposure strengthens the inference of a causal association between exposure to the agent and the development of neoplasms.

The form of the dose-response relationship can vary widely, depending on the particular agent under study and the target organ. Since many chemicals require metabolic activation before being converted into their reactive intermediates, both metabolic and pharmaco-kinetic aspects are important in determining the dose-response pattern. Saturation of steps such as absorption, activation, inactivation and elimination of the carcinogen may produce nonlinearity in the dose-response relationship, as could saturation of processes such as DNA repair(12,13).

(c) Statistical analysis of long-term experiments in animals

Factors considered by the Working Group include the adequacy of the information given for each treatment group: (i) the number of animals on study and the number examined histologically, (ii) the number of animals with a given tumour type and (iii) length of survival. The statistical methods used should be clearly stated and should be the generally accepted techniques refined for this purpose(13,14). When there is no difference in survival between control and treatment groups, the Working Group usually compares the proportions of animals developing each tumour type in each of the groups. Otherwise, consideration is given as to whether or not appropriate adjustments have been made for differences in survival. These adjustments can include: comparisons of the proportions of tumour-bearing animals among the 'effective number' of animals alive at the time the first tumour is discovered, in the case where most differences in survival occur before tumours appear; life-table methods, when tumours are visible or when they may be considered 'fatal' because mortality rapidly follows tumour development; and the Mantel-Haenszel test or logistic regression, when occult tumours do not affect the animals' risk of dying but are 'incidental' findings at autopsy.

In practice, classifying tumours as fatal or incidental may be difficult. Several survival-adjusted methods have been developed that do not require this distinction(13), although they have not been fully evaluated.

10. OTHER RELEVANT DATA IN EXPERIMENTAL SYSTEMS AND HUMANS

(a) Structure-activity considerations

This section describes structure-activity correlations that are relevant to an evaluation of the carcinogenicity of an agent.

(b) Absorption, distribution, excretion and metabolism

Concise information is given on absorption, distribution (including placental transfer) and excretion. Kinetic factors that may affect the dose-reponse relationship, such as saturation of uptake, protein binding, metabolic activation, detoxification and DNA-repair processes, are mentioned. Studies that indicate the metabolic fate of the agent in experimental animals and humans are summarized briefly, and comparisons of data from animals and humans are made when possible. Comparative information on the relationship between exposure and the dose that reaches the target site may be of particular importance for extrapolation between species.

(c) Toxicity

Data are given on acute and chronic toxic effects (other than cancer), such as organ toxicity, immunotoxicity, endocrine effects and preneoplastic lesions. Effects on reproduction, teratogenicity, feto- and embryotoxicity are also summarized briefly.

(d) Genetic and related effects

Tests of genetic and related effects may indicate possible carcinogenic activity. They can also be used in detecting active metabolites of known carcinogens in human or animal body fluids, in detecting active components in complex mixtures and in the elucidation of possible mechanisms of carcinogenesis.

The available data are interpreted critically by phylogenetic group according to the endpoints detected, which may include DNA damage, gene mutation, sister chromatid exchange, micronuclei, chromosomal aberrations, aneuploidy and cell transformation. The concentrations (doses) employed are given and mention is made of whether an exogenous metabolic system was required. When appropriate, these data may be represented by bar graphs (activity profiles), with corresponding summary tables and listings of test systems, data and references. Detailed information on the preparation of these profiles is given in an appendix to those volumes in which they are used.

Positive results in tests using prokaryotes, lower eukaryotes, plants, insects and cultured mammalian cells suggest that genetic and related effects (and therefore possibly carcinogenic effects) could occur in mammals. Results from such tests may also give information about the types of genetic effects produced by an agent and about the involvement of metabolic activation. Some endpoints described are clearly genetic in nature (e.g., gene mutations and chromosomal aberrations), others are to a greater or lesser degree associated with genetic effects (e.g., unscheduled DNA synthesis). In-vitro tests for tumour-promoting activity and for cell transformation may detect changes that are not necessarily the result of genetic alterations but that may have specific relevance to the process of carcinogenesis. A critical appraisal of these tests has been published(11).

Genetic or other activity detected in the systems mentioned above is not always manifest in whole mammals. Positive indications of genetic effects in experimental mammals and in humans are regarded as being of greater relevance than those in other organisms. The demonstration that an agent can induce gene and chromosomal mutations in whole mammals indicates that it may have the potential for carcinogenic activity, although this activity may not be detectably expressed in any or all species tested. The relative potency of agents in tests for mutagenicity and related effects is not a reliable indicator of carcinogenic potency. Negative results in tests for mutagenicity in selected tissues from animals treated *in vivo* provide less weight, partly because they do not exclude the possibility of an effect in tissues other than those examined. Moreover, negative results in short-term tests with genetic endpoints cannot be considered to provide evidence to rule out carcinogenicity of agents that act through other mechanisms. Factors may arise in many tests that could give misleading results; these have been discussed in detail elsewhere(11).

The adequacy of epidemiological studies of reproductive outcomes and genetic and related effects in humans is evaluated by the same criteria as are applied to epidemiological studies of cancer.

11. EVIDENCE FOR CARCINOGENICITY IN HUMANS

(a) *Types of studies considered*

Three types of epidemiological studies of cancer contribute data to the assessment of carcinogenicity in humans — cohort studies, case-control studies and correlation studies. Rarely, results from randomized trials may be available. Case reports of cancer in humans exposed to particular agents are also reviewed.

Cohort and case-control studies relate individual exposure to the agent under study to the occurrence of cancer in individuals, and provide an estimate of relative risk (ratio of incidence in those exposed to incidence in those not exposed) as the main measure of association.

In correlation studies, the units of investigation are usually whole populations (e.g., in particular geographical areas or at particular times), and cancer incidence is related to a summary measure of the exposure of the population to the agent under study. Because individual exposure is not documented, however, a causal relationship is less easy to infer from correlation studies than from cohort and case-control studies.

Case reports generally arise from a suspicion, based on clinical experience, that the concurrence of two events — that is, exposure to a particular agent and occurrence of a cancer — has happened rather more frequently than would be expected by chance. Case reports usually lack complete ascertainment of cases in any population, definition or enumeration of the population at risk and estimation of the expected number of cases in the absence of exposure.

The uncertainties surrounding interpretation of case reports and correlation studies make them inadequate, except in rare instances, to form the sole basis for inferring a causal relationship. When taken together with case-control and cohort studies, however, relevant case reports or correlation studies may add materially to the judgement that a causal relationship is present.

Epidemiological studies of benign neoplasms and presumed preneoplastic lesions are also reviewed by working groups. They may, in some instances, strengthen inferences drawn from studies of cancer itself.

(b) Quality of studies considered

It is necessary to take into account the possible roles of bias, confounding and chance in the interpretation of epidemiological studies. By 'bias' is meant the operation of factors in study design or execution that lead erroneously to a stronger or weaker association between an agent and disease than in fact exists. By 'confounding' is meant a situation in which the relationship between an agent and a disease is made to appear stronger or to appear weaker than it truly is as a result of an association between the agent and another agent that is associated with either an increase or decrease in the incidence of the disease. In evaluating the extent to which these factors have been minimized in an individual study, working groups consider a number of aspects of design and analysis as described in the report of the study. Most of these considerations apply equally to case-control, cohort and correlation studies. Lack of clarity of any of these aspects in the reporting of a study can decrease its credibility and its consequent weighting in the final evaluation of the exposure.

Firstly, the study population, disease (or diseases) and exposure should have been well defined by the authors. Cases in the study population should have been identified in a way that was independent of the exposure of interest, and exposure should have been assessed in a way that was not related to disease status.

Secondly, the authors should have taken account in the study design and analysis of other variables that can influence the risk of disease and may have been related to the exposure of interest. Potential confounding by such variables should have been dealt with either in the design of the study, such as by matching, or in the analysis, by statistical adjustment. In cohort studies, comparisons with local rates of disease may be more appropriate than those with national rates. Internal comparisons of disease frequency among individuals at different levels of exposure should also have been made in the study.

Thirdly, the authors should have reported the basic data on which the conclusions are founded, even if sophisticated statistical analyses were employed. At the very least, they should have given the numbers of exposed and unexposed cases and controls in a case-control study and the numbers of cases observed and expected in a cohort study. Further tabulations by time since exposure began and other temporal factors are also important. In a cohort study, data on all cancer sites and all causes of death should have been given, to avoid the possibility of reporting bias. In a case-control study, the effects of investigated factors other than the agent of interest should have been reported.

Finally, the statistical methods used to obtain estimates of relative risk, absolute cancer rates, confidence intervals and significance tests, and to adjust for confounding should have been clearly stated by the authors. The methods used should preferably have been the generally accepted techniques that have been refined since the mid-1970s. These methods have been reviewed for case-control studies(15) and for cohort studies(16).

(c) Quantitative considerations

Detailed analyses of both relative and absolute risks in relation to age at first exposure and to temporal variables, such as time since first exposure, duration of exposure and time since exposure ceased, are reviewed and summarized when available. The analysis of temporal relationships can provide a useful guide in formulating models of carcinogenesis. In particular, such analyses may suggest whether a carcinogen acts early or late in the process of carcinogenesis(5), although such speculative inferences cannot be used to draw firm conclusions concerning the mechanism of action of the agent and hence the shape (linear or otherwise) of the dose-response relationship below the range of observation.

(d) Criteria for causality

After the quality of individual epidemiological studies has been summarized and assessed, a judgement is made concerning the strength of evidence that the agent in question is carcinogenic for humans. In making their judgement, the Working Group considers several criteria for causality. A strong association (i.e., a large relative risk) is more likely to indicate causality than a weak association, although it is recognized that relative risks of small magnitude do not imply lack of causality and may be important if the disease is common. Associations that are replicated in several studies of the same design or using different epidemiological approaches or under different circumstances of exposure are more likely to represent a causal relationship than isolated observations from single studies. If there are inconsistent results among investigations, possible reasons are sought (such as differences in amount of exposure), and results of studies judged to be of high quality are given more weight than those from studies judged to be methodologically less sound. When suspicion of carcinogenicity arises largely from a single study, these data are not combined with those from later studies in any subsequent reassessment of the strength of the evidence.

If the risk of the disease in question increases with the amount of exposure, this is considered to be a strong indication of causality, although absence of a graded response is not necessarily evidence against a causal relationship. Demonstration of a decline in risk after cessation of or reduction in exposure in individuals or in whole populations also supports a causal interpretation of the findings.

Although the same carcinogenic agent may act upon more than one target, the specificity of an association (i.e., an increased occurrence of cancer at one anatomical site or of one morphological type) adds plausibility to a causal relationship, particularly when excess cancer occurrence is limited to one morphological type within the same organ.

Although rarely available, results from randomized trials showing different rates among exposed and unexposed individuals provide particularly strong evidence for causality.

When several epidemiological studies show little or no indication of an association between an agent and cancer, the judgement may be made that, in the aggregate, they show evidence of lack of carcinogenicity. Such a judgement requires first of all that the studies giving rise to it meet, to a sufficient degree, the standards of design and analysis described above. Specifically, the possibility that bias, confounding or misclassification of exposure or outcome could explain the observed results should be considered and excluded with reasonable certainty. In addition, all studies that are judged to be methodologically sound should be consistent with a relative risk of unity for any observed level of exposure to the agent and, when considered together, should provide a pooled estimate of relative risk which is at or near unity and has a narrow confidence interval, due to sufficient population size. Moreover, no individual study nor the pooled results of all the studies should show any consistent tendency for relative risk of cancer to increase with increasing amount of exposure to the agent. It is important to note that evidence of lack of carcinogenicity obtained in this way from several epidemiological studies can apply only to the type(s) of cancer studied and to dose levels of the agent and intervals between first exposure to it and observation of disease that are the same as or less than those observed in all the studies. Experience with human cancer indicates that, for some agents, the period from first exposure to the development of clinical cancer is seldom less than 20 years; latent periods substantially shorter than 30 years cannot provide evidence for lack of carcinogenicity.

12. SUMMARY OF DATA REPORTED

In this section, the relevant experimental and epidemiological data are summarized. Only reports, other than in abstract form, that meet the criteria outlined on pp. 18-19 are considered for evaluating carcinogenicity. Inadequate studies are generally not summarized: such studies are usually identified by a square-bracketed comment in the text.

(a) Exposures

Human exposure is summarized on the basis of elements such as production, use, occurrence in the environment and determinations in human tissues and body fluids. Quantitative data are given when available.

(b) Experimental carcinogenicity data

Data relevant to the evaluation of the carcinogenicity of the agent in animals are summarized. For each animal species and route of administration, it is stated whether an increased incidence of neoplasms was observed, and the tumour sites are indicated. If the agent produced tumours after prenatal exposure or in single-dose experiments, this is also indicated. Dose-response and other quantitative data may be given when available. Negative findings are also summarized.

(c) Human carcinogenicity data

Results of epidemiological studies that are considered to be pertinent to an assessment of human carcinogenicity are summarized. When relevant, case reports and correlation studies are also considered.

(d) Other relevant data

Structure-activity correlations are mentioned when relevant.

Toxicological information and data on kinetics and metabolism in experimental animals are given when considered relevant. The results of tests for genetic and related effects are summarized for whole mammals, cultured mammalian cells and nonmammalian systems.

Data on other biological effects in humans of particular relevance are summarized. These may include kinetic and metabolic considerations and evidence of DNA binding, persistence of DNA lesions or genetic damage in humans exposed to the agent.

When available, comparisons of such data for humans and for animals, and particularly animals that have developed cancer, are described.

13. EVALUATION

Evaluations of the strength of the evidence for carcinogenicity arising from human and experimental animal data are made, using standard terms.

It is recognized that the criteria for these evaluations, described below, cannot encompass all of the factors that may be relevant to an evaluation of the carcinogenicity of an agent. In considering all of the relevant data, the Working Group may assign the agent to a higher or lower category than a strict interpretation of these criteria would indicate.

(a) Degrees of evidence for carcinogenicity to humans and to experimental animals and supporting evidence

It should be noted that these categories refer only to the strength of the evidence that these agents are carcinogenic and not to the extent of their carcinogenic activity (potency) nor to the mechanism involved. The classification of some agents may change as new information becomes available.

(i)   *Human carcinogenicity data*

The evidence relevant to carcinogenicity from studies in humans is classified into one of the following categories:

Sufficient evidence of carcinogenicity: The Working Group considers that a causal relationship has been established between exposure to the agent and human cancer. That is, a positive relationship has been observed between exposure to the agent and cancer in studies in which chance, bias and confounding could be ruled out with reasonable confidence.

Limited evidence of carcinogenicity: A positive association has been observed between exposure to the agent and cancer for which a causal interpretation is considered by the Working Group to be credible, but chance, bias or confounding could not be ruled out with reasonable confidence.

Inadequate evidence of carcinogenicity: The available studies are of insufficient quality, consistency or statistical power to permit a conclusion regarding the presence or absence of a causal association.

Evidence suggesting lack of carcinogenicity: There are several adequate studies covering the full range of doses to which human beings are known to be exposed, which are mutually consistent in not showing a positive association between exposure to the agent and any studied cancer at any observed level of exposure. A conclusion of 'evidence suggesting lack of carcinogenicity' is inevitably limited to the cancer sites, circumstances and doses of exposure and length of observation covered by the available studies. In addition, the possibility of a very small risk at the levels of exposure studied can never be excluded.

In some instances, the above categories may be used to classify the degree of evidence for the carcinogenicity of the agent for specific organs or tissues.

(ii)   *Experimental carcinogenicity data*

The evidence relevant to carcinogenicity in experimental animals is classified into one of the following categories:

Sufficient evidence of carcinogenicity: The Working Group considers that a causal relationship has been established between the agent and an increased incidence of malignant neoplasms or of an appropriate combination of benign and malignant neoplasms (as described on p.23) in (a) two or more species of animals or (b) in two or more independent studies in one species carried out at different times or in different laboratories or under different protocols.

Exceptionally, a single study in one species might be considered to provide sufficient evidence of carcinogenicity when malignant neoplasms occur to an unusual degree with regard to incidence, site, type of tumour or age at onset.

In the absence of adequate data on humans, it is biologically plausible and prudent to regard agents for which there is *sufficient evidence* of carcinogenicity in experimental animals as if they presented a carcinogenic risk to humans.

Limited evidence of carcinogenicity: The data suggest a carcinogenic effect but are limited for making a definitive evaluation because, e.g., (a) the evidence of carcinogenicity is restricted to a single experiment; or (b) there are unresolved questions regarding the adequacy of the design, conduct or interpretation of the study; or (c) the agent increases the incidence only of benign neoplasms or lesions of uncertain neoplastic potential, or of certain neoplasms which may occur spontaneously in high incidences in certain strains.

Inadequate evidence of carcinogenicity: The studies cannot be interpreted as showing either the presence or absence of a carcinogenic effect because of major qualitative or quantitative limitations.

Evidence suggesting lack of carcinogenicity: Adequate studies involving at least two species are available which show that, within the limits of the tests used, the agent is not carcinogenic. A conclusion of evidence suggesting lack of carcinogenicity is inevitably limited to the species, tumour sites and doses of exposure studied.

(iii) *Supporting evidence of carcinogenicity*

The other relevant data judged to be of sufficient importance as to affect the making of the overall evaluation are indicated.

(*b*) *Overall evaluation*

Finally, the total body of evidence is taken into account; the agent is described according to the wording of one of the following categories, and the designated group is given. The categorization of an agent is a matter of scientific judgement, reflecting the strength of the evidence derived from studies in humans and in experimental animals and from other relevant data.

Group 1 — The agent is carcinogenic to humans.

This category is used only when there is *sufficient evidence* of carcinogenicity in humans.

Group 2

This category includes agents for which, at one extreme, the degree of evidence of carcinogenicity in humans is almost sufficient, as well as agents for which, at the other extreme, there are no human data but for which there is experimental evidence of carcinogenicity. Agents are assigned to either 2A (probably carcinogenic) or 2B (possibly carcinogenic) on the basis of epidemiological, experimental and other relevant data.

Group 2A — The agent is probably carcinogenic to humans.

This category is used when there is *limited evidence* of carcinogenicity in humans and *sufficient evidence* of carcinogenicity in experimental animals. Exceptionally, an agent may be classified into this category solely on the basis of *limited evidence* of carcinogenicity in humans or of *sufficient evidence* of carcinogenicity in experimental animals strengthened by supporting evidence from other relevant data.

Group 2B — The agent is possibly carcinogenic to humans.

This category is generally used for agents for which there is *limited evidence* in humans in the absence of *sufficient evidence* in experimental animals. It may also be used when there is *inadequate evidence* of carcinogenicity in humans or when human data are nonexistent but there is *sufficient evidence* of carcinogenicity in experimental animals. In some instances, an agent for which there is inadequate evidence or no data in humans but *limited evidence* of carcinogenicity in experimental animals together with supporting evidence from other relevant data may be placed in this group.

Group 3 — The agent is not classifiable as to its carcinogenicity to humans.

Agents are placed in this category when they do not fall into any other group.

Group 4 — The agent is probably not carcinogenic to humans.

This category is used for agents for which there is *evidence suggesting lack of carcinogenicity* in humans together with *evidence suggesting lack of carcinogenicity* in experimental animals. In some circumstances, agents for which there is *inadequate evidence* of or no data on carcinogenicity in humans but *evidence suggesting lack of carcinogenicity* in experimental animals, consistently and strongly supported by a broad range of other relevant data, may be classified in this group.

References

1. IARC (1977) *IARC Monographs Programme on the Evaluation of the Carcinogenic Risk of Chemicals to Humans. Preamble (IARC intern. tech. Rep. No. 77/002)*, Lyon

2. IARC (1978) *Chemicals with* Sufficient Evidence *of Carcinogenicity in Experimental Animals —* IARC Monographs *Volumes 1-17 (IARC intern. tech. Rep. No. 78/003)*, Lyon

3. IARC (1979) *Criteria to Select Chemicals for* IARC Monographs (*IARC intern. tech. Rep. No. 79/003*), Lyon

4. IARC (1982) *IARC Monographs on the Evaluation of the Carcinogenic Risk of Chemicals to Humans*, Supplement 4, *Chemicals, Industrial Processes and Industries Associated with Cancer in Humans (IARC Monographs, Volumes 1 to 29)*, Lyon

5. IARC (1983) *Approaches to Classifying Chemical Carcinogens According to Mechanism of Action (IARC intern. tech. Rep. No. 83/001)*, Lyon

6. IARC (1973-1984) *Information Bulletin on the Survey of Chemicals Being Tested for Carcinogenicity*, Numbers 1-12, Lyon

    Number 1 (1973)   52 pages
    Number 2 (1973)   77 pages
    Number 3 (1974)   67 pages
    Number 4 (1974)   97 pages
    Number 5 (1975)   88 pages
    Number 6 (1976)   360 pages

Number 7 (1978) 460 pages
Number 8 (1979) 604 pages
Number 9 (1981) 294 pages
Number 10 (1983) 326 pages
Number 11 (1984) 370 pages
Number 12 (1986) 385 pages

7.   Muir, C. & Wagner, G., eds (1977-87) *Directory of On-going Studies in Cancer Epidemiology 1977-87 (IARC Scientific Publications)*, Lyon, International Agency for Research on Cancer

8.   IARC (1984) *Chemicals and Exposures to Complex Mixtures Recommended for Evaluation in IARC Monographs and Chemicals and Complex Mixtures Recommended for Long-term Carcinogenicity Testing (IARC intern. tech. Rep. No. 84/002)*, Lyon

9.   *Environmental Carcinogens. Selected Methods of Analysis:*

Vol. 1. *Analysis of Volatile Nitrosamines in Food (IARC Scientific Publications No. 18).* Edited by R. Preussmann, M. Castegnaro, E.A. Walker & A.E. Wassermann (1978)

Vol. 2. *Methods for the Measurement of Vinyl Chloride in Poly(vinyl chloride), Air, Water and Foodstuffs (IARC Scientific Publications No. 22).* Edited by D.C.M. Squirrell & W. Thain (1978)

Vol. 3. *Analysis of Polycycic Aromatic Hydrocarbons in Environmental Samples (IARC Scientific Publications No. 29).* Edited by M. Castegnaro, P. Bogovski, H. Kunte & E.A. Walker (1979)

Vol. 4. *Some Aromatic Amines and Azo Dyes in the General and Industrial Environment (IARC Scientific Publications No. 40).* Edited by L. Fishbein, M. Castegnaro, I.K. O'Neill & H. Bartsch (1981)

Vol. 5. *Some Mycotoxins (IARC Scientific Publications No. 44).* Edited by L. Stoloff, M. Castegnaro, P. Scott, I.K. O'Neill & H. Bartsch (1982)

Vol. 6. N-*Nitroso Compounds (IARC Scientific Publications No. 45).* Edited by R. Preussmann, I.K. O'Neill, G. Eisenbrand, B. Spiegelhalder & H. Bartsch (1983)

Vol. 7. *Some Volatile Halogenated Hydrocarbons (IARC Scientific Publications No. 68).* Edited by L. Fishbein & I.K. O'Neill (1985)

Vol. 8. *Some Metals: As, Be, Cd, Cr, Ni, Pb, Se, Zn (IARC Scientific Publications No. 71).* Edited by I.K. O'Neill, P. Schuller & L. Fishbein (1986)

Vol. 9. *Passive Smoking (IARC Scientific Publications No. 81).* Edited by I.K. O'Neill, K.D. Brunnemann, B. Dodet & D. Hoffmann (1987)

10. Wilbourn, J., Haroun, L., Heseltine, E., Kaldor, J., Partensky, C. & Vainio, H. (1986) Response of experimental animals to human carcinogens: an analysis based upon the IARC Monographs Programme. *Carcinogenesis, 7*, 1853-1863

11. Montesano, R., Bartsch, H., Vainio, H., Wilbourn, J. & Yamasaki, H., eds (1986) *Long-term and Short-term Assays for Carcinogenesis — A Critical Appraisal (IARC Scientific Publications No. 83)*, Lyon, International Agency for Research on Cancer

12. Hoel, D.G., Kaplan, N.L. & Anderson, M.W. (1983) Implication of nonlinear kinetics on risk estimation in carcinogenesis. *Science, 219*, 1032-1037

13.   Gart, J.J., Krewski, D., Lee, P.N., Tarone, R.E. & Wahrendorf, J. (1986) *Statistical Methods in Cancer Research, Vol. 3, The Design and Analysis of Long-term Animal Experiments (IARC Scientific Publications No.79)*, Lyon, International Agency for Research on Cancer

14.   Peto, R., Pike, M.C., Day, N.E., Gray, R.G., Lee, P.N., Parish, S., Peto, J., Richards, S. & Wahrendorf, J. (1980) *Guidelines for simple, sensitive significance tests for carcinogenic effects in long-term animal experiments.* In: *IARC Monographs on the Evaluation of the Carcinogenic Risk of Chemicals to Humans,* Supplement 2, *Long-term and Short-term Screening Assays for Carcinogens: A Critical Appraisal,* Lyon, pp. 311-426

15.   Breslow, N.E. & Day, N.E. (1980) *Statistical Methods in Cancer Research, Vol. 1, The Analysis of Case-control Studies (IARC Scientific Publications No. 32)*, Lyon, International Agency for Research on Cancer

16.   Breslow, N.E. & Day, N.E. (1987) *Statistical Methods in Cancer Research, Vol. 2, The Design and Analysis of Cohort Studies (IARC Scientific Publications No. 82)*, Lyon, International Agency for Research on Cancer

OVERALL EVALUATIONS OF CARCINOGENICITY

INTRODUCTION

An international group of experts in cancer research met in Lyon in February 1982 to re-evaluate the epidemiological and experimental carcinogenicity data, as well as other relevant data, on 155 chemicals, groups of chemicals and exposures to complex mixtures that had been evaluated in Volumes 1-29 of the *IARC Monographs*, for which there were some data on carcinogenicity in humans. The background, purpose and overall conclusions of the Working Group and the evidence on which the evaluation for each agent was based were issued as Supplement 4 to the *IARC Monographs* (IARC, 1982).

This volume, Supplement 7, of the *IARC Monographs* is an updating of Supplement 4 to the *IARC Monographs* and represents the conclusions of two IARC Working Groups —one which met in December 1986 and another which met in March 1987.

The aim of the Working Group that met in December 1986 was to summarize and bring up to date the findings from tests for genetic and related effects and from studies of DNA damage, chromosomal effects and mutation in humans for all the agents (chemicals, groups of chemicals, industrial processes, occupational exposures and cultural habits) that had been evaluated in Volumes 1-42 of the *Monographs* and for which some data on carcinogenicity in humans were available. Other data considered particularly relevant to evaluations of carcinogenicity were also included. The conclusions of the December Working Group are presented in full in Supplement 6 of the *IARC Monographs* (IARC, 1987). Summaries of their conclusions are given in the sections on other relevant data for each compound and in Appendix 1 to this volume.

The aim of the Working Group that met in March 1987 was two-fold. The first was to summarize and bring up to date the data on carcinogenicity in humans and in experimental animals for all 189 agents that had been evaluated in Volumes 1-42 of the *Monographs* and for which some data on carcinogenicity in humans were available. The second was to make overall evaluations of carcinogenicity to humans for all 628 agents (comprising more than 700 chemicals, groups of chemicals, industrial processes, occupational exposures and cultural habits) that had been evaluated in Volumes 1-42 of the *Monographs*, on the basis of all the available data, as described below.

METHODS

The data on animal and human carcinogenicity for each of the agents for which information on carcinogenicity in humans was available were reviewed and evaluated before the meeting by members of the Working Group, who prepared draft summaries of the findings. During the meeting of the Working Group, these summaries and evaluations were discussed, modified as appropriate and adopted. Overall evaluations of carcinogenicity to humans for these agents were made by the Working Group on the basis of the combined evidence from: human carcinogenicity data, animal carcinogenicity data, the conclusions of the December 1986 Working Group on studies on genetic and related effects, and other relevant data judged to be of sufficient importance to affect the making of the overall evaluation.

The criteria for evaluating the degree of evidence for carcinogenicity in humans and in experimental animals and for making the overall evaluation of carcinogenicity to humans are those described in the Preamble to this volume (see pp. 29-32), which represents the conclusions of two working groups which met in September/October 1986 and in January 1987.

Some closely-related chemicals were evaluated as groups, as at previous meetings, when such an approach was biologically plausible and when the available evidence did not permit separate evaluation of each individual chemical within the group. For groups of chemicals categorized into Group 1 ('The agent is carcinogenic to humans'), the evaluation was considered to apply to the group as a whole and not necessarily to all chemicals within the group. If and when further evidence is obtained, separate evaluations may be made for individual chemicals, possibly into different categories.

Evaluations of carcinogenicity to humans were sometimes made for a group of human exposures, e.g., industrial processes and therapeutic combinations. Under such circumstances, the composition of different mixtures, and consequently their biological effects, are likely to vary with settings and conditions. Although the degree of evidence for carcinogenicity has been characterized with all possible specificity, it is difficult to be specific for such variable human exposures, which are also likely to change considerably over time, e.g., with the introduction of new processes. The Working Group therefore recognizes that the evaluation of a complex situation may not apply to all constituents or to every combination or to every point in time.

Other relevant data, including the results of tests for genetic and related effects (see Supplement 6 [IARC, 1987]), were used by the Working Group in making the overall evaluation of carcinogenicity to humans of an agent when one of the following sets of information was available:

(1)   the agent produces genetic or related effects in exposed humans (i.e., indicative of DNA or chromosomal damage) and also gives positive results in a range of other types of assays;

or

(2)   the agent is active in a broad spectrum of assays for genetic and related effects, including those involving mammalian cells, and there is evidence from structure-activity and/or metabolism studies that the agent itself reacts covalently with DNA or is likely to be converted to a reactive form in humans.

This information was used in two ways:

(1)   to classify in Group 2A, as a probable human carcinogen, an agent for which there is *sufficient evidence* of carcinogenicity in experimental animals, which would otherwise have been classified in Group 2B as a possible human carcinogen; and

(2)   to classify in Group 2B, as a possible human carcinogen, an agent for which there is *limited evidence* of carcinogenicity in experimental animals, which would otherwise have been classified in Group 3.

In using the above information, it was recognized that certain known carcinogens are not detected in currently used assays for genetic and related effects.

Overall evaluations of carcinogenicity to humans for agents for which no data on carcinogenicity in humans were available were made on the basis of the combined evidence from animal carcinogenicity tests and from other relevant data that fell into one of the two categories described above. The overall evaluation was generally based on the summary and evaluation of the most recent monograph on that agent. The same procedure was used in the case of three agents (benzoyl peroxide, polyvinyl chloride and selenium and selenium compounds) for which a previous evaluation of *inadequate evidence* for carcinogenicity in humans had been made.

Prior to Volume 20 of the Monographs, the evaluations of *sufficient, limited, inadequate* and *no evidence* of carcinogenicity were not used. However, an ad-hoc group which was convened in 1978 re-evaluated all chemicals evaluated in Volumes 1-19 of the monographs and listed those for which there was considered to be *sufficient evidence* of carcinogenicity in experimental animals according to the criteria established at that time. All chemicals for which there is *sufficient evidence* of carcinogenicity in experimental animals were re-evaluated by the present group.

For agents for which there were no data on carcinogenicity in humans and which were evaluated in Volumes 1-19 of the *IARC Monographs*, prior to the development of criteria for defining *limited* and *inadequate evidence* of carcinogenicity, no formal re-evaluation was made. However, on the basis of data presented in the summaries in those volumes, an attempt was made in conjunction with the Secretariat to judge whether the available data at that time would have met the present criteria for *limited* and *inadequate evidence*.

With regard to compounds for which there are no data on carcinogenicity in humans, the Working Group also examined data from short-term tests and other relevant biological data in *Monographs* volumes 14-42. Only those compounds for which data were *limited* or *sufficient* in animal studies were considered for recategorization on the basis of the procedures described above for using data on genetic and related effects.

When additional published data of significant importance to affect the evaluation of *sufficient evidence* of carcinogenicity in experimental animals (upgrading to or downgrading from) were available to the Working Group, new summaries and evaluations of the data in experimental animals were prepared (see p. 389), and these were used in making the overall evaluations.

Only one agent was categorized as probably not carcinogenic to humans (Group 4). More agents did not fall into this category partly because one of the criteria used for selecting agents to be considered in the *Monographs* series is that there be a suspicion for the carcinogenicity of the agents on the basis of either epidemiological or experimental observations. Therefore, the monographs tend to represent a selection of agents for which positive findings have been reported in the literature.

The epidemiological evidence for diazepam, fluorides (inorganic, used in drinking-water) and prednisone appeared to be suitable for classification as 'suggesting lack of carcinogenicity' in humans. The different reasons why it could not be so described are given in the texts on each compound.

For two chemicals, ferric oxide and methyl parathion, there was considered to be 'evidence suggesting lack of carcinogenicity' in experimental animals, but there were insufficient supporting data to allow their classification into Group 4.

References

IARC (1982) *IARC Monographs on the Evaluation of the Carcinogenic Risk of Chemicals to Humans*, Supplement 4, *Chemicals, Industrial Processes and Industries Associated with Cancer in Humans (IARC Monographs, Volumes 1 to 29)*, Lyon

IARC (1987) *IARC Monographs on the Evaluation of Carcinogenic Risks to Humans*, Supplement 6, *Genetic and Related Effects: An Updating of Selected* IARC Monographs *from Volumes 1 to 42*, Lyon

RESULTS AND CONCLUSIONS

The assessments of degrees of evidence for carcinogenicity in humans and in experimental animals, as well as the overall evaluations of carcinogenicity to humans, are given in Table 1. A summary of the conclusions of the December 1986 Working Group on genetic and related effects is given in Appendix 1.

Group 1. The Working Group concluded that the following agents are carcinogenic to humans:

Aflatoxins
Aluminium production
4-Aminobiphenyl
Analgesic mixtures containing phenacetin

Arsenic and arsenic compounds*
Asbestos
Auramine, manufacture of
Azathioprine
Benzene
Benzidine
Betel quid with tobacco
N,N-Bis(2-chloroethyl)-2-naphthylamine (Chlornaphazine)
Bis(chloromethyl)ether and chloromethyl methyl ether (technical-grade)
Boot and shoe manufacture and repair
1,4-Butanediol dimethanesulphonate (Myleran)
Chlorambucil
1-(2-Chloroethyl)-3-(4-methylcyclohexyl)-1-nitrosourea (Methyl-CCNU)
Chromium compounds, hexavalent*
Coal gasification
Coal-tar pitches
Coal-tars
Coke production
Cyclophosphamide
Diethylstilboestrol
Erionite
Furniture and cabinet making
Haematite mining, underground, with exposure to radon
Iron and steel founding
Isopropyl alcohol manufacture, strong-acid process
Magenta, manufacture of
Melphalan
8-Methoxypsoralen (Methoxsalen) plus ultraviolet radiation
Mineral oils, untreated and mildly-treated
MOPP (combined therapy with nitrogen mustard, vincristine, procarbazine and prednisone) and other combined chemotherapy including alkylating agents
Mustard gas (Sulphur mustard)
2-Naphthylamine
Nickel and nickel compounds*
Oestrogen replacement therapy
Oestrogens, nonsteroidal*
Oestrogens, steroidal*
Oral contraceptives, combined[1]
Oral contraceptives, sequential
The rubber industry

---

*This evaluation applies to the group of chemicals as a whole and not necessarily to all individual chemicals within the group (see also Methods, p. 38).

[1]There is also conclusive evidence that these agents have a protective effect against cancers of the ovary and endometrium (see summary, p. 297).

Shale-oils
Soots
Talc containing asbestiform fibres
Tobacco products, smokeless
Tobacco smoke
Treosulphan
Vinyl chloride

Group 2A. The Working Group concluded that the following agents are probably carcinogenic to humans:

Acrylonitrile
Adriamycin
Androgenic (anabolic) steroids
Benz[*a*]anthracene
Benzidine-based dyes
Benzo[*a*]pyrene
Beryllium and beryllium compounds
Bischloroethyl nitrosourea (BCNU)
Cadmium and cadmium compounds
1-(2-Chloroethyl)-3-cyclohexyl-1-nitrosourea (CCNU)
Cisplatin
Creosotes
Dibenz[*a,h*]anthracene
Diethyl sulphate
Dimethylcarbamoyl chloride
Dimethyl sulphate
Epichlorohydrin
Ethylene dibromide
Ethylene oxide
N-Ethyl-*N*-nitrosourea
Formaldehyde
5-Methoxypsoralen
4,4′-Methylene bis(2-chloroaniline) (MOCA)
N-Methyl-*N*′-nitro-*N*-nitrosoguanidine (MNNG)
N-Methyl-*N*-nitrosourea
Nitrogen mustard
N-Nitrosodiethylamine
N-Nitrosodimethylamine
Phenacetin
Polychlorinated biphenyls
Procarbazine hydrochloride
Propylene oxide
Silica, crystalline

Styrene oxide
Tris(1-aziridinyl)phosphine sulphide (Thiotepa)
Tris(2,3-dibromopropyl) phosphate
Vinyl bromide

Group 2B. The Working Group concluded that the following agents are possibly carcinogenic to humans:

A-α-C (2-Amino-9*H*-pyrido[2,3-*b*]indole)
Acetaldehyde
Acetamide
Acrylamide
AF-2 [2-(2-Furyl)-3-(5-nitro-2-furyl)acrylamide]
para-Aminoazobenzene
ortho-Aminoazotoluene
2-Amino-5-(5-nitro-2-furyl)-1,3,4-thiadiazole
Amitrole
ortho-Anisidine
Aramite®
Auramine, technical-grade
Azaserine
Benzo[*b*]fluoranthene
Benzo[*j*]fluoranthene
Benzo[*k*]fluoranthene
Benzyl violet 4B
Bitumens, extracts of steam-refined and air-refined
Bleomycins
Bracken fern
1,3-Butadiene
Butylated hydroxyanisole (BHA)
β-Butyrolactone
Carbon-black extracts
Carbon tetrachloride
Carpentry and joinery
Carrageenan, degraded
Chloramphenicol
Chlordecone (Kepone)
α-Chlorinated toluenes
Chloroform
Chlorophenols
Chlorophenoxy herbicides
4-Chloro-*ortho*-phenylenediamine

para-Chloro-*ortho*-toluidine
Citrus Red No. 2
para-Cresidine
Cycasin
Dacarbazine
Daunomycin
DDT
N,*N*′-Diacetylbenzidine
2,4-Diaminoanisole
4,4′-Diaminodiphenyl ether
2,4-Diaminotoluene
Dibenz[*a,h*]acridine
Dibenz[*a,j*]acridine
7*H*-Dibenzo[*c,g*]carbazole
Dibenzo[*a,e*]pyrene
Dibenzo[*a,h*]pyrene
Dibenzo[*a,i*]pyrene
Dibenzo[*a,l*]pyrene
1,2-Dibromo-3-chloropropane
para-Dichlorobenzene
3,3′-Dichlorobenzidine
3,3′-Dichloro-4,4′-diaminodiphenyl ether
1,2-Dichloroethane
Dichloromethane
1,3-Dichloropropene (technical-grade)
Diepoxybutane
Di(2-ethylhexyl)phthalate
1,2-Diethylhydrazine
Diglycidyl resorcinol ether
Dihydrosafrole
3,3′-Dimethoxybenzidine (*ortho*-Dianisidine)
para-Dimethylaminoazobenzene
trans-2-[(Dimethylamino)methylimino]-5-[2-(5-nitro-2-furyl)vinyl]-1,3,4-oxadiazole
3,3′-Dimethylbenzidine (*ortho*-Tolidine)
1,1-Dimethylhydrazine
1,2-Dimethylhydrazine
1,4-Dioxane
Ethyl acrylate
Ethylene thiourea
Ethyl methanesulphonate
2-(2-Formylhydrazino)-4-(5-nitro-2-furyl)thiazole
Glu-P-1 (2-Amino-6-methyldipyrido[1,2-*a*:3′,2′-*d*]imidazole)
Glu-P-2 (2-Aminodipyrido[1,2-*a*:3′,2′-*d*]imidazole)

Glycidaldehyde
Griseofulvin
Hexachlorobenzene
Hexachlorocyclohexanes
Hexamethylphosphoramide
Hydrazine
Indeno[1,2,3-*cd*]pyrene
IQ (2-Amino-3-methylimidazo[4,5-*f*]quinoline)
Iron-dextran complex
Lasiocarpine
Lead and lead compounds, inorganic
MeA-*α*-C (2-Amino-3-methyl-9*H*-pyrido[2,3-*b*]indole)
Medroxyprogesterone acetate
Merphalan
2-Methylaziridine
Methylazoxymethanol and its acetate
5-Methylchrysene
4,4′-Methylene bis(2-methylaniline)
4,4′-Methylenedianiline
Methyl methanesulphonate
2-Methyl-1-nitroanthraquinone (uncertain purity)
N-Methyl-*N*-nitrosourethane
Methylthiouracil
Metronidazole
Mirex
Mitomycin C
Monocrotaline
5-(Morpholinomethyl)-3-[(5-nitrofurfurylidene)amino]-2-oxazolidinone
Nafenopin
Niridazole
5-Nitroacenaphthene
Nitrofen (technical-grade)
1-[(5-Nitrofurfurylidene)amino]-2-imidazolidinone
N-[4-(5-Nitro-2-furyl)-2-thiazolyl]acetamide
Nitrogen mustard *N*-oxide
2-Nitropropane
N-Nitrosodi-*n*-butylamine
N-Nitrosodiethanolamine
N-Nitrosodi-*n*-propylamine
3-(*N*-Nitrosomethylamino)propionitrile
4-(*N*-Nitrosomethylamino)-1-(3-pyridyl)-1-butanone (NNK)
N-Nitrosomethylethylamine
N-Nitrosomethylvinylamine

N-Nitrosomorpholine
N'-Nitrosonornicotine
N-Nitrosopiperidine
N-Nitrosopyrrolidine
N-Nitrososarcosine
Oil Orange SS
Panfuran S (containing dihydroxymethylfuratrizine)
Phenazopyridine hydrochloride
Phenobarbital
Phenoxybenzamine hydrochloride
Phenytoin
Polybrominated biphenyls
Ponceau MX
Ponceau 3R
Potassium bromate
Progestins
1,3-Propane sultone
β-Propiolactone
Propylthiouracil
Saccharin
Safrole
Sodium *ortho*-phenylphenate
Sterigmatocystin
Streptozotocin
Styrene
Sulfallate
2,3,7,8-Tetrachlorodibenzo-*para*-dioxin (TCDD)
Tetrachloroethylene
Thioacetamide
4,4'-Thiodianiline
Thiourea
Toluene diisocyanates
ortho-Toluidine
Toxaphene (Polychlorinated camphenes)
Trp-P-1 (3-Amino-1,4-dimethyl-5*H*-pyrido[4,3-*b*]indole)
Trp-P-2 (3-Amino-1-methyl-5*H*-pyrido[4,3-*b*]indole)
Trypan blue
Uracil mustard
Urethane

Group 3. The Working Group concluded that the following agents are not classifiable as to their carcinogenicity to humans:

Acridine orange
Acriflavinium chloride
Acrolein
Acrylic acid
Acrylic fibres
Acrylonitrile-butadiene-styrene copolymers
Actinomycin D
Agaritine
Aldrin
Allyl chloride
Allyl isothiocyanate
Allyl isovalerate
Amaranth
5-Aminoacenaphthene
2-Aminoanthraquinone
para-Aminobenzoic acid
1-Amino-2-methylanthraquinone
4-Amino-2-nitrophenol
2-Amino-5-nitrothiazole
11-Aminoundecanoic acid
Anaesthetics, volatile
Angelicin plus ultraviolet A radiation
Aniline
para-Anisidine
Anthanthrene
Anthracene
Anthranilic acid
Apholate
Attapulgite
Aurothioglucose
5-Azacytidine
Aziridine
2-(1-Aziridinyl)ethanol
Aziridyl benzoquinone
Azobenzene
Benz[*a*]acridine
Benz[*c*]acridine
Benzo[*ghi*]fluoranthene
Benzo[*a*]fluorene
Benzo[*b*]fluorene
Benzo[*c*]fluorene

Benzo[*ghi*]perylene
Benzo[*c*]phenanthrene
Benzo[*e*]pyrene
para-Benzoquinone dioxime
Benzoyl chloride
Benzoyl peroxide
Benzyl acetate
Betel quid without tobacco
Bis(1-aziridinyl)morpholinophosphine sulphide
Bis(2-chloroethyl)ether
1,2-Bis(chloromethoxy)ethane
1,4-Bis(chloromethoxymethyl)benzene
Bis(2-chloro-1-methylethyl)ether
Bitumens
Blue VRS
Brilliant Blue FCF
n-Butyl acrylate
Butylated hydroxytoluene (BHT)
Butyl benzyl phthalate
γ-Butyrolactone
Cantharidin
Captan
Carbaryl
Carbazole
3-Carbethoxypsoralen
Carbon blacks
Carmoisine
Carrageenan, native
Catechol
Chlordane/Heptachlor
Chlordimeform
Chlorinated dibenzodioxins (other than TCDD)
Chlorobenzilate
Chlorodifluoromethane
Chlorofluoromethane
4-Chloro-*meta*-phenylenediamine
Chloroprene
Chloropropham
Chloroquine
Chlorothalonil
2-Chloro-1,1,1-trifluoroethane
Cholesterol
Chromium compounds, trivalent

Chromium metal
Chrysene
Chrysoidine
CI Disperse Yellow 3
Cinnamyl anthranilate
Citrinin
Clofibrate
Clomiphene citrate
Copper 8-hydroxyquinoline
Coronene
Coumarin
meta-Cresidine
Cyclamates
Cyclochlorotine
Cyclopenta[*cd*]pyrene
D & C Red No. 9
Dapsone
Diacetylaminoazotoluene
Diallate
1,2-Diamino-4-nitrobenzene
1,4-Diamino-2-nitrobenzene
2,5-Diaminotoluene
Diazepam
Diazomethane
Dibenz[*a,c*]anthracene
Dibenz[*a,j*]anthracene
Dibenzo[*a,e*]fluoranthene
Dibenzo[*h,rst*]pentaphene
Dichloroacetylene
ortho-Dichlorobenzene
trans-1,4-Dichlorobutene
2,6-Dichloro-*para*-phenylenediamine
1,2-Dichloropropane
Dichlorvos
Dicofol
Dieldrin
Di(2-ethylhexyl)adipate
Dihydroxymethylfuratrizine
Dimethoxane
3,3'-Dimethoxybenzidine-4,4'-diisocyanate
para-Dimethylaminoazobenzenediazo sodium sulphonate
4,4'-Dimethylangelicin plus ultraviolet A radiation
4,5'-Dimethylangelicin plus ultraviolet A radiation

1,4-Dimethylphenanthrene
1,8-Dinitropyrene
Dinitrosopentamethylenetetramine
2,4'-Diphenyldiamine
Disulfiram
Dithranol
Dulcin
Endrin
Eosin
1-Epoxyethyl-3,4-epoxycyclohexane
3,4-Epoxy-6-methylcyclohexylmethyl-3,4-epoxy-6-methylcyclohexane carboxylate
cis-9,10-Epoxystearic acid
Ethionamide
Ethylene
Ethylene sulphide
Ethyl selenac
Ethyl tellurac
Eugenol
Evans blue
Fast Green FCF
Ferbam
Ferric oxide
Fluometuron
Fluoranthene
Fluorene
Fluorides (inorganic, used in drinking-water)
5-Fluorouracil
Furazolidone
Fusarenon-X
Glycidyl oleate
Glycidyl stearate
Guinea Green B
Gyromitrin
Haematite
Hexachlorobutadiene
Hexachloroethane
Hexachlorophene
Hycanthone mesylate
Hydralazine
Hydrogen peroxide
Hydroquinone
4-Hydroxyazobenzene
8-Hydroxyquinoline

Hydroxysenkirkine
Iron-dextrin complex
Iron sorbitol-citric acid complex
Isatidine
Isonicotinic acid hydrazide (Isoniazid)
Isophosphamide
Isopropyl alcohol
Isopropyl oils
Isosafrole
Jacobine
Kaempferol
Lauroyl peroxide
Lead compounds, organolead
Leather goods manufacture
Leather tanning and processing
Light Green SF
Lumber and sawmill industries (including logging)
Luteoskyrin
Magenta
Malathion
Maleic hydrazide
Malonaldehyde
Maneb
Mannomustine
Medphalan
MeIQ (2-Amino-3,4-dimethylimidazo[4,5-*f*]quinoline)
MeIQx (2-Amino-3,8-dimethylimidazo[4,5-*f*]quinoxaline)
Melamine
6-Mercaptopurine
Methotrexate
Methoxychlor
Methyl acrylate
5-Methylangelicin plus ultraviolet A radiation
Methyl bromide
Methyl carbamate
Methyl chloride
1-Methylchrysene
2-Methylchrysene
3-Methylchrysene
4-Methylchrysene
6-Methylchrysene
N-Methyl-*N*,4-dinitrosoaniline
4,4'-Methylenebis(*N*,*N*-dimethyl)benzenamine

4,4'-Methylenediphenyl diisocyanate
2-Methylfluoranthene
3-Methylfluoranthene
Methyl iodide
Methyl methacrylate
Methyl parathion
1-Methylphenanthrene
7-Methylpyrido[3,4-*c*]psoralen
Methyl red
Methyl selenac
Mineral oils, highly-refined
Modacrylic fibres
Monuron
1,5-Naphthalenediamine
1,5-Naphthalene diisocyanate
1-Naphthylamine
1-Naphthylthiourea (ANTU)
Nithiazide
5-Nitro-*ortho*-anisidine
9-Nitroanthracene
6-Nitrobenzo[*a*]pyrene
4-Nitrobiphenyl
6-Nitrochrysene
3-Nitrofluoranthene
5-Nitro-2-furaldehyde semicarbazone
1-Nitropyrene
N'-Nitrosoanabasine
N'-Nitrosoanatabine
N-Nitrosodiphenylamine
para-Nitrosodiphenylamine
N-Nitrosofolic acid
N-Nitrosoguvacine
N-Nitrosoguvacoline
N-Nitrosohydroxyproline
3-(*N*-Nitrosomethylamino)propionaldehyde
4-(*N*-Nitrosomethylamino)-4-(3-pyridyl)-1-butanal (NNA)
N-Nitrosoproline
Nitrovin
Nylon 6
Ochratoxin A
Oestradiol mustard
Oestrogen-progestin replacement therapy
Orange I

Orange G
Oxazepam
Oxyphenbutazone
Parasorbic acid
Parathion
Patulin
Penicillic acid
Pentachloroethane
Perylene
Petasitenine
Phenanthrene
Phenelzine sulphate
Phenicarbazide
Phenylbutazone
meta-Phenylenediamine
para-Phenylenediamine
N-Phenyl-2-naphthylamine
ortho-Phenylphenol
Piperonyl butoxide
Polyacrylic acid
Polychloroprene
Polyethylene
Polymethylene polyphenyl isocyanate
Polymethyl methacrylate
Polypropylene
Polystyrene
Polytetrafluoroethylene
Polyurethane foams
Polyvinyl acetate
Polyvinyl alcohol
Polyvinyl chloride
Polyvinyl pyrrolidone
Ponceau SX
Potassium bis(2-hydroxyethyl)dithiocarbamate
Prednisone
Proflavine salts
Pronetalol hydrochloride
Propham
n-Propyl carbamate
Propylene
Ptaquiloside
Pulp and paper manufacture
Pyrene
Pyrido[3,4-*c*]psoralen

Pyrimethamine
Quercetin
para-Quinone
Quintozene (Pentachloronitrobenzene)
Reserpine
Resorcinol
Retrorsine
Rhodamine B
Rhodamine 6G
Riddelliine
Rifampicin
Rugulosin
Saccharated iron oxide
Scarlet Red
Selenium and selenium compounds
Semicarbazide hydrochloride
Seneciphylline
Senkirkine
Sepiolite
Shikimic acid
Silica, amorphous
Sodium diethyldithiocarbamate
Spironolactone
Styrene-acrylonitrile copolymers
Styrene-butadiene copolymers
Succinic anhydride
Sudan I
Sudan II
Sudan III
Sudan Brown RR
Sudan Red 7B
Sulfafurazole (Sulphisoxasole)
Sulfamethoxazole
Sunset Yellow FCF
Symphytine
Talc not containing asbestiform fibres
Tannic acid and tannins
Terpene polychlorinates (Strobane®)
2,2′,5,5′-Tetrachlorobenzidine
1,1,1,2-Tetrachloroethane
1,1,2,2-Tetrachloroethane
Tetrachlorvinphos
Tetrafluoroethylene

Thiouracil
Thiram
Trichlorfon
1,1,1-Trichloroethane
1,1,2-Trichloroethane
Trichloroethylene
Trichlorotriethylamine hydrochloride
T_2-Trichothecene
Triethylene glycol diglycidyl ether
4,4′,6-Trimethylangelicin plus ultraviolet A radiation
2,4,5-Trimethylaniline
2,4,6-Trimethylaniline
4,5′,8-Trimethylpsoralen
Triphenylene
Tris(aziridinyl)-*para*-benzoquinone (Triaziquone)
Tris(1-aziridinyl)phosphine oxide
2,4,6-Tris(1-aziridinyl)-*s*-triazine
1,2,3-Tris(chloromethoxy)propane
Tris(2-methyl-1-aziridinyl)phosphine oxide
Vinblastine sulphate
Vincristine sulphate
Vinyl acetate
Vinyl chloride-vinyl acetate copolymers
4-Vinylcyclohexene
Vinyl fluoride
Vinylidene chloride
Vinylidene chloride-vinyl chloride copolymers
Vinylidene fluoride
N-Vinyl-2-pyrrolidone
Wollastonite
2,4-Xylidine
2,5-Xylidine
Yellow AB
Yellow OB
Zearalenone
Zectran
Zineb
Ziram

Group 4. The Working Group concluded that the following agent is probably not carcinogenic to humans:

Caprolactam

Table 1. Degrees of evidence for carcinogenicity in humans and in experimental animals, and overall evaluations of carcinogenicity to humans for agents evaluated in *IARC Monographs* volumes 1-42

Agent	Degree of evidence for carcinogenicity[a]		Overall evaluation[a]
	Human	Animal	
A-α-C (2-Amino-9*H*-pyrido[2,3-*b*]indole)[b] [40, 1986]	ND	S	2B
Acetaldehyde	I	S	2B
Acetamide[c]	ND	S	2B
Acridine orange[d] [16, 1978]	ND	I	3
Acriflavinium chloride[d] [13, 1977]	ND	I	3
Acrolein	I	I	3
Acrylamide[b] [39, 1986]	ND	S	2B
Acrylic acid[d] [19, 1979]	ND	ND	3
Acrylic fibres[d] [19, 1979]	ND	ND	3
Acrylonitrile	L	S	2A
Acrylonitrile-butadiene-styrene copolymers[d] [19, 1979]	ND	ND	3
Actinomycin D	I	L	3
Adriamycin[e]	I	S	2A
AF-2 [2-(2-Furyl)-3-(5-nitro-2-furyl)acrylamide][b] [31, 1983]	ND	S	2B
Aflatoxins	S	S	1
Agaritine[b] [31, 1983]	ND	I	3
Aldrin	I	L	3
Allyl chloride[b] [36, 1985]	ND	I	3
Allyl isothiocyanate[b] [36, 1985]	ND	L	3
Allyl isovalerate[b] [36, 1985]	ND	L	3
Aluminium production	S		1
Amaranth[d] [8, 1975]	ND	I	3
5-Aminoacenaphthene[d] [16, 1978]	ND	I	3
2-Aminoanthraquinone[b] [27, 1982]	ND	L	3
para-Aminoazobenzene[c]	ND	S	2B
ortho-Aminoazotoluene[b] [8, 1975]	ND	S	2B
para-Aminobenzoic acid[d] [16, 1978]	ND	I	3

[a]ND, no adequate data; ESL, evidence suggesting lack of carcinogenicity; I, inadequate evidence; L, limited evidence; S, sufficient evidence. For definitions of terms and overall evaluations, see Preamble, pp. 30-32.

[b]Overall evaluation based only on evidence of carcinogenicity in monograph [volume, year] (see Methods, p. 39) or in Supplement 4

[c]Degree of evidence in animals revised on the basis of data that appeared after the most recent monograph and/or on the basis of present criteria (see Methods, pp. 39-40)

[d]Degree of evidence not previously categorized; evaluation made according to present criteria on the basis of data in monograph [volume, year] (see Methods, p. 39)

[e]Other relevant data, as given in the summaries here or in monograph [volume, year], influenced the making of the overall evaluation (see Methods, pp. 38-39)

Table 1. (contd)

Agent	Degree of evidence for carcinogenicity[a]		Overall evaluation[a]
	Human	Animal	
4-Aminobiphenyl	S	S	1
1-Amino-2-methylanthraquinone[b] [27, 1982]	ND	L	3
2-Amino-5-(5-nitro-2-furyl)-1,3,4-thiadiazole[b] [7, 1974]	ND	S	2B
4-Amino-2-nitrophenol[d] [16, 1978]	ND	I	3
2-Amino-5-nitrothiazole[b] [31, 1983]	ND	L	3
11-Aminoundecanoic acid[b] [39, 1986]	ND	L	3
Amitrole	I	S	2B
Anaesthetics, volatile	I		3
Cyclopropane		ND	
Diethyl ether		ND	
Divinyl ether		ND	
Enflurane		I	
Fluroxene		ND	
Halothane		I	
Isoflurane		I	
Methoxyflurane		I	
Nitrous oxide		I	
Androgenic (anabolic) steroids	L		2A
Oxymetholone		ND	
Testosterone		S	
Angelicins[b] [40, 1986]			
Angelicin plus ultraviolet A radiation	ND	L	3
5-Methylangelicin plus ultraviolet A radiation	ND	L	3
4,4'-Dimethylangelicin plus ultraviolet A radiation	ND	ND	3
4,5'-Dimethylangelicin plus ultraviolet A radiation	ND	L	3
4,4',6-Trimethylangelicin plus ultraviolet A radiation	ND	ND	3
Aniline	I	L	3
ortho-Anisidine[b] [27, 1982]	ND	S	2B
para-Anisidine[b] [27, 1982]	ND	I	3
Anthanthrene[b] [32, 1982]	ND	L	3
Anthracene[c]	ND	I	3
Anthranilic acid[d] [16, 1978]	ND	I	3
Apholate[d] [9, 1975]	ND	I	3
Aramite®[b] [5, 1974]	ND	S	2B
Arsenic and arsenic compounds	S	L	1*
Asbestos	S	S	1
Attapulgite	I	L	3
Auramine (technical-grade)	I	S	2B
Manufacture of auramine	S		1
Aurothioglucose[d] [13, 1977]	ND	L	3
5-Azacytidine[b] [26, 1981]	ND	L	3
Azaserine[b] [10, 1976]	ND	S	2B

*This evaluation applies to the group of chemicals as a whole and not necessarily to all individual chemicals within the group (see also Methods, p. 38).

Table 1. (contd)

Agent	Degree of evidence for carcinogenicity[a]		Overall evaluation[a]
	Human	Animal	
Azathioprine	S	L	1
Aziridine[d] [9, 1975]	ND	L	3
2-(1-Aziridinyl)ethanol[d] [9, 1975]	ND	L	3
Aziridyl benzoquinone[d] [9, 1975]	ND	L	3
Azobenzene[d] [8, 1975]	ND	L	3
Benz[a]acridine[b] [32, 1983]	ND	I	3
Benz[c]acridine[b] [32, 1983]	ND	L	3
Benz[a]anthracene[b,e] [32, 1983]	ND	S	2A
Benzene	S	S	1
Benzidine	S	S	1
Benzidine-based dyes[e]	I		2A
Direct Black 38 (technical-grade)		S	
Direct Blue 6 (technical-grade)		S	
Direct Brown 95 (technical-grade)		S	
Benzo[b]fluoranthene[b] [32, 1983]	ND	S	2B
Benzo[j]fluoranthene[b] [32, 1983]	ND	S	2B
Benzo[k]fluoranthene[b] [32, 1983]	ND	S	2B
Benzo[ghi]fluoranthene[b] [32, 1983]	ND	I	3
Benzo[a]fluorene[b] [32, 1983]	ND	I	3
Benzo[b]fluorene[b] [32, 1983]	ND	I	3
Benzo[c]fluorene[b] [32, 1983]	ND	I	3
Benzo[ghi]perylene[b] [32, 1983]	ND	I	3
Benzo[c]phenanthrene[b] [32, 1983]	ND	I	3
Benzo[a]pyrene[b,e] [32, 1983]	ND	S	2A
Benzo[e]pyrene[b] [32, 1983]	ND	I	3
para-Benzoquinone dioxime[b] [29, 1982]	ND	L	3
Benzoyl chloride	I	I	3
Benzoyl peroxide[b] [36, 1985]	I	I	3
Benzyl acetate[b] [40, 1986]	ND	L	3
Benzyl violet 4B[b] [16, 1978]	ND	S	2B
Beryllium and beryllium compounds	L	S	2A
Betel quid			
With tobacco	S	L	1
Without tobacco	I	L	3
Bis(1-aziridinyl)morpholinophosphine sulphide[d] [9, 1975]	ND	L	3
Bis(2-chloroethyl)ether[d] [9, 1975]	ND	L	3
N,N-Bis(2-chloroethyl)-2-naphthylamine (Chlornaphazine)	S	L	1
1,2-Bis(chloromethoxy)ethane[d] [15, 1977]	ND	L	3
1,4-Bis(chloromethoxymethyl)benzene[d] [15, 1977]	ND	L	3
Bis(chloromethyl)ether and chloromethyl methyl ether (technical-grade)	S	S	1

Table 1. (contd)

Agent	Degree of evidence for carcinogenicity[a]		Overall evaluation[a]
	Human	Animal	
Bis(2-chloro-1-methylethyl)ether[b] [41, 1986]	ND	L	3
Bitumens	I		3
Steam-refined and cracking-residue bitumens		L	
Air-refined bitumens		I	
Extracts of steam-refined and air-refined bitumens		S	2B
Bleomycins[e]	I	L	2B
Blue VRS[d] [16, 1978]	ND	L	3
Bracken fern	I	S	2B
Brilliant Blue FCF[d] [16, 1978]	ND	L	3
1,3-Butadiene	I	S	2B
1,4-Butanediol dimethanesulphonate (Myleran)	S	L	1
n-Butyl acrylate[b] [39, 1986]	ND	I	3
Butylated hydroxyanisole (BHA)[b] [40, 1986]	ND	S	2B
Butylated hydroxytoluene (BHT)[b] [40, 1986]	ND	L	3
Butyl benzyl phthalate[b] [29, 1982]	ND	I	3
β-Butyrolactone[b] [11, 1976]	ND	S	2B
γ-Butyrolactone[b,c] [11, 1976]	ND	I	3
Cadmium and cadmium compounds	L	S	2A
Cantharidin[d] [10, 1976]	ND	L	3
Caprolactam[c]	ND	ESL	4
Captan[b] [30, 1983]	ND	L	3
Carbaryl[d] [12, 1976]	ND	I	3
Carbazole[b] [32, 1983]	ND	L	3
3-Carbethoxypsoralen[b,c] [40, 1986]	ND	I	3
Carbon blacks	I	I	3
Carbon-black extracts		S	2B
Carbon tetrachloride	I	S	2B
Carmoisine[d] [8, 1975]	ND	I	3
Carrageenan			
Native[b,c] [31, 1983]	ND	I	3
Degraded[b] [31, 1983]	ND	S	2B
Catechol[d] [15, 1977]	ND	I	3
Chlorambucil	S	S	1
Chloramphenicol	L	I	2B
Chlordane/Heptachlor	I	L	3
Chlordecone (Kepone)[b] [20, 1979]	ND	S	2B
Chlordimeform[b] [30, 1983]	ND	I	3
Chlorinated dibenzodioxins (other than TCDD)[d] [15, 1977]	ND	I	3

Table 1. (contd)

Agent	Degree of evidence for carcinogenicity[a]		Overall evaluation[a]
	Human	Animal	
α-Chlorinated toluenes	I		2B
Benzyl chloride		L	
Benzal chloride		L	
Benzotrichloride		S	
Chlorobenzilate[b] [30, 1983]	ND	L	3
Chlorodifluoromethane	I	L	3
Chloroethyl nitrosoureas			
Bischloroethyl nitrosourea (BCNU)	L	S	2A
1-(2-Chloroethyl)-3-cyclohexyl-1-nitrosourea (CCNU)[e]	I	S	2A
1-(2-Chloroethyl)-3-(4-methylcyclohexyl)-1-nitrosourea (Methyl-CCNU)	S	L	1
Chlorofluoromethane[b] [41, 1986]	ND	L	3
Chloroform	I	S	2B
Chlorophenols	L		2B
Pentachlorophenol		I	
2,4,5-Trichlorophenol		I	
2,4,6-Trichlorophenol		S	
Chlorophenoxy herbicides	L		2B
2,4-D		I	
2,4,5-T		I	
MCPA		ND	
4-Chloro-*ortho*-phenylenediamine[b] [27, 1982]	ND	S	2B
4-Chloro-*meta*-phenylenediamine[b] [27, 1982]	ND	I	3
Chloroprene	I	I	3
Chloropropham[d] [12, 1976]	ND	I	3
Chloroquine[d] [13, 1977]	ND	I	3
Chlorothalonil[b] [30, 1983]	ND	L	3
para-Chloro-*ortho*-toluidine[b] [30, 1983]	ND	S	2B
2-Chloro-1,1,1-trifluoroethane[b] [41, 1986]	ND	L	3
Cholesterol	I	I	3
Chromium and chromium compounds			
Chromium metal	I	I	3
Trivalent chromium compounds	I	I	3
Hexavalent chromium compounds	S	S	1[*]
Chrysene[b] [32, 1983]	ND	L	3
Chrysoidine	I	L	3
CI Disperse Yellow 3[d] [8, 1975]	ND	I	3
Cinnamyl anthranilate[b] [31, 1983]	ND	L	3
Cisplatin[e]	I	S	2A
Citrinin[b] [40, 1986]	ND	L	3
Citrus Red No. 2[b] [8, 1975]	ND	S	2B

[*]This evaluation applies to the group of chemicals as a whole and not necessarily to all individual chemicals within the group (see also Methods, p. 38).

Table 1. (contd)

Agent	Degree of evidence for carcinogenicity[a]		Overall evaluation[a]
	Human	Animal	
Clofibrate	I	L	3
Clomiphene citrate	I	I	3
Coal gasification	S		1
Coal-tar pitches	S	S	1
Coal-tars	S	S	1
Coke production	S		1
Copper 8-hydroxyquinoline[d] [15, 1977]	ND	I	3
Coronene[b] [32, 1983]	ND	I	3
Coumarin[d] [10, 1976]	ND	L	3
Creosotes	L	S	2A
meta-Cresidine[b] [27, 1982]	ND	I	3
para-Cresidine[b] [27, 1982]	ND	S	2B
Cycasin[b] [10, 1976] (see also Methylazoxymethanol and its acetate)	ND	S	2B
Cyclamates	I	L	3
Cyclochlorotine[d] [10, 1976]	ND	I	3
Cyclopenta[cd]pyrene[b] [32, 1983]	ND	L	3
Cyclophosphamide	S	S	1
Dacarbazine	I	S	2B
D & C Red No. 9[d] [8, 1975]	ND	I	3
Dapsone	I	L	3
Daunomycin[b] [10, 1976]	ND	S	2B
DDT	I	S	2B
Diacetylaminoazotoluene[d] [8, 1975]	ND	I	3
N,N'-Diacetylbenzidine[b] [16, 1978]	ND	S	2B
Diallate[b] [30, 1983]	ND	L	3
2,4-Diaminoanisole[b] [27, 1982]	ND	S	2B
4,4'-Diaminodiphenyl ether[b] [29, 1982]	ND	S	2B
1,2-Diamino-4-nitrobenzene[d] [16, 1978]	ND	I	3
1,4-Diamino-2-nitrobenzene[d] [16, 1978]	ND	I	3
2,4-Diaminotoluene[b] [16, 1978]	ND	S	2B
2,5-Diaminotoluene[d] [16, 1978]	ND	I	3
Diazepam	I	I	3
Diazomethane[d] [7, 1974]	ND	L	3
Dibenz[a,h]acridine[b] [32, 1983]	ND	S	2B
Dibenz[a,j]acridine[b] [32, 1983]	ND	S	2B
Dibenz[a,c]anthracene[b] [32, 1983]	ND	L	3
Dibenz[a,h]anthracene[b,e] [32, 1983]	ND	S	2A
Dibenz[a,j]anthracene[b] [32, 1983]	ND	L	3
7H-Dibenzo[c,g]carbazole[b] [32, 1983]	ND	S	2B
Dibenzo[a,e]fluoranthene[b] [32, 1983]	ND	L	3

Table 1. (contd)

Agent	Degree of evidence for carcinogenicity[a]		Overall evaluation[a]
	Human	Animal	
Dibenzo[h,rst]pentaphene[d] [3, 1973]	ND	L	3
Dibenzo[a,e]pyrene[b] [32, 1983]	ND	S	2B
Dibenzo[a,h]pyrene[b] [32, 1983]	ND	S	2B
Dibenzo[a,i]pyrene[b] [32, 1983]	ND	S	2B
Dibenzo[a,l]pyrene[b] [32, 1983]	ND	S	2B
1,2-Dibromo-3-chloropropane	I	S	2B
Dichloroacetylene[b] [39, 1986]	ND	L	3
ortho-Dichlorobenzene	I	I	3
para-Dichlorobenzene	I	S	2B
3,3'-Dichlorobenzidine	I	S	2B
trans-1,4-Dichlorobutene[d] [15, 1977]	ND	I	3
3,3'-Dichloro-4,4'-diaminodiphenyl ether[b] [16, 1978]	ND	S	2B
1,2-Dichloroethane[b] [20, 1979]	ND	S	2B
Dichloromethane	I	S	2B
2,6-Dichloro-para-phenylenediamine[b] [39, 1986]	ND	L	3
1,2-Dichloropropane[b] [41, 1986]	ND	L	3
1,3-Dichloropropene (technical-grade)	I	S	2B
Dichlorvos[b] [20, 1979]	ND	I	3
Dicofol[b] [30, 1983]	ND	L	3
Dieldrin	I	L	3
Diepoxybutane[b] [11, 1976]	ND	S	2B
Di(2-ethylhexyl)adipate[b] [29, 1982]	ND	L	3
Di(2-ethylhexyl)phthalate[b] [29, 1982]	ND	S	2B
1,2-Diethylhydrazine[b] [4, 1974]	ND	S	2B
Diethyl sulphate	L	S	2A
Diglycidyl resorcinol ether[b] [36, 1985]	ND	S	2B
Dihydrosafrole[b] [10, 1976]	ND	S	2B
Dihydroxymethylfuratrizine[b] [24, 1980] (see also Panfuran S)	ND	I	3
Dimethoxane[d] [15, 1977]	ND	L	3
3,3'-Dimethoxybenzidine (ortho-Dianisidine)	I	S	2B
3,3'-Dimethoxybenzidine-4,4'-diisocyanate[b] [39, 1986]	ND	L	3
para-Dimethylaminoazobenzene[b] [8, 1975]	ND	S	2B
para-Dimethylaminoazobenzenediazo sodium sulphonate[d] [8, 1975]	ND	I	3
trans-2-[(Dimethylamino)methylimino]-5-[2-(5-nitro-2-furyl)vinyl]-1,3,4-oxadiazole[b] [7, 1974]	ND	S	2B
3,3'-Dimethylbenzidine (ortho-Tolidine)[b] [1, 1972]	ND	S	2B
Dimethylcarbamoyl chloride[e]	I	S	2A
1,1-Dimethylhydrazine[b] [4, 1974]	ND	S	2B
1,2-Dimethylhydrazine[b] [4, 1974]	ND	S	2B
1,4-Dimethylphenanthrene[b] [32, 1983]	ND	I	3

Table 1. (contd)

Agent	Degree of evidence for carcinogenicity[a]		Overall evaluation[a]
	Human	Animal	
Dimethyl sulphate[e]	I	S	2A
1,8-Dinitropyrene[b] [33, 1984]	ND	I	3
Dinitrosopentamethylenetetramine[d] [11, 1976]	ND	I	3
1,4-Dioxane	I	S	2B
2,4'-Diphenyldiamine[d] [16, 1978]	ND	I	3
Disulfiram[d] [12, 1976]	ND	I	3
Dithranol[d] [13, 1977]	ND	I	3
Dulcin[d] [12, 1976]	ND	I	3
Endrin[d] [5, 1974]	ND	I	3
Eosin[d] [15, 1977]	ND	I	3
Epichlorohydrin[e]	I	S	2A
1-Epoxyethyl-3,4-epoxycyclohexane[d] [11, 1976]	ND	L	3
3,4-Epoxy-6-methylcyclohexylmethyl-3,4-epoxy-6-methylcyclohexane carboxylate[d] [11, 1976]	ND	L	3
cis-9,10-Epoxystearic acid[d] [11, 1976]	ND	I	3
Erionite	S	S	1
Ethionamide[d] [13, 1977]	ND	L	3
Ethyl acrylate[b] [39, 1986]	ND	S	2B
Ethylene[d] [19, 1979]	ND	ND	3
Ethylene dibromide[e]	I	S	2A
Ethylene oxide	L	S	2A
Ethylene sulphide[d] [11, 1976]	ND	L	3
Ethylene thiourea	I	S	2B
Ethyl methanesulphonate[b] [7, 1974]	ND	S	2B
N-Ethyl-N-nitrosourea[b,e] [17, 1978]	ND	S	2A
Ethyl selenac[d] [12, 1976]	ND	I	3
Ethyl tellurac[d] [12, 1976]	ND	I	3
Eugenol[b] [36, 1985]	ND	L	3
Evans blue[d] [8, 1975]	ND	L	3
Fast Green FCF[d] [16, 1978]	ND	L	3
Ferbam[d] [12, 1976]	ND	I	3
Fluometuron[b] [30, 1983]	ND	I	3
Fluoranthene[b,c] [32, 1983]	ND	I	3
Fluorene[b] [32, 1983]	ND	I	3
Fluorides (inorganic, used in drinking-water)	I	I	3
5-Fluorouracil	I	I	3
Formaldehyde	L	S	2A
2-(2-Formylhydrazino)-4-(5-nitro-2-furyl)thiazole[b] [7, 1974]	ND	S	2B
Furazolidone[b] [31, 1983]	ND	I	3

Table 1. (contd)

Agent	Degree of evidence for carcinogenicity[a]		Overall evaluation[a]
	Human	Animal	
Fusarenon-X[b] [*31*, 1983]	ND	I	3
Glu-P-1 (2-Amino-6-methyldipyrido[1,2-*a*:3′,2′-*d*]imidazole)[b] [*40*, 1986]	ND	S	2B
Glu-P-2 (2-Aminodipyrido[1,2-*a*:3′,2′-*d*]imidazole)[b] [*40*, 1986]	ND	S	2B
Glycidaldehyde[b] [*11*, 1976]	ND	S	2B
Glycidyl oleate[d] [*11*, 1976]	ND	I	3
Glycidyl stearate[d] [*11*, 1976]	ND	I	3
Griseofulvin[c]	ND	S	2B
Guinea Green B[d] [*16*, 1978]	ND	L	3
Gyromitrin[c]	ND	L	3
Haematite and ferric oxide			
Ferric oxide	I	ESL	3
Haematite	I	I	3
Underground haematite mining with exposure to radon	S		1
Hexachlorobenzene	I	S	2B
Hexachlorobutadiene[b] (*20*, 1979)	ND	L	3
Hexachlorocyclohexanes (HCH)	I		2B
Technical-grade HCH		S	
α-HCH		S	
β-HCH		L	
γ-HCH (Lindane)		L	
Hexachloroethane[b] [*20*, 1979]	ND	L	3
Hexachlorophene[b] [*20*, 1979]	ND	I	3
Hexamethylphosphoramide[b] [*15*, 1977]	ND	S	2B
Hycanthone mesylate[d] [*13*, 1977]	ND	I	3
Hydralazine	I	L	3
Hydrazine	I	S	2B
Hydrogen peroxide[b] [*36*, 1985]	ND	L	3
Hydroquinone[d] [*15*, 1977]	ND	I	3
4-Hydroxyazobenzene[d] [*8*, 1975]	ND	I	3
8-Hydroxyquinoline[d] [*13*, 1977]	ND	I	3
Hydroxysenkirkine[d] [*10*, 1976]	ND	I	3
Indeno[1,2,3-*cd*]pyrene[b] [*32*, 1983]	ND	S	2B
IQ (2-Amino-3-methylimidazo[4,5-*f*]quinoline)[b] [*40*, 1986]	ND	S	2B
Iron and steel founding	S		1
Iron-dextran complex	I	S	2B
Iron-dextrin complex[d] [*2*, 1973]	ND	L	3
Iron sorbitol-citric acid complex[d] [*2*, 1973]	ND	I	3

Table 1. (contd)

Agent	Degree of evidence for carcinogenicity[a]		Overall evaluation[a]
	Human	Animal	
Isatidine[d] [10, 1976]	ND	L	3
Isonicotinic acid hydrazide (Isoniazid)	I	L	3
Isophosphamide[b] [26, 1981]	ND	L	3
Isopropyl alcohol manufacture (strong-acid process)	S		1
Isopropyl alcohol	I	I	3
Isopropyl oils	I	I	3
Isosafrole[d] [10, 1976]	ND	L	3
Jacobine[d] [10, 1976]	ND	I	3
Kaempferol[b] [31, 1983]	ND	I	3
Lasiocarpine[b] [10, 1976]	ND	S	2B
Lauroyl peroxide[b] [36, 1985]	ND	I	3
Lead and lead compounds			
Inorganic	I	S	2B
Organolead	I	I	3
Leather industries			
Boot and shoe manufacture and repair	S		1
Leather goods manufacture	I		3
Leather tanning and processing	I		3
Light Green SF[d] [16, 1978]	ND	L	3
Luteoskyrin[d] [10, 1976]	ND	L	3
Magenta	I	I	3
Manufacture of magenta	S		1
Malathion[b,c] [30, 1983]	ND	I	3
Maleic hydrazide[d] [4, 1974]	ND	I	3
Malonaldehyde[b] [36, 1985]	ND	I	3
Maneb[d] [12, 1976]	ND	I	3
Mannomustine[d] [9, 1975]	ND	L	3
MeA-α-C (2-Amino-3-methyl-9H-pyrido[2,3-b]indole)[b] [40, 1986]	ND	S	2B
Medphalan[d] [9, 1975]	ND	I	3
MeIQ (2-Amino-3,4-dimethylimidazo[4,5-f]quinoline)[b] [40, 1986]	ND	I	3
MeIQx (2-Amino-3,8-dimethylimidazo[4,5-f]quinoxaline)[b] [40, 1986]	ND	I	3
Melamine[b] [39, 1986]	ND	I	3
Melphalan	S	S	1
6-Mercaptopurine	I	I	3
Merphalan[b] [9, 1975]	ND	S	2B
Methotrexate	I	I	3

Table 1. (contd)

Agent	Degree of evidence for carcinogenicity[a]		Overall evaluation[a]
	Human	Animal	
Methoxychlor[b,c] [20, 1979]	ND	I	3
5-Methoxypsoralen[e]	I	S	2A
8-Methoxypsoralen (Methoxsalen) plus ultraviolet radiation	S	S	1
Methyl acrylate[b] [39, 1986]	ND	I	3
2-Methylaziridine[b] [9, 1975]	ND	S	2B
Methylazoxymethanol and its acetate[b] [10, 1976]	ND	S	2B
Methyl bromide	I	L	3
Methyl carbamate[d] [12, 1976]	ND	I	3
Methyl chloride	I	I	3
1-Methylchrysene[b] [32, 1983]	ND	I	3
2-Methylchrysene[b] [32, 1983]	ND	L	3
3-Methylchrysene[b] [32, 1983]	ND	L	3
4-Methylchrysene[b] [32, 1983]	ND	L	3
5-Methylchrysene[b] [32, 1983]	ND	S	2B
6-Methylchrysene[b] [32, 1983]	ND	L	3
N-Methyl-N,4-dinitrosoaniline[d] [1, 1972]	ND	L	3
4,4'-Methylene bis(2-chloroaniline) (MOCA)[e]	I	S	2A
4,4'-Methylenebis(N,N-dimethyl)benzenamine[b] [27, 1982]	ND	L	3
4,4'-Methylene bis(2-methylaniline)	I	S	2B
4,4'-Methylenedianiline[b] [39, 1986]	ND	S	2B
4,4'-Methylenediphenyl diisocyanate[d] [19, 1979]	ND	ND	3
2-Methylfluoranthene[b] [32, 1983]	ND	L	3
3-Methylfluoranthene[b] [32, 1983]	ND	I	3
Methyl iodide[b] [41, 1986]	ND	L	3
Methyl methacrylate[d] [19, 1979]	ND	I	3
Methyl methanesulphonate[b] [7, 1974]	ND	S	2B
2-Methyl-1-nitroanthraquinone (uncertain purity)[b] [27, 1982]	ND	S	2B
N-Methyl-N'-nitro-N-nitrosoguanidine (MNNG)[e]	I	S	2A
N-Methyl-N-nitrosourea[b,e] [17, 1978]	ND	S	2A
N-Methyl-N-nitrosourethane[b] [4, 1974]	ND	S	2B
Methyl parathion[c]	ND	ESL	3
1-Methylphenanthrene[b] [32, 1983]	ND	I	3
Methyl red[d] [8, 1975]	ND	I	3
Methyl selenac[d] [12, 1976]	ND	I	3
Methylthiouracil[b] [7, 1974]	ND	S	2B
Metronidazole	I	S	2B
Mineral oils			
Untreated and mildly-treated oils	S	S	1
Highly-refined oils	I	I	3
Mirex[b] [20, 1979]	ND	S	2B

Table 1. (contd)

Agent	Degree of evidence for carcinogenicity[a]		Overall evaluation[a]
	Human	Animal	
Mitomycin C[b] [10, 1976]	ND	S	2B
Modacrylic fibres[d] [19, 1979]	ND	ND	3
Monocrotaline[b] [10, 1976]	ND	S	2B
Monuron[d] [12, 1976]	ND	L	3
MOPP[1] and other combined chemotherapy including alkylating agents	S	I	1
5-(Morpholinomethyl)-3-[(5-nitrofurfurylidene)amino]-2-oxazolidinone[b] [7, 1974]	ND	S	2B
Mustard gas (Sulphur mustard)	S	L	1
Nafenopin[b] [24, 1980]	ND	S	2B
1,5-Naphthalenediamine[b] [27, 1982]	ND	L	3
1,5-Naphthalene diisocyanate[d] [19, 1979]	ND	ND	3
1-Naphthylamine	I	I	3
2-Naphthylamine	S	S	1
1-Naphthylthiourea (ANTU)	I	I	3
Nickel and nickel compounds	S	S	1*
Niridazole[b] [13, 1977]	ND	S	2B
Nithiazide[b] [31, 1983]	ND	L	3
5-Nitroacenaphthene[b] [16, 1978]	ND	S	2B
5-Nitro-ortho-anisidine[b] [27, 1982]	ND	L	3
9-Nitroanthracene[b] [33, 1984]	ND	ND	3
6-Nitrobenzo[a]pyrene[b] [33, 1984]	ND	I	3
4-Nitrobiphenyl[d] [4, 1974]	ND	I	3
6-Nitrochrysene[b] [33, 1984]	ND	I	3
Nitrofen (technical-grade)[b] [30, 1983]	ND	S	2B
3-Nitrofluoranthene[b] [33, 1984]	ND	I	3
5-Nitro-2-furaldehyde semicarbazone[d] [7, 1974]	ND	I	3
1-[(5-Nitrofurfurylidene)amino]-2-imidazolidinone[b] [7, 1974]	ND	S	2B
N-[4-(5-Nitro-2-furyl)-2-thiazolyl]acetamide[b] [7, 1974]	ND	S	2B
Nitrogen mustard	L	S	2A
Nitrogen mustard N-oxide[b] [9, 1975]	ND	S	2B
2-Nitropropane[b] [29, 1982]	ND	S	2B
1-Nitropyrene[b] [33, 1984]	ND	L	3
N'-Nitrosoanabasine[b] [37, 1985]	ND	L	3
N'-Nitrosoanatabine[b] [37, 1985]	ND	I	3
N-Nitrosodi-n-butylamine[b] [17, 1978]	ND	S	2B
N-Nitrosodiethanolamine[b] [17, 1978]	ND	S	2B
N-Nitrosodiethylamine[b,e] [17, 1978]	ND	S	2A
N-Nitrosodimethylamine[b,e] [17, 1978]	ND	S	2A
N-Nitrosodiphenylamine[b] [27, 1982]	ND	L	3

[1]Combined therapy with nitrogen mustard, vincristine, procarbazine and prednisone

*This evaluation applies to the group of chemicals as a whole and not necessarily to all individual chemicals within the group (see also Methods, p. 38).

Table 1. (contd)

Agent	Degree of evidence for carcinogenicity[a]		Overall evaluation[a]
	Human	Animal	
para-Nitrosodiphenylamine[b] [*27*, 1982]	ND	I	3
N-Nitrosodi-*n*-propylamine[b] [*17*, 1978]	ND	S	2B
N-Nitrosofolic acid[d] [*17*, 1978]	ND	I	3
N-Nitrosoguvacine[b] [*37*, 1985]	ND	ND	3
N-Nitrosoguvacoline[b] [*37*, 1985]	ND	I	3
N-Nitrosohydroxyproline[d] [*17*, 1978]	ND	I	3
3-(*N*-Nitrosomethylamino)propionaldehyde[b] [*37*, 1985]	ND	ND	3
3-(*N*-Nitrosomethylamino)propionitrile[b] [*37*, 1985]	ND	S	2B
4-(*N*-Nitrosomethylamino)-4-(3-pyridyl)-1-butanal (NNA)[b] [*37*, 1985]	ND	I	3
4-(*N*-Nitrosomethylamino)-1-(3-pyridyl)-1-butanone (NNK)[b] [*37*, 1985]	ND	S	2B
N-Nitrosomethylethylamine[b] [*17*, 1978]	ND	S	2B
N-Nitrosomethylvinylamine[b] [*17*, 1978]	ND	S	2B
N-Nitrosomorpholine[b] [*17*, 1978]	ND	S	2B
N'-Nitrosonornicotine[b] [*37*, 1985]	ND	S	2B
N-Nitrosopiperidine[b] [*17*, 1978]	ND	S	2B
N-Nitrosoproline[d] [*17*, 1978]	ND	I	3
N-Nitrosopyrrolidine[b] [*17*, 1978]	ND	S	2B
N-Nitrososarcosine[b] [*17*, 1978]	ND	S	2B
Nitrovin[b] [*31*, 1983]	ND	I	3
Nylon 6[d] [*19*, 1979]	ND	I	3
Ochratoxin A	I	L	3
Oestradiol mustard[d] [*9*, 1975]	ND	L	3
Oestrogens, progestins and combinations			
Oestrogens			
Nonsteroidal oestrogens	S		1*
Diethylstilboestrol	S	S	1
Dienoestrol		L	
Hexoestrol		S	
Chlorotrianisene		I	
Steroidal oestrogens	S		1*
Oestrogen replacement therapy	S		1
Conjugated oestrogens		L	
Oestradiol-17β and esters		S	
Oestriol		L	
Oestrone		S	
Ethinyloestradiol		S	
Mestranol		S	

*This evaluation applies to the group of chemicals as a whole and not necessarily to all individual chemicals within the group (see also Methods, p. 38).

Table 1. (contd)

Agent	Degree of evidence for carcinogenicity[a]		Overall evaluation[a]
	Human	Animal	
Progestins	I		2B
Medroxyprogesterone acetate	I	S	2B
Chlormadinone acetate		L	
Dimethisterone		I	
Ethynodiol diacetate		L	
17α-Hydroxyprogesterone caproate		I	
Lynoestrenol		I	
Megestrol acetate		L	
Norethisterone		S	
Norethynodrel		L	
Norgestrel		I	
Progesterone		S	
Oestrogen-progestin combinations			
Sequential oral contraceptives	S		1
Dimethisterone and oestrogens		I	
Combined oral contraceptives	S		1[1]
Chlormadinone acetate and oestrogens		L	
Ethynodiol diacetate and oestrogens		L	
Lynoestrenol and oestrogens		I	
Megestrol acetate and oestrogens		L	
Norethisterone and oestrogens		L	
Norethynodrel and oestrogens		S	
Norgestrel and oestrogens		I	
Progesterone and oestrogens		L	
Investigational oral contraceptives		L	
Oestrogen-progestin replacement therapy	I		3
Oil Orange SS[b] [8, 1975]	ND	S	2B
Orange I[d] [8, 1975]	ND	I	3
Orange G[d] [8, 1975]	ND	I	3
Oxazepam[d] [13, 1977]	ND	L	3
Oxyphenbutazone[d] [13, 1977]	ND	ND	3
Panfuran S (containing dihydroxymethylfuratrizine)[b] [24, 1980]	ND	S	2B
Parasorbic acid[d] [10, 1976]	ND	L	3
Parathion[b] [30, 1983]	ND	I	3
Patulin[b] [40, 1986]	ND	I	3
Penicillic acid[d] [10, 1976]	ND	L	3
Pentachloroethane[b] [41, 1986]	ND	L	3
Perylene[b] [32, 1983]	ND	I	3
Petasitenine[b] [31, 1983]	ND	L	3
Phenacetin	L	S	2A
Analgesic mixtures containing phenacetin	S	L	1
Phenanthrene[b] [32, 1983]	ND	I	3

[1]There is also conclusive evidence that these agents have a protective effect against cancers of the ovary and endometrium (see summary, p. 297).

Table 1. (contd)

Agent	Degree of evidence for carcinogenicity[a]		Overall evaluation[a]
	Human	Animal	
Phenazopyridine hydrochloride	I	S	2B
Phenelzine sulphate	I	L	3
Phenicarbazide[d] [12, 1976]	ND	L	3
Phenobarbital	I	S	2B
Phenoxybenzamine hydrochloride[b] [24, 1980]	ND	S	2B
Phenylbutazone	I	ND	3
meta-Phenylenediamine[d] [16, 1978]	ND	I	3
para-Phenylenediamine[d] [16, 1978]	ND	I	3
N-Phenyl-2-naphthylamine	I	L	3
ortho-Phenylphenol[b] [30, 1983]	ND	I	3
Phenytoin	L	L	2B
Piperonyl butoxide[b,c] [30, 1983]	ND	I	3
Polyacrylic acid[d] [19, 1979]	ND	ND	3
Polybrominated biphenyls	I	S	2B
Polychlorinated biphenyls	L	S	2A
Polychloroprene[d] [19, 1979]	ND	ND	3
Polyethylene[d] [19, 1979]	ND	I	3
Polymethylene polyphenyl isocyanate[d] [19, 1979]	ND	ND	3
Polymethyl methacrylate[d] [19, 1979]	ND	I	3
Polypropylene[d] [19, 1979]	ND	I	3
Polystyrene[d] [19, 1979]	ND	I	3
Polytetrafluoroethylene[d] [19, 1979]	ND	I	3
Polyurethane foams[d] [19, 1979]	ND	I	3
Polyvinyl acetate[d] [19, 1979]	ND	I	3
Polyvinyl alcohol[d] [19, 1979]	ND	I	3
Polyvinyl chloride[d] [19, 1979]	I	I	3
Polyvinyl pyrrolidone[d] [19, 1979]	ND	L	3
Ponceau MX[b] [8, 1975]	ND	S	2B
Ponceau 3R[b] [8, 1975]	ND	S	2B
Ponceau SX[d] [8, 1975]	ND	I	3
Potassium bis(2-hydroxyethyl)dithiocarbamate[d] [12, 1976]	ND	L	3
Potassium bromate[b] [40, 1986]	ND	S	2B
Prednisone	I	I	3
Procarbazine hydrochloride[e]	I	S	2A
Proflavine salts[b] [24, 1980]	ND	I	3
Pronetalol hydrochloride[d] [13, 1977]	ND	L	3
1,3-Propane sultone[b] [4, 1974]	ND	S	2B
Propham[d] [12, 1976]	ND	I	3
β-Propiolactone[b] [4, 1974]	ND	S	2B
n-Propyl carbamate[d] [12, 1976]	ND	L	3

Table 1. (contd)

Agent	Degree of evidence for carcinogenicity[a]		Overall evaluation[a]
	Human	Animal	
Propylene[d] [*19*, 1979]	ND	ND	3
Propylene oxide[e]	I	S	2A
Propylthiouracil	I	S	2B
Ptaquiloside[b] [*40*, 1986]	ND	L	3
Pyrene[b,c] [*32*, 1983]	ND	I	3
Pyrido[3,4-*c*]psoralen[b] [*40*, 1986]	ND	I	3
7-Methylpyrido[3,4-*c*]psoralen[b] [*40*, 1986]	ND	I	3
Pyrimethamine[d] [*13*, 1977]	ND	L	3
Quercetin[b] [*31*, 1983]	ND	L	3
para-Quinone[d] [*15*, 1977]	ND	I	3
Quintozene (Pentachloronitrobenzene)[d] [*5*, 1974]	ND	L	3
Reserpine	I	L	3
Resorcinol[d] [*15*, 1977]	ND	I	3
Retrorsine[d] [*10*, 1976]	ND	L	3
Rhodamine B[d] [*16*, 1978]	ND	L	3
Rhodamine 6G[d] [*16*, 1978]	ND	L	3
Riddelliine[d] [*10*, 1976]	ND	I	3
Rifampicin[b] [*24*, 1980]	ND	L	3
Rubber industry	S	I	1
Rugulosin[b] [*40*, 1986]	ND	I	3
Saccharated iron oxide[d] [*2*, 1973]	ND	L	3
Saccharin	I	S	2B
Safrole[b] [*10*, 1976]	ND	S	2B
Scarlet Red[d] [*8*, 1975]	ND	I	3
Selenium and selenium compounds[d] [*9*, 1975]	I	I	3
Semicarbazide hydrochloride[d] [*12*, 1976]	ND	L	3
Seneciphylline[d] [*10*, 1976]	ND	ND	3
Senkirkine[b] [*31*, 1983]	ND	L	3
Sepiolite[b] [*42*, 1987]	ND	I	3
Shale-oils	S	S	1
Shikimic acid[b] [*40*, 1986]	ND	I	3
Silica			
Crystalline silica	L	S	2A
Amorphous silica	I	I	3
Sodium diethyldithiocarbamate[d] [*12*, 1976]	ND	I	3
Sodium *ortho*-phenylphenate[c]	ND	S	2B
Soots	S	I	1
Spironolactone	I	L	3

Table 1. (contd)

Agent	Degree of evidence for carcinogenicity[a]		Overall evaluation[a]
	Human	Animal	
Sterigmatocystin[b] [*10*, 1976]	ND	S	2B
Streptozotocin[b] [*17*, 1978]	ND	S	2B
Styrene[e]	I	L	2B
Styrene-acrylonitrile copolymers[d] [*19*, 1979]	ND	ND	3
Styrene-butadiene copolymers[d] [*19*, 1979]	ND	ND	3
Styrene oxide[b,e] [*36*, 1985]	ND	S	2A
Succinic anhydride[d] [*15*, 1977]	ND	L	3
Sudan I[d] [*8*, 1975]	ND	L	3
Sudan II[d] [*8*, 1975]	ND	L	3
Sudan III[d] [*8*, 1975]	ND	I	3
Sudan Brown RR[d] [*8*, 1975]	ND	I	3
Sudan Red 7B[d] [*8*, 1975]	ND	I	3
Sulfafurazole (Sulphisoxazole)	I	I	3
Sulfallate[b] [*30*, 1983]	ND	S	2B
Sulfamethoxazole	I	L	3
Sunset Yellow FCF[d] [*8*, 1975]	ND	I	3
Symphytine[b] [*31*, 1983]	ND	I	3
Talc			
Not containing asbestiform fibres	I	I	3
Containing asbestiform fibres	S	I	1
Tannic acid and tannins[d] [*10*, 1976]	ND	L	3
Terpene polychlorinates (Strobane®)[d] [*5*, 1974]	ND	L	3
2,2′,5,5′-Tetrachlorobenzidine[b] [*27*, 1982]	ND	I	3
2,3,7,8-Tetrachlorodibenzo-*para*-dioxin (TCDD)	I	S	2B
1,1,1,2-Tetrachloroethane[b] [*41*, 1986]	ND	L	3
1,1,2,2-Tetrachloroethane	I	L	3
Tetrachloroethylene	I	S	2B
Tetrachlorvinphos[b] [*30*, 1983]	ND	L	3
Tetrafluoroethylene[d] [*19*, 1979]	ND	ND	3
Thioacetamide[b] [*7*, 1974]	ND	S	2B
4,4′-Thiodianiline[b] [*27*, 1982]	ND	S	2B
Thiouracil[d] [*7*, 1974]	ND	L	3
Thiourea[b] [*7*, 1974]	ND	S	2B
Thiram[d] [*12*, 1976]	ND	I	3
Tobacco products, smokeless	S	I	1
Tobacco smoke	S	S	1
Toluene diisocyanates[b] [*39*, 1986]	ND	S	2B
ortho-Toluidine	I	S	2B
Toxaphene (Polychlorinated camphenes)[b] [*20*, 1979]	ND	S	2B

Table 1. (contd)

Agent	Degree of evidence for carcinogenicity[a]		Overall evaluation[a]
	Human	Animal	
Treosulphan	S	ND	1
Trichlorfon[b] [30, 1983]	ND	I	3
1,1,1-Trichloroethane[b] [20, 1979]	ND	I	3
1,1,2-Trichloroethane[b] [20, 1979]	ND	L	3
Trichloroethylene	I	L	3
Trichlorotriethylamine hydrochloride[d] [9, 1975]	ND	I	3
T$_2$-Trichothecene[b] [31, 1983]	ND	I	3
Triethylene glycol diglycidyl ether[d] [11, 1976]	ND	L	3
2,4,5-Trimethylaniline[b] [27, 1982]	ND	L	3
2,4,6-Trimethylaniline[b] [27, 1982]	ND	I	3
4,5',8-Trimethylpsoralen	I	I	3
Triphenylene[b] [32, 1983]	ND	I	3
Tris(aziridinyl)-para-benzoquinone (Triaziquone)	I	L	3
Tris(1-aziridinyl)phosphine oxide[d] [9, 1975]	ND	I	3
Tris(1-aziridinyl)phosphine sulphide (Thiotepa)[e]	I	S	2A
2,4,6-Tris(1-aziridinyl)-s-triazine[d] [9, 1975]	ND	L	3
1,2,3-Tris(chloromethoxy)propane[d] [15, 1977]	ND	L	3
Tris(2,3-dibromopropyl) phosphate[e]	I	S	2A
Tris(2-methyl-1-aziridinyl)phosphine oxide[d] [9, 1975]	ND	I	3
Trp-P-1 (3-Amino-1,4-dimethyl-5H-pyrido[4,3-b]indole)[b] [31, 1983]	ND	S	2B
Trp-P-2 (3-Amino-1-methyl-5H-pyrido[4,3-b]indole)[b][31, 1983]	ND	S	2B
Trypan blue[b] [8, 1975]	ND	S	2B
Uracil mustard	I	S	2B
Urethane[b] [7, 1974]	ND	S	2B
Vinblastine sulphate	I	I	3
Vincristine sulphate	I	I	3
Vinyl acetate[b] [39, 1986]	ND	I	3
Vinyl bromide[b,e] [39, 1986]	ND	S	2A
Vinyl chloride	S	S	1
Vinyl chloride-vinyl acetate copolymers[d] [19, 1979]	ND	I	3
4-Vinylcyclohexene[b] [39, 1986]	ND	L	3
Vinyl fluoride[b] [39, 1986]	ND	ND	3
Vinylidene chloride	I	L	3
Vinylidene chloride-vinyl chloride copolymers[d] [19, 1979]	ND	ND	3
Vinylidene fluoride[b] [39, 1986]	ND	I	3
N-Vinyl-2-pyrrolidone[d] [19, 1979]	ND	ND	3

Table 1. (contd)

Agent	Degree of evidence for carcinogenicity[a]		Overall evaluation[a]
	Human	Animal	
Wollastonite	I	L	3
Wood industries			
Carpentry and joinery	L		2B
Furniture and cabinet making	S	I	1
Lumber and sawmill industries (including logging)	I		3
Pulp and paper manufacture	I		3
2,4-Xylidine[d] [*16*, 1978]	ND	I	3
2,5-Xylidine[d] [*16*, 1978]	ND	I	3
Yellow AB[d] [*8*, 1975]	ND	I	3
Yellow OB[d] [*8*, 1975]	ND	L	3
Zearalenone[b] [*31*, 1983]	ND	L	3
Zectran[d] [*12*, 1976]	ND	I	3
Zineb[d] [*12*, 1976]	ND	I	3
Ziram[d] [*12*, 1976]	ND	I	3

SUMMARIES AND EVALUATIONS OF EVIDENCE FOR CARCINOGENICITY IN HUMANS AND IN EXPERIMENTAL ANIMALS, AND SUMMARIES OF OTHER RELEVANT DATA, FOR AGENTS FOR WHICH THERE ARE DATA ON CARCINOGENICITY IN HUMANS

ACETALDEHYDE (Group 2B)

A. Evidence for carcinogenicity to humans (*inadequate*)

In a survey of chemical plants (without prior hypothesis) in the German Democratic Republic, nine cancer cases were found in a factory where the main process was dimerization of acetaldehyde and where the main exposures were to acetaldol, acetaldehyde, butyraldehyde, crotonaldehyde and other higher, condensed aldehydes, as well as to traces of acrolein (see p. 78). Of the cancer cases, five were bronchial tumours and two were carcinomas of the oral cavity. All nine patients were smokers. The relative frequencies of these tumours were reported to be higher than those expected in the German Democratic Republic[1]. The study is inconclusive because of mixed exposure, the small number of cases and the poorly defined exposed population.

B. Evidence for carcinogenicity to animals (*sufficient*)

Acetaldehyde was tested for carcinogenicity in rats by inhalation and in hamsters by inhalation and by intratracheal instillation. It produced tumours of the respiratory tract following its inhalation, particularly adenocarcinomas and squamous-cell carcinomas of the nasal mucosa in rats[1,2] and laryngeal carcinomas in hamsters[1]. In hamsters, it did not result in an increased incidence of tumours following intratracheal instillation[1]. Inhalation of acetaldehyde enhanced the incidence of respiratory-tract tumours induced by intratracheal instillation of benzo[a]pyrene in hamsters[1].

C. Other relevant data

No data were available on the genetic and related effects of acetaldehyde in humans.

Acetaldehyde increased the incidence of sister chromatid exchanges in bone-marrow cells of mice and hamsters treated *in vivo* and induced chromosomal aberrations in rat embryos exposed *in vivo*. It induced DNA cross-links, chromosomal aberrations and sister chromatid exchanges in human cells *in vitro* and chromosomal aberrations, micronuclei and sister chromatid exchanges in cultured rodent cells. It induced chromosomal aberrations, micronuclei and sister chromatid exchanges in plants and DNA damage and mutation in bacteria. Acetaldehyde induced cross-links in isolated DNA[3].

References

[1] IARC Monographs, *36*, 101-132, 1985

[2] Woutersen, R.A., Appelman, L.M., van Garderen-Hoetmer, A. & Feron, V.J. (1986) Inhalation toxicity of acetaldehyde in rats. III. Carcinogenicity study. *Toxicology, 41*, 213-231

[3] *IARC Monographs, Suppl. 6*, 21-23, 1987

ACROLEIN (Group 3)

A. Evidence for carcinogenicity to humans (*inadequate*)

Exposure to traces of acrolein was reported to have occurred in a chemical plant in the German Democratic Republic, where the main exposures were to acetaldol, acetaldehyde (see p. 77), butyraldehyde and crotonaldehyde. Nine cancer cases occurred in the plant; the relative frequencies of the tumours observed were reported to be higher than those expected in the German Democratic Republic. Acrolein was a relatively minor component of the exposure[1]. Because of the mixed exposure pattern, the small number of cases and the poorly defined exposed population, this study is inconclusive.

B. Evidence for carcinogenicity to animals (*inadequate*)

Acrolein was tested in mice by skin application and in hamsters by inhalation. The study in mice was inadequate for an evaluation of carcinogenicity. No carcinogenic effect was detected in hamsters[1].

C. Other relevant data

No data were available on the genetic and related effects of acrolein in humans. It did not induce dominant lethal mutations in mice. It induced sister chromatid exchanges in Chinese hamster ovary cells *in vitro*. In yeast, it did not cause DNA cross-links or strand breaks and was not mutagenic. Acrolein was mutagenic to bacteria[2].

References

[1] *IARC Monographs, 36*, 133-161, 1985
[2] *IARC Monographs, Suppl. 6*, 24-26, 1987

ACRYLONITRILE (Group 2A)

A. Evidence for carcinogenicity to humans (*limited*)

In the USA, 1345 male workers potentially exposed to acrylonitrile in a textile fibre plant and observed for 20 or more years had a greater than expected incidence of lung cancer (8 observed, 4.4 expected). The risk was greater among workers with more than five years' exposure (6 observed, 2.3 expected) or with jobs where exposure was likely to have been heavier (6 observed, 2.7 expected) than among workers with shorter duration of exposure (2 observed, 1.4 expected) or low levels of exposure (2 observed, 1.4 expected)[1,2]. Further follow-up of this cohort until 1981 revealed a continued excess of lung cancer (10 observed, 7.2 expected), although during the actual follow-up period (1976-1981) there was no excess (2 observed, 2.8 expected). The updating also showed, however, a significant excess of cancer of the prostate (6 observed, 1.8 expected)[3]. In a similar study at another US textile fibre plant, an excess of prostatic cancer (5 cases observed, 1.9 expected) was observed, but there was no excess of lung cancer[4]. In the UK, a study of 1111 male workers exposed to acrylonitrile during polymerization between 1950 and 1968 and followed for ten years or more revealed five stomach cancers (1.9 expected), two colon cancers (1.1 expected), two brain cancers (0.7 expected) and nine cancers of the respiratory tract (7.6 expected)[5]. Among 327 rubber workers exposed to acrylonitrile in the USA, excesses were noted for cancers of the lung (9 observed, 5.9 expected), bladder (2 observed, 0.5 expected) and of the lymphatic and haematopoietic system (4 observed, 1.8 expected). The risk for lung cancer was greatest among workers with five to 14 years' exposure and $\geqslant$15 years of latency (4 observed, 0.8 expected)[6]. Another study of rubber workers in the USA, however, showed no association between exposure to acrylonitrile and lung cancer[7]. In the Federal Republic of Germany, one study of 1469 workers exposed to acrylonitrile in 12 different plants showed excesses of bronchial cancer (11 observed, 5.7 expected) and of tumours of the lymphatic system (4 observed, 1.7 expected)[8].

B. Evidence for carcinogenicity to animals (*sufficient*)

Acrylonitrile was tested for carcinogenicity in rats by oral administration and by inhalation. Following its oral administration, it induced neoplasms of the brain, squamous-cell papillomas of the stomach and Zymbal-gland carcinomas; tumours of the tongue, small intestine and mammary gland were also reported[1,9,10]. Following its inhalation, neoplasms of the central nervous system, mammary gland, Zymbal gland and forestomach were observed[1,11].

C. Other relevant data

Acrylonitrile did not enhance the frequency of chromosomal aberrations in lymphocytes of exposed workers in one study[12].

In animals treated *in vivo*, acrylonitrile did not induce dominant lethal mutations, chromosomal aberrations (in bone-marrow cells or spermatogonia) or micronuclei in mice, or chromosomal aberrations in rat bone-marrow cells. It bound covalently to rat liver DNA *in vivo* and induced unscheduled DNA synthesis in rat liver but not brain. It induced sister chromatid exchanges, mutation and unscheduled DNA synthesis but not chromosomal aberrations in human cells *in vitro*. Acrylonitrile induced cell transformation in several test systems and inhibited intercellular communication in Chinese hamster V79 cells. It did not induce aneuploidy but induced chromosomal aberrations, micronuclei and sister chromatid exchanges in Chinese hamster cells; in one study, it did not induce chromosomal aberrations or sister chromatid exchanges in rat cells *in vitro*. It induced mutation and DNA strand breaks in rodent cells *in vitro*. It induced somatic mutation in *Drosophila* and was weakly mutagenic in plants. It induced aneuploidy, mutation, mitotic crossing-over and gene conversion in fungi. Acrylonitrile was mutagenic to bacteria. Urine from treated mice and rats, but not bile from rats, was mutagenic to bacteria. It bound covalently to isolated DNA[12].

References

[1]*IARC Monographs*, *19*, 73-113, 1979

[2]O'Berg, M.T. (1980) Epidemiologic study of workers exposed to acrylonitrile. *J. occup. Med.*, *22*, 245-252

[3]O'Berg, M.T., Chen, J.L., Burke, C.A., Walrath, J. & Pell, S. (1985) Epidemiologic study of workers exposed to acrylonitrile: an update. *J. occup. Med.*, *27*, 835-840

[4]Chen, J.L., Walrath, J., O'Berg, M.T., Burke, C.A. & Pell, S. (1987) Cancer incidence and mortality among workers exposed to acrylonitrile. *Am. J. ind. Med.*, *11*, 157-163

[5]Werner, J.B. & Carter, J.T. (1981) Mortality of United Kingdom acrylonitrile polymerisation workers. *Br. J. ind. Med.*, *38*, 247-253

[6]Delzell, E. & Monson, R.R. (1982) Mortality among rubber workers: VI. Men with potential exposure to acrylonitrile. *J. occup. Med.*, *24*, 767-769

[7]Waxweiler, R.J., Smith, A.H., Falk, H. & Tyroler, H.A. (1981) Excess lung cancer risk in a synthetic chemicals plant. *Environ. Health Perspect.*, *41*, 159-165

[8]Thiess, A.M., Frentzel-Beyme, R., Link, R. & Wild, H. (1980) Mortality study of chemical workers in different plants with exposure to acrylonitrile (Ger.). *Zbl. Arbeitsmed.*, *30*, 259-267

[9]Bigner, D.D., Bigner, S.H., Burger, P.C., Shelburne, J.D. & Friedman, H.S. (1986) Primary brain tumours in Fischer 344 rats chronically exposed to acrylonitrile in their drinking-water. *Food chem Toxicol.*, *24*, 129-137

[10]Quast, J.F., Humiston, C.G., Wade, C.E., Carreon, R.M., Hermann, E.A., Park, C.N. & Schwetz, B.A. 1981) Results of a chronic toxicity and oncogenicity study in rats maintained on water containing acrylonitrile for 24 months (Abstract No. 467). *Toxicologist*, *1*, 129

[11]Maltoni, C., Ciliberti, A. & Carretti, D. (1982) Experimental contributions in identifying brain potential carcinogens in the petrochemical industry. *Ann. N.Y. Acad. Sci.*, *381*, 216-249

[12]*IARC Monographs*, *Suppl. 6*, 27-31, 1987

ACTINOMYCIN D (Group 3)

A. Evidence for carcinogenicity to humans (*inadequate*)

A comparison was made in the USA between survivors of childhood cancer who developed second malignant neoplasms and controls, also survivors, matched on hospital, primary diagnosis, length of follow-up, site and dose of radiotherapy, and chronological period. Subjects who had received no radiotherapy, or who were believed to have some 'predisposing genetic syndrome', and whose second tumour had been diagnosed within six months of the first diagnosis, or with tumours that lay outside the field previously treated with radiation were excluded. Unexpectedly, cases had been treated much less often with actinomycin D than controls (relative risk, 0.13; upper 95% confidence limit, 0.47), and those who had been treated had received fewer courses of treatment (median, 2, compared to 6.5). For each type of primary childhood malignancy, except for bone tumours, the majority of cases had not been treated with actinomycin D. Second malignancies included soft-tissue sarcomas, haematological malignancies and various solid tumours. A relationship is plausible in view of the radiomimetic properties of actinomycin D, the simultaneous exposure of the treated patients to radiation, and the modal shape of radiation dose-effect curves in some laboratory systems[1].

A single attempt to confirm this finding covered only eight second malignancies (meeting criteria comparable to those in the first study) occurring among 412 patients who had been treated with radiation for Wilms' tumour of whom 222 had also received actinomycin D. No similar reduction in risk was observed. This study differed from the original in the small sample size, the uniformity with respect to primary diagnosis and that the comparison was made with historical controls[2].

B. Evidence for carcinogenicity to animals (*limited*)

Actinomycin D was tested for carcinogenicity in rats by intraperitoneal injection and by intragastric administration and in mice by repeated subcutaneous injections. It produced peritoneal sarcomas in rats following intraperitoneal injections[3,4], and a low incidence of subcutaneous sarcomas occurred in mice following repeated subcutaneous injections[3]. No tumour was observed in rats after intragastric administration of actinomycin D, but the duration of the experiment was short[5].

C. Other relevant data

Actinomycin D did not induce sister chromatid exchanges in peripheral blood lymphocytes of treated patients in one study[6].

Actinomycin D induced chromosomal aberrations and DNA strand breaks in human cells *in vitro*. It transformed mouse C3H 10T1/2 cells and induced chromosomal aberrations, sister chromatid exchanges, mutation, DNA strand breaks and unscheduled DNA synthesis, but not aneuploidy, in rodent cells *in vitro*. It induced sex-linked recessive lethal mutations in *Drosophila*. Actinomycin D did not cause chromosomal aberrations in plants. It was mutagenic to *Neurospora crassa* but not to *Saccharomyces cerevisiae*, and conflicting results were obtained for gene conversion and mitotic recombination. It did not induce DNA damage in *Schizosaccharomyces pombe*. It was not mutagenic to bacteria and did not induce prophage[6].

References

[1]D'Angio, G.J., Meadows, A., Miké, V., Harris, C., Evans, A., Jaffe, N., Newton, W., Schweisguth, O., Sutow, W. & Morris-Jones, P. (1976) Decreased risk of radiation-associated second malignant neoplasms in actinomycin-D-treated patients. *Cancer, 37*, 1177-1185

[2]Li, F.P., Yan, J.C., Sallan, S:, Cassady, J.R., Jr, Danahy, J., Fine, W., Gelber, R.D. & Green, D.M. (1983) Second neoplasms after Wilms' tumor in childhood. *J. natl Cancer Inst., 71*, 1205-1209

[3]*IARC Monographs, 10*, 29-41, 1976

[4]Weisburger, J.H., Griswold, D.P., Prejean, J.D., Casey, A.E., Wood, H.B. & Weisburger, E.K. (1975) The carcinogenic properties of some of the principal drugs used in clinical cancer chemotherapy. *Recent Results Cancer Res., 52*, 1-17

[5]Philips, F.S. & Sternberg, S.S. (1975) Tests for tumor induction by antitumor agents. *Recent Results Cancer Res., 52*, 29-35

[6]*IARC Monographs, Suppl. 6*, 32-34, 1987

ADRIAMYCIN (Group 2A)

A. Evidence for carcinogenicity to humans (*inadequate*)

No epidemiological study of adriamycin as a single agent was available to the Working Group. Occasional case reports, especially in the presence of concurrent therapy with other putative carcinogens, such as ionizing radiation, alkylating agents and other potent oncotherapeutic drugs, do not constitute evidence of carcinogenesis.

In a large systematic follow-up of patients with Hodgkin's disease treated with an intensive chemotherapeutic combination including adriamycin [plus vinblastine (see p. 371), bleomycin (see p. 134) and dacarbazine (see p. 184)] but no alkylating agent, preliminary evidence suggested no excess of acute nonlymphocytic leukaemia in the first decade after therapy[1].

B. Evidence for carcinogenicity to animals (*sufficient*)

Adriamycin was tested for carcinogenicity in rats by a single intravenous injection, producing mammary tumours[2-5], and by single or repeated subcutaneous injections, producing local sarcomas and mammary tumours[6,7]. Intravesicular instillation of adriamycin in rats resulted in a low incidence of bladder papillomas and enhanced the incidence of bladder tumours induced by N-nitroso-N-(4-hydroxybutyl)-N-butylamine[8].

C. Other relevant data

Adriamycin induced chromosomal aberrations in treated patients in one of two studies and sister chromatid exchanges in both studies. In another study, cisplatin-adriamycin combination chemotherapy induced sister chromatid exchanges in peripheral blood lymphocytes of treated patients. DNA strand breaks were induced in the cells of treated patients in one study[9].

Adriamycin has been tested extensively for genetic effects in a wide variety of tests *in vivo* and *in vitro*, giving consistently positive results. It induced chromosomal aberrations, micronuclei, sister chromatid exchanges and DNA damage in rodents *in vivo* and chromosomal aberrations, micronuclei, sister chromatid exchanges and DNA damage in human cells *in vitro*. It transformed virus-infected Fischer rat embryo cells and induced chromosomal aberrations, sister chromatid exchanges, mutation and DNA damage in cultured rodent cells. Adriamycin induced sex-linked recessive lethal mutations in *Drosophila*, chromosomal aberrations in plants and mutation in fungi. It was mutagenic to bacteria and induced DNA damage[9].

References

[1]Valagussa, P., Santoro, A., Kenda, R., Fossati Bellani, F., Franchi, F., Banfi, A., Rilke, F. & Bonadonna, G. (1980) Second malignancies in Hodgkin's disease: a complication of certain forms of treatment. *Br. med. J.*, *i*, 216-219

[2]*IARC Monographs*, *10*, 43-49, 1976

[3]Marquardt, H., Philips, F.S. & Sternberg, S.S. (1976) Tumorigenicity *in vivo* and induction of malignant transformation and mutagenesis in cell cultures by adriamycin and daunomycin. *Cancer Res.*, *36*, 2065-2069

[4]Solcia, E., Ballerini, L., Bellini, O., Sala, L. & Bertazolli, C. (1978) Mammary tumors induced in rats by adriamycin and daunomycin. *Cancer Res.*, *38*, 1444-1446

[5]Bucciarelli, E. (1981) Mammary tumor induction in male and female Sprague-Dawley rats by adriamycin and daunomycin. *J. natl Cancer Inst.*, *66*, 81-84

[6]Maltoni, C. & Chieco, P. (1975) Adriamycin: a new potent carcinogen (Ital.). *Osp. Vita*, *2*, 107-109

[7]Casazza, A.M., Bellini, O., Formelli, F., Giuliani, F., Lenaz, L. & Magrini, U. (1977) Tumors and dental and ocular abnormalities after treatment of infant rats with adriamycin. *Tumori*, *63*, 331-338

[8]Ohtani, M., Fukushima, S., Okamura, T., Sakata, T., Ito, N., Koiso, K. & Niijima, T. (1984) Effects of intravesical instillation of antitumor chemotherapeutic agents on bladder carcinogenesis in rats treated with *N*-butyl-*N*-(4-hydroxybutyl)nitrosamine. *Cancer*, *54*, 1525-1529

[9]*IARC Monographs*, *Suppl. 6*, 35-39, 1987

AFLATOXINS (Group 1)

A. Evidence for carcinogenicity to humans (*sufficient*)

A positive correlation between estimated aflatoxin intake or level of aflatoxin contamination of market food samples and cooked food and incidence of hepatocellular cancer was observed in early studies in Uganda, Swaziland, Thailand and Kenya[1-4]. Similar correlations between aflatoxin intake and hepatocellular cancer incidence and mortality have been reported from Mozambique and China, where there is considerable geographical variation in the occurrence of this cancer[5-8]. Summary analysis of the data obtained from studies conducted in different regions of Africa and Asia where hepatocellular cancer incidence or mortality and aflatoxin intake were measured revealed a highly significant correlation between these variables[5].

In south-eastern USA, in an area with a high average daily intake of aflatoxin B_1 (13-197 ng/kg bw), a 10% excess (6% for the 30-49 age group) in hepatocellular cancer incidence was observed compared to 'northern' and 'western' areas with low aflatoxin B_1 intake (0.2-0.3 ng/kg bw)[9].

A case-control study in the Philippines, where mean aflatoxin contamination levels in dietary items were established and individual levels of aflatoxin consumption were determined retrospectively, demonstrated an increased, dose-related relative risk of developing hepatocellular cancer in persons with higher ingestion of aflatoxin. Relative risks of developing hepatocellular cancer by category of overall mean load of aflatoxin in the diet, e.g., very heavy *versus* light and moderately heavy *versus* light, were 17.0 and 13.9 (both significant at the 0.05 level). The effect of aflatoxin on relative risk was increased by alcohol consumption, and heavy aflatoxin/heavy alcohol consumption gave a relative risk of 35.0[10].

In a case-control study conducted in Hong Kong where 107 hepatocellular cancer patients and 107 controls were studied, the relative risk of hepatocellular cancer was not related to dietary intake of corn or beans, which are the chief sources of aflatoxin contamination in Hong Kong. The relative risk was increased (2.2), but not significantly, for consumption of 'other grains', including wheat, barley and oats[11]; however, among 878 market food samples, only 22 contained aflatoxins[12].

One major difficulty in interpreting these studies is potential confounding due to hepatitis virus B infection, which is endemic in many areas where the relationship between aflatoxin intake and hepatocellular carcinoma has been examined. However, in three recent studies, both factors have been taken into account. In China, both dietary and urinary levels of aflatoxins were found to be related to hepatocellular cancer incidence. Levels of aflatoxin M_1 as high as 35 ng were found in urine in high-incidence areas, whereas levels of <2 ng were observed in low-risk areas. Serological surveys did not show corresponding differences in the prevalence of the hepatitis B virus-carrier state[13]. In another area of China, the mortality rate for hepatocellular cancer was 9.9 times higher in villages with high aflatoxin contamination of foodstuffs than in villages with lightly contaminated foods. In this area, aflatoxin contamination of foods appeared to be a risk factor over and above hepatitis B infection[14]. In Swaziland, in a study based on surveys of levels of aflatoxin intake across four broad geographic regions, liver cancer incidence was strongly associated with estimated levels of aflatoxin. In a multivariate analysis involving ten smaller subregions, aflatoxin exposure emerged as a more important determinant of the variation in liver cancer incidence than the prevalence of hepatitis B infection. This analysis was based on 52 cases spread over ten subareas, and estimations of aflatoxin intake and prevalence of hepatitis B infection were based on surveys conducted among the general population and on samples from blood donors, respectively. Imprecision in measuring intake of aflatoxin or in establishing hepatitis B infection, or the presence of unmeasured confounders, seem unlikely to account for the five-fold differences in hepatocellular cancer incidence seen in association with aflatoxin intake[15].

Additional evidence for a causative association between aflatoxin exposure and human cancer was found in a retrospective cohort study of 71 workers in a plant in the Netherlands where oil was extracted from linseeds and from peanuts. In the aflatoxin-exposed group, the observed mortality over the entire 18-year study period was higher than expected for all cancers (standardized mortality ratio [SMR], 250; 95% confidence interval, 140-400) and for the first six years of observation (SMR, 438; 180-870). An increase in mortality from respiratory cancer in the exposed group was also evident (SMR, 253; 100-500)[16].

A few case reports of cancer other than hepatocellular in aflatoxin-exposed workers have been published[1,17-19].

B. Evidence for carcinogenicity to animals (*sufficient*)

Aflatoxins produce liver tumours in mice, rats, fish, ducks, marmosets, tree shrews and monkeys after administration by several routes, including the mouth. In rats, cancers of the colon and kidney were also seen[1]. Recent studies have extended these findings. In hamsters, aflatoxin B_1 produced cholangiocellular but not hepatocellular tumours[20]. In mice, aflatoxin B_1 administered orally or intraperitoneally resulted in an increased incidence of lung adenomas[1,21]. All rats fed 5 mg/kg of diet aflatoxin B_1 for six weeks developed hepatocellular carcinomas[22]; neoplastic hepatic nodules were produced in rats by oral administration of a single dose of 5 mg/kg bw aflatoxin B_1[23]; rats fed peanut oil containing 5-7 μg/kg aflatoxin B_1 developed parenchymal liver damage but no liver-cell tumour[24]. Aflatoxin B_1 can induce liver tumours in monkeys[25,26]; osteogenic sarcoma, adeno-carcinoma of the gall-bladder or bile duct and carcinomas of the pancreas were also observed[26]. Aflatoxin B_1 also induced liver tumours in the subhuman primate tree shrew, *Tupaia glis*[27]. Intraperitoneal administration of aflatoxin B_1 to pregnant rats induced liver and other tumours in the mothers and in the progeny[28]. Aflatoxin M_1, a hydroxy metabolite of aflatoxin B_1, produced fewer hepatocellular carcinomas following its oral administration to rats than aflatoxin B_1 given at the same dose level and by the same route[29].

C. Other relevant data

In one study, aflatoxin B_1-DNA adducts were excreted in human urine. No data were available on the genetic and related effects of aflatoxins B_2, G_1, G_2 or M_1 in humans[30].

Aflatoxin B_1 has been tested extensively for genetic effects in a wide variety of tests *in vivo* and *in vitro*, giving consistently positive results. It induced chromosomal aberrations, micronuclei, sister chromatid exchanges, unscheduled DNA synthesis and DNA strand breaks, and bound covalently to DNA in cells of rodents treated *in vivo*; it was reported to be weakly active in a dominant-lethal mutation assay in mice. In human cells *in vitro*, it induced chromosomal aberrations, micronuclei, sister chromatid exchanges and unscheduled DNA synthesis and bound covalently to DNA. It induced cell transformation in several test systems, and induced chromosomal aberrations, sister chromatid exchanges, mutation, unscheduled DNA synthesis and DNA strand breaks in rodent cells *in vitro*. It induced sex-linked recessive lethal mutations and somatic mutation and recombination in *Drosophila*. In fungi, aflatoxin B_1 was mutagenic and induced gene conversion and mitotic recombination. It was mutagenic and induced DNA damage in bacteria and bound covalently to isolated DNA[30].

Aflatoxin B_2 bound covalently to DNA in hepatocytes of rats treated *in vivo*. It transformed Syrian hamster embryo cells and induced sister chromatid exchanges in Chinese hamster cells *in vitro* and induced unscheduled DNA synthesis in rat hepatocytes, but not in human fibroblasts, *in vitro*. It was not mutagenic to fungi in the absence of a metabolic system and did not induce gene conversion or mitotic recombination in yeast. Aflatoxin B_2 induced mutation but not DNA damage in bacteria[30].

Aflatoxin G_1 induced chromosomal aberrations in bone-marrow cells of Chinese hamsters treated *in vivo* and bound to DNA in kidney and liver cells of treated rats. It induced unscheduled DNA synthesis in human fibroblasts and rat hepatocytes *in vitro* and caused chromosomal aberrations and sister chromatid exchanges in Chinese hamster cells *in vitro*. It induced mutation in *Neurospora crassa* but neither mutation nor gene conversion in *Saccharomyces cerevisiae*. Aflatoxin G_1 induced mutation and DNA damage in bacteria and bound covalently to isolated DNA[30].

Aflatoxin G_2 did not induce unscheduled DNA synthesis in human fibroblasts *in vitro*. It induced sister chromatid exchanges in Chinese hamster cells and unscheduled DNA synthesis in rat and hamster hepatocytes *in vitro*. It did not induce mutation in cultured rodent cells or in fungi in the absence of a metabolic system. Aflatoxin G_2 gave conflicting results for mutation in bacteria and did not cause DNA damage[30].

Aflatoxin M_1 induced unscheduled DNA synthesis in rat hepatocytes *in vitro* and was mutagenic to bacteria[30].

References

[1]*IARC Monographs*, *10*, 51-72, 1976

[2]Linsell, C.A. & Peers, F.G. (1977) Aflatoxin and liver cell cancer. *Trans. R. Soc. trop. Med. Hyg.*, *71*, 471-473

[3]van Rensburg, S.J. (1977) *Role of epidemiology in the elucidation of mycotoxin health risks*. In: Rodricks, J.V., Hesseltine, C.W. & Mehlman, M.A., eds, *Mycotoxins in Human and Animal Health*, Park Forest South, IL, Pathotox, pp. 699-711

[4]Peers, F.G., Gilman, G.A. & Linsell, C.A. (1976) Dietary aflatoxins and human liver cancer. A study in Swaziland. *Int. J. Cancer*, *17*, 167-176

[5]van Rensburg, S.J., Cook-Mozaffari, P., van Schalkwyk, D.J., van der Watt, J.J., Vincent, T.J. & Purchase, I.F. (1985) Hepatocellular carcinoma and dietary aflatoxin in Mozambique and Transkei. *Br. J. Cancer*, *51*, 713-726

[6]Armstrong, B. (1980) The epidemiology of cancer in the People's Republic of China. *Int. J. Epidemiol.*, *9*, 305-315

[7]Yaobin, W., Lizun, L., Benfa, Y., Yaochu, X., Yunyuan, L. & Wenguang, L. (1983) Relation between geographical distribution of liver cancer and climate-aflatoxin B_1 in China. *Sci. sin.* (*Ser. B*), *26*, 1166-1175

[8]Yeh, F.S., Yan, R.C., Mor, C.C., Liu, Y.K. & Yang, K.C. (1982) *Research on etiological factors of hepatocellular carcinoma in Guangxi, China* (Abstract no. 1935). In: *Proceedings of the XIII International Cancer Congress, Seattle, September 1982*, Seattle, WA, Cancer Research Center, p. 340

[9]Stoloff, L. (1983) Aflatoxin as a cause of primary liver-cell cancer in the United States: a probability study. *Nutr. Cancer*, *5*, 165-186

[10]Bulatao-Jayme, J., Almero, E.M., Castro, M.C.A, Jardeleza, M.T.R. & Salamat, L.A. (1982) A case-control dietary study of primary liver cancer risk from aflatoxin exposure. *Int. J. Epidemiol.*, *11*, 112-119

[11]Lam, K.C., Yu, M.C., Leung, J.W.C. & Henderson, B.E. (1982) Hepatitis B virus and cigarette smoking: risk factors for hepatocellular carcinoma in Hong Kong. *Cancer Res.*, *42*, 5246-5248

[12]Shank, R.C., Wogan, G.N., Gibson, J.B. & Nondasuta, A. (1972) Dietary aflatoxins and human liver cancer. II. Aflatoxins in market foods and foodstuffs of Thailand and Hong Kong. *Food Cosmet. Toxicol.*, *10*, 61-69

[13]Sun, T.-T. & Chu, Y.-Y. (1984) Carcinogenesis and prevention strategy of liver cancer in areas of prevalence. *J. cell. Physiol., Suppl. 3*, 39-44

[14]Yeh, F.-S., Mo, C.-C. & Yen, R.-C. (1985) Risk factors for hepatocellular carcinoma in Guangxi, People's Republic of China. *Natl Cancer Inst. Monogr.*, *69*, 47-48

[15]Peers, F., Bosch, X., Kaldor, J., Linsell, A. & Pluijmen, M. (1987) Aflatoxin exposure, hepatitis B virus infection and liver cancer in Swaziland. *Int. J. Cancer*, *39*, 545-553

[16]Hayes, R.B., van Nieuwenhuize, J.P., Raatgever, J.W. & ten Kate, F.J.W. (1984) Aflatoxin exposures in the industrial setting: an epidemiological study of mortality. *Food chem. Toxicol.*, *22*, 39-43

[17]Deger, G.E. (1976) Aflatoxin — human colon carcinogenesis? *Ann. intern. Med.*, *85*, 204-205

[18]Dvořáčková, I. (1976) Aflatoxin inhalation and alveolar cell carcinoma. *Br. med. J.*, *i*, 691

[19]Dvořáčková, I., Stora, C. & Ayraud, N. (1981) Evidence for aflatoxin B_1 in two cases of lung cancer in man. *J. Cancer Res. clin. Oncol.*, *100*, 221-224

[20]Moore, M.R., Pitot, H.C., Miller, E.C. & Miller, J.A. (1982) Cholangiocellular carcinomas induced in Syrian golden hamsters administered aflatoxin B_1 in large doses. *J. natl Cancer Inst.*, *68*, 271-278

[21]Stoner, G.D., Conran, P.B., Greisiger, E.A., Stober, J., Morgan, M. & Pereira, M.A. (1986) Comparison of two routes of chemical administration on the lung adenoma response in strain A/J mice. *Toxicol. appl. Pharmacol.*, *82*, 19-31

[22]Butler, H.W. & Hempsall, V. (1981) Histochemical studies of hepatocellular carcinomas in the rat induced by aflatoxin. *J. Pathol.*, *134*, 157-170

[23]Bannasch, P., Benner, U., Enzmann, H. & Hacker, H.J. (1985) Tigroid cell foci and neoplastic nodules in the liver of rats treated with a single dose of aflatoxin B_1. *Carcinogenesis*, *6*, 1641-1648

[24]Fong, L.Y.Y. & Chan, W.C. (1981) Long-term effects of feeding aflatoxin-contaminated market peanut oil to Sprague-Dawley rats. *Food Cosmet. Toxicol.*, *19*, 179-183

[25]Adamson, R.H., Correa, P., Sieber, S.M., McIntire, K.R. & Dalgard, D.W. (1976) Carcinogenicity of aflatoxin B_1 in rhesus monkeys: two additional cases of primary liver cancer. *J. natl Cancer Inst.*, *57*, 67-78

[26]Sieber, S.M., Correa, P., Dalgard, D.W. & Adamson, R.H. (1979) Induction of osteogenic sarcomas and tumors of the hepatobiliary system in nonhuman primates with aflatoxin B_1. *Cancer Res.*, *39*, 4545-4554

[27]Reddy, J.K., Svoboda, D.J. & Rao, M.S. (1976) Induction of liver tumors by aflatoxin B_1 in the tree shrew (*Tupaia glis*), a nonhuman primate. *Cancer Res.*, *36*, 151-160

[28]Goerttler, K., Löhrke, H., Schweizer, H.-J. & Hesse, B. (1980) Effects of aflatoxin B_1 on pregnant inbred Sprague-Dawley rats and their F_1 generation. A contribution to transplacental carcinogenesis. *J. natl Cancer Inst.*, *64*, 1349-1354

[29]Hsieh, D.P.H., Cullen, J.M. & Ruebner, B.H. (1984) Comparative hepatocarcinogenicity of aflatoxins B_1 and M_1 in the rat. *Food chem. Toxicol.*, *22*, 1027-1028

[30]*IARC Monographs, Suppl. 6*, 40-56, 1987

ALDRIN (Group 3)

A. Evidence for carcinogenicity to humans (*inadequate*)

Specific mention of aldrin in analytical epidemiological studies is limited to reports of follow-up of two cohorts of men employed in its manufacture in plants where dieldrin (see p. 196) and endrin (and, in one, telodrin) were also manufactured[1-4]. In the most recent report of the first of these cohorts[3], 232 of 233 exposed workers were successfully followed from four to 29 (mean, 24) years, with duration of exposure to pesticides varying between four and 27 (mean, 11) years. There were nine deaths from cancer with 12 expected (standardized mortality ratio [SMR], 75; 95% confidence interval, 25-125). In the second cohort[4], 90% of 1155 men were followed for 13 years or more. Mortality from all cancers was not increased (SMR, 82; 56-116), although there were apparent increases in mortality from cancers of the oesophagus, rectum and liver, based on very small numbers.

B. Evidence for carcinogenicity to animals (*limited*)

Aldrin was tested for carcinogenicity by the oral route in mice and rats. In mice, it produced malignant liver neoplasms[1,5]. In rats, the incidence of thyroid tumours was increased in exposed animals in one study[5], but this could not be clearly associated with treatment; three other studies in rats gave negative results[1,6] and one was inadequate[1].

C. Other relevant data

No data were available on the genetic and related effects of aldrin in humans. It did not induce dominant lethal mutations in mice. In single studies, it induced chromosomal aberrations in bone-marrow cells of rats and mice, but no micronuclei in bone-marrow cells of mice treated *in vivo*. It induced chromosomal aberrations in cultured human lymphocytes; studies of DNA damage in human and rodent cells *in vitro* were inconclusive. Aldrin inhibited intercellular communication in both human and rodent cell systems. It did not induce sex-linked recessive lethal mutations in *Drosophila* but was mutagenic to yeast. It was not mutagenic to bacteria and did not induce breakage of plasmid DNA[7].

References

[1]*IARC Monographs*, 5, 25-38, 1974

[2]Van Raalte, H.G.S. (1977) Human experience with dieldrin in perspective. *Ecotoxicol. environ. Saf.*, 1, 203-210

[3]Ribbens, P.H. (1985) Mortality study of industrial workers exposed to aldrin, dieldrin and endrin. *Int. Arch. occup. environ. Health*, 56, 75-79

[4]Ditraglia, D., Brown, D.P., Namekata, T. & Iverson, N. (1981) Mortality study of workers employed at organochlorine pesticide manufacturing plants. *Scand. J. Work Environ. Health*, 7 (*Suppl. 4*), 140-146

[5]National Cancer Institute (1978) *Bioassays of Aldrin and Dieldrin for Possible Carcinogenicity (Tech. Rep. Ser. No. 21; DHEW Publ. No. (NIH) 78-821)*, Bethesda, MD, US Department of Health, Education, and Welfare

[6]Deichmann, W.B., MacDonald, W.E. & Lu, F.C. (1979) *Effects of chronic aldrin feeding in two strains of female rats and a discussion on the risks of carcinogens in man*. In: Deichmann, W.B., ed., *Toxicology and Occupational Medicine*, New York, Elsevier/North-Holland, pp. 407-413
[7]*IARC Monographs, Suppl. 6*, 57-59, 1987

ALUMINIUM PRODUCTION (Group 1)

A. Evidence for carcinogenicity to humans (*sufficient*)

The lung has been the most common site identified for which there is an excess cancer risk in populations of aluminium production workers. Overall, early studies showed a borderline excess in relative risk, with some studies showing a doubling of risk and some showing no excess. Smoking histories were not given in any of these studies. In one study in which populations in the industry were compared on the basis of their exposures to pitch volatiles, there was a relationship between incidence of lung cancer and length of exposure, and there was a significant excess of cancer among workers who had worked for 21 years or more[1].

In three studies in the same aluminium-producing area, an increased risk of bladder cancer was associated with work in aluminium production in plants where primarily the Söderberg process was used. In one study in which smoking was controlled for, while there was a borderline excess in risk for nonsmokers, the risk for smokers was markedly increased[1].

Excess mortality from lymphosarcoma/reticulosarcoma was noted in two cohort studies, which covered partially the same population[1].

Statistically significant excess risks for pancreatic cancer and for leukaemia were noted as isolated findings in two studies and in one study, respectively[1].

Some of these studies have been updated. In Canada, the mortality of a large group of men employed in aluminium production using the Söderberg process was examined between 1950 and 1977, and compared with the pertinent rates for the Province of Quebec. Workers 'ever' exposed to condensed pitch volatiles ('tar') exhibited significantly increased mortality from all cancers (304 observed, 246.6 expected), and from oesophageal and stomach cancer (50 observed, 32.8 expected), lung cancer (101 observed, 70.7 expected) and other malignancies (60 observed, 45.3 expected). Analysis of lung cancer mortality by increasing years of exposure, tar-years of exposure and years since first exposure to tar revealed a steady, statistically significant, increasing trend. No similarly clear-cut pattern was noted for cancers of the oesophagus or stomach. Deaths from cancer of the urinary organs (20 observed, 13.7 expected) and bladder (12 observed, 7.5 expected) were more numerous than expected, but not significantly so. Nonetheless, when mortality from cancer at each of these sites was analysed according to tar-years of exposure, significantly increasing trends were noted. Among workers 'never' exposed to tar, mortality was not elevated above expectancy for any cancer site[2].

The risk for bladder cancer was further investigated in a case-control study based on 488 bladder cancer cases occurring in 1970-1979 in regions of the Province of Quebec where five aluminium plants were operating using the Söderberg production process. A statistically significant odds ratio of 2.7, based on 45 exposed cases, was found for employment in Söderberg reactor rooms. The risk increased steadily with time worked in this department, with odds ratios ranging from 1.9 for those who had worked for one to nine years, up to 4.5 for those who had worked in the department for over 30 years. This trend was statistically significant. The risk also increased steadily with increasing estimated exposure to 'tar' and polycyclic aromatic hydrocarbons and remained almost unchanged after adjusting for cigarette smoking, length of employment and age[3]. This set of data was later reanalysed in an attempt to quantify the noted exposure-response relationship. More refined quantitative estimates of historical workplace exposure and more complete information on smoking habits were used. Estimates of bladder cancer risk were highly statistically significantly related to three exposure indices: years spent in the Söderberg potroom; cumulative exposure to benzene-soluble material, an indicator of overall exposure to tar volatiles; and cumulative exposure to benzo[a]pyrene, an indicator of exposure to polycyclic aromatic hydrocarbons. It was estimated that an aluminium smelter worker exposed to 0.2 mg/m³ benzene-soluble material for 40 years has a likelihood of contracting bladder cancer approximately 2.5-fold that of a nonexposed person. Workers exposed to 5 μg/m³ benzo[a]pyrene for 40 years had a likelihood of contracting bladder cancer approximately five-fold that of an unexposed person. Smoking did not confound the relationship[4].

There is sufficient evidence that certain exposures occurring during aluminium production cause cancer. Pitch volatiles have fairly consistently been suggested in epidemiological studies as being possible causative agents. Dose-response relationships have been clarified, and confounding by smoking controlled for.

B. Other relevant data

No effect on the incidence of sister chromatid exchanges in peripheral blood lymphocytes of workers in the aluminium industry was observed in one study. No increase in the incidence of structural chromosomal aberrations was observed in the lymphocytes of workers in an aluminium reduction plant exposed to coal-tar pitch volatiles (anode production area); analyses of the semen showed no effect on sperm morphology, sperm count or double-Y bodies, when compared to matched controls from the same area, but there was an excess of mutagenic urine samples among these workers as compared to controls. Urine samples from workers in an anode manufacturing plant were not mutagenic to *Salmonella typhimurium* in the presence of a metabolic system. Methanol extracts of sputum and bronchial expectorates, pooled separately for smoking and for nonsmoking workers in a Söderberg process potroom, were tested for mutagenicity to *S. typhimurium* in the presence of an exogenous metabolic system. Expectorates from smokers were mutagenic, while those from nonsmokers yielded inconclusive results; samples from pooled controls were inactive[5].

References

[1]*IARC Monographs, 34*, 37-64, 1984

[2]Gibbs, G.W. (1985) Mortality of aluminum reduction plant workers, 1950 through 1977. *J. occup. Med., 27*, 761-770

[3]Thériault, G., Tremblay, C., Cordier, S. & Gingras, S. (1984) Bladder cancer in the aluminium industry. *Lancet, i*, 947-950

[4]Armstrong, B.G., Tremblay, C.G., Cyr, D. & Thériault, G.P. (1986) Estimating the relationship between exposure to tar volatiles and the incidence of bladder cancer in aluminum smelter workers. *Scand. J. Work Environ. Health, 12*, 486-493

[5]*IARC Monographs, Suppl. 6*, 60, 1987

4-AMINOBIPHENYL (Group 1)

A. Evidence for carcinogenicity to humans (*sufficient*)

The extent of bladder cancer risk associated with exposure to 4-aminobiphenyl was first documented by a descriptive study in the mid-1950s: of 171 men exposed to 4-amino-biphenyl between 1935 and 1955, 19 developed bladder tumours[1]. This observation appears to have been sufficient to prompt discontinuation of production and to prevent widespread use of the chemical. In 1955, a surveillance programme was initiated on workers reported to have been exposed to the chemical: during the following 14 years, 541 men were kept under surveillance by clinical and laboratory examinations; 86 had positive or suspicious cytology of the urinary sediment some time during the observation period, and 43 developed histologically confirmed carcinoma of the urinary bladder[2].

The hypothesis that another potential carcinogen, 4-nitrobiphenyl, was actually associated with the increased bladder cancer risk among these workers was raised but was dismissed by careful reconsideration of the processes involved and the possible exposures of the workers under surveillance[3].

In a survey of cancer mortality among workers at a chemical plant producing a variety of chemicals, a ten-fold increase in mortality from bladder cancer was reported. All of the nine cases on which the excess was based had started work in the plant before 1949, and 4-aminobiphenyl was known to have been used from 1941 until 1952[4].

B. Evidence for carcinogenicity to animals (*sufficient*)

4-Aminobiphenyl was tested for carcinogenicity by oral administration in rabbits, dogs and mice and by subcutaneous administration in rats. Following its oral administration, it induced bladder papillomas and carcinomas in rabbits[1] and dogs[1,5], and neoplasms at various sites in mice, including dose-related increases in the incidences of angiosarcomas[6], hepatocellular tumours[1,6] and bladder carcinomas[1,6]. Following its subcutaneous administration to rats, it induced tumours of the mammary gland and intestine[1].

C. Other relevant data

No data were available on the genetic and related effects of 4-aminobiphenyl in humans. It formed DNA adducts in the bladder epithelium of dogs and protein adducts in serum albumin of rats treated *in vivo*. It induced mutation in human fibroblasts and mutation, DNA strand breaks and unscheduled DNA synthesis in cultured rodent cells. 4-Aminobiphenyl was mutagenic to bacteria and induced prophage[7].

References

[1]*IARC Monographs*, *1*, 74-79, 1972

[2]Melamed, M.R. (1972) Diagnostic cytology of urinary tract carcinoma. A review of experience with spontaneous and carcinogen induced tumors in man. *Eur. J. Cancer*, *8*, 287-292

[3]Melick, W.F. (1972) Bladder carcinoma and xenylamine. *New Engl. J. Med.*, *287*, 1103

[4]Zack, J.A. & Gaffey, W.R. (1983) A mortality study of workers employed at the Monsanto Company plant in Nitro, West Virginia. *Environ. Sci. Res.*, *26*, 575-591

[5]Block, N.L., Sigel, M.M., Lynne, C.M., Ng, A.B. & Grosberg, R.A. (1978) The initiation, progress, and diagnosis of dog bladder cancer induced by 4-aminobiphenyl. *Invest. Urol.*, *16*, 50-54

[6]Schieferstein, G.J., Littlefield, N.A., Gaylor, D.W., Sheldon, W.G. & Burger, G.T. (1985) Carcinogenesis of 4-aminobiphenyl in BALB/cStCr1fC3Hf/Nctr mice. *Eur. J. Cancer clin. Oncol.*, *21*, 865-873

[7]*IARC Monographs, Suppl. 6*, 60-63, 1987

AMITROLE (Group 2B)

A. Evidence for carcinogenicity to humans (*inadequate*)

In a small cohort study of 348 Swedish railroad workers exposed for 45 days or more to amitrole, 2,4-D or 2,4,5-T (see p. 256) and to other organic (e.g., monuron and diuron) and inorganic chemicals (e.g., potassium chlorate), there was an excess of deaths from malignant neoplasms (17 observed, 11.9 expected). There was a statistically significant excess of all cancers among those exposed to amitrole and chlorophenoxy herbicides: six deaths from cancer with 2.9 expected, of which all six — with 1.8 expected ($p < 0.005$) — occurred in those first exposed ten years or more before death. No significant excess was seen among those exposed mainly to amitrole: five deaths from cancer with 3.3 expected, three deaths with two expected occurring in those first exposed ten years or more before death[1]. The role of amitrole exposure is therefore not possible to evaluate.

B. Evidence for carcinogenicity to animals (*sufficient*)

Amitrole was tested for carcinogenicity in mice by oral administration, skin application and transplacental exposure, in rats by oral and subcutaneous administration and in hamsters by oral administration. After oral administration, it produced thyroid tumours and benign and malignant liver tumours in mice of each sex, benign and malignant thyroid tumours in male and female rats and benign pituitary tumours in female rats[1].

C. Other relevant data

No data were available on the genetic and related effects of amitrole in humans.

Amitrole did not induce micronuclei in bone-marrow cells of mice or unscheduled DNA synthesis in hepatocytes of rats treated *in vivo*. It induced transformation of Syrian hamster embryo cells and increased the incidence of sister chromatid exchanges in Chinese hamster ovary cells; both positive and negative results were reported for mutation in cultured rodent cells. Amitrole did not induce sex-linked recessive lethal mutations or aneuploidy in *Drosophila*; it induced chromosomal aberrations in plants. Both positive and negative results were obtained in assays for gene conversion and mutation in fungi, but amitrole induced aneuploidy. It was not mutagenic to bacteria and did not induce DNA damage[2].

References

[1]*IARC Monographs*, *41*, 293-317, 1986
[2]*IARC Monographs*, *Suppl. 6*, 64-67, 1987

ANAESTHETICS, VOLATILE (Group 3)

A. Evidence for carcinogenicity to humans (*inadequate*)

Data from postal surveys of cancer incidence among working populations showed a higher rate of cancer among female operating-room personnel than among controls[1-4], partly reflecting an excess of leukaemia and lymphoma[2]. In one of the studies[4], a higher rate of cancer was reported among dental assistants with relatively heavy exposure to anaesthetics, reflecting a higher prevalence of cervical and uterine cancer in women with heavier exposure to anaesthetics than in those with a lighter exposure (significant only for cancer of the cervix). All of these postal surveys had major shortcomings[5], with response rates varying from 40-82%. Five mortality studies were carried out on anaesthetists[6-10]. A deficiency of deaths from cancer was seen in four[6,8-10]; however, in one study[6], there was an excess of deaths from lymphoma and myeloma (17 observed, 8.9 expected, with a ratio of 1.9 [95% confidence interval, 1.2-2.6]) and, in another, a possible excess of cancer of the pancreas[7]. Cancer incidence was also studied in 28 235 registered nurses. Minor excesses of breast cancer, lymphoma and acute myelogenous leukaemia were balanced by deficits in cancers at other sites. No significant difference was found for active operation and anaesthetic nurses as compared to the female Norwegian population[11]. In a study of the incidence of cancer among offspring born to nurse anaesthetists, three neoplasms occurred in two of 434 children born to anaesthetists who had worked during pregnancy (a neuroblastoma and a carcinoma of the thyroid in one, and a carcinoma of the parotid in the other) and one leukaemia among the 261 children born to anaesthetists who had not worked during pregnancy[12].

It is not possible to consider exposure to different volatile anaesthetics separately, although the study of US anaesthesiologists working during 1930-1946[10] concerned the period before fluorinated anaesthetic agents were introduced in the 1950s.

B. Evidence for carcinogenicity to animals (*inadequate* for enflurane, halothane, isoflurane, methoxyflurane and nitrous oxide)

Enflurane was tested for carcinogenicity by inhalation in one strain of mice at the maximum tolerated dose[13] and at several dose levels in a limited study in which treatment started *in utero*[14]. No treatment-related neoplasm was observed.

Halothane was tested for carcinogenicity by inhalation in mice and rats. When mice were exposed *in utero* and then three times weekly for 78 weeks at the maximum tolerated dose[15] or 24 times at several dose levels[14], no treatment-related neoplasm was observed. No carcinogenic effect was seen in rats exposed to a low level of halothane alone or in combination with nitrous oxide[16].

Isoflurane was tested for carcinogenicity by inhalation in one strain of mice. It induced liver tumours in one experiment[1] but no treatment-related neoplasm in another[14]. Both experiments had limitations.

Methoxyflurane was tested for carcinogenicity in mice by inhalation *in utero* in one limited study. No treatment-related neoplasm was observed[14].

Nitrous oxide was tested for carcinogencity by inhalation in mice and rats. In one limited study in mice in which exposure started *in utero*, no treatment-related neoplasm was observed[14]. No carcinogenic effect was seen in rats exposed chronically to a low dose of nitrous oxide alone or in combination with halothane[16].

C. Other relevant data

Studies in hospital personnel exposed to inhalation anaesthetics showed an increased frequency of chromosomal aberrations but not of sister chromatid exchanges in peripheral blood lymphocytes[17,18].

Neither enflurane nor halothane induced dominant lethal mutations in rodents *in vivo*, and halothane did not induce chromosomal aberrations, micronuclei or sister chromatid exchanges in rodents treated *in vivo*[19].

Divinyl ether and fluroxene induced sister chromatid exchanges in cultured Chinese hamster ovary cells and mutation in bacteria. Negative results were obtained in these tests with halothane, enflurane, diethyl ether, isoflurane, methoxyflurane and nitrous oxide. Halothane caused gene conversion and mutation in yeast under conditions that enhanced endogenous levels of cytochrome P450. Diethyl ether was not mutagenic to fungi. Cyclopropane was not mutagenic to bacteria[19].

References

[1]*IARC Monographs*, *11*, 285-293, 1976

[2]American Society of Anesthesiologists Ad Hoc Committee on the Effect of Trace Anesthetics on the Health of Operating Room Personnel (1974) Occupational disease among operating room personnel: a national study. *Anesthesiology*, *41*, 321-340

[3]Spence, A.A., Cohen, E.N., Brown, B.W., Jr, Knill-Jones, R.P. & Himmelberger, D.U. (1977) Occupational hazards for operating room-based physicians. Analysis of data from the United States and the United Kingdom. *J. Am. med. Assoc.*, *238*, 955-959

[4]Cohen, E.N., Brown, B.W., Wu, M.L., Whitcher, C.E., Brodsky, J.B., Gift, H.C., Greenfield, W., Jones, T.W. & Driscoll, E.J. (1980) Occupational disease in dentistry and chronic exposure to trace anesthetic gases. *J. Am. dent. Assoc.*, *101*, 21-31

[5]Vessey, M.P. (1978) Epidemiological studies of the occupational hazards of anaesthesia — a review. *Anaesthesia*, *33*, 430-438

[6]Bruce, D.L., Eide, K.A., Linde, H.W. & Eckenhoff, J.E. (1968) Causes of death among anesthesiologists: a 20-year survey. *Anesthesiology*, *29*, 565-569

[7]Doll, R. & Peto, R. (1977) Mortality among doctors in different occupations. *Br. med. J.*, *i*, 1433-1436

[8]Bruce, D.L., Eide, K.A., Smith, N.J., Seltzer, F. & Dykes, M.H.M. (1974) A prospective survey of anesthesiologist mortality, 1967-1971. *Anesthesiology*, *41*, 71-74

[9]Lew, E.A. (1979) Mortality experience among anesthesiologists, 1954-1976. *Anesthesiology*, *51*, 195-199

[10]Linde, H.W., Mesnick, P.S. & Smith, N.J. (1981) Causes of death among anesthesiologists: 1930-1946. *Anesth. Analg.*, *60*, 1-7

[11]Lund, E. (1985) Cancer among nurses especially in relation to exposure to anaesthetic gases (Norv.). *Tidsskr. Loeg.*, *105*, 572-575

[12]Corbett, T.H., Cornell, R.G., Endres, J.L. & Lieding, K. (1974) Birth defects among children of nurse-anesthetists. *Anesthesiology*, *41*, 341-344

[13]Baden, J.M., Egbert, B. & Mazze, R.I. (1982) Carcinogen bioassay of enflurane in mice. *Anaesthesiology*, *56*, 9-13

[14]Eger, E.I., II, White, A.E., Brown, C.L., Biava, C.G., Corbett, T.H. & Stevens, W.C. (1978) A test of the carcinogenicity of enflurane, isoflurane, halothane, methoxyflurane, and nitrous oxide in mice. *Anesth. Analg.*, *57*, 678-694

[15]Baden, J.M., Mazze, R.I., Wharton, R.S., Rice, S.A. & Kosek, J.C. (1979) Carcinogenicity of halothane in Swiss/ICR mice. *Anesthesiology*, *51*, 20-26

[16]Coate, W.B., Ulland, B.M. & Lewis, T.R. (1979) Chronic exposure to low concentrations of halothane-nitrous oxide: lack of carcinogenic effect in the rat. *Anesthesiology*, *50*, 306-309

[17]Bigatti, P., Lamberti, L., Ardito, G., Armellino, F. & Malanetto, C. (1985) Chromosome aberrations and sister chromatid exchanges in occupationally exposed workers. *Med. Lav.*, *76*, 334-339

[18]Husum, B. & Wulf, H.C. (1980) Sister chromatid exchanges in peripheral lymphocytes in operating room personnel. *Acta anaesth. scand.*, *24*, 22-24

[19]*IARC Monographs*, *Suppl. 6*, 68, 206-207, 248-249, 282-285, 319-320, 325-327, 345-346, 375-376, 425-426, 1987

ANDROGENIC (ANABOLIC) STEROIDS (Group 2A)

A. Evidence for carcinogenicity to humans (*limited*)

Cases of benign hepatoma, peliosis hepatis, primary hepatocellular carcinoma and hepatic cholangiocarcinoma have all been linked to the use of androgenic steroids, mostly oxymetholone[1-13]. At least 25 cases of liver-cell tumour have been reported in patients with Fanconi's anaemia[1-6,11,12], aplastic anaemia[1,4,7,8], paroxysmal nocturnal haemoglobinuria[1,12,13], panmyelopathy[9] or megaloblastic anaemia[10] treated with oxymetholone alone or in combination with other androgenic steroid drugs. Usually, treatment was given for years, but cancer has occurred within as little as two months of therapy[6], and there have been well-documented instances of remission following the withdrawal of oxymetholone treatment[8,9,11]. Hepatocellular carcinomas were also reported after extended treatment with oxymetholone of one patient with nephrolithiasis[14] and of another with chronic renal failure[15]; and hepatocellular carcinomas[1,16], cholangiocarcinomas[15] and adenomas[16] were reported after extended treatment of patients with methyltestosterone, testosterone oenanthate and nandrolone decanoate for hypogonadism[16], hypopituitarism[13], chronic renal failure[15] and generalized weakness[15].

The fact that castration palliates prostatic cancers suggests that testosterone may be involved in the genesis of these tumours[17], and a number of epidemiological observations suggest that increased testosterone levels may increase the risk for prostatic cancer. In addition, patients with cirrhosis, who have depressed testosterone levels[18], have low rates of prostatic cancer[19], and prostatic cancer is seemingly unknown among castrates[20]. There have also been a number of case reports[21-23] of prostatic cancer developing after androgen therapy; there was only one, unusual case, however, in which the cancer developed in a 'body-builder' at the age of 40 who had taken anabolic steroids for 18 years[23].

Blacks in the USA have the highest prostatic cancer rates in the world. Their two-fold increased risk, compared to US whites, is evident at the earliest age at which prostatic cancer occurs. Ross *et al.*[24] showed that young US blacks have a 15% higher mean testosterone serum level than young US whites, and argued that this difference could readily explain the two-fold difference in rates.

In one study[25], prostatic cancer cases were found to have higher mean levels of serum testosterone than healthy controls of the same age. Prostatic cancer cases in this study had a clear excess of high testosterone values. Another study [26] showed significantly higher levels of serum testosterone in prostatic cancer cases than in age-matched controls among US blacks, but not among African blacks. A number of case-control studies, however, showed no significant difference between cases and controls[27-29]. At present, there are insufficient data to permit firm conclusions to be drawn.

The development of myeloid leukaemia as a complication of Fanconi's anaemia has been reported in association with the use of oxymetholone[11,30,31], and there has been one case report of paroxysmal nocturnal haemoglobinuria in which a myeloproliferative disorder developed after oxymetholone therapy[32].

The evidence that anabolic steroids can cause both benign and malignant liver tumours is quite strong. However, because no analytical epidemiological study has been done, the Working Group felt constrained to classify the evidence for carcinogenicity in humans as no more than 'limited'.

B. Evidence for carcinogenicity to animals (*sufficient* for testosterone)

Testosterone propionate was tested for carcinogenicity in mice and rats by subcutaneous implantation, producing cervical-uterine tumours in female mice and prostatic adenocarcinomas in male rats. Neonatal treatment of female mice by subcutaneous injection of testosterone induced hyperplastic epithelial lesions of the genital tract and increased the incidence of mammary tumours. 5β-Dihydrotestosterone, which is considered hormonally inactive in adults, also increased the incidence of mammary tumours in mice when given neonatally by subcutaneous injection[33]. Depots of testosterone propionate implanted in rats resulted in an increased incidence of prostatic adenocarcinomas[34]. Subcutaneous administration of testosterone propionate following intravenous treatment with *N*-methyl-*N*-nitrosourea produced a high incidence of prostatic adenocarcinoma not seen with the individual compounds[35].

No data were available to the Working Group on oxymetholone.

C. Other relevant data

No data were available on the genetic and related effects of oxymetholone or testosterone in humans.

Testosterone did not induce sperm abnormalities or micronuclei in mice treated *in vivo* and was not mutagenic to bacteria[36].

References

[1]*IARC Monographs*, *13*, 131-139, 1977

[2]Port, R.B., Petasnick, J.P. & Ranniger, K. (1971) Angiographic demonstration of hepatoma in association with Fanconi's anemia. *Am. J. Roentgenol.*, *113*, 82-83

[3]Kew, M.C., Van Coller, B., Prowse, C.M., Skikne, B., Wolfsdorf, J.I., Isdale, J., Krawitz, S., Altman, H., Levin, S.E. & Bothwell, T.H. (1976) Occurrence of primary hepatocellular cancer and peliosis hepatis after treatment with androgenic steroids. *S.A. med. J.*, *50*, 1233-1237

[4]Sweeney, E.C. & Evans, D.J. (1976) Hepatic lesions in patients treated with synthetic anabolic steroids. *J. clin. Pathol.*, *29*, 626-633

[5]Shapiro, P., Ikeda, R.M., Ruebner, B.H., Connors, M.H., Halsted, C.C. & Abildgaard, C.F. (1977) Multiple hepatic tumors and peliosis hepatis in Fanconi's anemia treated with androgens. *Am. J. Dis. Child.*, *131*, 1104-1106

[6]Mokrohisky, S.T., Ambruso, D.R. & Hathaway, W.E. (1977) Fulminant hepatic neoplasia after androgen therapy. *New Engl. J. Med.*, *296*, 1411-1412

[7]Sale, G.E. & Lerner, K.G. (1977) Multiple tumors after androgen therapy. *Arch. Pathol. Lab. Med.*, *101*, 600-603

[8]Montgomery, R.R., Ducore, J.M., Githens, J.H., August, C.S. & Johnson, M.L. (1980) Regression of oxymetholone-induced hepatic tumors after bone marrow transplantation in aplastic anemia. *Transplantation, 30,* 90-96

[9]Treuner, J., Niethammer, D., Flach, A., Fischbach, H. & Schenck, W. (1980) Hepatocellular carcinoma following oxymetholone treatment (Ger.). *Med. Welt, 31,* 952-955

[10]Stromeyer, F.W., Smith, D.H. & Ishak, K.G. (1979) Anabolic steroid therapy and intrahepatic cholangiocarcinoma. *Cancer, 43,* 440-443

[11]Obeid, D.A., Hill, F.G.H., Harnden, D., Mann, J.R. & Wood, B.S.B. (1980) Fanconi anemia. Oxymetholone hepatic tumors, and chromosome aberrations associated with leukemic transition. *Cancer, 46,* 1401-1404

[12]Čáp, J., Ondruš, B. & Danihel, L. (1983) Focal nodular hyperplasia of the liver and hepatocellular carcinoma in children with Fanconi's anaemia after long-term treatment with androgen (Czech.). *Bratisl. lek. Listy., 79,* 73-81

[13]McCaughan, G.W., Bilous, M.J. & Gallagher, N.D. (1985) Long-term survival with tumor regression in androgen-induced liver tumors. *Cancer, 56,* 2622-2626

[14]Zevin, D., Turani, H., Cohen, A. & Levi, J. (1981) Androgen-associated hepatoma in a hemodialysis patient. *Nephron, 29,* 274-276

[15]Turani, H., Levi, J., Zevin, D. & Kessler, E. (1983) Hepatic lesions in patients on anabolic androgenic therapy. *Isr. J. med. Sci., 19,* 332-337

[16]Westaby, D., Portmann, B. & Williams, R. (1983) Androgen related primary hepatic tumors in non-Fanconi patients. *Cancer, 51,* 1947-1952

[17]Huggins, C. & Hodges, C.V. (1941) Studies on prostatic cancer. I. The effect of castration, of estrogen, and of androgen injection on serum phosphatases in metastatic carcinoma of the prostate. *Cancer Res., 1,* 293-297

[18]Gordon, G.G., Altman, K., Southren, A.L., Rubin, E. & Lieber, C.S. (1976) Effect of alcohol (ethanol) administration on sex-hormone metabolism in normal men. *New Engl. J. Med., 295,* 793-797

[19]Glantz, G.M. (1964) Cirrhosis and carcinoma of the prostate gland. *J. Urol., 91,* 291-293

[20]Hovenanian, M.S. & Deming, C.L. (1948) The heterologous growth of cancer of the human prostate. *Surg. Gynecol. Obstet., 86,* 29-35

[21]Sandeman, T.F. (1975) The possible dangers of androgens used for male climacteric. *Med. J. Aust., i,* 634-635

[22]Guinan, P.D., Sadoughi, W., Alsheik, H., Ablin, R.J., Alrenga, D. & Bush, I.M. (1976) Impotence therapy and cancer of the prostate. *Am. J. Surg., 131,* 599-600

[23]Roberts, J.T. & Essenhigh, D.M. (1986) Adenocarcinoma of prostate in a 40-year-old body-builder. *Lancet, ii,* 742

[24]Ross, R., Bernstein, L., Judd, H., Hanisch, R., Pike, M. & Henderson, B. (1986) Serum testosterone levels in healthy young black and white men. *J. natl Cancer Inst., 76,* 45-48

[25]Ghanadian, R., Puah, C.M. & O'Donoghue, E.P.N. (1979) Serum testosterone and dihydro-testosterone in carcinoma of the prostate. *Br. J. Cancer, 39,* 696-699

[26]Ahluwalia, B., Jackson, M.A., Jones, G.W., Williams, A.O., Rao, M.S. & Rajguru, S. (1981) Blood hormone profiles in prostate cancer patients in high-risk and low-risk populations. *Cancer, 48,* 2267-2273

[27]Hammond, G.L., Kontturi, M., Vihko, P. & Vihko, R. (1978) Serum steroids in normal males and patients with prostatic diseases. *Clin. Endocrinol.*, *9*, 113-121

[28]Bartsch, W., Steins, P. & Becker, H. (1977) Hormone blood levels in patients with prostatic carcinoma and their relation to the type of carcinoma growth differentiation. *Eur. Urol.*, *3*, 47-52

[29]Harper, M.E., Peeling, W.B., Cowley, T., Brownsey, B.G., Phillips, M.E.A., Groom, G., Fahmy, D.R. & Griffiths, K. (1976) Plasma steroid and protein hormone concentrations in patients with prostatic carcinoma, before and during oestrogen therapy. *Acta endocrinol.*, *81*, 409-426

[30]Sarna, G., Tomasulo, P., Lotz, M.J., Bubinak, J.F. & Shulman, N.R. (1975) Multiple neoplasms in two siblings with a variant form of Fanconi's anemia. *Cancer*, *36*, 1029-1033

[31]Bourgeois, C.A. & Hill, F.G.H. (1977) Fanconi's anemia leading to acute myelomonocytic leukemia. Cytogenetic studies. *Cancer*, *39*, 1163-1167

[32]Boyd, A.W., Parkin, J.D. & Castaldi, P.A. (1979) A case of paroxysmal nocturnal haemoglobinuria terminating in a myeloproliferative syndrome. *Aust. N.Z. J. Med.*, *9*, 181-183

[33]*IARC Monographs*, *21*, 519-547, 1979

[34]Pollard, M. & Luckert, P.H. (1986) Promotional effects of testosterone and high fat diet on the development of autochthonous prostate cancer in rats. *Cancer Lett.*, *32*, 223-227

[35]Pollard, M. & Luckert, P.H. (1986) Production of autochthonous prostate cancer in Lobund-Wistar rats by treatments with *N*-nitroso-*N*-methylurea and testosterone. *J. natl Cancer Inst.*, *77*, 583-587

[36]*IARC Monographs*, *Suppl. 6*, 506-507, 1987

ANILINE (Group 3)

A. Evidence for carcinogenicity to humans (*inadequate*)

The excess of bladder cancer deaths observed in clusters of cases of workers in the aniline-dye industry has been attributed to exposure to chemicals other than aniline. Epidemiological studies of workers exposed to aniline but not to other known bladder carcinogens have shown little evidence of increased risk. These studies are generally methodologically inadequate due to incomplete follow-up of workers who left the industry and to absence of estimates of expected numbers of bladder cancers. In the most methodologically vigorous study, one death from bladder cancer was reported among 1223 men who had produced or used aniline, with 0.83 deaths expected from population rates[1]. A recent mortality study of 342 men employed in the manufacture of organic dyes, in which two of the three processes involved aniline as a raw material, showed no death from bladder cancer[2].

B. Evidence for carcinogenicity to animals (*limited*)

Aniline hydrochloride was tested for carcinogenicity in single experiments in mice and rats by oral administration. No increase in tumour incidence was observed in mice. In rats, it produced fibrosarcomas, sarcomas and haemangiosarcomas of the spleen and peritoneal cavity[1]. In several limited studies, largely negative results were obtained following oral administration to rats[1], subcutaneous injection of mice[1] and hamsters[3], and after single intraperitoneal injection of mice[4].

C. Other relevant data

No data were available on the genetic and related effects of aniline in humans.

Aniline induced sister chromatid exchanges, but not micronuclei, in bone-marrow cells of mice treated *in vivo*, and DNA strand breakage was induced in liver and kidney of rats *in vivo*. Sister chromatid exchange assays in human cells *in vitro* gave negative results. Syrian hamster embryo cells and virus-infected Fischer rat embryo cells were not transformed by aniline, but BALB/c 3T3 cells were. It induced sister chromatid exchanges and chromosomal aberrations but not DNA strand breaks or unscheduled DNA synthesis in mammalian cells *in vitro*. Aniline did not induce sex-linked recessive lethal mutations in *Drosophila* and did not induce mutation or mitotic recombination in fungi. It was not mutagenic to bacteria and did not cause DNA damage. Urine from rats treated with aniline was reported to be mutagenic to bacteria[5].

References

[1]*IARC Monographs*, 27, 39-61, 1982

[2]Ott, M.G. & Langner, R.R. (1983) A mortality survey of men engaged in the manufacture of organic dyes. *J. occup. med.*, 25, 763-768

[3]Hecht, S.S., El-Bayoumy, K., Rivenson, A. & Fiala, E.S. (1983) Bioassay for carcinogenicity of 3,2′-dimethyl-4-nitrosobiphenyl, *o*-nitrosotoluene, nitrosobenzene and the corresponding amines in Syrian golden hamsters. *Cancer Lett.*, 20, 349-354

[4]Delclos, K.B., Tarpley, W.G., Miller, E.C. & Miller, J.A. (1984) 4-Aminoazobenzene and *N,N*-dimethyl-4-aminoazobenzene as equipotent hepatic carcinogens in male C57BL/6 × C3H/He F₁ mice and characterization of *N*-(deoxyguanosin-8-yl)-4-aminoazobenzene as the major persistent hepatic DNA-bound dye in these mice. *Cancer Res.*, 44, 2540-2550

[5]*IARC Monographs*, Suppl. 6, 68-70, 1987

ARSENIC AND ARSENIC COMPOUNDS (Group 1*)

A. Evidence for carcinogenicity to humans (*sufficient*)

Many cases of skin cancer have been reported among people exposed to arsenic through medical treatment with inorganic trivalent arsenic compounds, particularly Fowler's

*This evaluation applies to the group of chemicals as a whole and not necessarily to all individual chemicals within the group (see also Methods, p. 38).

solution[1], and further reports have confirmed these findings[2-9]. In some instances, skin cancers have occurred in combination with other cancers, such as liver angiosarcoma (after six months' treatment with Fowler's solution giving a total intake of 0.24 g arsenic)[6], intestinal and bladder cancers[7] and meningioma[9]. Liver angiosarcomas have also been associated with medicinal exposure to arsenic[1,6,10].

Epidemiological studies of cancer following medical treatment with arsenic have shown an excess of skin cancers, but no clear association with other cancers has been obtained[1], as confirmed by a recent cohort study on individuals treated with Fowler's solution[11]. No relation was found between prostatic cancer and treatment of syphilis with arsenicals[12].

An association between environmental exposure to arsenic through drinking-water and skin cancer has been observed[1] and confirmed[13,14]; two cases of bladder cancer were also described, with latent periods of eight to 20 years[15]. The latent periods for two cases of skin cancer related to arsenic in drinking-water were 20 and 23 years, and the concentrations or uptake of arsenic were reported to be 1.2 and 1 mg per day, respectively, with an estimated total ingested dose of about 8 g in one study[14].

Epidemiological studies in areas with different frequencies of black-foot disease and where drinking-water contained 0.35-1.14 mg/l arsenic revealed elevated risks for cancers of the bladder, kidney, skin, lung, liver and colon in both men and women[16,17].

A case of liver angiosarcoma was reported in the 20-month-old child of an exposed worker living in the vicinity of a copper mine and smelter[18]. Four rather inconsistent studies describing the effect of air pollutants containing arsenic[1,19,20] were followed by further reports that indicated an effect on lung cancer incidence of arsenic in polluted air from smelters and pesticide production, with risk ratios of 2.0-2.5 near smelters[21,22]. Two further studies near smelters showed no clear effect[23,24].

Occupational exposure to inorganic arsenic, especially in mining and copper smelting, has quite consistently been associated with an increased risk of cancer[1]. A number of studies of smelter workers relate to populations that have been reported previously[1] and represent both partial[25-27] and total[28,29] updates. An almost ten-fold increase in the incidence of lung cancer was found in workers most heavily exposed to arsenic, and relatively clear dose-response relationships have been obtained with regard to cumulative exposure[29] and especially with 30-day ceiling levels[27]. Sulphur dioxide in the smelter environment appeared to play a minor role, if any, in the development of lung cancer[27]. Other forms of cancer were considered, but their incidences were not found to be consistently increased[28]. Other US smelter worker populations have been shown to have consistent increases in lung cancer incidence, as well as increases of about 20% in the incidence of gastrointestinal cancer and of 30% for renal cancer and haematolymphatic malignancies[30,31]. The observation in an earlier study of an increase in lung cancer risk among a population of Swedish smelter workers[1] has been confirmed, with a risk of six to eight fold among roasters[32].

A decrease in lung cancer risk after cessation of exposure to arsenic has been observed in some studies[30,33], possibly indicating a late-stage effect of arsenic[34,35].

With regard to histological type of lung cancer, a significant, relative excess of adeno-carcinomas and a slight excess of oat-cell cancers were seen among smelter workers[36].

A multiplicative effect of arsenic exposure and smoking was observed among Swedish smelter workers[37]. A slightly increased risk was also indicated for exposure to sulphur dioxide in this study. Other studies have shown a lesser influence of smoking[25,33].

Relatively high concentrations of arsenic, as well as of antimony, cadmium, lead and lanthanum, were found in lung tissue of lung cancer cases, whereas the concentrations of selenium were low[38,39].

An approximately two-fold risk for lung and stomach cancers has been observed among (fine) glass workers with some exposure to arsenic but who were also exposed to other potentially carcinogenic metals and to asbestos. Stomach cancer was especially frequent among glass blowers, suggesting an association with oral contact with contaminated pipes[40].

Some excess of lung cancer was seen among female hat makers exposed to arsenic, but also to mercury[41].

Additional reports have suggested an increased risk of skin and lung cancers in vineyard workers[42,43] and have also suggested that ingestion of arsenic in wine byproducts may have contributed to this increase[42]. One case of lung cancer was reported in an individual involved in the production of lead arsenate and calcium arsenate[44]; multiple skin keratoses and chronic lymphatic leukaemia were reported in one person involved in the production of copper acetoarsenate[45].

Three studies of two populations of workers in pesticide production showed an increased risk ratio for lung cancer — up to about 3 — and some excess of malignant neoplasms of the lymphatic and haematopoietic tissues[1,46]. In a study of liver angiosarcomas, two of 26 cases had been in contact with arsenical pesticides occupationally[1].

B. Evidence for carcinogenicity to animals (*limited*)

Various arsenic compounds have been tested for carcinogenicity by perinatal treatment of mice, by intratracheal instillation in hamsters and rats and by implantation into the stomach of rats. Arsenic trioxide produced lung adenomas in mice after perinatal treatment[47], and induced low incidences of carcinomas, adenomas, papillomas and adenomatoid lesions of the respiratory tract in hamsters after its intratracheal instillation[48,49]. It induced a low incidence of adenocarcinomas at the site of its implantation into the stomach of rats[50]. A high incidence of lung carcinomas was induced in rats following a single intratracheal instillation of a pesticide mixture containing calcium arsenate[1]. Intratracheal instillations of calcium arsenate into hamsters resulted in a borderline increase in the incidence of lung adenomas, while no such effect was observed with arsenic trisulphide[51]. Oral administration of sodium arsenite enhanced the incidence of renal tumours induced in rats by intraperitoneal injection of N-nitrosodiethylamine[52].

No adequate data on the carcinogenicity of organic arsenicals were available to the Working Group.

C. Other relevant data

In one study of people exposed to trivalent arsenic in drinking-water, no increase in the incidence of sister chromatid exchanges or chromosomal aberrations was observed. A number of other studies published on people occupationally exposed to arsenic or patients treated with arsenic have shown increased levels of chromosomal aberrations or sister chromatid exchanges. The interpretation of these results remains uncertain because of methodological problems[53].

Trivalent arsenic did not induce dominant lethal mutations in mice, but it produced a small increase in the incidence of chromosomal aberrations and micronuclei in bone-marrow cells of mice treated *in vivo*. It induced chromosomal aberrations and sister chromatid exchanges in human and rodent cells *in vitro*, and transformation of Syrian hamster embryo cells; it did not induce mutation in rodent cells *in vitro*. It induced gene conversion in yeast but did not cause mutation or induce prophage in bacteria[53].

Pentavalent arsenic induced chromosomal aberrations in human and rodent cells *in vitro*; equivocal results were obtained in assays for the induction of sister chromatid exchanges. It induced transformation in Syrian hamster embryo cells but did not induce mutation or DNA strand breaks in rodent cells *in vitro*. It induced gene conversion in yeast but did not induce mutation in bacteria[53].

References

[1]*IARC Monographs, 23*, 39-141, 1980

[2]Heddle, R. & Bryant, G.D. (1983) Small cell lung carcinoma and Bowen's disease 40 years after arsenic ingestion. *Chest, 84*, 776-777

[3]Cowlishaw, J.L., Pollard, E.J., Cowen, A.E. & Powell, L.W. (1979) Liver disease associated with chronic arsenic ingestion. *Aust. N.Z. J. Med., 9*, 310-313

[4]Kastl, J. & Horáček, J. (1980) Arning's carcinoids in a psoriatic receiving long-term arsenic treatment (Czech.). *Čs. Dermatol., 55*, 89-93

[5]Kastl, J. & Horáček, J. (1985) Multiple basal cell carcinomas after long-term intake of arsenic (Ger.). *Dermatol. Monatsschr., 171*, 158-161

[6]Roat, J.W., Wald, A., Mendelow, H. & Pataki, K.I. (1982) Hepatic angiosarcoma associated with short-term arsenic ingestion. *Am. J. Med., 73*, 933-936

[7]von Roemeling, R., Hartwich, G. & König, H. (1979) Occurrence of tumours at different locations after arsenic therapy (Ger.). *Med. Welt, 30*, 1928-1929

[8]Southwick, G.J. & Schwartz, R.A. (1979) Arsenically associated cutaneous squamous cell carcinoma with hypercalcemia. *J. surg. Oncol., 12*, 115-118

[9]Weiss, J. & Jänner, M. (1980) Multiple basal cell carcinomas and meningioma after long-term arsenic therapy (Ger.). *Hautarzt, 31*, 654-656

[10]Falk, H., Caldwell, G.G., Ishak, K.G., Thomas, L.B. & Popper, H. (1981) Arsenic-related hepatic angiosarcoma. *Am. J. ind. Med., 2*, 43-50

[11]Cuzick, J., Evans, S., Gillman, M. & Price Evans, D.A. (1982) Medicinal arsenic and internal malignancies. *Br. J. Cancer, 45*, 904-911

[12]Lees, R.E.M., Steele, R. & Wardle, D. (1985) Arsenic, syphilis, and cancer of the prostate. *J. Epidemiol. Commun. Health, 39*, 227-230

[13]Armando, V.L. & Angel, A.O. (1979) Chronical arsenicism (Span.). *Bol. med. Hosp. Infant.*, *36*, 849-861

[14]Zaldívar, R., Prunés, L. & Ghai, G.L. (1981) Arsenic dose in patients with cutaneous carcinomata and hepatic haemangio-endothelioma after environmental and occupational exposure. *Arch. Toxicol.*, *47*, 145-154

[15]Nagy, G., Németh, A., Bodor, F. & Ficsór, E. (1980) Urinary bladder cancer induced by chronic arsenic poisoning (Hung.). *Orv. Hetil.*, *121*, 1009-1011

[16]Chen, C.-J., Chuang, Y.-C., Lin, T.-M. & Wu, H.-Y. (1985) Malignant neoplasms among residents of a blackfoot disease-endemic area in Taiwan: high-arsenic artesian well water and cancers. *Cancer Res.*, *45*, 5895-5899

[17]Chen, C.-J., Chuang, Y.-C., You, S.-L., Lin, T.-M. & Wu, H.-Y. (1986) A retrospective study on malignant neoplasms of bladder, lung and liver in blackfoot disease endemic area in Taiwan. *Br. J. Cancer*, *53*, 399-405

[18]Falk, H., Herbert, J.T., Edmonds, L., Heath, C.W., Jr, Thomas, L.B. & Popper, H. (1981) Review of four cases of childhood hepatic angiosarcoma — elevated environmental arsenic exposure in one case. *Cancer*, *47*, 382-391

[19]Brown, L.M., Pottern, L.M. & Blot, W.J. (1984) Lung cancer in relation to environmental pollutants emitted from industrial sources. *Environ. Res.*, *34*, 250-261

[20]Pershagen, G. (1985) Lung cancer mortality among men living near an arsenic-emitting smelter. *Am. J. Epidemiol.*, *122*, 684-694

[21]Matanoski, G.M., Landau, E., Tonascia, J., Lazar, C., Elliott, E.A., McEnroe, W. & King, K. (1981) Cancer mortality in an industrial area of Baltimore. *Environ. Res.*, *25*, 8-28

[22]Matanoski, G.M., Landau, E., Tonascia, J. & Elliott, E.A. (1983) Epidemiologic approach to arsenic pollution. *J. Univ. occup. environ. Health*, *5 (Suppl.)*, 117-124

[23]Greaves, W.W., Rom, W.N., Lyon, J.L., Varley, G., Wright, D.D. & Chiu, G. (1981) Relationship between lung cancer and distance of residence from nonferrous smelter stack effluent. *Am. J. ind. Med.*, *2*, 15-23

[24]Rom, W.N., Varley, G., Lyon, J.L. & Shopkow, S. (1982) Lung cancer mortality among residents living near the El Paso smelter. *Br. J. ind. Med.*, *39*, 269-272

[25]Higgins, I., Welch, K., Oh, M., Bond, G. & Hurwitz, P. (1981) Influence of arsenic exposure and smoking on lung cancer among smelter workers: a pilot study. *Am. J. ind. Med.*, *2*, 33-41

[26]Lubin, J.H., Pottern, L.M., Blot, W.J., Tokudome, S., Stone, B.J. & Fraumeni, J.R., Jr (1981) Respiratory cancer among copper smelter workers: recent mortality statistics. *J. occup. Med.*, *23*, 779-784

[27]Welch, K., Higgins, I., Oh, M. & Burchfiel, C. (1982) Arsenic exposure, smoking, and respiratory cancer in copper smelter workers. *Arch. environ. Health*, *37*, 325-335

[28]Lee-Feldstein, A. (1983) Arsenic and respiratory cancer in humans: follow-up of copper smelter employees in Montana. *J. natl Cancer Inst.*, *70*, 601-609

[29]Lee-Feldstein, A. (1986) Cumulative exposure to arsenic and its relationship to respiratory cancer among copper smelter employees. *J. occup. Med.*, *28*, 296-302

[30]Enterline, P.E. & Marsh, G.M. (1980) Mortality studies of smelter workers. *Am. J. ind. Med.*, *1*, 251-259

[31]Enterline, P.E. & Marsh, G.M. (1982) Cancer among workers exposed to arsenic and other substances in a copper smelter. *Am. J. Epidemiol.*, *116*, 895-911

[32]Wall, S. (1980) Survival and mortality pattern among Swedish smelter workers. *Int. J. Epidemiol.*, *9*, 73-87

[33]Pinto, S.S., Henderson, V. & Enterline, P.E. (1978) Mortality experience of arsenic-exposed workers. *Arch. environ. Health*, *33*, 325-331

[34]Brown, C.C. & Chu, K.C. (1983) Implications of the multistage theory of carcinogenesis applied to occupational arsenic exposure. *J. natl Cancer Inst.*, *70*, 455-463

[35]Brown, C.C. & Chu, K.C. (1983) A new method for the analysis of cohort studies: implications of the multistage theory of carcinogenesis applied to occupational arsenic exposure. *Environ. Health Perspect.*, *50*, 293-308

[36]Wicks, M.J., Archer, V.E., Auerbach, O. & Kuschner, M. (1981) Arsenic exposure in a copper smelter as related to histological type of lung cancer. *Am. J. ind. Med.*, *2*, 25-31

[37]Pershagen, G., Wall, S., Taube, A. & Linnman, L. (1981) On the interaction between occupational arsenic exposure and smoking and its relationship to lung cancer. *Scand. J. Work Environ. Health*, *7*, 302-309

[38]Wester, P.O., Brune, D. & Nordberg, G. (1981) Arsenic and selenium in lung, liver, and kidney tissue from dead smelter workers. *Br. J. ind. Med.*, *38*, 179-184

[39]Gerhardsson, L., Brune, D., Nordberg, I.G.F. & Wester, P.O. (1985) Protective effect of selenium on lung cancer in smelter workers. *Br. J. ind. Med.*, *42*, 617-626

[40]Wingren, G. & Axelson, O. (1985) Mortality pattern in a glass producing area in SE Sweden. *Br. J. ind. Med.*, *42*, 411-414

[41]Buiatti, E., Kriebel, D., Geddes, M., Santucci, M. & Pucci, N. (1985) A case control study of lung cancer in Florence, Italy. I. Occupational risk factors. *J. Epidemiol. Commun. Health*, *39*, 244-250

[42]Lüchtrath, H. (1983) The consequences of chronic arsenic poisoning among Moselle wine growers. Pathoanatomical investigations of post-mortem examinations between 1960 and 1977. *J. Cancer Res. clin. Oncol.*, *105*, 173-182

[43]Thiers, H., Colomb, D., Moulin, G. & Colin, L. (1967) Arsenical skin cancer in vineyards in the Beaujolais (Fr.). *Ann. Dermatol.*, *94*, 133-158

[44]Horiguchi, S. (1979) A case of lung cancer due to exposure to arsenical compounds in an insecticides factory. (Studies on lead arsenate poisoning. Part 4). *Osaka City med. J.*, *25*, 45-51

[45]Leyh, F. & Rothlaender, J.P. (1985) Multiple bowenoid keratoses due to arsenic (Ger.). *Dermatosen*, *33*, 99-101

[46]Mabuchi, K., Lilienfeld, A.M. & Snell, L.M. (1980) Cancer and occupational exposure to arsenic: a study of pesticide workers. *Prev. Med.*, *9*, 51-77

[47]Rudnay, P. & Börzsönyi, M. (1981) The tumorigenic effect of treatment with arsenic trioxide (Hung.). *Magyar Onkol.*, *25*, 73-77

[48]Ishinishi, N., Yamamoto, A., Hisanaga, A. & Inamasu, T. (1983) Tumorigenicity of arsenic trioxide to the lung in Syrian golden hamsters by intermittent instillations. *Cancer Lett.*, *21*, 141-147

[49]Pershagen, G., Nordberg, G. & Björklund, N.-E. (1984) Carcinomas of the respiratory tract in hamsters given arsenic trioxide and/or benzo[a]pyrene by the pulmonary route. *Environ. Res.*, *34*, 227-241

[50]Katsnelson, B.A., Neizvestnova, Y.M. & Blokhin, V.A. (1986) Stomach carcinogenesis induction by chronic treatment with arsenic (Russ.). *Vopr. Onkol.*, *32*, 68-73

[51]Pershagen, G. & Björklund, N.-E. (1985) On the pulmonary tumorigenicity of arsenic trisulfide and calcium arsenate in hamsters. *Cancer Lett.*, *27*, 99-104

[52]Shirachi, D.Y., Johansen, M.G., McGowan, J.P. & Tu, S.-H. (1983) Tumorigenic effect of sodium arsenite in rat kidney. *Proc. West. pharmacol. Soc.*, *26*, 413-415

[53]*IARC Monographs*, *Suppl. 6*, 71-76, 1987

ASBESTOS* (Group 1)

A. Evidence for carcinogenicity to humans (*sufficient*)

Numerous reports from several countries have described cases or series of pleural and peritoneal mesotheliomas in relation to occupational exposure to various types and mixtures of asbestos (including talc containing asbestos), although occupational exposures have not been identified in all cases[1-21]. Mesotheliomas of the tunica vaginalis testis and of the pericardium have been reported in persons occupationally exposed to asbestos[22-24].

Environmental exposure either in the houses of asbestos workers or in the neighbourhood of asbestos mines or factories has been noted in some of the cases[1,2,4-6,9,11,25,26]. It has been estimated that a third of the mesotheliomas occurring in the USA may be due to nonoccupational exposure[27]. In a study from Israel, the incidence of mesothelioma was found to be higher among those born in the USA or in Europe relative to those born in Israel[9].

In some of these case reports and in other studies, asbestos fibres were identified in the lung[5,6,11,28-32]. Amphibole fibres usually predominated, but in a few cases mainly or only chrysotile fibres were found[6,28].

The long latency required for mesothelioma to develop after asbestos exposure has been documented in a number of publications[11,13,26,28,33-37]. An increasing proportion of cases has been seen with increasing duration of exposure[36].

A number of epidemiological studies of respiratory cancer and mesothelioma have been reported in relation to exposure to unspecified or complex mixtures of asbestos in shipyard work[38-45]. The risk ratio for lung cancer has usually been moderately increased, both in these studies and in studies on various other occupational groups with similarly job-related but unspecified or complex asbestos exposures[35,46-54]. Risk ratios of about 2-5 have been reported in some studies, but the ratio was considerably higher in one rather small study[55] and did not exceed unity in another[42]. In one study, individuals suffering from asbestosis had a considerably greater risk for lung cancer, with a risk ratio of 9.0[56]. In some of the studies referred to, a number of mesotheliomas were also observed[41,42,44,47,51,53,55]. Abdominal mesotheliomas have sometimes been mistaken for pancreatic cancer[57]. Mesothelioma cases have been observed to have a relatively lower fibre content in the lungs than lung cancer cases[32].

---

*Actinolite, amosite, anthophyllite, chrysotile, crocidolite, tremolite

Laryngeal cancer has been considered in two case-control studies, resulting in risk ratios of 2.4 and 2.3 that relate to shipyard work and unspecified exposure, respectively[40,58]. A cohort study of insulation workers showed a relative risk of 1.9, based on nine cases[57]. A case series indicated a high frequency of exposure to asbestos, especially in low-grade smokers[59]. A risk ratio of 3.2 for laryngeal cancer was reported among chrysotile miners in an area with generally high incidence[60], but no increased risk was seen in a cohort of workers with exposure to crocidolite[61]. Two correlation studies have also indicated a relationship between laryngeal cancer and exposure to asbestos[39,62].

Mesotheliomas related to shipyard work and other exposures, including household contact with asbestos workers, have also been subject to epidemiological studies[36,63-67], resulting in risk ratios of about 3-15 in comparison with background rates not clearly referable to asbestos exposure.

Some studies have specifically considered environmental exposures with reference to mesotheliomas[66,67]. Three correlation studies and one case-control study considering exposure to piped drinking-water[68-71] did not show consistently increased risks for any type of cancer, whereas another study[72] considering chrysotile contamination mainly from natural sources gave some indication of an increase in the incidence of peritoneal and stomach cancers in persons of each sex, although no other cancer site was consistent in this respect.

Exposure to crocidolite has been studied with regard to risk of lung cancer[61,73-76], and risk ratios of about 2-3 have been reported. Three lung cancers and two mesotheliomas occurred in 20 individuals after one year of high exposure to crocidolite; at least 17 of the cases had asbestos-induced lung changes on X-ray films[77].

One study[78] of histological types of lung cancers showed that among persons exposed to crocidolite 45.7% of cases were squamous-cell carcinomas, as compared to 35.2% among unexposed persons. In the context of unspecified and complex exposures, small-cell carcinoma was found to be relatively more prevalent than other forms[50].

Exposure to chrysotile was found in some studies to result in virtually no increase in risk ratio[60,79-81], or a slightly elevated relative risk of lung cancer[82-86]. Somewhat higher risk ratios, up to 2.5, 3.5 and 2, respectively, were obtained in one study of chrysotile miners[87] and in two independent studies from one asbestos [chrysotile] textile plant[88,89], the latter being the more comprehensive. With regard to mesotheliomas, one study suggested a particularly high risk of combined exposure to chrysotile and amphiboles (risk ratio, 61), thus almost multiplying the risk ratios (6 and 12, respectively) of exposures to chrysotile and to amphiboles alone[90]. Another study showed no mesothelioma among a large worker population with exposure to chrysotile only[91].

A slight excess of lung cancer and some mesotheliomas appeared in some groups with mixed exposures involving amosite, chrysotile and crocidolite[92-94]. Exposure predominantly to amosite, but also to chrysotile, was reported to be the probable cause of at least four of five mesotheliomas (one peritoneal) observed in a UK insulation-board factory[95]. One cohort with exposure to cummingtonite-grunerite, which is closely related to amosite, had no clear excess of lung cancer, although one case of mesothelioma was observed[96].

Exposure to tremolite and actinolite has been the subject of a few studies in investigations of vermiculite mining and milling[97,98] and environmental exposure[99]. The studies of miners indicated a risk ratio for lung cancer of up to approximately six fold. Deaths from mesothelioma were found in the occupational studies, whereas the study of environmental exposure showed no increased risk, although pleural plaques were reported. Publication of one case report of a mesothelioma after environmental exposure suggests that tremolite was of etiological importance[31].

Cancers other than of the lung or mesothelioma have been considered in many studies[1,17,35,39,41–44,48,51,55,60–62,68–70,72–74,76,83,87,89,92,93,96,97,99–108]. Some indicated an approximately two-fold risk with regard to gastrointestinal cancer in connection with shipyard work[41,43], and some increased risk was also seen in association with exposure to both chrysotile and crocidolite[103], to crocidolite[61,74] or to chrysotile[87]. Cancer of the colon and rectum was associated with asbestos exposure during chrysotile production, with an approximately two-fold risk[87]; a similar excess was found for unspecified asbestos exposure[104]. Some excess of ovarian cancer has been reported in two studies[73,76] but not in another[92]; exposure to crocidolite was probably more predominant in the studies that showed excesses. Bile-duct cancer appeared in excess in one study based on record-linking[105], and large-cell lymphomas of the gastrointestinal tract and oral cavity appeared to be strongly related to asbestos exposure in one small study covering 28 cases and 28 controls, giving a risk ratio of 8; however, ten cases and one control also had a history of malaria[106]. An excess of lymphopoietic and haematopoietic malignancies has been reported in plumbers, pipe-fitters, sheet-metal workers and others with asbestos exposure[17,54,107,108].

The relationship between asbestos exposure and smoking indicates a synergistic effect of smoking with regard to lung cancer[1]. Further evaluations indicate that this synergistic effect is close to a multiplicative model[52,109]. As noted previously[1], the risk of mesothelioma appears to be independent of smoking[47,66], and a significantly decreasing trend in risk was observed with the amount smoked in one study[65].

The studies of the carcinogenic effect of asbestos exposure, including evidence reviewed earlier[1], show that occupational exposure to chrysotile, amosite and anthophyllite asbestos and to mixtures containing crocidolite results in an increased risk of lung cancer, as does exposure to minerals containing tremolite and actinolite and to tremolitic material mixed with anthophyllite and small amounts of chrysotile. Mesotheliomas have been observed after occupational exposure to crocidolite, amosite, tremolitic material and chrysotile asbestos. Gastrointestinal cancers occurred at an increased incidence in groups occupationally exposed to crocidolite, amosite, chrysotile or mixed fibres containing crocidolite, although not all studies are consistent in this respect. An excess of laryngeal cancer has also been observed in some groups of exposed workers. No clear excess of cancer has been associated with the presence of asbestos fibres in drinking-water. Mesotheliomas have occurred in individuals living in the neighbourhood of asbestos factories and mines and in people living with asbestos workers.

B. Evidence for carcinogenicity to animals (*sufficient*)

Asbestos has been tested for carcinogenicity by inhalation in rats, by intrapleural administration in rats and hamsters, by intraperitoneal injection in mice, rats and hamsters and by oral administration in rats and hamsters. Chrysotile, crocidolite, amosite, anthophyllite and tremolite produced mesotheliomas and lung carcinomas in rats after inhalation[1,110,111] and mesotheliomas following intrapleural administration[1,112]. Chrysotile, crocidolite, amosite and anthophyllite induced mesotheliomas in hamsters following intrapleural administration[1]. Intraperitoneal administration of chrysotile, crocidolite and amosite induced peritoneal tumours, including mesotheliomas, in mice[1,113] and rats[1,111,114]. Given by the same route, crocidolite produced abdominal tumours in hamsters[115], and tremolite and actinolite produced abdominal tumours in rats[110,116-118]. A statistically significant increase in the incidence of malignant tumours was observed in rats given filter material containing chrysotile orally[1]. In more recent studies, tumour incidence was not increased by oral administration of amosite or tremolite in rats[119], of amosite in hamsters[120,121] or of chrysotile in hamsters[121]. In two studies in rats, oral administration of chrysotile produced a low incidence of benign adenomatous polyps of the large intestine in males (9/250 *versus* 3/254 pooled controls)[122] and of mesenteric haemangiomas (4/22 *versus* 0/47 controls)[123]. Synergistic effects were observed following intratracheal administration of chrysotile and benzo[*a*]pyrene to rats and hamsters[1] and of intratracheal administration of chrysotile and subcutaneous or oral administration of *N*-nitrosodiethylamine to hamsters[124].

C. Other relevant data

Insulation workers exposed to asbestos 'displayed a marginal increase' in the incidence of sister chromatid exchanges in lymphocytes in one study[125].

Chrysotile did not induce micronuclei in bone-marrow cells of mice or chromosomal aberrations in bone-marrow cells of rhesus monkeys treated *in vivo*. In cultured human cells, conflicting results were reported for the induction of chromosomal aberrations and negative results for the induction of sister chromatid exchanges by chrysotile and crocidolite; amosite and crocidolite did not induce DNA strand breaks, and crocidolite was not mutagenic. Amosite, anthophyllite, chrysotile and crocidolite induced transformation of Syrian hamster embryo cells, chrysotile and crocidolite transformed BALB/c 3T3 mouse cells, and chrysotile transformed rat mesothelial cells. Neither amosite nor crocidolite transformed CH3 10T1/2 cells. In cultured rodent cells, amosite, anthophyllite, chrysotile and crocidolite induced chromosomal aberrations, and amosite, chrysotile and crocidolite induced sister chromatid exchanges; chrysotile and crocidolite induced aneuploidy and micronuclei. Chrysotile induced unscheduled DNA synthesis in rat hepatocytes. Amosite, chrysotile and crocidolite were inactive or weakly active in inducing mutation in rodent cells *in vitro*; none was mutagenic to bacteria[125].

References

[1]*IARC Monographs, 14*, 1977

[2]Armstrong, B.K., Musk, A.W., Baker, J.E., Hunt, J.M., Newall, C.C., Henzell, H.R., Blunsdon, B.S., Clarke-Hundley, M.D., Woodward, S.D. & Hobbs, M.S.T. (1984) Epidemiology of malignant mesothelioma in Western Australia. *Med. J. Aust., 141*, 86-88

[3]Beck, B. & Irmscher, G. (1979) Extrathoracic mesotheliomas after inhalation of asbestos dust (Ger.). *Z. Erkrank. Atm.-Org., 152*, 282-293

[4]Biava, P.M., Fiorito, A., Canciani, L. & Bovenzi, M. (1983) Epidemiology of mesothelioma of the pleura in the province of Trieste: role of occupational exposure to asbestos (Ital.). *Med. Lav., 74*, 260-265

[5]Edge, J.R. & Choudhury, S.L. (1978) Malignant mesothelioma of the pleura in Barrow-in-Furness. *Thorax, 33*, 26-30

[6]Emonot, A., Marquet, M., Baril, A., Berardj & Braillon (1979) Epidemiology of asbestos mesotheliomas in the region of St Etienne (Fr.). *Ann. Med. intern., 130*, 71-74

[7]Griffiths, M.H., Riddell, R.J. & Xipell, J.M. (1980) Malignant mesothelioma: a review of 35 cases with diagnosis and prognosis. *Pathology, 12*, 591-603

[8]Kovarik, J.L. (1976) Primary pleural mesothelioma. *Cancer, 38*, 1816-1825

[9]Lemesch, C., Steinitz, R. & Wassermann, M. (1976) Epidemiology of mesothelioma in Israel. *Environ. Res., 12*, 255-261

[10]McDonald, A.D. (1980) *Malignant mesothelioma in Quebec.* In: Wagner, J.C., ed., *Biological Effects of Mineral Fibres (IARC Scientific Publications No. 30)*, Lyon, International Agency for Research on Cancer, pp. 673-680

[11]Mowé, G. & Gylseth, B. (1986) Occupational exposure and regional variation of malignant mesothelioma in Norway, 1970-79. *Am. J. ind. Med., 9*, 323-332

[12]Paur, R., Woitowitz, H.-J., Rödelsperger, K. & Jahn, H. (1985) Pleural mesothelioma after asbestos exposure in brake repair work in automobile repair workshop: case observations (Ger.). *Prax. klin. Pneumol., 39*, 362-366

[13]Sheers, G. & Coles, R.M. (1980) Mesothelioma risks in a naval dockyard. *Arch. environ. Health, 35*, 276-282

[14]Vande Weyer, R., Groetenbriel, C., Lauwers, D. & Yernault, J.C. (1982) Evolution of deaths by bronchial carcinoma and pleural mesothelioma among two groups of Belgian workers who died between 1973 and 1981: the role of asbestosis and coalworkers' pneumoconiosis (Abstract No. 5). *Eur. J. respir. Dis., 63 (Suppl. 125)*, 10

[15]Xu, Z., Armstrong, B.K., Blundson, B.J., Rogers, J.M., Musk, A.W. & Shilkin, K.B. (1985) Trends in mortality from malignant mesothelioma of the pleura, and production and use of asbestos in Australia. *Med. J. Aust., 143*, 185-187

[16]Ben-Dror, G., Suprun, H. & Shkolnik, T. (1985) Peritoneal mesotheliomas and exposure to asbestos (Arabic). *Harefuah, 108*, 435-437

[17]Cantor, K.P., Sontag, J.M. & Heid, M.F. (1986) Patterns of mortality among plumbers and pipefitters. *Am. J. ind. Med., 10*, 73-89

[18]Gardner, M.J., Jones, R.D., Pippard, E.C. & Saitoh, N. (1985) Mesothelioma of the peritoneum during 1967-82 in England and Wales. *Br. J. Cancer, 51*, 121-126

[19]Mancuso, T.F. (1983) Mesothelioma among machinists in railroad and other industries. *Am. J. ind. Med.*, *4*, 501-513

[20]Newhouse, M.L., Oakes, D. & Woolley, A.J. (1985) Mortality of welders and other craftsmen at a shipyard in NE England. *Br. J. ind. Med.*, *42*, 406-410

[21]Sera, Y. & Kang, K.-Y. (1981) Asbestos and cancer in the Sennan district of Osaka. *Tohoku J. exp. Med.*, *133*, 313-320

[22]Fligiel, Z. & Kaneko, M. (1976) Malignant mesothelioma of the tunica vaginalis propria testis in a patient with asbestos exposure. *Cancer*, *37*, 1478-1484

[23]Beck, B., Konetzke, G., Ludwig, V., Röthig, W. & Sturm, W. (1982) Malignant pericardial mesotheliomas and asbestos exposure: a case report. *Am. J. ind. Med.*, *3*, 149-159

[24]Kahn, E.I., Rohl, A., Barrett, E.W. & Suzuki, Y. (1980) Primary pericardial mesothelioma following exposure to asbestos. *Environ. Res.*, *23*, 270-281

[25]Arul, K.J. & Holt, P.F. (1977) Mesothelioma possibly due to environmental exposure to asbestos in childhood. *Int. Arch. occup. environ. Health*, *40*, 141-143

[26]Bignon, J., Sébastien, P., di Menza, L., Nebut, M. & Payan, H. (1979) French registry of mesotheliomas 1965-1978 (Fr.). *Rev. fr. Mal. respir.*, *7*, 223-242

[27]Enterline, P.E. (1983) Cancer produced by nonoccupational asbestos exposure in the United States. *J. Air Pollut. Control Assoc.*, *33*, 318-322

[28]Greenberg, M. & Davies, T.A.L. (1974) Mesothelioma register 1967-68. *Br. J. ind. Med.*, *31*, 91-104

[29]Chen, W.-J. & Mottet, N.K. (1978) Malignant mesothelioma with minimal asbestos exposure. *Hum. Pathol.*, *9*, 253-258

[30]Gylseth, B., Mowé, G. & Wannag, A. (1983) Fibre type and concentration in the lungs of workers in an asbestos cement factory. *Br. J. ind. Med.*, *40*, 375-379

[31]Magee, F., Wright, J.L., Chan, N., Lawson, L. & Churg, A. (1986) Malignant mesothelioma caused by childhood exposure to long-fiber low aspect ratio tremolite. *Am. J. ind. Med.*, *9*, 529-533

[32]Wagner, J.C., Moncrieff, C.B., Coles, R., Griffiths, D.M. & Munday, D.E. (1986) Correlation between fibre content of the lungs and disease in naval dockyard workers. *Br. J. ind. Med.*, *43*, 391-395

[33]Browne, K. (1983) Asbestos-related mesothelioma: epidemiological evidence for asbestos as a promoter. *Arch. environ. Health*, *38*, 261-266

[34]Churg, A., Warnock, M.L. & Bensch, K.G. (1978) Malignant mesothelioma arising after direct application of asbestos and fiber glass to the pericardium. *Am. Rev. respir. Dis.*, *118*, 419-424

[35]Beck, E.G. & Schmidt, P. (1985) Epidemiological investigations of deceased employees of the asbestos cement industry in the Federal Republic of Germany. *Zbl. Bakt. Hyg., I. Abt. Orig. B*, *181*, 207-215

[36]Hughes, J.M., Hammad, Y.Y. & Weill, H. (1986) Mesothelioma risk in relation to duration and type of asbestos fiber exposure (Abstract). *Am. Rev. respir. Dis.*, *133* (*Suppl. 4*), A33

[37]Selikoff, I.J., Hammond, E.C. & Seidman, H. (1980) Latency of asbestos disease among insulation workers in the United States and Canada. *Cancer*, *46*, 2736-2740

[38]Blot, W.J., Harrington, J.M., Toledo, A., Hoover, R., Heath, C.W., Jr & Fraumeni, J.F., Jr (1978) Lung cancer after employment in shipyards during World War II. *New Engl. J. Med.*, *299*, 620-624

[39]Blot, W.J., Stone, B.J., Fraumeni, J.F., Jr & Morris, L.E. (1979) Cancer mortality in US counties with shipyard industries during World War II. *Environ. Res., 18*, 281-290

[40]Blot, W.J., Morris, L.E., Stroube, R., Tagnon, I. & Fraumeni, J.F., Jr (1980) Lung and laryngeal cancers in relation to shipyard employment in coastal Virginia. *J. natl Cancer Inst., 65*, 571-575

[41]Kolonel, L.N., Yoshizawa, C.N., Hirohata, T. & Myers, B.C. (1985) Cancer occurrence in shipyard workers exposed to asbestos in Hawaii. *Cancer Res., 45*, 3924-3928

[42]Rossiter, C.E. & Coles, R.M. (1980) *HM Dockyard, Devonport: 1947 mortality study.* In: Wagner, J.C., ed., *Biological Effects of Mineral Fibres (IARC Scientific Publications No. 30)*, Lyon, International Agency for Research on Cancer, pp. 713-721

[43]Sandén, Å., Näslund, P.-E. & Järvholm, B. (1985) Mortality in lung and gastrointestinal cancer among shipyard workers. *Int. Arch. occup. environ. Health, 55*, 277-283

[44]Lumley, K.P.S. (1976) A proportional study of cancer registrations of dockyard workers. *Br. J. ind. Med., 33*, 108-114

[45]Nicholson, W.J., Lilis, R., Frank, A.L. & Selikoff, I.J. (1980) Lung cancer prevalence among shipyard workers. *Am. J. ind. Med., 1*, 191-203

[46]Alies-Patin, A.M. & Valleron, A.J. (1985) Mortality of workers in a French asbestos cement factory 1940-82. *Br. J. ind. Med., 42*, 219-225

[47]Berry, G., Newhouse, M.L. & Antonis, P. (1985) Combined effect of asbestos and smoking on mortality from lung cancer and mesothelioma in factory workers. *Br. J. ind. Med., 42*, 12-18

[48]Hodgson, J.T. & Jones, R.D. (1986) Mortality of asbestos workers in England and Wales. *Br. J. ind. Med., 43*, 158-164

[49]Coggon, D., Pannett, B. & Acheson, E.D. (1984) Use of job-exposure matrix in an occupational analysis of lung and bladder cancers on the basis of death certificates. *J. natl Cancer Inst., 72*, 61-65

[50]Kjuus, H., Skjaerven, R., Langård, S., Lien, J.T. & Aamodt, T. (1986) A case-referent study of lung cancer, occupational exposures and smoking. II. Role of asbestos exposure. *Scand. J. Work Environ. Health, 12*, 203-209

[51]Newhouse, M.L., Berry, G. & Wagner, J.C. (1985) Mortality of factory workers in East London 1933-80. *Br. J. ind. Med., 42*, 4-11

[52]Hilt, B., Langård, S., Andersen, A. & Rosenberg, J. (1985) Asbestos exposure, smoking habits, and cancer incidence among production and maintenance workers in an electrochemical plant. *Am. J. ind. Med., 8*, 565-577

[53]Woitowitz, H.-J., Lange, H.-J., Beierl, L., Rathgeb, M., Schmidt, K., Ulm, K., Giesen, T., Woitowitz, R.H., Pache, L. & Rödelsperger, K. (1986) Mortality rates in the Federal Republic of Germany following previous occupational exposure to asbestos dust. *Int. Arch. occup. environ. Health, 57*, 161-171

[54]Zoloth, S. & Michaels, D. (1985) Asbestos disease in sheet metal workers: the results of a proportional mortality analysis. *Am. J. ind. Med., 7*, 315-321

[55]Elmes, P.C. & Simpson, M.J.C. (1977) Insulation workers in Belfast. A further study of mortality due to asbestos exosure (1940-75). *Br. J. ind. Med., 34*, 174-180

[56]Huuskonen, M.S. (1980) Asbestos and cancer in Finland. *J. Toxicol. environ. Health, 6*, 1261-1265

[57]Selikoff, I.J. & Seidman, H. (1981) Cancer of the pancreas among asbestos insulation workers. *Cancer, 47 (Suppl.)*, 1469-1473

[58]Burch, J.D., Howe, G.R., Miller, A.B. & Semenciw, R. (1981) Tobacco, alcohol, asbestos, and nickel in the etiology of cancer of the larynx: a case-control study. *J. natl Cancer Inst.*, *67*, 1219-1224

[59]von Bittersohl, G. (1977) On the problem of asbestos-induced carcinoma of the larynx (Ger.). *Z. ges. Hyg.*, *23*, 27-30

[60]Rubino, G.F., Piolatto, G., Newhouse, M.L., Scansetti, G., Aresini, G.A. & Murray, R. (1979) Mortality of chrysotile asbestos workers at the Balangero mine, Northern Italy. *Br. J. ind. Med.*, *36*, 187-194

[61]Musk, A.W., de Klerk, N., Hobbs, M.S.T. & Armstrong, B.K. (1986) Mortality in crocidolite miners and millers from Wittenoom, Western Australia (Abstract). *Am. Rev. respir. Dis.*, *133* (*Suppl. 4*), A34

[62]Graham, S., Blanchet, M. & Rohrer, T. (1977) Cancer in asbestos-mining and other areas of Quebec. *J. natl Cancer Inst.*, *59*, 1139-1145

[63]Chiappino, G., Riboldi, L., Todaro, A. & Schulz, L. (1985) Survey of mesotheliomas in Lombardy in the period 1978-1982 (Ital.). *Med. Lav.*, *76*, 454-465

[64]Mowé, G., Gylseth, B., Hartveit, F. & Skaug, V. (1984) Occupational asbestos exposure, lung-fiber concentration and latency time in malignant mesothelioma. *Scand. J. Work Environ. Health*, *10*, 293-298

[65]Tagnon, I., Blot, W.J., Stroube, R.B., Day, N.E., Morris, L.E., Peace, B.B. & Fraumeni, J.F., Jr (1980) Mesothelioma associated with the shipbuilding industry in coastal Virginia. *Cancer Res.*, *40*, 3875-3879

[66]Thériault, G.P. & Grand-Bois, L. (1978) Mesothelioma and asbestos in the province of Quebec, 1969-1972. *Arch. environ. Health*, *33*, 15-19

[67]Vianna, N.J. & Polan, A.K. (1978) Non-occupational exposure to asbestos and malignant mesothelioma in females. *Lancet*, *i*, 1061-1063

[68]Meigs, J.W., Walter, S.D., Heston, J.F., Millette, J.R., Craun, G.F., Woodhull, R.S. & Flannery, J.T. (1980) Asbestos cement pipe and cancer in Connecticut 1955-1974. *J. environ. Health*, *42*, 187-191

[69]Wigle, D.T. (1977) Cancer mortality in relation to asbestos in municipal water supplies. *Arch. environ. Health*, *32*, 185-190

[70]Harrington, J.M., Craun, G.F., Meigs, J.W., Landrigan, P.J., Flannery, J.T. & Woodhull, R.S. (1978) An investigation of the use of asbestos cement pipe for public water supply and the incidence of gastrointestinal cancer in Connecticut, 1935-1973. *Am. J. Epidemiol.*, *107*, 96-103

[71]Polissar, L., Severson, R.K. & Boatman, E.S. (1984) A case-control study of asbestos in drinking water and cancer risk. *Am. J. Epidemiol.*, *119*, 456-471

[72]Kanarek, M.S., Conforti, P.M., Jackson, L.A., Cooper, R.C. & Murchio, J.C. (1980) Asbestos in drinking water and cancer incidence in the San Francisco Bay area. *Am. J. Epidemiol.*, *112*, 54-72

[73]Acheson, E.D., Gardner, M.J., Pippard, E.C. & Grime, L.P. (1982) Mortality of two groups of women who manufactured gas masks from chrysotile and crocidolite asbestos: a 40-year follow-up. *Br. J. ind. Med.*, *39*, 344-348

[74]Botha, J.L., Irwig, L.M. & Strebel, P.M. (1986) Excess mortality from stomach cancer, lung cancer, and asbestosis and/or mesothelioma in crocidolite mining districts in South Africa. *Am. J. Epidemiol.*, *123*, 30-40

[75]Hobbs, M.S.T., Woodward, S.D., Murphy, B., Musk, A.W. & Elder, J.E. (1980) *The incidence of pneumoconiosis, mesothelioma and other respiratory cancer in men engaged in mining and milling crocidolite in Western Australia.* In: Wagner, J.C., ed., *Biological Effects of Mineral Fibres (IARC Scientific Publications No. 30)*, Lyon, International Agency for Research on Cancer, pp. 615-625

[76]Wignall, B.K. & Fox, A.J. (1982) Mortality of female gas mask assemblers. *Br. J. ind. Med., 39,* 34-38

[77]Hilt, B., Rosenberg, J. & Langård, S. (1981) Occurrence of cancer in a small cohort of asbestos-exposed workers. *Scand. J. Work Environ. Health, 7,* 185-189

[78]Baker, J.E., Reutens, D.C., Graham, D.F., Sterrett, G.F., Musk, A.W., Hobbs, M.S.T., Armstrong, B.K. & de Klerk, N.H. (1986) Morphology of bronchogenic carcinoma in workers formerly exposed to crocidolite at Wittenoom Gorge in Western Australia. *Int. J. Cancer, 37,* 547-550

[79]Berry, G. & Newhouse, M.L. (1983) Mortality of workers manufacturing friction materials using asbestos. *Br. J. ind. Med., 40,* 1-7

[80]Gardner, M.J., Winter, P.D., Pannett, B. & Powell, C.A. (1986) Follow up study of workers manufacturing chrysotile asbestos cement products. *Br. J. ind. Med., 43,* 726-732

[81]Weiss, W. (1977) Mortality of a cohort exposed to chrysotile asbestos. *J. occup. Med., 19,* 737-740

[82]Haider, M. & Neuberger, M. (1980) *Comparison of lung cancer risks for dust workers, asbestos-cement workers and control groups.* In: Wagner, J.C., ed., *Biological Effects of Mineral Fibres (IARC Scientific Publications No. 30)*, Lyon, International Agency for Research on Cancer, pp. 973-977

[83]McDonald, A.D., Fry, J.S., Woolley, A.J. & McDonald, J.C. (1984) Dust exposure and mortality in an American chrysotile asbestos friction products plant. *Br. J. ind. Med., 41,* 151-157

[84]Peto, J. (1980) *Lung cancer mortality in relation to measured dust levels in an asbestos textile factory.* In: Wagner, J.C., ed., *Biological Effects of Mineral Fibres (IARC Scientific Publications No. 30)*, Lyon, International Agency for Research on Cancer, pp. 829-836

[85]Peto, J., Doll, R., Howard, S.V., Kinlen, L.J. & Lewinsohn, H.C. (1977) A mortality study among workers in an English asbestos factory. *Br. J. ind. Med., 34,* 169-173

[86]Peto, J., Doll, R., Hermon, C., Binns, W., Clayton, R. & Goffe, T. (1985) Relationship of mortality to measures of environmental asbestos pollution in an asbestos textile factory. *Ann. occup. Hyg., 29,* 305-355

[87]Liddell, F.D.K., Thomas, D.C., Gibbs, G.W. & McDonald, J.C. (1984) Fibre exposure and mortality from pneumoconiosis, respiratory and abdominal malignancies in chrysotile production in Quebec, 1926-75. *Ann. Acad. Med., 13,* 340-344

[88]Dement, J.M., Harris, R.L., Jr, Symons, M.J. & Shy, C. (1982) Estimates of dose-response for respiratory cancer among chrysotile asbestos textile workers. *Ann. occup. Hyg., 26,* 869-887

[89]McDonald, A.D., Fry, J.S., Woolley, A.J. & McDonald, J. (1983) Dust exposure and mortality in an American chrysotile textile plant. *Br. J. ind. Med., 40,* 361-367

[90]Acheson, E.D. & Gardner, M.J. (1979) Mesothelioma and exposure to mixtures of chrysotile and amphibole asbestos. *Arch. environ. Health, 34,* 240-242

[91]Browne, K. & Smither, W.J. (1983) Asbestos-related mesothelioma: factors discriminating between pleural and peritoneal sites. *Br. J. ind. Med., 40,* 145-152

[92]Newhouse, M.L., Berry, G. & Skidmore, J.W. (1982) A mortality study of workers manufacturing friction materials with chrysotile asbestos. *Ann. occup. Hyg., 26,* 899-909

[93] Ohlson, C.-G., Klaesson, B. & Hogstedt, C. (1984) Mortality among asbestos-exposed workers in a railroad workshop. *Scand. J. Work Environ. Health, 10,* 283-291

[94] McDonald, A.D. & Fry, J.S. (1982) Mesothelioma and fiber type in three American asbestos factories — preliminary report. *Scand. J. Work Environ. Health, 8 (Suppl. 1),* 53-58

[95] Acheson, E.D., Gardner, M.J., Bennett, C. & Winter, P.D. (1981) Mesothelioma in a factory using amosite and chrysotile asbestos. *Lancet, ii,* 1403-1405

[96] McDonald, J.C., Gibbs, G.W., Liddell, F.D.K. & McDonald, A.D. (1978) Mortality after long exposure to cummingtonite-grunerite. *Am. Rev. respir. Dis., 118,* 271-277

[97] McDonald, J.C., McDonald, A.D., Armstrong, B. & Sébastien, P. (1986) Cohort study of mortality in vermiculite miners exposed to tremolite. *Br. J. ind. Med., 43,* 436-444

[98] Amandus, H.E. & Wheeler, R. (1987) The morbidity and mortality of vermiculite miners and millers exposed to tremolite-actinolite: Part II. Mortality. *Am. J. ind. Med., 11,* 15-26

[99] Neuberger, M., Kundi, M. & Friedl, H.P. (1984) Environmental asbestos exposure and cancer mortality. *Arch. environ. Health, 39,* 261-265

[100] Ohlson, C.-G. & Hogstedt, C. (1985) Lung cancer among asbestos cement workers. A Swedish cohort study and a review. *Br. J. ind. Med., 42,* 397-402

[101] Thomas, H.F., Benjamin, I.T., Elwood, P.C. & Sweetnam, P.M. (1982) Further follow-up study of workers from an asbestos cement factory. *Br. J. ind. Med., 39,* 273-276

[102] Weill, H., Hughes, J. & Waggenspack, C. (1979) Influence of dose and fiber type on respiratory malignancy risk in asbestos cement manufacturing. *Am. Rev. respir. Dis., 120,* 345-354

[103] Finkelstein, M.M. (1984) Mortality among employees of an Ontario asbestos-cement factory. *Am. Rev. respir. Dis., 129,* 754-761

[104] Hardell, L. (1981) Relation of soft-tissue sarcoma, malignant lymphoma and colon cancer to phenoxy acids, chlorophenols and other agents. *Scand. J. Work Environ. Health, 7,* 119-130

[105] Malker, H.S.R., McLaughlin, J.K., Malker, B.K., Stone, B.J., Weiner, J.A., Ericsson, J.L.E. & Blot, W.J. (1986) Biliary tract cancer and occupation in Sweden. *Br. J. ind. Med., 43,* 257-262

[106] Ross, R., Nichols, P., Wright, W., Lukes, R., Dworsky, R., Paganini-Hill, A., Koss, M. & Henderson, B. (1982) Asbestos exposure and lymphomas of the gastrointestinal tract and oral cavity. *Lancet, ii,* 1118-1120

[107] Waxweiler, R.J. & Robinson, C. (1983) Asbestos and non-Hodgkin's lymphoma. *Lancet, i,* 189-190

[108] Spanedda, R., Barbieri, D. & La Corte, R. (1983) Asbestos and non-Hodgkin's lymphoma. *Lancet, i,* 190

[109] Saracci, R. (1977) Asbestos and lung cancer: an analysis of the epidemiological evidence on the asbestos-smoking interaction. *Int. J. Cancer, 20,* 323-331

[110] Davis, J.M.G., Addison, J., Bolton, R.E., Donaldson, K., Jones, A.D. & Miller, B.G. (1985) Inhalation studies on the effects of tremolite and brucite dust in rats. *Carcinogenesis, 6,* 667-674

111Davis, J.M.G., Addison, J., Bolton, R.E., Donaldson, K. & Jones, A.D. (1986) Inhalation and injection studies in rats using dust samples from chrysotile asbestos prepared by a wet dispersion process. *Br. J. exp. Pathol., 67,* 113-129

112Stanton, M.F., Layard, M., Tegeris, A., Miller, E., May, M., Morgan, E. & Smith, A. (1981) Relation of particle dimension to carcinogenicity in amphibole asbestoses and other fibrous minerals. *J. natl Cancer Inst., 67,* 965-975

113Suzuki, Y, & Kohyama, N. (1984) Malignant mesothelioma induced by asbestos and zeolite in the mouse peritoneal cavity. *Environ. Res., 35,* 277-292

114Bolton, R.E., Davis, J.M.G., Donaldson, K. & Wright, A. (1982) Variations in the carcinogenicity of mineral fibres. *Ann. occup. Hyg., 26,* 569-582

115Pott, F., Huth, F. & Spurny, K. (1980) *Tumour induction after intraperitoneal injection of fibrous dusts.* In: Wagner, J.C., ed., *Biological Effects of Mineral Fibres (IARC Scientific Publications No. 30),* Lyon, International Agency for Research on Cancer, pp. 337-342

116Spurny, K., Pott, F., Huth, F., Weiss, G. & Opiela, H. (1979) Identification and carcinogenic action of fibrous actinolite from a diabase rock (Ger.). *Staub-Reinhalt. Luft, 39,* 386-389

117Pott, F., Schlipköter, H.W., Ziem, U., Spurny, K. & Huth, F. (1982) *New results from implantation experiments with mineral fibres.* In: *Biological Effects of Man-made Fibres,* Vol. 2, Copenhagen, WHO Regional Office for Europe, pp. 286-302

118Pott, F., Matscheck, A., Ziem, U., Muhle, H. & Huth, F. (1987) Animal experiments with chemically treated fibres. *Ann. occup. Hyg.* (in press)

119McConnell, E.E., Rutter, H.A., Ulland, B.M. & Moore, J.A. (1983) Chronic effects of dietary exposure to amosite asbestos and tremolite in F344 rats. *Environ. Health Perspect., 53,* 27-44

120National Toxicology Program (1983) *Lifetime Carcinogenesis Studies of Amosite Asbestos (CAS No. 121-72-73-5) in Syrian Golden Hamsters (Feed Studies) (NIH Publ. No. 84-2505; NTP TR 249),* Research Triangle Park, NC

121McConnell, E.E., Shefner, A.M., Rust, J.H. & Moore, J.A. (1983) Chronic effects of dietary exposure to amosite and chrysotile asbestos in Syrian golden hamsters. *Environ. Health Perspect., 53,* 11-25

122National Toxicology Program (1985) *Toxicology and Carcinogenesis Studies of Chrysotile Asbestos (CAS No. 12001-29-5) in F344/N Rats (Feed Studies) (NIH Publ. No. 86-2551; NTP TR 295),* Research Triangle Park, NC

123Bolton, R.E., Davis, J.M.G. & Lamb, D. (1982) The pathological effects of prolonged asbestos ingestion in rats. *Environ. Res., 29,* 134-150

124Küng-Vösamäe, A. & Vinkmann, F. (1980) *Combined carcinogenic action of chrysotile asbestos dust and* N-*nitrosodiethylamine on the respiratory tract of Syrian golden hamsters.* In: Wagner, J.C., ed., *Biological Effects of Mineral Fibres (IARC Scientific Publications No. 30),* Lyon, International Agency for Research on Cancer, pp. 305-310

125*IARC Monographs, Suppl. 6,* 77-80, 1987

ATTAPULGITE (Group 3)

A. Evidence for carcinogenicity to humans (*inadequate*)

A cohort study of 2302 men employed for at least one month between 1940 and 1975 at an attapulgite mining and milling facility in the USA showed a statistically significant excess of lung cancer deaths for white men (16 observed, 8.3 expected), but not for black men. Lung cancer risk was not significantly associated with cumulative dust exposure level, induction-latent period or duration of employment, except that among men employed for five years or more in high-exposure jobs five lung cancer deaths were observed, with 1.6 expected[1]. Interpretation of the excess of lung cancer in this study is restricted because of a relatively small study population, the possibly incomplete identification of the study population, incomplete demographic information on original records, lack of information on smoking and the use of national mortality rates for comparison.

B. Evidence for carcinogenicity to animals (*limited*)

Attapulgite was tested for carcinogenicity in rats by intraperitoneal injection, by intrapleural administration and by inhalation. One sample of attapulgite with 30% of fibres longer than 5 μm and another with 50% of fibres longer than 1.3 μm produced mesotheliomas and sarcomas in the abdominal cavity of rats following its intraperitoneal injection. Three samples of shorter fibre length gave negative results[1,2]. One sample of attapulgite with some fibres longer than 4 μm and two samples with some fibres longer than 6 μm induced mesothelial tumours following intrapleural administration to rats[1,3], but one sample with fewer such fibres did not[1]. Rats administered particles (with a mean length of 0.77 μm, no fibres longer than 4 μm and a mean diameter of 0.06 μm) of 'French' attapulgite by intrapleural administration did not develop mesothelioma, whereas about 50% of rats treated similarly with various types of asbestos did[4]. One mesothelioma was observed in rats following inhalation of two samples of attapulgite[3].

C. Other relevant data

No data were available on the genetic and related effects of attapulgite in humans. It did not induce sister chromatid exchanges in rat mesothelial cells or unscheduled DNA synthesis in rat hepatocytes *in vitro*[5].

References

[1]*IARC Monographs*, *42*, 159-173, 1987

[2]Pott, F. (1987) The fibre as a carcinogenic agent (Ger.). *Zbl. Bakt. Hyg. B*, *184*, 1-23

[3]Wagner, J.C., Griffiths, D.M. & Munday, D.E. (1987) Experimental studies with polygorskite dusts. *Br. J. Cancer* (in press)

[4]Jaurand, M.-C., Fleury, J., Monchaux, G., Nebut, M. & Bignon, J. (1987) Pleural carcinogenic potency of mineral fibers (asbestos, attapulgite) and their cytotoxicity on cultured cells. *J. natl Cancer Inst.*, *79*, 797-804

[5]*IARC Monographs*, *Suppl. 6*, 81-82, 1987

AURAMINE (TECHNICAL-GRADE) (Group 2B) and MANUFACTURE OF AURAMINE (Group 1)

A. Evidence for carcinogenicity to humans (*inadequate* for auramine, technical-grade; *sufficient* for the manufacture of auramine)

The manufacture of auramine (which also involves exposure to other chemicals) was judged to be causally associated with an increased incidence of bladder cancer on the basis of one study dealing with experiences in the first half of the century in the UK[1]. Data reported later, in two studies dealing with one group of workers in the Federal Republic of Germany involved in the manufacture of auramine, were judged to show increased risks of both bladder cancer and prostatic cancer; however, these workers had also been exposed to other chemicals, including 2-naphthylamine (see p. 261)[2,3].

In a study of mortality and cancer incidence among hairdressers, the hypothesis was raised that the observed excess risk of bladder cancer was associated with exposure to colouring agents present in brilliantines used on men's hair. Auramine was reported to be one of the most commonly used dyes in brilliantines, at least in the 1930s; however, the occurrence of impurities, such as 2-naphthylamine could not be ruled out[4]. Data on exposure to auramine alone were considered to be inadequate for evaluation.

B. Evidence for carcinogenicity to animals (*sufficient* for auramine, technical-grade)

Auramine (technical-grade) was tested for carcinogenicity by oral administration in mice and rats and by subcutaneous injection in rats. Following its oral administration, it induced liver neoplasms in animals of each species[1,2]. After subcutaneous injection in one study in rats, it induced local sarcomas[1]. Studies in rabbits and dogs were inadequate for evaluation[1].

C. Other relevant data

No data were available on the genetic and related effects of auramine in humans. It did not induce micronuclei in bone-marrow cells of mice treated *in vivo*. It transformed Syrian hamster embryo cells and induced sister chromatid exchanges and DNA strand breaks in rodent cells in culture. It caused aneuploidy, mitotic recombination and DNA damage in yeast. Auramine was mutagenic to bacteria and induced prophage[5].

References

[1]*IARC Monographs*, *1*, 69-73, 1972

[2]Kirsch, P., Fleig, I., Frentzel-Beyme, R., Gembardt, C., Steinborn, J., Thiess, A.M., Koch, W., Seibert, W., Wellenreuther, G. & Zeller, H. (1978) Auramine. Toxicology and occupational health (Ger.). *Arbeitsmed. Sozialmed. Präventivmed.*, *13*, 1-28

[3]Thiess, A.M., Link, R. & Wellenreuther, G. (1982) *Mortality study of employees exposed to auramine*. In: El-Attal, M., Abdel-Gelil, S., Massoud, A. & Noweir, M., eds, *Proceedings of the 9th International Conference of Occupational Health in the Chemical Industry, Cairo, 1981*, pp. 197-208

[4]Gubéran, E., Raymond, L. & Sweetnam, P.M. (1985) Increased risk for male bladder cancer among a cohort of male and female hairdressers from Geneva. *Int. J. Epidemiol.*, *14*, 549-554

[5]*IARC Monographs, Suppl. 6*, 83-85, 1987

AZATHIOPRINE (Group 1)

A. Evidence for carcinogenicity to humans (*sufficient*)

Two large prospective epidemiological studies have shown that renal transplant patients, who usually receive azathioprine as an immunosuppressant, become at high risk for non-Hodgkin's lymphoma, squamous-cell cancers of the skin, hepatobiliary carcinomas and mesenchymal tumours. While this is true for each of the various etiological entities resulting in the need for a transplant, these patients also have in common heavy exposure to foreign antigens[1]. Other patients who have received azathioprine as an immunosuppressant, including those with rheumatoid arthritis, systemic lupus and other 'collagen' disorders, inflammatory bowel disease and certain skin and renal diseases, have also been studied: the same array of malignancies was found to be in excess, although to a lesser extent[1,2]. For these patients, however, the picture is still not completely clear, because patients with rheumatoid arthritis constituted the largest category in the latter study[2], and some[3], but not all studies[4], have found that this disease conveys a risk for non-Hodgkin's lymphoma in the absence of treatment.

B. Evidence for carcinogenicity to animals (*limited*)

Suggestive evidence was obtained that lymphomas were induced in mice after intraperitoneal, subcutaneous or intramuscular injection of azathioprine, and that thymic lymphomas and squamous-cell carcinomas of the ear duct were induced in rats after oral administration, but there were limitations in the design and reporting of these studies[1,5].

C. Other relevant data

There are conflicting reports of effects on the incidence of chromosomal aberrations in lymphocytes and bone-marrow cells of patients treated with azathioprine. In one study, the incidence of sister chromatid exchanges in lymphocytes of treated patients was not increased[6].

In animals treated *in vivo*, azathioprine induced dominant lethal mutations in mice, chromosomal aberrations in rabbit lymphocytes and Chinese hamster bone-marrow cells, and micronuclei in mice, rats and hamsters; it did not induce sister chromatid exchanges in

Chinese hamster bone-marrow cells. Azathioprine induced chromosomal aberrations but not sister chromatid exchanges in human lymphocytes *in vitro*. It induced chromosomal aberrations in *Drosophila*, was weakly mutagenic to fungi and was mutagenic to bacteria[6].

References

[1]*IARC Monographs*, *26*, 47-78, 1981

[2]Kinlen, L.J. (1985) Incidence of cancer in rheumatoid arthritis and other disorders after immunosuppressive treatment. *Am. J. Med.*, *78 (Suppl. 1A)*, 44-49

[3]Isomäki, H.A., Hakulinen, T. & Joutsenlahti, U. (1978) Excess risk of lymphomas, leukemia and myeloma in patients with rheumatoid arthritis. *J. chron. Dis.*, *31*, 691-696

[4]Fries, J.F., Bloch, D., Spitz, P. & Mitchell, D.M. (1985) Cancer in rheumatoid arthritis: a prospective long-term study of mortality. *Am. J. Med.*, *78 (Suppl. 1A)*, 56-59

[5]Cohen, S.M., Erturk, E., Skibba, J.L. & Bryan, G.T. (1983) Azathioprine induction of lymphomas and squamous cell carcinomas in rats. *Cancer Res.*, *43*, 2768-2772

[6]*IARC Monographs*, *Suppl. 6*, 86-88, 1987

BENZENE (Group 1)

A. Evidence for carcinogenicity to humans (*sufficient*)

Numerous case reports and series have suggested a relationship between exposure to benzene and the occurrence of various types of leukaemia[1]. Several case-control studies have also shown increased odds ratios for exposure to benzene, but mixed exposure patterns and poorly defined exposures render their interpretation difficult[1,2].

Three independent cohort studies have demonstrated an increased incidence of acute nonlymphocytic leukaemia in workers exposed to benzene[1,3]. An updating of a cohort study published earlier on benzene-exposed workers[1] confirmed the previous findings and added a further case of myelogenous leukaemia, giving a standardized mortality ratio (SMR) of 194 (95% confidence interval, 52-488), based on four cases; the difference was statistically significant when only myelogenous leukaemia was considered (4 observed, 0.9 expected; $p = 0.011$)[4]. A further cohort study found an excess of acute myeloid leukaemia (SMR, 394; 172-788) among refinery workers, based on eight cases; however, the patients had not worked in jobs identified as having the highest benzene exposure[5]. Another study of refinery workers showed no death from leukaemia (0.4 expected); however, the median exposure intensity for benzene was 0.14 ppm (0.45 mg/m³), and only 16% of 1394 personal samples, taken between 1973 and 1982 inclusive, contained more than 1 ppm (3.19 mg/m³). The median exposure intensity in 'benzene-related units' was 0.53 ppm (1.7 mg/m³)[6].

In a Chinese retrospective cohort study, encompassing 28 460 workers exposed to benzene in 233 factories, 30 cases of leukaemia (23 acute, seven chronic) were found, as compared to four cases in a reference cohort of 28 257 workers in 83 machine production, textile and cloth factories. The mortality rate from leukaemia was 14/100 000 person-years among the exposed and 2/100 000 person-years among the unexposed (SMR, 574; $p < 0.01$). Mortality was especially high for workers engaged in organic synthesis, painting and rubber production. The mortality from leukaemia for cases that had previously had benzene poisoning was 701/100 000 person-years. 'Grab' samples of benzene in air were taken during the time of the survey in workplaces where cases of leukaemia were observed; the mean concentrations varied in a wide range, from 10 to 1000 mg/m[3], but the range 50-500 mg/m[3] covered most of them[7].

B. Evidence for carcinogenicity to animals (*sufficient*)

Benzene was tested for carcinogenicity in mice and rats by several routes of administration. Following its oral administration at several dose levels, it induced neoplasms at multiple sites in males and females of both species[1,8-11]. After mice were exposed to benzene by inhalation, a tendency towards induction of lymphoid neoplasms was observed[1,12,13]. Exposure of rats by inhalation increased the incidence of neoplasms, mainly carcinomas, at various sites[9,10,14-16]. Skin application or subcutaneous injection of benzene to mice did not produce evidence of carcinogenicity, but most of the experiments were inadequate for evaluation[1]. In a mouse-lung tumour bioassay by intraperitoneal injection, an increase in the incidence of lung adenomas was observed in males[17].

C. Other relevant data

Chromosomal aberrations in human peripheral lymphocytes have been associated with occupational exposure to benzene, although many of the studies are very difficult to interpret[18].

Benzene induced chromosomal aberrations, micronuclei and sister chromatid exchanges in bone-marrow cells of mice, chromosomal aberrations in bone-marrow cells of rats and Chinese hamsters and sperm-head anomalies in mice treated *in vivo*. It induced chromosomal aberrations and mutation in human cells *in vitro* but did not induce sister chromatid exchanges in cultured human lymphocytes, except in one study in which high concentrations of an exogenous metabolic system were used. In some test systems, benzene induced cell transformation. It did not induce sister chromatid exchanges in rodent cells *in vitro*, but did induce aneuploidy and, in some studies, chromosomal aberrations in cultured Chinese hamster ovary cells. Benzene induced mutation and DNA damage in some studies in rodent cells *in vitro*[18].

In *Drosophila*, benzene was reported to be weakly positive in assays for somatic mutation and for crossing-over in spermatogonia; in single studies, it did not induce sex-linked recessive lethal mutations or translocations. It induced aneuploidy, mutation and gene conversion in fungi. Benzene was not mutagenic to bacteria[18].

References

[1]*IARC Monographs*, *29*, 93-148, 391-398, 1982

[2]Arp, E.W., Jr, Wolf, P.H. & Checkoway, H. (1983) Lymphocytic leukemia and exposures to benzene and other solvents in the rubber industry. *J. occup. Med.*, *25*, 598-602

[3]Decouflé, P., Blattner, W.A. & Blair, A. (1983) Mortality among chemical workers exposed to benzene and other agents. *Environ. Res.*, *30*, 16-25

[4]Bond, G.G., McLaren, E.A., Baldwin, C.L. & Cook, R.R. (1986) An update of mortality among chemical workers exposed to benzene. *Br. J. ind. Med.*, *43*, 685-691

[5]McCraw, D.S., Joyner, R.E. & Cole, P. (1985) Excess leukemia in a refinery population. *J. occup. Med.*, *27*, 220-222

[6]Tsai, S.P., Wen, C.P., Weiss, N.S., Wong, O., McClellan, W.A. & Gibson, R.L. (1983) Retrospective mortality and medical surveillance studies of workers in benzene areas of refineries. *J. occup. Med.*, *25*, 685-692

[7]Yin, S.-N., Li, G.-L., Tain, F.-D., Fu, Z.-I., Jin, C., Chen, Y.-J., Luo, S.-J., Ye, P.-Z., Zhang, J.-Z., Wang, G.-C., Zhang, X.-C., Wu, H.-N. & Zhong, Q.-C. (1987) Leukaemia in benzene workers: a retrospective cohort study. *Br. J. ind. Med.*, *44*, 124-128

[8]Maltoni, C., Conti, B. & Scarnato, C. (1982) Squamous cell carcinomas of the oral cavity in Sprague Dawley rats, following exposure to benzene by ingestion. First experimental demonstration. *Med. Lav.*, *4*, 441-445

[9]Maltoni, C., Conti, B. & Cotti, G. (1983) Benzene: a multi-potential carcinogen. Results of long-term bioassays performed at the Bologna Institute of Oncology. *Am. J. ind. Med.*, *4*, 589-630

[10]Maltoni, C., Conti, B., Cotti, G. & Belpoggi, F. (1985) Experimental studies on benzene carcinogenicity at the Bologna Institute of Oncology: current results and ongoing research. *Am. J. ind. Med.*, *7*, 415-446

[11]National Toxicology Program (1986) *Toxicology and Carcinogenesis Studies of Benzene (CAS No. 71-43-2) in F344/N rats and B6C3F$_1$ Mice (Gavage Studies) (NTP Technical Report 289; NIH Publ. No. 86-2545)*, Research Triangle Park, NC

[12]Cronkite, E.P., Bullis, J.E., Inoue, T. & Drew, R.T. (1984) Benzene inhalation produces leukemia in mice. *Toxicol. appl. Pharmacol.*, *75*, 358-361

[13]Cronkite, E.P., Drew, R.T., Inoue, T. & Bullis, J.E. (1985) Benzene hematotoxicity and leukemogenesis. *Am. J. ind. Med.*, *7*, 447-456

[14]Maltoni, C., Cotti, G., Valgimigli, L. & Mandrioli, A. (1982) Zymbal gland carcinomas in rats following exposure to benzene by inhalation. *Am. J. ind. Med.*, *3*, 11-16

[15]Maltoni, C., Cotti, G., Valgimigli, L. & Mandrioli, A. (1982) Hepatocarcinomas in Sprague-Dawley rats, following exposure to benzene by inhalation. First experimental demonstration. *Med. Lav.*, *4*, 446-450

[16]Snyder, C.A., Goldstein, B.D., Sellakumar, A.R. & Albert, R.E. (1984) Evidence for hematotoxicity and tumorigenesis in rats exposed to 100 ppm benzene. *Am. J. ind. Med.*, *5*, 429-434

[17]Stoner, G.D., Conran, P.B., Greisiger, E.A., Stober, J., Morgan, M. & Pereira, M.A. (1986) Comparison of two routes of chemical administration on the lung adenoma response in strain A/J mice. Toxicol. appl. Pharmacol., *82*, 19-31

[18]*IARC Monographs, Suppl. 6*, 91-95, 1987

BENZIDINE (Group 1)

A. Evidence for carcinogenicity to humans (*sufficient*)

Case reports and follow-up studies of workers in many countries have demonstrated that occupational exposure to benzidine is causally associated with an increased risk of bladder cancer. In one extreme instance, all five of a group of workers continuously employed in the manufacture of benzidine for 15 years or more developed bladder cancer[1]. Earlier data suggesting that the incidence of this cancer in workers decreased after a reduction in industrial exposure[1] have been supported by a study of a cohort of workers at a US benzidine-manufacturing facility, in which major preventive measures were instituted in 1950 to minimize worker exposure. The study period covered 1945-1979, and, overall, there was a clearly significant excess of bladder cancer incidence, which, however, declined in those first employed after 1950[2]. Although a longer follow-up is required to evaluate fully the effect of preventive measures on cancer risks, the causal association is strengthened by these two independent observations. Few other epidemiological studies have examined the cancer risk associated with exposure to benzidine alone. In a study at a dyestuffs factory in Italy, it was possible to distinguish a very high bladder cancer risk (5 deaths observed, 0.06 expected) associated with benzidine production[3]. The study was extended and updated, but the role of exposure to benzidine alone in the dramatically increased bladder cancer risk could not be examined further[4]. Of 25 benzidine 'operators' at a plant in the USA, 13 developed bladder cancer; all cases had been exposed for six years or more[5]. A surveillance programme of 179 active and 65 retired workers in a dyestuffs manufacturing plant in Japan revealed nine cases of bladder cancer that occurred between 1968 and 1981; all of the cases had been engaged in benzidine production[6].

Other investigations have shown high incidences of cancer of the bladder and urinary tract after concomitant exposure to benzidine and 2-naphthylamine (see p. 261) [7,8]. Exposure to these two compounds was also associated with an increase in the occurrence of second primary cancers at sites other than the bladder, including the liver[9].

Among 1601 workers in the chemical-dye industry in China who were exposed to benzidine, methylnaphthylamine and dianisidine (see p. 198), 21 cases of bladder carcinoma were found. All had a history of exposure to benzidine, while no carcinoma was found among workers exposed to methylnaphthylamine or dianisidine. Suggestions of a dose-response relationship were provided by analysis according to length of exposure[10].

Bladder cancer was also found to be increased in ecological studies of areas where benzidine (as well as 2-naphthylamine and other compounds) was used, manufactured or stored[11,12].

B. Evidence for carcinogenicity to animals (*sufficient*)

Benzidine and/or its salts were tested for carcinogenicity by oral administration in mice, rats, hamsters and dogs and by subcutaneous and intraperitoneal injection and inhalation in rats. Following oral administration of benzidine and its hydrochloride, significant increases in the incidences of benign and malignant liver neoplasms were observed in mice and hamsters[1,13-17] and of mammary cancer in rats; benzidine induced bladder carcinomas in dogs. Following subcutaneous administration of benzidine and its sulphate to rats, a high incidence of Zymbal-gland tumours was observed. After intraperitoneal administration of benzidine to rats, a marked increase in the incidence of mammary-gland and Zymbal-gland neoplasms was observed. The results of one study in rats by inhalation could not be evaluated[1].

Two metabolites of benzidine, N,N'-diacetylbenzidine and N-hydroxy-N,N'-diacetylbenzidine, produced mammary-gland and Zymbal-gland tumours in rats following their intraperitoneal injection[1].

C. Other relevant data

No data were available on the genetic and related effects of benzidine in humans.

Covalent binding products of benzidine with DNA have been described in the liver of mice and rats treated *in vivo*. Benzidine induced micronuclei, sister chromatid exchanges, DNA strand breaks and unscheduled DNA synthesis in cells of rodents treated *in vivo*. It induced unscheduled DNA synthesis in humans cells *in vitro*. It caused transformation of Syrian hamster embryo and BALB/c 3T3 cells and induced chromosomal aberrations, sister chromatid exchanges, unscheduled DNA synthesis and DNA strand breaks in rodent cells *in vitro*; conflicting results were obtained for mutation. Benzidine induced aneuploidy, gene conversion and DNA damage in yeast, but not mutation. It was mutagenic to plants and bacteria[18].

References

[1]*IARC Monographs*, 29, 149-183, 391-398, 1982

[2]Meigs, J.W., Marrett, L.D., Ulrich, F.U. & Flannery, J.T. (1986) Bladder tumor incidence among workers exposed to benzidine: a thirty-year follow-up. *J. natl Cancer Inst.*, 76, 1-8

[3]Rubino, G.F., Scansetti, G., Piolatto, G. & Pira, E. (1982) The carcinogenic effect of aromatic amines: an epidemiological study on the role of o-toluidine and 4,4'-methylene bis(2-methylaniline) in inducing bladder cancer in man. *Environ. Res.*, 27, 241-254

[4]Decarli, A., Peto, J., Piolatto, G. & La Vecchia, C. (1985) Bladder cancer mortality of workers exposed to aromatic amines: analysis of models of carcinogenesis. *Br. J. Cancer*, 51, 707-712

[5]Horton, A.W. & Bingham, E.L. (1977) Risk of bladder tumors among benzidine workers and their serum properdin levels. *J. natl Cancer Inst.*, 58, 1225-1228

[6]Yamaguchi, N., Tazaki, H., Okubo, T. & Toyama, T. (1982) Periodic urine cytology surveillance of bladder tumor incidence in dyestuff workers. *Am. J. ind. Med.*, 3, 139-148

[7]Tsuchiya, K., Okubo, T. & Ishizu, S. (1975) An epidemiological study of occupational bladder tumours in the dye industry of Japan. *Br. J. ind. Med.*, 32, 203-209

[8]Nakamura, J., Takamatsu, M., Doi, J., Ohkawa, T., Fujinaga, T., Ebisuno, S. & Sone, M. (1980) Clinical study on the occupational urinary tract tumor in Wakayama (Jpn.). *Jpn. J. Urol.*, 71, 945-951

[9]Morinaga, K., Oshima, A. & Hara, I. (1982) Multiple primary cancers following exposure to benzidine and beta-naphthylamine. *Am. J. ind. Med.*, 3, 243-246

[10]Sun, L.D. & Deng, X.M. (1980) An epidemiologic survey of bladder carcinoma in chemical dye industry (Chin.). *Chin. J. Surg., 18*, 491-493

[11]Segnan, N. & Tanturri, G. (1976) Study on the geographical pathology of laryngeal, bladder and childhood cancer in the province of Torino (Ital.). *Tumori, 62*, 377-386

[12]Budnick, L.D., Sokal, D.C., Falk, H., Logue, J.N. & Fox, J.M. (1984) Cancer and birth defects near the Drake superfund site, Pennsylvania. *Arch. environ. Health, 39*, 409-413

[13]Littlefield, N.A., Nelson, C.J. & Frith, C.H. (1983) Benzidine dihydrochloride: toxicological assessment in mice during chronic exposures. *J. Toxicol. environ. Health, 12*, 671-685

[14]Littlefield, N.A., Nelson, C.J. & Gaylor, D.W. (1984) Benzidine dihydrochloride: risk assessment. *Fundam. appl. Toxicol., 4*, 69-80

[15]Littlefield, N.A., Wolff, G.L. & Nelson, C.J. (1985) Influence of genetic composition of test-animal populations on chronic toxicity studies used for risk estimation. *J. Toxicol. environ. Health, 15*, 357-367

[16]Nelson, C.J., Baetcke, K.P., Frith, C.H., Kodell, R.L. & Schieferstein, G. (1982) The influence of sex, dose, time, and cross on neoplasia in mice given benzidine dihydrochloride. *Toxicol. appl. Pharmacol., 64*, 171-186

[17]Vesselinovitch, S.D. (1983) Perinatal hepatocarcinogenesis. *Biol. Res. Pregn. Perinatol., 4*, 22-25

[18]*IARC Monographs, Suppl. 6*, 96-100, 1987

BENZIDINE-BASED DYES (Group 2A)

A. Evidence for carcinogenicity to humans (*inadequate*)

The epidemiological data were inadequate to evaluate the carcinogenicity of three benzidine-based dyes, Direct Black 38, Direct Blue 6 and Direct Brown 95, to humans. However, a study of silk dyers and painters who had had multiple exposure to benzidine-based and other dyes indicated that those exposures were strongly associated with the occurrence of bladder cancer[1].

B. Evidence for carcinogenicity to animals (*sufficient* for technical-grade Direct Black 38, technical-grade Direct Blue 6 and technical-grade Direct Brown 95)

Direct Black 38 was tested for carcinogenicity in mice by administration in drinking-water, producing liver and mammary tumours. Commercial Direct Black 38 produced hepatocellular carcinomas within 13 weeks after administration in the diet to rats and small numbers of carcinomas in the urinary bladder, liver and colon after administration to rats in drinking-water[1].

In a single study, commercial Direct Blue 6 produced hepatocellular carcinomas in rats within 13 weeks after its oral administration.

Commercial Direct Brown 95 produced neoplastic nodules in the livers of 4/8 female rats, and a hepatocellular carcinoma in one, after its oral administration in a single study terminated after 13 weeks. The finding of preneoplastic lesions after such a short exposure prior indicates a carcinogenic effect similar to that of Direct Black 38 and Direct Blue 6[1].

C. Other relevant data

Benzidine-based dyes are structurally related to benzidine, exposure to which is causally associated with cancer in humans (see p. 123), and commercial material may contain small amounts of benzidine. Commercial Direct Black 38 may contain small quantities of 4-aminobiphenyl (see p. 91) and 2,4-diaminobenzene (the hydrochloride of which is chrysoidine [see p. 169])[1].

Benzidine has been detected in the urine of workers exposed to benzidine-based azo dyes. No data were available on the genetic and related effects of Direct Black 38, Direct Blue 6 or Direct Brown 95, in humans[1].

In experimental animals, Direct Black 38, Direct Blue 6 and Direct Brown 95 undergo reduction of the azo bonds with the appearance in the urine of benzidine and monoacetyl-benzidine. The reductive cleavage of the azo bond has been attributed to the activities of intestinal microflora and/or liver azoreductases[2]

Direct Black 38 was mutagenic to bacteria. Urine from rodents treated with Direct Black 38 was mutagenic to bacteria in the presence of an exogenous metabolic system, and human intestinal microflora metabolized Direct Black 38 to highly mutagenic metabolites[2].

DNA adducts (including covalent binding products of benzidine) have been described in the livers of rats treated with Direct Blue 6 *in vivo*. Direct Blue 6 is mutagenic to bacteria only in the presence of an exogenous metabolic system and the cofactor flavine mononucleotide[2].

Direct Brown 95 induced unscheduled DNA synthesis in rat hepatocytes in an in-vivo/in-vitro assay but not in hepatocytes *in vitro*. It was mutagenic to bacteria in the presence of an exogenous metabolic system; this activity was enhanced by the cofactor flavine mononucleotide. The urine from rats treated with Direct Brown 95 was mutagenic to bacteria in the presence of an exogenous metabolic system[2].

References

[1]*IARC Monographs*, *29*, 295-310, 311-320, 321-330, 1982
[2]*IARC Monographs*, *Suppl. 6*, 275-281, 1987

BENZOYL CHLORIDE (Group 3)

A. Evidence for carcinogenicity to humans (*inadequate*)

Six cases of respiratory cancer were reported among workers in two small factories where benzoyl chloride and its chlorinated precursors were produced[1].

B. Evidence for carcinogenicity to animals (*inadequate*)

Benzoyl chloride was tested in two sets of experiments by skin application to female mice. A few skin carcinomas were observed, but their incidence was not statistically significant[1].

C. Other relevant data

No data were available on the genetic and related effects of benzoyl chloride in humans. It did not induce mutation or DNA damage in bacteria[2].

References

[1]*IARC Monographs*, *29*, 83-91, 1982
[2]*IARC Monographs*, *Suppl. 6*, 103-104, 1987

BERYLLIUM AND BERYLLIUM COMPOUNDS (Group 2A)

A. Evidence for carcinogenicity to humans (*limited*)

Observations, reviewed elsewhere[1,2], on beryllium-exposed subjects cover two industrial populations and a registry of berylliosis cases. Workers at beryllium extraction, production and fabrication facilities in the USA were followed up and their causes of mortality compared with those of both the general population and a cohort of viscose-rayon workers. Ratios of observed to expected deaths for lung cancer in the two industrial populations (65 observed) were found to be elevated in both comparisons (1.4 in respect of both the general population [95% confidence interval (CI), 1.1-1.8] and the viscose-rayon workers [1.0-2.0]) and tended to be concentrated in workers who had been employed for less than five years. Data from the US Beryllium Case Registry, in which cases of beryllium-related lung diseases were collected from a wide variety of sources (including the two facilities previously mentioned), indicate an approximately three-fold (six deaths observed, 2.1 expected; ratio of observed:expected, 2.9 [95% CI, 1.0-6.2]) increase in mortality from lung cancer among subjects who had suffered from acute berylliosis, which usually follows heavy exposure to beryllium, but not among those who had had chronic berylliosis (one death observed, 1.4 expected; ratio of observed:expected, 0.7; 95% CI, 0.1-3.7).

B. Evidence for carcinogenicity to animals (*sufficient*)

Beryllium metal, beryllium-aluminium alloy, beryl ore, beryllium chloride, beryllium fluoride, beryllium hydroxide, beryllium sulphate (and its tetrahydrate) and beryllium oxide[1,3,4] all produced lung tumours in rats exposed by inhalation or intratracheally. Single intratracheal instillations or one-hour inhalation exposures were effective[3]. Beryllium oxide and beryllium sulphate produced lung tumours in monkeys after intrabronchial implantation or inhalation[1]. Beryllium metal, beryllium carbonate, beryllium oxide, beryllium phosphate, beryllium silicate and zinc beryllium silicate all produced osteosarcomas in rabbits following their intravenous and/or intramedullary administration[1].

C. Other relevant data

No data were available on the genetic and related effects of beryllium and beryllium compounds in humans.

All of the available experimental studies considered by the Working Group were carried out with water-soluble beryllium salts. In one study, beryllium sulphate increased the frequency of chromosomal aberrations and sister chromatid exchanges in human lymphocytes and in Syrian hamster cells *in vitro*; in another study, chromosomal aberrations were not seen in human lymphocytes. It caused transformation of cultured rodent cells in several test systems. In one study, beryllium chloride induced mutation in cultured Chinese hamster cells. Beryllium sulphate did not induce unscheduled DNA synthesis in rat hepatocytes *in vitro*, mitotic recombination in yeast or mutation in bacteria. Beryllium chloride was mutagenic to bacteria[5].

References

[1]*IARC Monographs*, *23*, 143-204, 1980

[2]Saracci, R. (1985) *Beryllium: epidemiological evidence.* In: Wald, N.J. & Doll, R., eds, *Interpretation for Negative Epidemiological Evidence for Carcinogenicity (IARC Scientific Publications No. 65)*, Lyon, International Agency for Research on Cancer, pp. 203-219

[3]Litvinov, N.N., Kazenashev, V.K. & Bugryshev, P.F. (1983) Blastomogenic activities of various beryllium compounds (Russ.). *Eksp. Oncol.*, *5*, 23-26

[4]Ishinishi, N., Mizunoe, M., Inamasu, T. & Hisanaga, A. (1980) Experimental study on carcinogenicity of beryllium oxide and arsenic trioxide to the lung of rats by an intratracheal instillation (Jpn.). *Fukuoka Acta med.*, *71*, 19-26

[5]*IARC Monographs, Suppl. 6*, 110-112, 1987

BETEL QUID WITH TOBACCO (Group 1) and BETEL QUID WITHOUT TOBACCO (Group 3)

A. Evidence for carcinogenicity to humans (*sufficient* for betel quid with tobacco; *inadequate* for betel quid without tobacco)

Many descriptive studies and case reports have shown an association between the habit of chewing betel quid with tobacco and oral cancer. A significant increase in the risk of oral cancer has been observed in chewers of betel quid with tobacco in several case-control studies and in one large-scale cohort study. In chewers of betel quid with tobacco, a statistically significant increase in risk was also observed for cancers of the oropharynx, hypopharynx, larynx and oesophagus[1].

Several descriptive studies from Papua-New Guinea and a number of case-control studies have suggested an association between the habit of chewing betel quid without tobacco and oral cancer. In one of the case-control studies, in which smoking was not controlled for, a statistically significant increase in risk was also observed for cancers of the oropharynx, hypopharynx, larynx and oesophagus. In another case-control study of oral cancer, in which a clear effect of chewing betel with tobacco was found, no such effect was found for chewing betel without tobacco[1].

B. Evidence for carcinogenicity to animals (*limited* for betel quid with and without tobacco)

Aqueous extracts of betel quid containing tobacco were tested for carcinogenicity in mice by gastric intubation, skin painting and subcutaneous injection; some malignant tumours occurred at the site of skin or subcutaneous administration. In hamsters, forestomach carcinomas occurred after painting of the cheek-pouch mucosa with aqueous extracts or implantation of wax pellets containing powdered betel quid with tobacco in the cheek pouch; carcinomas occurred in the cheek pouch following implantation of wax pellets[1].

Aqueous extracts of betel quid without tobacco were tested in mice by gastric intubation and by subcutaneous administration; an increased incidence of local tumours was observed after subcutaneous injection. In hamsters, painting of the cheek-pouch mucosa or implantation of wax pellets into the cheek pouch resulted in the induction of forestomach carcinomas; carcinomas occurred in the cheek pouch following implantation of wax pellets[1].

Aqueous or dimethyl sulphoxide extracts of areca nut with tobacco were tested in mice by skin application; a low incidence of skin tumours was reported in a study lacking controls. In hamsters, applications of such extracts to cheek-pouch mucosa produced squamous-cell carcinomas of the cheek pouch and forestomach carcinomas[1].

Areca nut and aqueous extracts of areca nut were tested in mice by oral intubation, dietary administration, skin application and intraperitoneal and subcutaneous injection. Local tumours were produced following subcutaneous injection. In rats, areca nut was inadequately tested by oral administration; aqueous extracts tested by subcutaneous injection produced local mesenchymal tumours. In hamsters, administration of areca nut and application of aqueous or dimethyl sulphoxide extracts to the cheek-pouch mucosa resulted in squamous-cell carcinomas of the cheek pouch and carcinomas of the forestomach[1]. Oral administration of a diet containing 20% betel-nut powder enhanced the incidences of preneoplastic and neoplastic lesions of the tongue in rats pretreated with 4-nitroquinoline-1-oxide and of preneoplastic liver lesions in rats pretreated with 2-acetylaminofluorene[2].

Aqueous extracts of betel leaf were tested in mice by oral intubation and by intraperitoneal injection, in hamsters by application to the cheek-pouch mucosa[1] and in rats by oral administration[3]. Betel leaf was tested in rats by dietary administration and in hamsters by implantation in beeswax pellets into the cheek pouch[1]. All of these studies were inadequate for evaluation.

C. Other relevant data

Chewing of betel quid with or without tobacco increased the frequencies of micro-nucleated cells in the buccal mucosa of chewers; dose-dependence was observed in relation to the number of betel quids chewed per day. Chewing of betel quid with or without tobacco increased the frequency of sister chromatid exchanges in peripheral blood lymphocytes of chewers. Increased frequencies of sister chromatid exchanges were observed in peripheral blood lymphocytes of chewers of areca nut with slaked lime and tobacco, either alone or wrapped in betel leaf, particularly among chewers who had developed oral submucous fibrosis. Extracts of urine from chewers of betel quid with tobacco were mutagenic to *Salmonella typhimurium* in the presence of an exogenous metabolic system[4].

An aqueous extract of betel quid (containing tobacco) induced micronuclei in bone-marrow cells of mice treated *in vivo* and was mutagenic to Chinese hamster V79 cells. No such effect was observed with extracts of betel quids not containing tobacco. Aqueous extracts of betel quids (both with and without tobacco) were mutagenic to *S. typhimurium*[4].

References

[1]*IARC Monographs, 37*, 141-200, 1985

[2]Tanaka, T., Kuniyasu, T., Shima, H., Sugie, S., Mori, H., Takahashi, M. & Hirono, I. (1986) Carcinogenicity of betel quid. III. Enhancement of 4-nitroquinoline-1-oxide and *N*-2-fluorenylacetamide-induced carcinogenesis in rats by subsequent administration of betel nut. *J. natl Cancer Inst., 77*, 777-781

[3]Rao, A.R., Sinha, A. & Selvan, R.S. (1985) Inhibitory action of *Piper betle* on the initiation of 7,12-dimethylbenz[*a*]anthracene-induced mammary carcinogenesis in rats. *Cancer Lett., 26*, 207-214

[4]*IARC Monographs, Suppl. 6*, 113, 1987

N,N-BIS(2-CHLOROETHYL)-2-NAPHTHYLAMINE (CHLORNAPHAZINE) (Group 1)

A. Evidence for carcinogenicity to humans (*sufficient*)

Among 61 patients with polycythaemia vera treated with chlornaphazine in 1954-1962 and followed until 1974, eight developed invasive carcinoma of the bladder, five developed papillary carcinomas of the bladder and eight had abnormal urinary cytology. The invasive carcinomas were seen in four of five patients treated with a cumulative dose of 200 g or more, in two of 15 patients given 100-199 g, in one of ten patients given 50-99 g and in one of 31 patients given less than 50 g. No noncausal explanation can be suggested[1].

B. Evidence for carcinogenicity to animals (*limited*)

Chlornaphazine produced lung tumours in mice following its intraperitoneal injection, and local sarcomas in rats after its subcutaneous administration[2].

C. Other relevant data

No data were available on the genetic and related effects of chlornaphazine in humans.

Rats administered chlornaphazine excreted metabolites of 2-naphthylamine (see p. 261) in the urine. Chlornaphazine induced chromosomal aberrations in Chinese hamster cells, mutation in mouse lymphoma cells and unscheduled DNA synthesis in rat hepatocytes *in vitro*. A single study of cell transformation in virus-infected Syrian hamster embryo cells was inconclusive. It induced sex-linked recessive lethal mutations and chromosomal aberrations in *Drosophila* and was mutagenic to bacteria[3].

References

[1]Thiede, T. & Christensen, B.C. (1975) Tumours of the bladder induced by chlornaphazine (Norw.). *Ugesk. Laeger, 137*, 661-666

[2]*IARC Monographs, 4*, 119-124, 1974

[3]*IARC Monographs, Suppl. 6*, 113-115, 1987

BIS(CHLOROMETHYL)ETHER AND CHLOROMETHYL METHYL ETHER (TECHNICAL-GRADE) (Group 1)

A. Evidence for carcinogenicity to humans (*sufficient*)

Numerous epidemiological studies[1-9] and case reports[10-13] from around the world have demonstrated that workers exposed to chloromethyl methyl ether and/or bis(chloromethyl)-ether have an increased risk for lung cancer. Among heavily exposed workers, the relative risks are ten fold or more. Risks increase with duration and cumulative exposure. Histological evaluation indicates that exposure results primarily in lung cancer of the small-cell type[8]. Maximal relative risks appear to occur 15-20 years after first exposure[6], and latency is shortened among workers with heavier exposure[5,11].

B. Evidence for carcinogenicity to animals (*sufficient*)

Bis(chloromethyl)ether produced tumours at the site of its administration to mice after exposure by inhalation[1,14], skin application[1] or subcutaneous injection[1,15] and was an initiator of mouse skin tumours[15]; it also increased the incidence of lung tumours after its subcutaneous administration[1]. In rats, it produced tumours of the respiratory tract (lung tumours and nasal-cavity carcinoma) after exposure by inhalation[14,16-18].

Technical-grade chloromethyl methyl ether produced local sarcomas in mice after its subcutaneous administration and was an initiator of mouse skin tumours[1]; in rats and hamsters, it produced a low incidence of tumours of the respiratory tract after exposure by inhalation[19].

C. Other relevant data

A slight increase in the incidence of chromosomal aberrations was observed in peripheral lymphocytes of workers exposed to bis(chloromethyl)ether or chloromethyl methyl ether in the preparation of ion-exchange resins[20].

Bis(chloromethyl)ether did not cause chromosomal aberrations in bone-marrow cells of rats treated *in vivo*. It induced unscheduled DNA synthesis in human fibroblasts *in vitro* and was mutagenic to bacteria[20].

Chloromethyl methyl ether enhanced virus-induced transformation of Syrian hamster embryo cells and was mutagenic to bacteria[20].

References

[1]*IARC Monographs*, 4, 231-238, 239-245, 1974

[2]Albert, R.E., Pasternack, B.S., Shore, R.E., Lippmann, M., Nelson, N. & Ferris, B. (1975) Mortality patterns among workers exposed to chloromethyl ethers — a preliminary report. *Environ. Health Perspect.,* 11, 209-214

[3]DeFonso, L.R. & Kelton, S.C., Jr (1976) Lung cancer following exposure to chloromethyl methyl ether. An epidemiological study. *Arch. environ. Health*, 31, 125-130

[4]Pasternack, B.S., Shore, R.E. & Albert, R.E. (1977) Occupational exposure to chloromethyl ethers. A retrospective cohort mortality study (1948-1972). *J. occup. Med.*, 19, 741-746

[5]Pasternack, B.S. & Shore, R.E. (1981) *Lung cancer following exposure to chloromethyl ethers.* In: Chwat, M. & Dror, K., eds, *Proceedings of the International Conference on Critical Current Issues in Environmental Health Hazards, Tel-Aviv, Israel*, pp. 76-85

[6]Weiss, W. (1982) Epidemic curve of respiratory cancer due to chloromethyl ethers. *J. natl Cancer Inst.*, 69, 1265-1270

[7]McCallum, R.I., Woolley, V. & Petrie, A. (1983) Lung cancer associated with chloromethyl methyl ether manufacture: an investigation at two factories in the United Kingdom. *Br. J. ind. Med.*, 40, 384-389

[8]Weiss, W. & Boucot, K.R. (1975) The respiratory effects of chloromethyl methyl ether. *J. Am. med. Assoc.*, 234, 1139-1142

[9]Weiss, W., Moser, R.L. & Auerbach, O. (1979) Lung cancer in chloromethyl ether workers. *Am. Rev. respir. Dis.*, 120, 1031-1037

[10]Sakabe, H. (1973) Lung cancer due to exposure to bis(chloromethyl)ether. *Ind. Health*, 11, 145-148

[11]Weiss, W. & Figueroa, W.G. (1976) The characteristics of lung cancer due to chloromethyl ethers. *J. occup. Med.*, 18, 623-627

[12]Reznik, G., Wagner, H.H. & Atay, Z. (1977) Lung cancer following exposure to bis(chloromethyl)-ether: a case report. *J. environ. Pathol. Toxicol.*, 1, 105-111

[13]Bettendorf, U. (1977) Occupational lung carcinoma after inhalation of alkylating agents. Dichloro-dimethyl ether, monochlorodimethylether and dimethylsulphate (Ger.). *Dtsch. med. Wochenschr.*, 102, 396-398

[14]Leong, B.K.J., Kociba, R.J. & Jersey, G.C. (1981) A lifetime study of rats and mice exposed to vapors of bis(chloromethyl)ether. *Toxicol. appl. Pharmacol.*, 58, 269-281

[15]Zajdela, F., Croisy, A., Barbin, A., Malaveille, C., Tomatis, L. & Bartsch, H. (1980) Carcinogenicity of chloroethylene oxide, an ultimate reactive metabolite of vinyl chloride, and bis(chloromethyl)-ether after subcutaneous administration and in initiation-promotion experiments in mice. *Cancer Res., 40*, 352-356

[16]Dulak, N.C. & Snyder, C.A. (1980) The relationship between the chemical reactivity and the inhalation carcinogenic potency of direct-acting chemical agents (Abstract No. 426). *Proc. Am. Assoc. Cancer Res., 21*, 106

[17]Kuschner, M., Laskin, S., Drew, R.T., Cappiello, V. & Nelson, N. (1975) Inhalation carcinogenicity of alpha halo ethers. III. Lifetime and limited period inhalation studies with bis(chloromethyl)-ether at 0.1 ppm. *Arch. environ. Health, 30*, 73-77

[18]Leong, B.K.J., Kociba, R.J., Jersey, G.C. & Gehring, P.J. (1975) Effects of repeated inhalation of parts per billion of bis(chloromethyl)ether in rats (Abstract No. 131). *Toxicol. appl. Pharmacol., 33*, 175

[19]Laskin, S., Drew, R.T., Cappiello, V., Kuschner, M. & Nelson, N. (1975) Inhalation carcinogenicity of alpha halo ethers. II. Chronic inhalation studies with chloromethyl methyl ether. *Arch. environ. Health, 30*, 70-72

[20]*IARC Monographs, Suppl. 6*, 119-120, 159-160, 1987

BITUMENS (Group 3) and
EXTRACTS OF STEAM-REFINED AND AIR-REFINED BITUMENS (Group 2B)

A. Evidence for carcinogenicity to humans (*inadequate* for bitumens)

No epidemiological study of workers exposed only to bitumens is available. A cohort study of US roofers indicates an increased risk for cancer of the lung and suggests increased risks for cancers of the oral cavity, larynx, oesophagus, stomach, skin and bladder and for leukaemia. Some evidence of excess risks for lung, oral cavity and laryngeal cancers is provided by other epidemiological studies of roofers. As roofers may be exposed not only to bitumens but also to coal-tar pitches (see p. 174) and other materials, the excess cancer risk cannot be attributed specifically to bitumens[1]. Several case reports of skin cancer among workers exposed to bitumens are available; however, exposure to coal-tars (see p. 175) or products derived from them cannot be ruled out[1-3].

B. Evidence for carcinogenicity to animals (*limited* for undiluted steam-refined and cracking-residue bitumens; *inadequate* for undiluted air-refined bitumens; *sufficient* for extracts of steam-refined and air-refined bitumens)

In several studies, application to the skin of mice of various extracts of steam- and air-refined bitumens and mixtures of the two resulted in tumours at the sites of application[1,4]. Undiluted steam-refined bitumens and cracking-residue bitumens produced skin tumours when applied to the skin of mice. No skin tumour was found in mice after application of an undiluted air-refined bitumen. In limited studies, subcutaneous injection into mice and intramuscular injection into mice and rats of steam- and air-refined bitumens produced sarcomas at the injection sites[1].

C. Other relevant data

Antigenicity against benzo[a]pyrene diol epoxide-DNA adducts has been demonstrated in peripheral blood lymphocytes of roofers[5].

Both an extract of road-surfacing bitumen and its emissions were mutagenic to *Salmonella typhimurium*, whereas, in another study, 'asphalt tar' extracted from an asphalt concrete used for road surfacing was not. Bitumen-based paints for pipe coating were not mutagenic to *S. typhimurium*[5].

References

[1]*IARC Monographs*, *35*, 39-81, 1985

[2]Jørgensen, N.K. (1984) Exposure to asphalt as the cause of development of skin cancer (Dan.). *Ugeskr. Laeger*, *146*, 2832-2833

[3]Tsyrkunov, L.P. (1985) Multiple basalioma in a worker laying asphalt (Russ.). *Vestn. Dermatol. Venerol.*, *2*, 48-51

[4]Niemeier, R.W., Thayer, P.S., Menzies, K.T., von Thuna, P., Moss, C.E. & Burg, J. (1987) *A comparison of the skin carcinogenicity of condensed roofing asphalt and coal tar pitch fumes.* In: Cooke, M. & Dennis, A.J., eds, *Proceedings of the 10th International Symposium on Polynuclear Aromatic Hydrocarbons, Chemistry, Characterization and Carcinogenesis*, Columbus, OH, Battelle, pp. 609-647

[5]*IARC Monographs, Suppl. 6*, 121, 1987

BLEOMYCINS (Group 2B)

A. Evidence for carcinogenicity to humans (*inadequate*)

No epidemiological study of bleomycins alone was available to the Working Group. Occasional case reports of exposure to bleomycins, especially in the presence of concurrent therapy with other putative carcinogens such as ionizing radiation, alkylating agents and other potent oncotherapeutic drugs, do not constitute evidence of carcinogenesis[1].

In a large systematic follow-up of patients with Hodgkin's disease treated with an intensive chemotherapeutic combination including bleomycins (plus adriamycin [see p. 82], vinblastine [see p. 371] and dacarbazine [see p. 184]) but no alkylating agent, preliminary evidence suggested no excess of acute nonlymphocytic leukaemia in the first decade after therapy[2].

B. Evidence for carcinogenicity to animals (*limited*)

Bleomycin has been tested in mice by subcutaneous and intramuscular injection and in rats transplacentally. These studies could not be evaluated because of incomplete reporting[1]. A study in rats by repeated subcutaneous injections showed that bleomycin produced renal tumours (adenomas, adenocarcinomas, sarcomas) and fibrosarcomas at the site of application at significantly dose-related incidences[3].

C. Other relevant data

Bleomycins induced chromosomal aberrations in lymphocytes of treated patients in one study[4].

In mice treated *in vivo*, bleomycin induced chromosomal aberrations (including heritable translocations) and sister chromatid exchanges but gave conflicting results in tests for micronuclei. It induced chromosomal aberrations and DNA strand breaks in human cells *in vitro* but gave conflicting results in tests for unscheduled DNA synthesis and sister chromatid exchange. It induced transformation of mouse C3H 10T1/2 cells, and induced aneuploidy, chromosomal aberrations, mutation and DNA damage in rodent cells *in vitro*; a weakly positive response was observed for the induction of sister chromatid exchanges. In *Drosophila*, bleomycin induced aneuploidy, chromosomal aberrations, sex-linked recessive lethal mutations, somatic mutations, genetic crossing-over and recombination, but not heritable translocations. It induced chromosomal aberrations but not sister chromatid exchanges in plants. Bleomycin was mutagenic to fungi and induced gene conversion, recombination and genetic crossing-over. It was mutagenic and caused DNA damage in bacteria[4].

References

[1]*IARC Monographs*, 26, 97-113, 1981

[2]Santoro, A., Viviani, S., Villarreal, C.J.R., Bonfante, V., Delfino, A., Valagussa, P. & Bonadonna, G. (1986) Salvage chemotherapy in Hodgkin's disease irradiation failures: superiority of doxorubicin-containing regimens over MOPP. *Cancer Treat. Rep.*, 70, 343-348

[3]Habs, M. & Schmähl, D. (1984) Carcinogenicity of bleomycin sulfate and peplomycin sulfate after repeated subcutaneous application to rats. *Oncology*, 41, 114-119

[4]*IARC Monographs*, Suppl. 6, 121-125, 1987

BRACKEN FERN (Group 2B)

A. Evidence for carcinogenicity to humans (*inadequate*)

In a case-control study of 98 oesophageal cancer patients and 476 controls in Japan, a relative risk of 2.7 was found for daily consumption of bracken fern. Interpretation of this study is hampered by the absence of detail about the survey and the method of selecting controls, and by failure to take account of consumption of alcohol, a risk factor for cancer of the oesophagus[1].

B. Evidence for carcinogenicity to animals (*sufficient*)

Bracken fern was tested for carcinogenicity in mice, rats, guinea-pigs, cows and toads by oral administration, producing leukaemia, intestinal tumours, lung adenomas and gastric tumours in mice, small-intestinal tumours, urinary bladder carcinomas and mammary adenocarcinomas in rats, urinary bladder tumours in guinea-pigs, alimentary-tract and bladder cancers in cows, and intestinal carcinomas and hepatomas in toads. Processed bracken fern produced intestinal tumours in rats; boiling-water extracts of bracken fern produced intestinal and bladder tumours in rats; and hot-ethanol extracts produced intestinal tumours in quails[1].

Shikimic acid isolated from bracken fern induced neoplasms of the glandular stomach in mice after a single intraperitoneal injection. Ptaquiloside derived from bracken fern induced mammary and small-intestinal carcinomas in female rats after administration by gavage[1].

Most of these studies involved small numbers of animals and were incompletely reported; however, they indicate that bracken fern is associated with cancers of the intestine and urinary bladder in many different species.

C. Other relevant data

No data were available on the genetic and related effects of bracken fern in humans.

An acetone extract of bracken fern was mutagenic to *Salmonella typhimurium* in the presence of an exogenous metabolic system. Light-petroleum and methanol extracts of bracken fern activated by alkaline treatment were also mutagenic to *S. typhimurium*[2].

References

[1]*IARC Monographs*, *40*, 47-65, 1986
[2]*IARC Monographs*, *Suppl. 6*, 126, 1987

1,3-BUTADIENE (Group 2B)

A. Evidence for carcinogenicity to humans (*inadequate*)

A retrospective cohort study conducted in two styrene-butadiene rubber plants showed a slight excess of lymphatic and haematopoietic tissue cancers in one plant but not in the other, where exposure levels had been ten-fold higher. Concomitant exposure to styrene (see p. 345) and to traces of benzene (see p. 120) had occurred at least in the first plant[1].

Another cohort study comprised 13 920 men who had worked in eight styrene-butadine rubber polymer manufacturing plants in the USA and Canada for at least one year and who had been followed for deaths from 1943 to 1979. There was no excess of mortality from all cancers or from cancer at any specific site, either in the total cohort or in subcohorts defined on the basis of major work area or salaried and hourly pay grade[2].

Several studies have shown elevated standardized mortality ratios for cancers at various sites among workers in the rubber industry (see p. 332), where there is potential exposure to 1,3-butadiene, among other chemicals[3].

B. Evidence for carcinogenicity to animals (*sufficient*)

1,3-Butadiene was tested for carcinogenicity in mice by inhalation. It was carcinogenic to animals of each sex, producing haemangiosarcomas of the heart, malignant lymphomas, alveolar/bronchiolar adenomas and carcinomas, papillomas and carcinomas of the stomach, hepatocellular adenomas and carcinomas, mammary-gland carcinomas and granulosa-cell tumours of the ovary[1]. Exposure of rats to 1,3-butadiene by inhalation resulted in increased incidences of tumours of the mammary gland, thyroid and pancreas[4].

C. Other relevant data

No data were available on the genetic and related effects of 1,3-butadiene in humans. It induced micronuclei and sister chromatid exchanges in bone-marrow cells of mice but not of rats treated *in vivo*. It was mutagenic to bacteria[5].

References

[1]*IARC Monographs, 39*, 155-179, 1986

[2]Matanoski, G.M. & Schwartz, L. (1987) Mortality of workers in styrene-butadiene polymer production. *J. occup. Med., 29*, 675-680

[3]*IARC Monographs, 28*, 183-230, 1982

[4]Owen, P.E., Glaister, J.R., Gaunt, I.F. & Pullinger, D.H. (1987) Inhalation toxicity studies with 1,3-butadiene. 3. Two year toxicity/carcinogenicity study in rats. *Am. ind. Hyg. Assoc. J., 48*, 407-413

[5]*IARC Monographs, Suppl. 6*, 126-128, 1987

1,4-BUTANEDIOL DIMETHANESULPHONATE (MYLERAN) (Group 1)

A. Evidence for carcinogenicity to humans (*sufficient*)

Leukaemia patients who had been treated with Myleran developed many different cytological abnormalities, and some developed carcinomas[1-8]. A follow-up study of patients with bronchial carcinoma who were randomized to chemotherapy after pulmonary resection showed that of 69 who had been given Myleran and had survived five years, four developed acute nonlymphocytic leukaemia (three myelomonocytic leukaemias and one erythroleukaemia) and 15 others developed pancytopenia in the succeeding four years; among 148 other survivors at five years who had not been given Myleran, one case of pancytopenia appeared. Risk was not dose-related, although the cases were confined to those who had received no radiation and no other cytotoxic agent[9].

B. Evidence for carcinogenicity to animals (*limited*)

Myleran was tested for carcinogenicity by intraperitoneal injection and by intravenous injection in mice and rats and by oral administration to rats. Intraperitoneal administration of Myleran to mice did not increase the incidence of tumours in two studies[1,10], but leukaemia[11] and hypoplastic marrow[11,12] were induced in further studies and T-cell lymphoma in another, in which the effect was markedly enhanced by combined administration of chloramphenicol[13]. Leukaemia/lymphosarcoma was also reported in one study[12], but the experiment could not be evaluated due to incomplete reporting. No mammary tumour was seen in rats after intraperitoneal injection, but near-lethal doses were used and the animals were followed for only five months[14]. Intravenous administration of Myleran to mice significantly increased the incidences of thymic and ovarian tumours[1]. Intravenous administration of 7% of the LD_{50} dose to rats for one year was reported to induce a variety of tumours in male rats, but the experiments could not be evaluated due to incomplete reporting[15]. Oral administration to rats of Myleran did not increase the incidence of tumours over that seen in untreated animals[1].

C. Other relevant data

Myleran is a bifunctional alkylating agent. Patients treated with Myleran for chronic myeloid leukaemia were found to have increased frequencies of sister chromatid exchanges and chromosomal aberrations (in a single study) in their peripheral blood lymphocytes[16].

Treatment of rodents *in vivo* with Myleran induced dominant lethal mutations and increased the frequency of chromosomal aberrations and micronuclei in bone-marrow cells; in single studies, it induced DNA damage but not mutation. Evidence for covalent binding to DNA, RNA and protein was obtained in mice treated *in vivo*. Myleran induced chromosomal aberrations and sister chromatid exchanges in human and rodent cells *in vitro*, and mutation in rodent cells *in vitro*. It induced sex-linked recessive lethal mutations in *Drosophila* and was mutagenic to bacteria[16].

References

[1]*IARC Monographs*, *4*, 247-252, 1974

[2]Waller, U. (1960) Giant nuclei after Myleran therapy and spleen irradiation for chronic myeloid leukaemia (Ger.). *Pathol. Microbiol.*, *23*, 283-290

[3]Güreli, N., Denham, S.W. & Root, S.W. (1963) Cytologic dysplasia related to busulfan (Myleran) therapy. Report of a case. *Obstet. Gynecol.*, *21*, 466-470

[4]Japp, H. (1974) Toxic effect of busulfan (Myleran) with irradiation for chronic myeloid leukaemia (Ger.). *Schweiz. med. Wochenschr.*, *104*, 1115-1119

[5]Diamond, I., Anderson, M.M. & McCreadie, S.R. (1960) Transplacental transmission of busulfan (Myleran®) in a mother with leukaemia. Production of fetal malformation and cytomegaly. *Pediatrics*, *25*, 85-90

[6]Feingold, M.L. & Koss, L.G. (1969) Effects of long-term administration of busulfan. Report of a patient with generalized nuclear abnormalities, carcinoma of vulva, and pulmonary fibrosis. *Arch. intern. Med.*, *124*, 66-71

[7]Pezzimenti, J.F., Kim, H.C. & Lindenbaum, J. (1976) Erythroleukemia-like syndrome due to busulfan toxicity in polycythemia vera. *Cancer*, *38*, 2242-2246

[8]Dittmar, K. (1979) Acute myeloblastic leukemia with polycythemia vera treated with busulfan and phlebotomy. *N.Y. State J. Med.*, *79*, 758-760

[9]Stott, H., Fox, W., Girling, D.J., Stephens, R.J. & Galton, D.A.G. (1977) Acute leukaemia after busulfan. *Br. med. J.*, *ii*, 1513-1517

[10]Stoner, G.D., Shimkin, M.B., Kniazeff, A.J., Weisburger, J.H., Weisburger, E.K. & Gori, G.B. (1973) Test for carcinogenicity of food additives and chemotherapeutic agents by the pulmonary tumor response in strain A mice. *Cancer Res.*, *33*, 3069-3085

[11]Chu, J., Cao, S., Ying, H. & Li, D. (1981) Experimental study of busulfan-induced leukemia in strain 615 mice (Chin.). *Zhonghua Xueyexue Zazhi*, *2*, 10-13

[12]Morley, A. & Blake, J. (1974) An animal model of chronic aplastic marrow failure. I. Late marrow failure after busulfan. *Blood*, *44*, 49-56

[13]Robin, E., Berman, M., Bhoopalam, N., Cohen, H. & Fried, W. (1981) Induction of lymphomas in mice by busulfan and chloramphenicol. *Cancer Res.*, *41*, 3478-3482

[14]Philips, F.S. & Sternberg, S.S. (1975) Tests for tumor induction by antitumor agents. *Recent Results Cancer Res.*, *52*, 29-35

[15]Schmähl, D. (1975) Experimental investigations with anti-cancer drugs for carcinogenicity with special reference to immunodepression. *Recent Results Cancer Res.*, *52*, 18-28

[16]*IARC Monographs, Suppl. 6*, 129-131, 1987

CADMIUM AND CADMIUM COMPOUNDS (Group 2A)

A. Evidence for carcinogenicity to humans (*limited*)

Exposure to cadmium (primarily as the oxide) has been associated with increased risks of prostatic and respiratory cancers[1,2]. In one follow up of an investigation of 269 cadmium-nickel battery workers (see also summary for nickel, p. 264) and 94 cadmium-copper alloy factory workers in Sweden, additional cases of nasopharyngeal, colorectal, prostatic and lung cancer were reported[3]. In another study, the mortality of 347 cadmium-copper alloy workers in the UK who were exposed to cadmium fume was compared with that of workers exposed indirectly to cadmium but also to arsenic (see p. 100). A third group of iron or brass founders was included, and the mortality rates were compared separately with statistics for the general population. Significantly increased mortality from prostatic, genito-urinary and lung cancers was seen in people working in the vicinity, but not in the cadmium workers themselves. Insufficient information was given regarding the movement of men between or out of the three adjacent plants to assess the relative contributions of arsenic, cadmium and smoking to the results (which run counter to those of most other studies)[4].

Follow-up studies of four populations of cadmium-exposed workers have been reported more recently. In the UK, excess lung cancer (16 observed, 11.3 expected) was noted among 6995 male workers employed at one of 17 plants in a group that had had 'ever medium' exposure for ten years or more; and an excess risk of prostatic cancer was seen in a group that had had 'always low' exposures for ten years or more (15 observed, 11.0 expected)[5].

Using a case-control approach for these cases of prostatic cancer and for those in two other UK cohorts (of cadmium-nickel battery and cadmium-copper alloy workers), 39 cases were reported to have an odds ratio for cadmium exposure of 1.6 for 'ever medium' compared to 'always low' exposure levels and 1.4 for 'ever high' compared to 'always low' exposures; a similar approach for nine renal cancer patients revealed no elevation of odds ratio[6]. In a cohort of 522 male Swedish cadmium workers, eight cases of lung cancer were reported, resulting in a statistically nonsignificantly elevated standardized mortality ratio (SMR) for five years' exposure and ten or more years' latency. For prostatic cancer, four cases resulted in a statistically nonsignificant excess for the same exposure and latent periods[7].

In the USA, a follow-up study of 602 white male cadmium smelter workers with at least six months of production work between 1940 and 1969 was extended to 1978. The SMR (95% confidence interval) for respiratory cancer deaths was 165 (101-254), based on 20 deaths, and that for lung cancer, 157 (93-249), based on 18 deaths. Concomitant exposure to arsenic was especially high up to 1925. Reanalysis of lung cancer mortality for workers employed before or after 1 January 1926 revealed SMRs of 714 (195-1829) for the pre-1926 group (four cases) and 229 (131-371) for the post-1926 group with two or more years employment (16 deaths). For the post-1926 group (576 workers), a significant trend was noted for cumulative cadmium exposure and lung cancer mortality. Although the data on smoking are inadequate, and arsenic exposure continued after 1926, albeit at a lower level, the authors contend that these factors do not account for the excess lung cancer rates noted in the study. The number of prostatic cancers was unchanged from the earlier study (3 observed, 2.2 expected)[8]. Further reports of a UK population of 3025 (2559 male and 466 female) cadmium-nickel battery workers showed an excess of lung cancer in groups exposed for 18 years or more[9]. The excess mortality from prostatic cancer was accounted for by the original four cases described in 1967[1].

Potential confounding factors in these studies, such as smoking and exposure to nickel and arsenic, do not appear to account for the excess of lung cancer deaths. For prostatic cancer, the risk appears to be debatable, especially when the four hypothesis-generating UK cases from 1967 are removed from the analysis.

B. Evidence for carcinogenicity to animals (*sufficient*)

Cadmium chloride, oxide, sulphate and sulphide produced local sarcomas in rats after their subcutaneous injection, and cadmium powder and cadmium sulphide produced local sarcomas in rats following their intramuscular administration. Cadmium chloride and cadmium sulphate produced testicular tumours in mice and rats after their subcutaneous administration[1,10]. In one experiment, cadmium chloride administered subcutaneously to rats produced local sarcomas, testicular tumours and a significant increase in the incidence of pancreatic islet-cell tumours[11]. Cadmium chloride produced a dose-dependent increase in the incidence of lung carcinomas in rats after exposure by inhalation[12,13] and a low incidence (5/100) of prostatic carcinomas after injection into the ventral prostate[14]. Administration of up to 50 mg/kg (ppm) cadmium chloride in the diet to rats did not increase the incidence of tumours[15]. Cadmium acetate was not carcinogenic in a mouse-lung adenoma assay[16].

C. Other relevant data

People exposed occupationally to cadmium (in an alkaline-battery factory and in the manufacture of cadmium pigments) did not exhibit increased frequencies of chromosomal aberrations in their peripheral lymphocytes. These findings contrast markedly with the positive results obtained on workers exposed in zinc smelting plants and on people environmentally intoxicated by cadmium; these people were also exposed to other compounds. In one study, sister chromatid exchanges were not induced in people exposed to cadmium in the environment[17].

Cadmium compounds did not produce dominant lethal effects in mice or rats nor did they increase the frequencies of chromosomal aberrations or micronuclei in mice treated *in vivo*. Cadmium compounds induced aneuploidy in hamsters but not in mice treated *in vivo*. They did not induce sister chromatid exchanges in human cells *in vitro*, and studies of chromosomal aberrations gave inconclusive results. They induced transformation of cultured rodent cells in several test systems and induced chromosomal aberrations but not sister chromatid exchanges in rodent cells *in vitro*. Cadmium compounds induced DNA single-strand breaks in human and rodent cells, and there is conflicting evidence that they produced mutation in rodent cells *in vitro*. Cadmium compounds did not induce aneuploidy or somatic or sex-linked recessive lethal mutations in *Drosophila*. They induced mitotic recombination in yeast, but they did not induce mutation in yeast or bacteria, nor did they induce prophage in bacteria[17].

References

[1]*IARC Monographs, 11*, 39-74, 1976

[2]Piscator, M. (1981) Role of cadmium in carcinogenesis with special reference to cancer of the prostate. *Environ. Health Perspect., 40*, 107-120

[3]Kjellström, T., Friberg, L. & Rahnster, B. (1979) Mortality and cancer morbidity among cadmium-exposed workers. *Environ. Health Perspect., 28*, 199-204

[4]Holden, H. (1980) *Further mortality studies on workers exposed to cadmium fume*. In: *Seminar on Occupational Exposure to Cadmium, March 1980*, London, Cadmium Association

[5]Kazantzis, G. & Armstrong, B.G. (1983) *A mortality study of cadmium workers in seventeen plants in England*. In: Wilson, D. & Volpe, R.A., eds, *Proceedings of the Fourth International Cadmium Conference, Munich, 1982*, London, Cadmium Association, pp. 139-142

[6]Armstrong, B.G. & Kazantzis, G. (1985) Prostatic cancer and chronic respiratory and renal disease in British cadmium workers: a case control study. *Br. J. ind. Med., 42*, 540-545

[7]Elinder, C.G., Kjellström, T., Hogstedt, C., Andersson, K. & Spång, G. (1985) Cancer mortality of cadmium workers. *Br. J. ind. Med., 42*, 651-655

[8]Thun, M.J., Schnorr, T.M., Smith, A.B., Halperin, W.E. & Lemen, R.A. (1985) Mortality among a cohort of US cadmium production workers — an update. *J. natl Cancer Inst., 74*, 325-333

[9]Sorahan, T. (1983) *A further mortality study of nickel-cadmium battery workers*. In: Wilson, D. & Volpe, R.A., eds, *Proceedings of the Fourth International Cadmium Conference, Munich, 1982*, London, Cadmium Association, pp. 143-148

[10]Reddy, J., Svoboda, D., Azarnoff, D. & Dawar, R. (1973) Cadmium-induced Leydig cell tumors of rat testis: morphologic and cytochemical study. *J. natl Cancer Inst., 51*, 891-903

[11]Poirier, L.A., Kasprzak, K.S., Hoover, K.L. & Wenk, M.L. (1983) Effects of calcium and magnesium acetates on the carcinogenicity of cadmium chloride in Wistar rats. *Cancer Res.*, *43*, 4575-4581

[12]Takenaka, S., Oldiges, H., König, H., Hochrainer, D. & Oberdörster, G. (1983) Carcinogenicity of cadmium chloride aerosols in W rats. *J. natl Cancer Inst.*, *70*, 367-373

[13]Oldiges, H., Hochrainer, D., Takenaka, S., Oberdörster, G. & König, H. (1984) Lung carcinomas in rats after low level cadmium inhalation. *Toxicol. environ. Chem.*, *9*, 41-51

[14]Hoffmann, L., Putzke, H.-P., Kampehl, H.-J., Russbült, R., Gase, P., Simonn, C., Erdmann, T. & Huckstorf, C. (1985) Carcinogenic effects of cadmium on the prostate of the rat. *J. Cancer Res. clin. Oncol.*, *109*, 193-199

[15]Löser, E. (1980) A 2 year oral carcinogenicity study with cadmium on rats. *Cancer Lett.*, *9*, 191-198

[16]Shimkin, M.B., Stoner, G.D. & Theiss, J.C. (1978) Lung tumor response in mice to metals and metal salts. *Adv. exp. Med. Biol.*, *91*, 85-91

[17]*IARC Monographs, Suppl. 6*, 132-135, 1987

CARBON BLACKS (Group 3) and
CARBON-BLACK EXTRACTS (Group 2B)

A. Evidence for carcinogenicity to humans (*inadequate* for carbon blacks)

One study of the carbon-black producing industry showed a high proportion of cancers of the skin, particularly melanomas, in equal numbers of carbon-black workers and of a comparison group consisting of other workers in the same plant[1]. A study from the UK in which workers were followed up beyond retirement showed excesses of cancers of the lung and bladder. The excess of lung cancer occurred in each of the five plants studied and was concentrated among persons with ten or more years of follow-up. The bladder cancer excess was based on only three deaths but was also concentrated in the group followed up longer[2]. Excesses of stomach cancer were reported in workers in other industries whose employment entailed exposure to dusts that included carbon blacks[1,3].

B. Evidence for carcinogenicity to animals (*inadequate* for carbon blacks; *sufficient* for carbon-black extracts)

In limited studies by oral administration in mice, carbon blacks were reported not to produce the gastrointestinal tumours seen after administration of solvent (benzene) extracts of one carbon black[1]. No increase in the development of colonic tumours occurred in mice or rats fed carbon black in the diet[4]. Skin-painting studies with carbon blacks showed them to have no tumorigenic activity in mice, while solvent (benzene) extracts induced benign and malignant skin tumours. Inhalation studies in mice, hamsters, guinea-pigs and monkeys with carbon blacks did not demonstrate tumorigenic activity; the studies suffered from many inadequacies, including poor characterization of the carbon-black aerosol. Studies in mice showed that materials extracted from carbon blacks were carcinogenic, producing local tumours after their subcutaneous injection. A carbon black containing demonstrable quantities of carcinogenic polynuclear aromatic compounds also produced local sarcomas when injected subcutaneously in tricaprylin. Administration of the same carbon black as pellets in the absence of that solvent produced a low incidence of subcutaneous tumours[1]. Carbon black given in the diet did not enhance the incidence of colonic tumours induced in mice and rats by intraperitoneal injection of 1,2-dimethylhydrazine[4].

C. Other relevant data

No data were available on the genetic and related effects of carbon blacks in humans. Extracts of various commercial carbon blacks were mutagenic to *Salmonella typhimurium* in the presence and absence of an exogenous metabolic system[5].

References

[1]*IARC Monographs*, *33*, 35-85, 1984

[2]Hodgson, J.T. & Jones, R.D. (1985) A mortality study of carbon black workers employed at five United Kingdom factories between 1947 and 1980. *Arch. environ. Health*, *40*, 261-266

[3]*IARC Monographs*, *28*, 183-230, 1982

[4]Pence, B.C. & Buddingh, F. (1985) The effect of carbon black ingestion on 1,2-dimethylhydrazine-induced colon carcinogenesis in rats and mice. *Toxicol. Lett.*, *25*, 273-277

[5]*IARC Monographs*, *Suppl. 6*, 136, 1987

CARBON TETRACHLORIDE (Group 2B)

A. Evidence for carcinogenicity to humans (*inadequate*)

Three case reports describe the occurrence of liver tumours associated with cirrhosis in people who had been exposed to carbon tetrachloride[1]. A mortality study of laundry and dry-cleaning workers exposed to a variety of solvents suggested excesses of respiratory cancers (17 observed, 10.0 expected), cervical cancers (10 observed, 4.8 expected), liver tumours (4 observed, 1.7 expected) and leukaemia (5 observed, 2.2 expected)[2].

B. Evidence for carcinogenicity to animals (*sufficient*)

Carbon tetrachloride produced liver neoplasms in mice and rats after its administration by various routes[1,3] and mammary neoplasms in rats following its subcutaneous injection[1]. It also produced liver tumours in trout and hamsters following its oral administration[1], although these studies were not adequate.

C. Other relevant data

No data were available on the genetic and related effects of carbon tetrachloride in humans.

It did not induce chromosomal aberrations, unscheduled DNA synthesis or DNA strand breaks in cells of rodents treated *in vivo*. It did not induce chromosomal aberrations or sister chromatid exchanges in rat cells *in vitro*, but anaphase abnormalities were induced in cultured Chinese hamster ovary cells. It induced mutation, gene conversion and mitotic recombination in *Saccharomyces cerevisiae*, under conditions in which endogenous levels of cytochrome P450 were enhanced; there was a weak induction of mitotic crossing-over and mutation in *Aspergillus*. It was not mutagenic to bacteria[4].

References

[1]*IARC Monographs*, 20, 371-399, 1979

[2]Blair, A., Decouflé, P. & Grauman, D. (1979) Causes of death among laundry and dry cleaning workers. *Am. J. public Health*, 69, 508-511

[3]Kalashnikova, M.M., Rubetskoy, L.S. & Zhuravleva, M.V. (1980) Electron-microscopic and histochemical characteristics of hepatomas arising after prolonged administration of carbon tetrachloride (Russ.). *Bjull. eksp. Biol. Med.*, 89, 744-747

[4]*IARC Monographs*, Suppl. 6, 136-138, 1987

CHLORAMBUCIL (Group 1)

A. Evidence for carcinogenicity to humans (*sufficient*)

Many case reports and a few small epidemiological studies of malignancy after therapy with chlorambucil have been reported among patients treated for breast cancer, juvenile arthritis, glomerulonephritis and ovarian cancer. Although in each study an excess of subsequent malignancy, especially acute nonlymphocytic leukaemia (ANLL), is inferred, these reports are difficult to interpret because the cases are few or because they had also received radiation or other putative carcinogens[1,2]. A randomized trial of therapy in 431 polycythemia vera patients[3] showed a significant, 13-fold increase in the incidence of ANLL in those receiving chlorambucil — 2.3 times higher than in patients receiving radioactive phosphorus. The excess was strongly related to dose and persisted throughout the first decade after treatment.

B. Evidence for carcinogenicity to animals (*sufficient*)

Chlorambucil has been tested for carcinogenicity in mice and rats by intraperitoneal injection and in female rats by oral gavage. It produced tumours of the lung and probably tumours of the haematopoietic system and ovaries in mice[1], and produced haematopoietic tumours in male rats and haematopoietic and lymphatic tumours in female rats[1,4]. It had an initiating effect in a two-stage skin carcinogenesis experiment in mice[1].

C. Other relevant data

Chlorambucil is a bifunctional alkylating agent. It induced sister chromatid exchanges in the lymphocytes of treated patients; studies of induction of chromosomal aberrations were inconclusive[5].

Chlorambucil induced chromosomal aberrations in embryo cells of rats treated *in vivo*. Sister chromatid exchanges and chromosomal aberrations were induced in human lymphocytes and sister chromatid exchanges and mutation in Chinese hamster cells *in vitro*. Chlorambucil induced sex-linked recessive lethal mutations in *Drosophila* and mutation and gene conversion in yeast. It was mutagenic to bacteria[5].

References

[1]*IARC Monographs*, *26*, 115-136, 1981

[2]Greene, M.H., Boice, J.D., Jr, Greer, B.E., Blessing, J.A. & Dembo, A.J. (1982) Acute nonlymphocytic leukemia after therapy with alkylating agents for ovarian cancer. A study of five randomized clinical trials. *New Engl. J. Med.*, *307*, 1416-1421

[3]Berk, P.D., Goldberg, J.D., Silverstein, M.N., Weinfeld, A., Donovan, P.B., Ellis, J.T., Landaw, S.A., Laszlo, J., Najean, Y., Pisciotta, A.V. & Wasserman, L.R. (1981) Increased incidence of acute leukemia in polycythemia vera associated with chlorambucil therapy. *New Engl. J. Med.*, *304*, 441-447

[4]Berger, M.R., Habs, M. & Schmähl, D. (1985) Comparative carcinogenic activity of prednimustine, chlorambucil, prenisolone and chlorambucil plus prednisolone in Sprague-Dawley rats. *Arch. Geschwulstforsch.*, *55*, 429-442

[5]*IARC Monographs*, *Suppl. 6*, 139-141, 1987

CHLORAMPHENICOL (Group 2B)

A. Evidence for carcinogenicity to humans (*limited*)

Aplastic anaemia has been associated with exposure to chloramphenicol[1,2], and case reports have described leukaemia in patients following chloramphenicol-induced aplastic anaemia[1,3]. A follow-up study showed three cases of leukaemia in 126 patients who had had bone-marrow depression following treatment with chloramphenicol[1].

B. Evidence for carcinogenicity to animals (*inadequate*)

Tests for the carcinogenicity of chloramphenicol in experimental animals were inadequate[1,4]. In a study reported only as an abstract, chloramphenicol administered in drinking-water increased the incidence of lymphomas in two strains of mice and of hepatocellular carcinomas in one strain[5].

C. Other relevant data

No data were available on the genetic and related effects of chloramphenicol in humans.

Contradictory results were obtained with respect to the ability of chloramphenicol to induce dominant lethal mutations in mice. It induced chromosomal aberrations in bone-marrow cells of mice, but not of rats, treated *in vivo*. Chloramphenicol induced chromosomal aberrations but not sister chromatid exchanges in cultured human lymphocytes and chromosomal aberrations in one study using cultured pig lymphocytes. It induced neither dominant lethal nor sex-linked recessive lethal mutations in *Drosophila*. It induced chromosomal aberrations but not mutation in plants. Chloramphenicol was not mutagenic and did not cause DNA damage in bacteria[6].

References

[1]*IARC Monographs*, *10*, 85-98, 1976

[2]Aoki, K. (1978) Aplastic anaemia induced by chloramphenicol — clinical studies (Jpn.). *Jpn. J. clin. Med.*, *36*, 30-37

[3]Schmitt-Gräff, A. (1981) Chloramphenicol-induced aplastic anemia terminating with acute non-lymphocytic leukemia. *Acta haematol.*, *66*, 267-268

[4]Robin, E., Berman, M., Bhoopalam, N., Cohen, H. & Fried, W. (1981) Induction of lymphomas in mice by busulfan and chloramphenicol. *Cancer Res.*, *41*, 3478-3482

[5]Sanguineti, M., Rossi, L., Ognio, E. & Santi, L. (1983) *Tumours induced in BALB/c and C57BL/6N mice following chronic administration of chloramphenicol* (Abstract No. 50) (Ital.). In: *Proceedings of a National Meeting on Experimental and Clinical Oncology, Parma 23-25 November, 1983*, Milan, Italian Society of Cancerology, p. 45

[6]*IARC Monographs*, *Suppl. 6*, 142-144, 1987

CHLORDANE/HEPTACHLOR (Group 3)

A. Evidence for carcinogenicity to humans (*inadequate*)

These compounds were evaluated together because they are structurally similar and because technical-grade chlordane contains 3-10% heptachlor.

Domestic use of chlordane has been reported to be associated with cases of neuroblastoma and acute leukaemia. Aplastic anaemia and blood dyscrasias have also been associated with exposure to chlordane and heptachlor[1]. Follow-up of 4411 pesticide applicators from Florida, USA, some of whom applied chlordane/heptachlor for treatment of termites, showed an excess of lung cancer deaths (34) which increased to nearly three fold (standardized mortality ratio, 267) among those who had been licensed for 20 years or more. The excess occurred in all licensing categories (termite, household pests, fumigants), except lawn and garden. There was also a slight, but nonsignificant excess of acute myeloid leukaemia (3 deaths)[2]. Follow-up of a group of 16 126 male pesticide applicators in the USA showed a deficit of deaths from all cancers but small excesses of deaths from cancers of the lung, skin and bladder, which did not appear to be related to intensity of exposure or to time since first exposure to pesticides. No excess of deaths from lung cancer was seen in termite-control workers (with particular exposure to chlordane and heptachlor) in comparison with other pesticide applicators[3]. Follow-up of 1403 men in two US factories where chlordane, and heptachlor and endrin were manufactured, respectively, also showed a deficit of deaths from all cancers and a small excess of lung cancer. The latter was not related to time since first exposure, and smoking habits were not documented[4]. In another study of four plants, including the two factories mentioned above, no significant excess in the incidence of lung cancer was observed. Slight excesses of lung cancer were noted in three of the four plants, and an excess of stomach cancer was seen, based on three deaths, in one plant[5]. A further study[6] of one plant included in these studies[4,5] has been reported, but the analyses were inappropriate and do not provide useful information.

B. Evidence for carcinogenicity to animals (*limited*)

Chlordane and heptachlor (containing about 20% chlordane) produced liver neoplasms in mice following their oral administration; results for rats were inconclusive[1]. Oral administration of chlordane or heptachlor enhanced the incidence of liver tumours induced in mice by oral administration of *N*-nitrosodiethylamine[7].

C. Other relevant data

No data were available on the genetic and related effects of chlordane or heptachlor in humans.

Chlordane did not induce dominant lethal mutations in mice; it induced sister chromatid exchanges in intestinal cells of fish treated *in vivo*. It was not mutagenic to cultured human fibroblasts, and studies on DNA damage in transformed human cells yielded conflicting results. It did not induce unscheduled DNA synthesis in cultured rodent hepatocytes; it was mutagenic to Chinese hamster V79 cells but not to rat liver cells. Evidence of inhibition of intercellular communication was obtained in rodent cell systems. Chlordane was mutagenic to plants and induced gene conversion in yeast. It was not mutagenic to bacteria and did not induce breakage of plasmid DNA[8].

Heptachlor did not induce dominant lethal mutations in mice. It induced unscheduled DNA synthesis in human fibroblast cultures but did not induce repair synthesis in cultured rodent cells. Heptachlor inhibited intercellular communication in rodent cell systems; it was not mutagenic to cultured rat liver cells. It did not induce sex-linked recessive lethal mutations in *Drosophila* or gene conversion in yeast. It was mutagenic to plants. It was not mutagenic to bacteria, but in one study, positive results were reported for technical-grade but not commercial-grade heptachlor. It did not produce breakage of plasmid DNA[8].

References

[1]*IARC Monographs*, 20, 45-65, 129-154, 1979

[2]Blair, A., Grauman, D.J., Lubin, J.H. & Fraumeni, J.F., Jr (1983) Lung cancer and other causes of death among licensed pesticide applicators. *J. natl Cancer Inst.*, 71, 31-37

[3]Wang, H.H. & MacMahon, B. (1979) Mortality of pesticide applicators. *J. occup. Med.*, 21, 741-744

[4]Wang, H.H. & MacMahon, B. (1979) Mortality of workers employed in the manufacture of chlordane and heptachlor. *J. occup. Med., 21*, 745-748

[5]Ditraglia, D., Brown, D.P., Namekata, T. & Iverson, N. (1981) Mortality study of workers employed at organochlorine pesticide manufacturing plants. *Scand. J. Work Environ. Health, 7 (Suppl. 4)*, 140-146

[6]Shindell, S. & Ulrich, S. (1986) Mortality of workers employed in the manufacture of chlordane: an update. *J. occup. Med., 28*, 497-501

[7]Williams, G.M. & Numoto, S. (1984) Promotion of mouse liver neoplasms by the organochlorine pesticides chlordane and heptachlor in comparison to dichlorodiphenyltrichloroethane. *Carcinogenesis, 5*, 1689-1696

[8]*IARC Monographs, Suppl. 6*, 145-147, 328-330, 1987

α-CHLORINATED TOLUENES (Group 2B)

A. Evidence for carcinogenicity to humans (*inadequate*)

Six cases of respiratory cancer were reported in two small factories in Japan where benzoyl chloride (see p. 126) and chlorinated toluenes were produced[1]. A mortality study in the UK of 163 workers exposed to benzoyl chloride and chlorinated toluenes showed excesses for cancers of the respiratory tract (5 observed, 1.8 expected) and digestive system (5 observed, 1.2 expected). The limited data did not, however, allow any differential risk estimation for the individual chlorinated toluenes[2].

B. Evidence for carcinogenicity to animals (*limited* for benzyl chloride and benzal chloride; *sufficient* for benzotrichloride)

Benzyl chloride was tested in mice by skin application and in rats by subcutaneous injection. Sarcomas at the injection site were observed in rats; a few skin carcinomas were observed in some mice, but their incidence was not statistically significant[1]. When mice and rats were administered benzyl chloride in corn oil by gavage, increased incidences of papillomas and carcinomas of the forestomach were observed in mice of each sex, and the incidence of thyroid C-cell tumours was increased in female rats but decreased in male rats; a few neoplasms of the forestomach were observed in male rats[3].

In one experiment in which benzal chloride was tested by skin application to female mice, it produced squamous-cell carcinomas of the skin. In a concurrent experiment in which it was tested for a shorter duration, a low incidence of skin papillomas was observed[1].

Benzotrichloride was tested in three studies by skin application to female mice. It produced squamous-cell carcinomas of the skin and lung tumours in all three experiments; upper digestive-tract tumours were also observed in two of the three experiments. Increases in the incidence of tumours at other sites were reported[1]. In a mouse-lung tumour bioassay, benzotrichloride increased the incidence of lung adenomas[4].

C. Other relevant data

No data were available on the genetic and related effects of benzal chloride, benzotrichloride or benzyl chloride in humans.

Benzyl chloride did not induce micronuclei in mice treated *in vivo*. It induced DNA strand breaks but not unscheduled DNA synthesis or chromosomal aberrations in cultured human cells; conflicting results were obtained for the induction of sister chromatid exchanges. Benzyl chloride induced sister chromatid exchanges, chromosomal aberrations, mutation and DNA strand breaks in cultured rodent cells. It induced somatic and sex-linked recessive lethal mutations in *Drosophila* and mitotic recombination, gene conversion, mutation and DNA damage in fungi. Benzyl chloride induced mutation and DNA damage in bacteria[5].

Benzal chloride and benzotrichloride induced mutation and DNA damage in bacteria[5].

References

[1]*IARC Monographs*, *29*, 49-63, 65-72, 73-82, 1982

[2]Sorahan, T., Waterhouse, J.A.H., Cooke, M.A., Smith, E.M.B., Jackson, J.R. & Temkin, L. (1983) A mortality study of workers in a factory manufacturing chlorinated toluenes. *Ann. occup. Hyg.*, *27*, 173-182

[3]Lijinsky, W. (1986) Chronic bioassay of benzyl chloride in F344 rats and (C57BL/6J×BALB/c)F₁ mice. *J. natl Cancer Inst.*, *76*, 1231-1236

[4]Stoner, G.D., You, M., Morgan, M.A. & Superczynski, M.J. (1986) Lung tumor induction in strain A mice with benzotrichloride. *Cancer Lett.*, *33*, 167-173

[5]*IARC Monographs*, *Suppl. 6*, 89-90, 101-102, 105-109, 1987

CHLORODIFLUOROMETHANE (Group 3)

A. Evidence for carcinogenicity to humans (*inadequate*)

A small study of 539 refrigeration workers exposed to a mixture of chlorofluorocarbons, including chlorodifluoromethane, for at least six months with up to 30 years' follow up was uninformative with regard to the carcinogenic hazard of this chemical (6 deaths due to cancer, 5.7 expected; 2 deaths from lung cancer, 1.0 expected)[1].

B. Evidence for carcinogenicity to animals (*limited*)

Chlorodifluoromethane was tested for carcinogenicity in rats by oral administration and in mice and rats by inhalation. Oral administration to rats yielded no increase in tumour incidence in one study. A study by inhalation in mice gave inconclusive results for males and negative results for females. One study by inhalation in rats was inadequate, while, in another, males exposed to the highest concentration had a marginal increase in the incidence of subcutaneous fibrosarcomas and Zymbal-gland tumours and negative results were obtained for females[1].

C. Other relevant data

No data were available on the genetic and related effects of chlorodifluoromethane in humans. It did not induce dominant lethal mutations in rats or chromosomal aberrations in bone-marrow cells of mice treated *in vivo*. It did not induce unscheduled DNA synthesis in human cells *in vitro* or mutation in cultured Chinese hamster V79 cells. It did not induce mutation or mitotic gene conversion in yeast, either after direct exposure or in a host-mediated assay. It was mutagenic to plants and bacteria[2].

References

[1]*IARC Monographs, 41*, 237-252, 1986

[2]*IARC Monographs, Suppl. 6*, 150-151, 1987

CHLOROETHYL NITROSOUREAS:
BISCHLOROETHYL NITROSOUREA (BCNU) (Group 2A)
1-(2-CHLOROETHYL)-3-CYCLOHEXYL-1-NITROSOUREA (CCNU) (Group 2A)
1-(2-CHLOROETHYL)-3-(4-METHYLCYCLOHEXYL)-1-NITROSOUREA (METHYL-CCNU) (Group 1)

A. Evidence for carcinogenicity to humans (*limited* for BCNU; *inadequate* for CCNU; *sufficient* for methyl-CCNU)

In seven randomized trials of treatment for brain tumours, two cases of acute nonlymphocytic leukaemia (ANLL) occurred among 1628 patients treated with BCNU (0.08 expected) within the first two years of treatment, whereas no such case occurred among 1028 patients not treated with BCNU[1].

No epidemiological study of CCNU as a single agent was available to the Working Group[2].

Adjuvant treatment with methyl-CCNU has been evaluated in 3633 patients with gastrointestinal cancer treated in nine randomized trials. Among 2067 patients treated with methyl-CCNU, 14 cases of ANLL occurred (relative risk, 12.4; 95% confidence interval, 1.7-250), whereas one occurred among 1566 patients treated with other therapies. Cumulative (actuarial) risk was 4% at six years and was not affected by concomitant radiotherapy or immunotherapy[3]. A subsequent report described a strong dose-response relationship, adjusted for survival time, giving a relative risk of almost 40 fold among patients who had received the highest dose[4].

B. Evidence for carcinogenicity to animals (*sufficient* for BCNU and CCNU; *limited* for methyl-CCNU)

BCNU produced malignant tumours of the lung and an increased risk for neurogenic tumours in rats after its repeated intraperitoneal or intravenous administration, and tumours in the peritoneal cavity after its intraperitoneal administration[2,5,6]. Tests in mice by intraperitoneal administration and in rats by oral administration could not be evaluated[2]. When tested in mice by skin application together with ultraviolet B irradiation, BCNU caused an earlier appearance of skin tumours[2]. Two studies by skin painting in mice were inadequate[2,7].

CCNU produced lung tumours in rats following its intraperitoneal or intravenous injection[2,5]. When tested in mice by intraperitoneal injection, it induced a slight increase in the incidence of lymphomas. Tests in rats by oral administration could not be evaluated[2]. In one study by skin application to mice, no skin tumour was observed, but the duration of the experiment was inadequate[7].

Data on methyl-CCNU were included in a report in which a large number of cancer chemotherapeutic agents were tested for carcinogenicity by intraperitoneal injection in Sprague-Dawley rats and Swiss mice. In male rats injected with methyl-CCNU thrice weekly for six months, total tumour incidence was reported to be increased 1.5-2 fold over that in controls at 18 months. A slight increase in tumour incidence was reported in mice[8]. Intravenous administration of methyl CCNU to rats induced lung tumours[5].

C. Other relevant data

BCNU, CCNU and Me-CCNU are directly-acting, bifunctional alkylating agents[9].

No data were available on the genetic and related effects of BCNU in humans. An increased frequency of sister chromatid exchanges was observed in a single study of peripheral blood lymphocytes of patients treated with CCNU.

BCNU induced chromosomal aberrations, micronuclei and sister chromatid exchanges in cells of mice treated *in vivo*, DNA damage in human cells *in vitro*, and aneuploidy, chromosomal aberrations, sister chromatid exchanges, mutation and DNA damage in rodent cells *in vitro*. It induced sex-linked recessive lethal mutations in *Drosophila* and gene conversion in yeast. It was mutagenic and caused DNA damage in bacteria[9].

CCNU induced dominant lethal mutations in rats and DNA damage in cells of mice and rats treated *in vivo*. It induced DNA damage in human and rodent cells *in vitro* and sister chromatid exchanges and mutation in cultured Chinese hamster cells. It induced mutation and DNA damage in bacteria[9].

References

[1]Greene, M.H., Boice, J.D., Jr & Strike, T.A. (1985) Carmustine as a cause of acute nonlymphocytic leukemia. *New Engl. J. Med., 313*, 579

[2]*IARC Monographs, 26*, 79-95, 137-149, 1981

[3]Boice, J.D., Jr, Greene, M.H., Killen, J.Y., Jr, Ellenberg, S.S. & Fraumeni, J.F., Jr (1986) Leukemia after adjuvant chemotherapy with semustine (methyl-CCNU). Evidence of a dose-response effect. *New Engl. J. Med., 314*, 119-120

[4]Boice, J.D., Jr, Greene, M.H., Killen, J.Y., Jr, Ellenberg, S.S., Keehn, R.J., McFadden, E., Chen, T.T. & Fraumeni, J.F., Jr (1983) Leukemia and preleukemia after adjuvant treatment of gastrointestinal cancer with semustine (methyl-CCNU). *New Engl. J. Med., 309*, 1079-1084

[5] Habs, M. & Schmähl, D. (1984) Long-term toxic and carcinogenic effects of cytostatic drugs. *Dev. Oncol.*, *15*, 201-209

[6] Eisenbrand, G. (1984) *Anticancer nitrosoureas: investigations on antineoplastic, toxic and neoplastic activities*. In: O'Neill, I.K., von Borstel, R.C., Miller, C.T., Long J. & Bartsch, H., eds, *N-Nitroso Compounds: Occurrence, Biological Effects and Relevance to Human Cancer* (*IARC Scientific Publications No. 57*), Lyon, International Agency for Research on Cancer, pp. 695-708

[7] Zackheim, H.S. & Smuckler, E.A. (1980) Tumorigenic effect of topical mechlorethamine, BCNU and CCNU in mice. *Experientia*, *36*, 1211-1212

[8] Weisburger, E.K. (1977) Bioassay program for carcinogenic hazards of cancer chemotherapeutic agents. *Cancer*, *40*, 1935-1951

[9] *IARC Monographs*, *Suppl. 6*, 116-118, 152-154, 1987

CHLOROFORM (Group 2B)

A. Evidence for carcinogenicity to humans (*inadequate*)

Two studies of trihalomethane levels in drinking-water supplies and community-based rates of cancer mortality have been reported. Correlations were found between these levels and various site-specific cancer mortality rates, especially those for bladder cancer, but also those for cancers of the rectum/large intestine, brain and kidney and lymphoma[1,2]. In one study in which trihalomethane levels in drinking-water at place of residence were compared directly for 395 matched pairs of female teachers with regard to colorectal cancer, no association with trihalomethane exposure was observed[3]. A mortality study of anaesthesiologists who worked at the time chloroform was used provided no significant information[4].

Several investigations have attempted to assess the effects of trihalomethanes in drinking-water indirectly by comparing risks of cancers at various sites with extent of chlorination. Although excesses of some cancers have been found, it is not possible to evaluate any effect of chloroform from such studies[5-16].

B. Evidence for carcinogenicity to animals (*sufficient*)

Chloroform produced benign and malignant tumours of the liver and kidney in mice following oral gavage[17,18]. Administration in drinking-water to female mice did not increase the incidence of liver tumours[19]. Administration of chloroform to rats by gavage or in drinking-water increased the incidences of kidney[17,19] and thyroid tumours[17] and of neoplastic nodules of the liver[20]. Chloroform was tested inadequately by subcutaneous and intraperitoneal injection in mice[17]. A study by oral administration in dogs gave negative results[21]. Oral administration of chloroform did not enhance the incidences of liver and lung tumours induced in mice by intraperitoneal injection of *N*-ethyl-*N*-nitrosourea[22], but it enhanced the incidence of liver preneoplastic foci induced in rats treated by gavage with a single dose of *N*-nitrosodiethylamine[23].

C. Other relevant data

No adequate data were available on the genetic and related effects of chloroform in humans.

Chloroform did not induce micronuclei in bone-marrow cells of mice or DNA damage in liver or kidney cells of rats treated *in vivo*. It did not induce chromosomal aberrations, sister chromatid exchanges or unscheduled DNA synthesis in human lymphocytes *in vitro*. Chloroform enhanced virus-induced cell transformation of Syrian hamster embryo cells. It did not induce sister chromatid exchanges or mutation in Chinese hamster cells or DNA damage in rat hepatocytes *in vitro*. Chloroform did not induce sex-linked recessive lethal mutations in *Drosophila* or aneuploidy, mutation or somatic segregation in *Aspergillus*. Chloroform induced DNA damage but not mutation, aneuploidy, mitotic recombination or gene conversion in *Saccharomyces cerevisiae*, whereas mutation, mitotic recombination and gene conversion were induced in *S. cerevisiae* under conditions in which endogenous levels of cytochrome P450 were enhanced. Chloroform did not induce mutation or DNA damage in bacteria[24].

References

[1]Hogan, M.D., Chi, P.-Y., Hoel, D.G. & Mitchell, T.J. (1979) Association between chloroform levels in finished drinking water supplies and various site-specific cancer mortality rates. *J. environ. Pathol. Toxicol., 2,* 873-887

[2]Cantor, K.P., Hoover, R., Mason, T.J., McCabe, L.J. (1978) Associations of cancer mortality with halomethanes in drinking water. *J. natl Cancer Inst., 61,* 979-985

[3]Lawrence, C.E., Taylor, P.R., Trock, B.J. & Reilly, A.A. (1984) Trihalomethanes in drinking water and human colorectal cancer. *J. natl Cancer Inst., 72,* 563-568

[4]Linde, H.W. & Mesnick, P.S. (1980) *Causes of Death of Anesthesiologists from the Chloroform Era* (PB 80-125172 (EPA/600/1-79-043)), Springfield VA, National Technical Information Service

[5]Cantor, K.P. (1982) Epidemiological evidence of carcinogenicity of chlorinated organics in drinking water. *Environ. Health Perspect., 46,* 187-195

[6]Carlo, G.L. & Mettlin, C.J. (1980) Cancer incidence and trihalomethane concentrations in a public drinking water system. *Am. J. public Health, 70,* 523-525

[7]Craun, G.F. (1985) Epidemiologic studies of organic micropollutants in drinking water. *Sci. total Environ., 47,* 461-472

[8]DeRouen, T.A. & Diem, J.E. (1977) *Relationships between cancer mortality in Louisiana drinking-water source and other possible causative agents.* In: Hiatt, H.H., Watson, J.D. & Winsten, J.A., eds, *Origins of Human Cancer,* Book A, *Incidence of Cancer in Humans,* Cold Spring Harbor, NY, CSH Press, pp. 331-345

[9]Gottlieb, M.S., Carr, J.K. & Morris, D.T. (1981) Cancer and drinking water in Louisiana: colon and rectum. *Int. J. Epidemiol., 10,* 117-125

[10]Alavanja, M., Goldstein, I. & Susser, M. (1978) *A case control study of gastrointestinal and urinary tract cancer mortality and drinking water chlorination.* In: Jolley, R.L., Gorchev, H. & Hamilton, D.H., Jr, eds, *Water Chlorination, Environmental Impact and Health Effects,* Vol. 2, Ann Arbor, MI, Ann Arbor Science, pp. 395-409

[11]Brenniman, G.R., Vasilomanolakis-Lagos, J., Amsel, J., Namekata, T. & Wolff, A.H. (1980) *Case-control study of cancer deaths in Illinois communities served by chlorinated or nonchlorinated water.* In: Jolly, R.J., Brungs, W.A., Cumming, R.B. & Jacobs, V.A., eds, *Water Chlorination, Environmental Impact and Health Effects*, Vol. 3, Ann Arbor, MI, Ann Arbor Science, pp. 1043-1057

[12]Crump, K.S. & Guess, H.A. (1982) Drinking water and cancer: review of recent epidemiological findings and assessment of risks. *Ann. Rev. public Health*, *3*, 339-357

[13]Gottlieb, M.S., Carr, J.K. & Clarkson, J.R. (1982) Drinking water and cancer in Louisiana. A retrospective mortality study. *Am. J. Epidemiol.*, *116*, 652-667

[14]Young, T.B., Kanarek, M.S. & Tsiatis, A.A. (1981) Epidemiologic study of drinking water chlorination and Wisconsin female cancer mortality. *J. natl Cancer Inst.*, *67*, 1191-1198

[15]Kanarek, M.S. & Young, T.B. (1982) Drinking water treatment and risk of cancer death in Wisconsin. *Environ. Health Perspect.*, *46*, 179-186

[16]Wilkins, J.R., III & Comstock, G.W. (1981) Source of drinking water at home and site-specific cancer incidence in Washington county, Maryland. *Am. J. Epidemiol.*, *114*, 178-190

[17]*IARC Monographs*, *20*, 401-427, 1979

[18]Roe, F.J.C., Palmer, A.K., Worden, A.N. & Van Abbé, N.J. (1979) Safety evaluation of toothpaste containing chloroform. I. Long-term studies in mice. *J. environ. Pathol. Toxicol.*, *2*, 799-819

[19]Jorgenson, T.A., Meierhenry, E.F., Rushbrook, C.J., Bull, R.J. & Robinson, M. (1985) Carcinogenicity of chloroform in drinking water to male Osborne-Mendel rats and female B6C3F$_1$ mice. *Fundam. appl. Toxicol.*, *5*, 760-769

[20]Tumasonis, C.F., McMartin, D.N. & Bush, B. (1985) Lifetime toxicity of chloroform and bromodichloromethane when administered over a lifetime in rats. *Ecotoxicol. environ. Saf.*, *9*, 233-240

[21]Heywood, R., Sortwell, R.J., Noel, P.R.B., Street, A.E., Prentice, D.E., Roe, F.J.C., Wadsworth, P.F., Worden, A.N. & Van Abbé, N.J. (1979) Safety evaluation of toothpaste containing chloroform. III. Long-term study in beagle dogs. *J. environ. Pathol. Toxicol.*, *2*, 835-851

[22]Pereira, M.A., Knutsen, G.L. & Herren-Freund, S.L. (1985) Effect of subsequent treatment of chloroform or phenobarbital on the incidence of liver and lung tumors initiated by ethylnitrosourea in 15 day old mice. *Carcinogenesis*, *6*, 203-207

[23]Deml, E. & Oesterle, D. (1985) Dose-dependent promoting activity of chloroform in rat liver foci bioassay. *Cancer Lett.*, *29*, 59-63

[24]*IARC Monographs*, *Suppl. 6*, 155-158, 1987

CHLOROPHENOLS (Group 2B)

A. Evidence for carcinogenicity to humans (*limited*)

Several cohort studies have concerned workers in the chemical industry with potential exposure to 2,4,5-trichlorophenol, 2,3,7,8-tetrachlorodibenzo-*para*-dioxin (TCDD) and other chemicals. Mortality rates for all cancers combined were not elevated over those expected. A Danish cohort with potential exposure to 2,4-dichlorophenol, present as an intermediate during the production of chlorophenoxy herbicides, had no increase in the incidence of cancers at all sites combined, but there were statistically significantly increased risks of soft-tissue sarcoma and lung cancer in some subcohorts. Two case-control studies conducted in different regions of Sweden showed a statistically significant association between soft-tissue sarcoma and exposure to chlorophenols; studies from New Zealand have not clearly confirmed the results from Sweden, although slightly but nonsignificantly elevated risks were seen for non-Hodgkin's lymphoma with respect to chlorophenol exposure[1,2]. A case-control study from Washington State, USA, briefly reported an increased risk of soft-tissue sarcoma in connection with exposure to chlorophenols, but only in persons of Scandinavian descent[3].

A case-control study in Sweden detected a significant association between nasal and nasopharyngeal cancer and exposure to chlorophenols, independent of exposure to wood dust[1].

B. Evidence for carcinogenicity to animals (*inadequate* for pentachlorophenol and 2,4,5-trichlorophenol; *sufficient* for 2,4,6-trichlorophenol)

Pentachlorophenol was tested in one experiment in two strains of mice and in one experiment in rats by oral administration at dose levels sufficiently high to cause mild toxicity; no carcinogenic effect was seen in either species. Pentachlorophenol was also tested in two strains of mice by subcutaneous injection of single doses; it produced hepatomas in males of one strain[4].

2,4,6-Trichlorophenol was tested in one experiment in two strains of mice by oral administration, and 2,4,5- and 2,4,6-trichlorophenols were tested in one experiment by subcutaneous injection in two strains of mice. 2,4,5-Trichlorophenol was also tested in one experiment for its promoting activity in female mice. All three experiments were considered to be inadequate[5]. In a further experiment, oral administration of 2,4,6-trichlorophenol to rats and mice caused increased incidences of hepatocellular carcinomas or adenomas in mice of each sex and increased incidences of lymphomas and leukaemias in male rats[6].

C. Other relevant data

No data were available on the genetic and related effects of 2,4-dichlorophenol, 2,3,4,6-tetrachlorophenol or 2,4,6-trichlorophenol in humans. In one study, the frequency of chromosomal aberrations but not of sister chromatid exchanges was increased in the lymphocytes of men exposed occupationally to pentachlorophenol; in a smaller study, no increase in chromosomal aberrations was observed. Neither chromosomal aberrations nor sister chromatid exchanges were observed in a single study of workers exposed to 2,4,5-trichlorophenol[7].

2,4-Dichlorophenol did not induce unscheduled DNA synthesis in rat hepatocytes *in vitro* or mutation in bacteria[7].

Pentachlorophenol was mutagenic in the mouse spot test. It did not induce aneuploidy or sex-linked recessive lethal mutations in *Drosophila*. It induced mutation and gene conversion but not mitotic crossing-over in yeast. There were conflicting data for mutagenicity in bacteria. Pentachlorophenol did not induce strand breaks in DNA from bacteriophage. It gave negative results in a host-mediated assay with mice using bacteria as indicators[7].

2,4,6-Trichlorophenol induced somatic mutations in the spot test in mice *in vivo*. It induced mutation but not gene conversion or crossing-over in yeast and was not mutagenic to bacteria[7].

Neither 2,3,4,6-tetrachlorophenol nor 2,4,5-trichlorophenol was mutagenic to bacteria[7].

References

[1]*IARC Monographs*, *41*, 319-356, 1986

[2]Pearce, N.E., Sheppard, R.A., Smith, A.H. & Teague, C.A. (1987) Non-Hodgkin's lymphoma and farming: an expanded case-control study. *Int. J. Cancer*, *39*, 155-161

[3]Woods, J.S., Polissar, L., Severson, R.K., Heuser, L.S. & Kulander, B.G. (1987) Soft tissue sarcoma and non-Hodgkin's lymphoma in relation to phenoxy herbicide and chlorinated phenol exposure in western Washington. *J. natl Cancer Inst*, *78*, 899-910

[4]*IARC Monographs*, *20*, 303-325, 1979

[5]*IARC Monographs*, *20*, 349-367, 1979

[6]National Cancer Institute (1979) *Bioassay of 2,4,6-Trichlorophenol for Possible Carcinogenicity (Tech. Rep. Ser. No. 155; DHEW Publ. No. (NIH) 79-1711)*, Washington DC, US Department of Health, Education, and Welfare

[7]*IARC Monographs*, *Suppl. 6*, 231-232, 445-447, 517-518, 533-537, 1987

CHLOROPHENOXY HERBICIDES (Group 2B)

A. Evidence for carcinogenicity to humans (*limited*)

In a Danish cohort study of chemical workers exposed to chlorophenoxy herbicides [particularly (4-chloro-2-methylphenoxy)acetic acid (MCPA), 2-(4-chloro-2-methylphenoxy)-propanoic acid (mecoprop), 2,4-dichlorophenoxyacetic acid (2,4-D) and 2-(2,4-dichloro-phenoxy)propanoic acid (dichlorprop)], as well as other chemicals, no overall increase in cancer incidence rate was observed, but there were significantly increased risks for soft-tissue sarcoma and lung cancer in some subcohorts, which were not necessarily those with the highest exposures to chlorophenoxy herbicide preparations[1].

A recently reported cohort of 5784 male employees in a UK company that manufactured, formulated and sprayed MCPA and other pesticides, but only small amounts of 2,4,5-trichlorophenoxyacetic acid (2,4,5-T), had no general excess mortality from cancer. Three potentially exposed workers died from nasal carcinoma, however. One death due to soft-tissue sarcoma approximately equalled the expected rate. No excess of lymphoma was seen[2].

A Finnish cohort study of brush control workers with short follow-up time showed no increased cancer risk. A small Swedish cohort study of railroad workers who sprayed herbicides showed an increased risk of cancers at all sites combined for those exposed to chlorophenoxy herbicide preparations and other herbicides. An excess incidence of all cancers was also reported from a very small cohort of Swedish forestry foremen exposed to chlorophenoxy herbicide preparations and other herbicides. A study of long-term pesticide applicators in the German Democratic Republic, heavily exposed to a number of chemicals, including 2,4-D and MCPA, demonstrated an increased risk of bronchial carcinoma[1].

Two population-based case-control studies conducted in northern and southern Sweden, respectively, showed a statistically significant association between exposure to chlorophenoxy herbicides, especially in forestry and agriculture, and the occurrence of soft-tissue sarcomas. An increased risk of soft-tissue sarcoma was described among highly exposed Italian rice weeders in a population-based case-control study. However, a case-control study from New Zealand did not demonstrate any increased risk of soft-tissue sarcoma in people exposed to chlorophenoxy herbicides[1]. Nor did a recently reported population-based case-control study of soft-tissue sarcoma and lymphoma in Kansas, USA, find any association between soft-tissue sarcoma and exposure to 2,4-D[3].

A statistically significant association between malignant lymphoma (Hodgkin's and non-Hodgkin's) and exposure to chlorophenoxy herbicides was found in a Swedish case-control study[1]. The population-based case-control study of soft-tissue sarcoma and Hodgkin's and non-Hodgkin's lymphoma in Kansas showed that use of 2,4-D was associated with non-Hodgkin's lymphoma, especially among farmers who had been exposed for more than 20 days per year, among whom there was an approximately six-fold excess, and among those who had mixed or applied the herbicides themselves. Hodgkin's lymphoma was not, however, found to be associated with herbicide exposure[3]. No significant or consistent association was seen in a case-control study of these tumours from New Zealand, and in a Danish cohort of chemical workers exposed to chlorophenoxy herbicides there was also no significantly increased risk of malignant lymphoma[1,4]. Farmers and forestry workers in Washington State, USA, with exposure to phenoxy herbicides had a significantly increased risk of non-Hodgkin's lymphoma. People of Scandinavian descent in the area had an increased risk of soft-tissue sarcoma in connection with phenoxy herbicide exposure, but no increased risk of non-Hodgkin's lymphoma[5].

Three Swedish case-control studies of colon, liver, and nasal and nasopharyngeal cancer, which used the same study design and methods as in the studies on soft-tissue sarcoma and malignant lymphoma, did not demonstrate significantly increased risks, although a risk ratio of 2.1 was reached for nasal and nasopharyngeal cancer[1].

A record-linkage study using census data on occupation and cancer registry information in Sweden did not reveal any excess of soft-tissue sarcoma among agricultural and forestry workers[6,7]. However, on the basis of occupational titles, the elevated risks seen in Swedish case-control studies of soft-tissue sarcoma and lymphoma were reduced to 1.4 or less[8]. A UK study based on data from cancer registration showed a slightly but significantly increased risk of soft-tissue sarcoma among farmers, farm managers and market gardeners, but not in other subgroups in forestry and farming[9]. No association with soft-tissue sarcoma has been found with military service in Viet Nam, despite potential exposure to phenoxy herbicides[1,10], although there is a case report in this respect[1].

B. Evidence for carcinogenicity to animals (*inadequate* for 2,4-D and 2,4,5-T)

2,4-D and several of its esters were tested in rats and mice by oral administration and in mice by subcutaneous administration. All of these studies had limitations, due either to inadequate reporting or to the small number of animals used. Therefore, although increased incidences of tumours were observed in one study in which rats received 2,4-D orally and in another in which mice received its isooctyl ester by subcutaneous injection, no evaluation of the carcinogenicity of this compound could be made[11].

2,4,5-T was tested in mice by oral and subcutaneous administration. All of the studies had limitations due to the small numbers of animals used. Therefore, although an increased incidence of tumours at various sites was observed in one study in which 2,4,5-T (containing less than 0.05 mg/kg chlorinated dibenzodioxins) was given orally, no evaluation of the carcinogenicity of this compound could be made on the basis of the available data[12]. In rats fed diets containing three different concentrations of 2,4,5-T, the incidences of all tumour types were comparable to those in the control groups, with the exception that the incidence of interfollicular C-cell adenomas of the thyroid was increased significantly in female rats receiving the lowest dose. This increase was not considered to be related to treatment since it was not dose-related and the female control group had an unusually low incidence of thyroid adenomas[13].

A study of the incidence of small-intestinal adenocarcinoma in groups of sheep from different farms showed an association with use of phenoxy herbicides, as elicited by farmers' responses to a questionnaire. However, other herbicides were in use, and there was no documentation of exposures[14].

No adequate data were available on the carcinogenicity of MCPA[15].

C. Other relevant data

In single studies, lymphocytes of persons occupationally exposed to chlorophenoxy herbicides, including 2,4-D, did not show increased frequencies of sister chromatid exchanges or chromosomal aberrations. Other studies could not be assessed since workers were also exposed to other formulations. A single study of herbicide and pesticide sprayers exposed to 2,4,5-T, in which a small increase in the incidence of sister chromatid exchanges was reported, could not be assessed since workers were also exposed to other formulations. Persons occupationally exposed to MCPA did not have increased frequencies of sister chromatid exchanges (one study) or chromosomal aberrations in their lymphocytes[16].

2,4-D did not induce dominant lethal mutations, micronuclei or sister chromatid exchanges in rodents treated *in vivo*. Pure 2,4-D did not induce chromosomal aberrations in human lymphocytes *in vitro*, whereas a commercial formulation did. 2,4-D induced sister chromatid exchanges and unscheduled DNA synthesis in human cells *in vitro*. It did not induce sister chromatid exchanges but did induce mutation and inhibited intercellular communication in Chinese hamster cells *in vitro*. 2,4-D induced somatic mutation in *Drosophila*, but conflicting results were obtained for induction of sex-linked recessive lethal mutations; it did not induce aneuploidy. 2,4-D caused chromosomal aberrations and was mutagenic in plants. It induced mutation, gene conversion and mitotic recombination in yeast. It was not mutagenic to bacteria or bacteriophage. The *n*-butyl and *iso*-octyl esters of 2,4-D were also not mutagenic to bacteria[16].

2,4,5-T induced chromosomal aberrations in bone-marrow cells of Mongolian gerbils, but not in spermatogonia of Chinese hamsters, and aneuploidy in oocytes of rats treated *in vivo*. It did not induce micronuclei in mice or dominant lethal mutations in mice or rats *in vivo*. 2,4,5-T inhibited intercellular communication in Chinese hamster V79 cells *in vitro*. There was weak evidence for the induction of sex-linked recessive lethal mutations in *Drosophila*; it did not induce aneuploidy or somatic mutation. It induced chromosomal aberrations in plants. It was mutagenic to yeast, but neither 2,4,5-T nor the *n*-butyl-, *iso*-butyl or *iso*-octyl ester of 2,4,5-T was mutagenic to bacteria[16].

MCPA did not induce structural chromosomal aberrations or micronuclei in mice treated *in vivo*; weakly positive results were obtained for sister chromatid exchanges in cells of Chinese hamsters treated *in vivo* and *in vitro*. It was weakly active in inducing sex-linked recessive lethal mutations but did not induce aneuploidy in *Drosophila*. MCPA and its methyl ester were mutagenic to yeast but not to bacteria[16].

References

[1]*IARC Monographs, 41*, 357-406, 1986

[2]Coggon, D., Pannett, B., Winter, P.D., Acheson, E.D. & Bonsall, J. (1986) Mortality of workers exposed to 2-methyl-4-chlorophenoxyacetic acid. *Scand. J. Work Environ. Health, 12,* 448-454

[3]Hoar, S.K., Blair, A., Holmes, F.F., Boysen, C.D., Robel, R.J., Hoover, R. & Fraumeni, J.F., Jr (1986) Agricultural herbicide use and risk of lymphoma and soft-tissue sarcoma. *J. Am. med. Assoc., 256,* 1141-1147

[4]Pearce, N.E., Sheppard, R.A., Smith, A.H. & Teague, C.A. (1987) Non-Hodgkin's lymphoma and farming: an expanded case-control study. *Int. J. Cancer, 39,* 155-161

[5]Woods, J.S., Polissar, L., Severson, R.K., Heuser, L.S. & Kulander, B.G. (1987) Soft tissue sarcoma and non-Hodgkin's lymphoma in relation to phenoxy herbicide and chlorinated phenol exposure in western Washington. *J. natl Cancer Inst., 78,* 899-910

[6]Wirklund, K. & Holm, L.-E. (1986) Soft tissue sarcoma risk in Swedish agricultural and forestry workers. *J. natl Cancer Inst., 76,* 229-234

[7]Wirklung, K., Holm, L.-E. & Dich, J. (1987) Soft tissue sarcoma risk among agricultural and forestry workers in Sweden. *Chemosphere* (in press)

[8]Hardell, L. & Axelson, O. (1986) *Phenoxyherbicides and other pesticides in the etiology of cancer: some comments on Swedish experiences.* In: Becker, C.E. & Coye, M.J., eds, *Cancer Prevention. Strategies in the Workplace*, Washington DC, Hemisphere, pp. 107-119

[9]Balarajan, R. & Acheson, E.D. (1984) Soft tissue sarcomas in agriculture and forestry workers. *J. Epidemiol. Commun. Health, 38,* 113-116

[10]Kang, H.K., Weatherbee, L., Breslin, P.P., Lee, Y. & Shepard, B.M. (1986) Soft tissue sarcomas and military service in Vietnam: a case comparison group analysis of hospital patients. *J. occup. Med., 28,* 1215-1218

[11]*IARC Monographs, 15*, 111-138, 1977

[12]*IARC Monographs, 15*, 273-299, 1977

[13]Kociba, R.J., Keyes, D.G., Lisowe, R.W., Kalnins, R.P., Dittenber, D.D., Wade, C.E., Gorzinski, S.J., Mahle, N.H. & Schwetz, B.A. (1979) Results of a two-year chronic toxicity and oncogenic study of rats ingesting diets containing 2,4,5-trichlorophenoxyacetic acid (2,4,5-T). *Food Cosmet. Toxicol.*, *17*, 205-221

[14]Newell, K.W., Ross, A.D. & Renner, R.M. (1984) Phenoxy and picolinic acid herbicides and small intestinal adenocarcinoma in sheep. *Lancet*, *ii*, 1301-1305

[15]*IARC Monographs*, *30*, 255-269, 1983

[16]*IARC Monographs*, *Suppl. 6*, 161-163, 233-236, 538-540, 1987

CHLOROPRENE (Group 3)

A. Evidence for carcinogenicity to humans (*inadequate*)

In one study, an excess of lung and skin cancers was related to occupational exposure to chloroprene. In another investigation, no excess of lung or other type of cancer was reported among chloroprene workers. There is one case report of an angiosarcoma of the liver in a worker exposed to chloroprene[1].

B. Evidence for carcinogenicity to animals (*inadequate*)

A number of experimental studies were considered to be inadequate for an evaluation of the carcinogenicity of chloroprene[1]. In a further study[2] in which chloroprene was given orally to pregnant rats and their offspring were treated for life by stomach tube, the total incidence of tumours was similar in treated and untreated animals.

C. Other relevant data

An increased incidence of chromosomal aberrations was found in the lymphocytes of workers exposed to chloroprene[3].

Chloroprene induced dominant lethal mutations in rats and chromosomal aberrations in bone-marrow cells of mice treated *in vivo*. It induced transformation in one hamster cell line but did not induce mutation in Chinese hamster cells. It induced sex-linked recessive lethal mutations in *Drosophila* and was mutagenic to bacteria[3].

References

[1]*IARC Monographs*, *19*, 131-156, 1979

[2]Ponomarkov, V. & Tomatis, L. (1980) Long-term testing of vinylidene chloride and chloroprene for carcinogenicity in rats. *Oncology*, *37*, 136-141

[3]*IARC Monographs*, *Suppl. 6*, 164-165, 1987

CHOLESTEROL (Group 3)

A. Evidence for carcinogenicity to humans (*inadequate*)

Intake of dietary cholesterol was greater in premenopausal cases than controls in a case-control study of diet and breast cancer; however, this finding was not statistically significant, and the association was less strong than that with dietary fat[1]. In a reanalysis of the same data, dietary cholesterol did not have an effect independent of saturated fat intake[2]. Further, in a cohort study of 89 538 US nurses, there was no increased risk of breast cancer associated with dietary fat or dietary cholesterol[3]. Dietary cholesterol intake was greater in cases than in controls in a case-control study of colorectal cancer, but the risk ratios were lower than for saturated fat intake[4]. Risk ratios were also elevated for dietary cholesterol and colon cancer in a second case-control study, although they were lower for rectal cancer and risk ratios were elevated to a greater extent for dietary protein[5]. In a study in which cholesterol intake of Seventh-Day Adventists was compared with that of lacto-ovo-vegetarians and nonvegetarians, differences for colon cancer risk were not 'striking'[6]. However, a study using food disappearance data from 20 countries showed that, when dietary cholesterol was controlled for, the partial correlations of dietary fat and fibre with colon cancer mortality were no longer significant. Cross-classification showed a significant, main effect for cholesterol but not for fat or fibre[7].

Dietary cholesterol was associated with increased risk of lung cancer in a case-control study. The association was found in all subjects, in smoking subjects and in males, but not in females[8]. Dietary cholesterol was also found to be weakly associated with increased risk of bladder cancer in a further case-control study[9]. These studies involved the use of relatively restricted dietary questionnaires, and it was not possible to determine whether the association with dietary cholesterol was part of a stronger association with other dietary factors with which the intake of cholesterol is associated.

Dietary cholesterol was analysed in relation to cancer mortality in a ten-year follow-up of the Honolulu Heart Program in the USA. There was no significant association, but data for individual cancer sites were not reported[10].

The available data on serum cholesterol levels and cancer have been considered[11], and subsequently reported independently[12]. It was concluded that observational studies afford substantial evidence that preclinical cancer causes a lowering of blood cholesterol, and limited, but biologically plausible evidence that males with naturally low blood cholesterol levels are at increased risk of colon cancer. Since then, there have been reports of seven studies primarily related to follow-up of cohorts established for the study of cardiovascular disease[13-20]. A study of 4035 residents of California, USA, aged 40-89, showed no association between plasma cholesterol and cancer morbidity or mortality over a seven-year period for either men or women for any cancer site[13]. In a five-year follow-up of 10 940 participants in the Hypertension Detection and Follow-up Program in the USA, a small but statistically significant inverse relationship was found between baseline serum cholesterol level and cancer incidence. When cases diagnosed in the first two years were excluded, the association was similar in magnitude but no longer statistically significant. The numbers of cases did not permit analysis by cancer site[14]. Up to six years of follow-up (mean, three years) were reported for 10 000 middle-aged men in the Malmö Preventive Program in Sweden[15]. Serum cholesterol was inversely related to cancer mortality (44 deaths) — a relationship seen also for the 25 cancer deaths that occurred more than 2.5 years after screening[15]. Serum urate levels at screening were correlated with early but not late (more than 2.5 years after screening) cancer mortality. As urate levels might indicate proliferation of cancer cells, the association of raised serum cholesterol with late deaths may be due to another mechanism than cancer present at the time of screening[16].

In the Busselton community study in Western Australia, 1564 subjects have been followed for 13 years. In men aged 60-74, but not in men aged 40-59 or in women, a negative association between serum cholesterol level and cancer mortality was found[17]. It was not indicated if the association persisted when early cancer deaths were excluded. In New Zealand, 630 Maoris aged 25-74 were followed for over 17 years. A significant inverse relationship between cancer mortality and serum cholesterol was found for men and women considered together. The relative risk in the pooled data, derived by comparing the approximate 10th and 90th percentiles of serum cholesterol concentration, decreased from 3.0 to 2.4 after excluding deaths in the first five years[18]. Fifteen years of follow-up of 11 325 healthy men aged 40-59 in the Seven Countries Study has also been reported. Among 477 cancer deaths five or more years after cholesterol measurement, there was a significant excess of deaths from lung cancer in the lower 20% of the cholesterol distribution in the populations. Nevertheless, regional comparisons of cancer mortality showed highest cancer rates in northern Europe, where the cholesterol levels were highest[19]. In contrast, in a cohort study in Sweden of 92 000 subjects less than 75 years old examined in 1963-1965 and followed by linkage to the Swedish Cancer Registry until 1979, there was a positive association between serum cholesterol level and risk of rectal cancer in men. When serum cholesterol and β-lipoprotein levels were considered together, the risk for men with elevated serum cholesterol ($\geqslant$ 2.5 g/l) and β-lipoprotein ($\geqslant$ 2.2 g/l), relative to those with lower levels, was 1.6 for colon cancer (95% confidence interval, 1.2-2.2) and 1.7 for rectal cancer (1.2-2.4)[20]. In the largest study so far reported, the incidence of cancer was determined in 160 135 male and female members of a prepaid health plan in California, USA, for whom serum cholesterol levels were determined as part of a multiphasic health examination. Follow-up was for eight to 16 years. No consistent association of low cholesterol with cancer incidence was found, although cancer incidence was highest in those in the lowest quintile of serum cholesterol levels in the first two years after the measurement[21].

Five case-control studies have been reported in which serum cholesterol was assessed[22-26]. A case-control study of 37 cases of primary brain tumours and two controls per case found elevated levels of serum cholesterol in the cases compared to the controls. The difference was not reduced by controlling for potential confounders (including weight)[22]. In the second study, serum cholesterol was measured in 244 patients with adenomatous polyps of the colon, 182 patients with Dukes' A or B colon cancer and 688 hospital controls. The mean serum cholesterol levels were lower for the Dukes' B cases, accounting for most of the difference. There was no difference in mean levels between those with adenomatous polyps and their controls. After adjustment for nutritional status using serum albumin level, however, there was no difference between any of the groups[23]. In a nested case-control study within a cohort, 245 newly-diagnosed cases of large-bowel cancer in members of a prepaid health care plan and five matched controls for each case were compared, on the basis of serum cholesterol measurements performed as part of a multiphasic health examination prior to the diagnosis of the cases. No direct or inverse relationship between serum cholesterol and large-bowel cancer was found[24]. A fourth case-control study was based on a cohort of 18 995 people examined at a health centre between 1970-1973, where medical records were found for 100 of 176 cancer cases who had died by 1979, for 393 of 900 control subjects still alive in 1979, and for 69 of 153 people who had died of cardiovascular disease in the same period. Serum cholesterol levels in the cancer cases were significantly lower than those in controls only in the two-year period prior to death and were inconsistently depressed three to six or seven to 16 years prior to death[25]. In a fifth study, a positive association was found between serum cholesterol levels and the prevalence of adenomatous polyps at colonoscopy performed in 842 patients. The odds ratio for large-bowel adenoma between the highest and lowest quintiles of serum cholesterol was 1.9 (95% confidence interval, 1.1-3.5) after adjustment for age and 2.0 (1.1-3.6) after adjustment for body-mass index[26]. Serum cholesterol was assessed in relation to disease-free survival of 279 colon cancer patients. There was an 11% (nonsignificant) lower cumulative disease-free survival at five years in those with serum cholesterol levels below the median than in those with levels above the median[27]. In a further study, family history of cancer was found to be positively associated with serum cholesterol levels in young adults[28].

Thus, although studies of cohorts assembled to study cardiovascular disease risk continue to show associations of low serum cholesterol with cancer incidence and mortality, the studies designed specifically to assess the relationship do not in general confirm the association. When site-specific data are available, they are not consistent. Nevertheless, a plausible mechanism exists — namely, that those who maintain a low serum cholesterol in face of a possibly elevated fat intake increase the concentration of cholesterol metabolites (especially bile acids) in the intestine and thus increase their risk for colon cancer[29].

B. Evidence for carcinogenicity to animals (*inadequate*)

Cholesterol was tested for carcinogenicity in mice by administration in the diet, by subcutaneous administration and by bladder implantation. These studies were all inadequate for evaluation. Cholesterol has also been tested in combination with various carcinogens, but the results were inadequate to assess the carcinogenesis-enhancing potential of the compound[11]. Feeding of cholesterol to rats exposed to a mammary carcinogen did not affect the incidence of mammary tumours[30], while feeding after administration of a colon carcinogen resulted in a lower incidence of colon tumours[31].

C. Other relevant data

No data were available on the genetic and related effects of cholesterol in humans. It did not transform Syrian hamster embryo cells and was not mutagenic to bacteria[32].

References

[1] Miller, A.B., Kelley, A., Choi, N.W., Matthews, V., Morgan, R.W., Munan, L., Burch, J.D., Feather, J., Howe, G.R. & Jain, M. (1978) A study of diet and breast cancer. *Am. J. Epidemiol.*, *107*, 499-509

[2] Howe, G.R. (1985) The use of polytomous dual response data to increase power in case-control studies: an application to the association between dietary fat and breast cancer. *J. chron. Dis.*, *38*, 663-670

[3] Willett, W.C., Stampfer, M.J., Colditz, G.A., Rosner, B.A., Hennekens, C.H. & Speizer, F.E. (1987) Dietary fat and the risk of breast cancer. *New Engl. J. Med.*, *316*, 22-28

[4] Jain, M., Cook, G.M., Davis, F.G., Grace, M.G., Howe, G.R. & Miller, A.B. (1980) A case-control study of diet and colo-rectal cancer. *Int. J. Cancer*, *26*, 757-768

[5] Potter, J.D. & McMichael, A.J. (1986) Diet and cancer of the colon and rectum: a case-control study. *J. natl Cancer Inst.*, *76*, 557-569

[6] Turjman, N., Calkins, B., Phillips, R., Goodman, G.T. & Nair, P.P. (1984) Dietary intake of plant sterols and cholesterol among population groups at different risks for colon cancer (Abstract No. 3330). *Fed. Proc.*, *43*, 855

[7] Liu, K., Stamler, J., Moss, D., Garside, D., Persky, V. & Soltero, I. (1979) Dietary cholesterol, fat and fibre, and colon-cancer mortality. An analysis of international data. *Lancet*, *ii*, 782-785

[8] Hinds, M.W., Kolonel, L.N., Hankin, J.H. & Lee, J. (1983) Dietary cholesterol and lung cancer risk in a multiethnic population in Hawaii. *Int. J. Cancer*, *32*, 727-732

[9] Risch, H.A., Burch, J.D., Miller, A.B., Hill, G.B., Steele, R. & Howe, G.R. (1987) Dietary factors and the incidence of cancer of the urinary bladder. *Am. J. Epidemiol.* (in press)

[10] McGee, D., Reed, D., Stemmerman, G., Rhoads, G., Yano, K. & Feinleib, M. (1985) The relationship of dietary fat and cholesterol to mortality in 10 years: the Honolulu Heart Program. *Int. J. Epidemiol.*, *14*, 97-105

[11] *IARC Monographs*, *31*, 95-132, 1983

[12] McMichael, A.J., Jensen, O.M., Parkin, D.M. & Zaridze, D.G. (1984) Dietary and endogenous cholesterol and human cancer. *Epidemiol. Rev.*, *6*, 192-216

[13] Wingard, D.L., Criqui, M.H., Holdbook, M.J. & Barrett-Connor, E. (1984) Plasma cholesterol and cancer morbidity and mortality in an adult community. *J. chron. Dis.*, *37*, 401-406

[14] Morris, D.L., Borhani, N.O., Fitzsimons, E., Hardy, R.J., Hawkins, C.M., Kraus, J.F., Labarthe, D.R., Mastbaum, L. & Payne, G.H. (1983) Serum cholesterol and cancer in the hypertension detection and follow-up program. *Cancer*, *52*, 1754-1759

[15] Petersson, B. & Trell, E. (1983) Premature mortality in middle-aged men: serum cholesterol as risk factor. *Klin. Wochenschr.*, *63*, 795-801

[16] Petersson, B. & Trell, E. (1983) Raised serum urate concentration as risk factor for premature mortality in middle aged men: relation to death from cancer. *Br. med. J.*, *287*, 7-9

[17] Cullen, K., Stenhouse, N.S., Wearne, K.L. & Welborn, T.A. (1983) Multiple regression analysis of risk factors for cardiovascular disease and cancer mortality in Busselton, Western Australia — 13-year study. *J. chron. Dis.*, *36*, 371-377

[18] Salmond, C.E., Beaglehole, R. & Prior, I.A.M. (1985) Are low cholesterol values associated with excess mortality? *Br. med. J.*, *290*, 422-424

[19]Keys, A., Aravanis, C., Blackburn, H., Buzina, R., Dontas, A.S., Fidanza, F., Karvonen, M.J., Menotti, A., Nedeljkovič, S., Punsar, S. & Toshima, H. (1985) Serum cholesterol and cancer mortality in the Seven Countries Study. *Am. J. Epidemiol.*, *121*, 870-883

[20]Törnberg, S.A., Holm, L.-E., Cartensen, J.M. & Eklund, G.A. (1986) Risks of cancer of the colon and rectum in relation to serum cholesterol and beta-lipoprotein. *New Engl. J. Med.*, *315*, 1629-1633

[21]Hiatt, R.A. & Fireman, B.H. (1986) Serum cholesterol and the incidence of cancer in a large cohort. *J. chron. Dis.*, *39*, 861-870

[22]Abramson, Z.H. & Kark, J.D. (1985) Serum cholesterol and primary brain tumours: a case-control study. *Br. J. Cancer*, *52*, 93-98

[23]Neugut, A.I., Johnsen, C.M. & Fink, D.J. (1986) Serum cholesterol levels in adenomatous polyps and cancer of the colon. A case-control study. *J. Am. med. Assoc.*, *255*, 365-367

[24]Sidney, S., Friedman, G.D. & Hiatt, R.A. (1986) Serum cholesterol and large bowel cancer. A case-control study. *Am. J. Epidemiol.*, *124*, 33-38

[25]Gerhardsson, M., Rosenqvist, U., Ahlbom, A. & Carlson, L.A. (1986) Serum cholesterol and cancer — a retrospective case-control study. *Int. J. Epidemiol.*, *15*, 155-159

[26]Mannes, G.A., Maier, A., Thieme, C., Wiebecke, B. & Paumgartner, G. (1986) Relation between the frequency of colorectal adenoma and the serum cholesterol level. *New Engl. J. Med.*, *315*, 1634-1638

[27]Tartter, P.I., Slater, G., Papatestas, A.E. & Aufses, A.H., Jr (1984) Cholesterol, weight, height, Quetelet's index, and colon cancer recurrence. *J. surg. Oncol.*, *27*, 232-235

[28]Reed, T., Wagener, D.K., Donahue, R.P. & Kuller, L.H. (1986) Family history of cancer related to cholesterol level in young adults. *Genet. Epidemiol.*, *3*, 63-71

[29]Broitman, S.A. (1981) Cholesterol excretion and colon cancer. *Cancer Res.*, *41*, 3738-3740

[30]Cohen, L.A. & Chan, P.-C. (1982) Dietary cholesterol and experimental mammary cancer development. *Nutr. Cancer*, *4*, 99-106

[31]Cohen, B.I., Raicht, R.F. & Fazzini, E. (1982) Reduction of N-methyl-N-nitrosourea-induced colon tumors in the rat by cholesterol. *Cancer Res.*, *42*, 5050-5052

[32]*IARC Monographs, Suppl. 6*, 166-167, 1987

CHROMIUM AND CHROMIUM COMPOUNDS:
CHROMIUM METAL (Group 3)
TRIVALENT CHROMIUM COMPOUNDS (Group 3)
HEXAVALENT CHROMIUM COMPOUNDS (Group 1*)

A. Evidence for carcinogenicity to humans (*inadequate* for chromium metal and trivalent chromium compounds; *sufficient* for hexavalent chromium compounds)

An increased incidence of lung cancer has been observed among workers in both the bichromate-producing industry and chromate-pigment manufacturing. There is evidence of

---

*This evaluation applies to the group of chemicals as a whole and not necessarily to all individual chemicals within the group (see also Methods, p. 38).

a similar risk among chromium platers and chromium alloy workers. The incidences of cancers at other sites may also be increased in such populations. However, a clear distinction between the relative carcinogenicity of chromium compounds of different oxidation states or solubilities has been difficult to achieve[1].

Recent studies of chromate-pigment makers and users[2-10], chrome platers[11], welders[12-16] and chrome-alloy foundry workers[17] have shed some light on this problem. For chromate-pigment makers and users, respiratory cancer excesses have usually been found. Chromium pigments are usually hexavalent and commonly include zinc, lead (see p. 230) or strontium chromate. A small Norwegian study identified 24 workers primarily exposed to zinc chromate out of a total chromium-pigment worker population of 133. All six lung cancer cases, with more than three years' exposure, occurred among the zinc chromate group (0.14 expected)[9]. One report from the UK contrasts the mortality experience of three plants, in one of which only lead chromate was used. The lung cancer excess was restricted to the plants in which there was mixed exposure to lead and zinc chromate. In the lead chromate plant, there was no lung cancer excess, whereas in the other two the observed:expected ratios for high-/medium-exposed workers ranged from 13:5.9 to 5:0.9[10].

Chrome platers have also been found to have excess lung cancer[11]. Stainless-steel welding involves the greatest exposure to hexavalent chromium, as well as to nickel[14] (see p. 264), and observed:expected ratios for lung cancer for this subgroup of welders ranged from 4.4 (based on three cases)[12] to 1.7 (based on six cases)[13]. One study of chromium-nickel alloy foundry workers showed a statistically significant excess of lung cancer in the 65-99-year age group only[17].

Excess ratios for tumours at other sites are an unusual finding, but they have been reported for chromate paint workers (gastrointestinal tract)[1,18], chromate-pigment users (stomach and pancreas)[6] and chrome platers (gastrointestinal tract)[11]. The observed numbers are, however, small, and the observed:expected ratios do not reach statistical significance. In a post-mortem investigation of lung cancer deaths, it was found that, of the cases diagnosed as small-cell carcinoma, many had been exposed mainly to hexavalent chromium compounds[19].

B. Evidence for carcinogenicity to animals (*inadequate* for chromium metal and trivalent chromium compounds; *sufficient* for hexavalent chromium compounds)

Chromium metal and chromium compounds have been tested for carcinogenicity by a wide variety of routes in mice, rats and rabbits. Calcium chromate produced bronchial carcinomas after implantation of an intrabronchial pellet in rats[1,20] and injection-site sarcomas after intramuscular implantation in rats and mice and after intrapleural injection in rats[1]. Bronchial carcinomas were produced in rats after intrabronchial implantation of strontium chromate and zinc chromate[20]. Injection-site sarcomas were produced in rats and mice after intramuscular, intrapleural and subcutaneous injections of chromite ore, strontium chromate, chromium trioxide, lead chromate and zinc chromate, but few or no sarcomas were induced by barium chromate, sodium chromate or dichromate, or chromic acetate. Chromium powder has been tested inadequately in mice, rats and rabbits[1].

C. Other relevant data

The available evidence indicates that the carcinogenicity of chromium-containing materials can be related to both valency and bioavailability. Trivalent and hexavalent chromium have markedly different chemical and biological properties. Trivalent chromium is the more stable oxidation state, and under physiological conditions it may form complexes with ligands such as nucleic acids, proteins and organic acids. Biological membranes are thought to be impermeable to trivalent chromium, although phagocytosis of particulate trivalent chromium can occur. Hexavalent chromium usually forms strongly oxidizing chromate and dichromate ions, which readily cross biological membranes and are easily reduced under physiological conditions to trivalent chromium. Trivalent chromium compounds may be contaminated with hexavalent chromium compounds (and *vice versa*)[21]. Chromium compounds that are sparingly soluble in water appear to have greater carcinogenic activity than those substances that are either highly soluble or insoluble.

People occupationally exposed to hexavalent chromium compounds (in chromate production and in electroplating factories) had elevated incidences of chromosomal aberrations in their peripheral blood lymphocytes; reports on sister chromatid exchange induction were conflicting. Workers exposed to chromium compounds during stainless-steel welding did not show increased incidences of chromosomal aberrations, micronuclei or sister chromatid exchanges in peripheral blood lymphocytes[21].

No data were available on the genetic and related effects of trivalent chromium compounds in humans.

Hexavalent chromium induced dominant lethal mutations, chromosomal aberrations and micronuclei in rodents treated *in vivo*. In human cells *in vitro*, it caused chromosomal aberrations, sister chromatid exchanges and DNA damage. In cultured rodent cells, it induced transformation, chromosomal aberrations, sister chromatid exchanges, mutation and DNA damage. It induced aneuploidy in *Drosophila* and mitotic recombination in yeast. It was mutagenic and caused DNA damage in bacteria[21].

There is no consistent evidence that water-soluble trivalent chromium has genetic activity. The few positive results were obtained only with doses about 100 times higher than those of hexavalent chromium required to produce such effects[21].

Trivalent chromium did not induce micronuclei in bone-marrow cells of mice treated *in vivo*. Conflicting results were obtained for the induction of chromosomal aberrations in human lymphocytes *in vitro*, and neither sister chromatid exchange nor unscheduled DNA synthesis was induced in human cells *in vitro*. Conflicting results were obtained concerning the induction of chromosomal aberrations, mutation and sister chromatid exchanges in rodent cells in culture. Trivalent chromium did not induce mutation in bacteria, but it induced DNA damage[21].

Insoluble crystalline chromium oxide (Cr_2O_3) induced sister chromatid exchanges and mutation in cultured Chinese hamster cells, which were shown to contain particles of the test material[21].

References

[1]*IARC Monographs*, 23, 205-323, 1980

[2]Dalager, N.A., Mason, T.J., Fraumeni, J.F., Jr, Hoover, R. & Payne, W.W. (1980) Cancer mortality among workers exposed to zinc chromate paints. *J. occup. Med., 22*, 25-29

[3]Satoh, K., Fukuda, Y., Torii, K. & Katsuno, N. (1981) Epidemiological study of workers engaged in the manufacture of chromium compounds. *J. occup. Med., 23*, 835-838

[4]Alderson, M.R., Rattan, N.S. & Bidstrup, L. (1981) Health of workmen in the chromate-producing industry in Britain. *Br. J. ind. Med., 38*, 117-124

[5]Bertazzi, P.A., Zocchetti, C., Terzaghi, G.F., Riboldi, L., Guercilena, S. & Beretta, F. (1981) Carcinogenic risk in the production of paints. A mortality study (Ital.). *Med. Lav., 6*, 465-472

[6]Sheffet, A., Thind, I., Miller, A.M. & Louria, D.B. (1982) Cancer mortality in a pigment plant utilizing lead and zinc chromates. *Arch. environ. Health, 37*, 44-52

[7]Korallus, U., Lange, H.-J., Neiss, A., Wüstefeld, E. & Zwingers, T. (1982) The relationship between active environmental measures taken in the chromate producing industry and lung carcinoma mortality (Ger.). *Arbeitsmed. Sozialmed. Prävent. Med., 17*, 159-167

[8]Frentzel-Beyme, R. (1983) Lung cancer mortality of workers employed in chromate pigment factories. A multicentric European epidemiological study. *J. Cancer Res. clin. Oncol., 105*, 183-188

[9]Langård, S. & Vigander, T. (1983) Occurrence of lung cancer in workers producing chromium pigments. *Br. J. ind. Med., 40*, 71-74

[10]Davies, J.M. (1984) Lung cancer mortality among workers making lead chromate and zinc chromate pigment at three English factories. *Br. J. ind. Med., 41*, 158-169

[11]Franchini, I., Magnani, F. & Mutti, A. (1983) Mortality experience among chromeplating workers. Initial findings. *Scand. J. Work Environ. Health, 9*, 247-252

[12]Sjögren, B. (1980) A retrospective cohort study of mortality among stainless steel welders. *Scand. J. Work Environ. Health, 6*, 197-200

[13]Becker, N., Claude, J. & Frentzel-Beyme, R. (1985) Cancer risk of arc welders exposed to fumes containing chromium and nickel. *Scand. J. Work Environ. Health, 11*, 75-82

[14]Stern, R.M. (1983) Assessment of risk of lung cancer for welders. *Arch. environ. Health, 38*, 148-155

[15]Hernberg, S., Westerholm, P., Schultz-Larsen, K., Degerth, R., Kuosma, E., Englund, A., Engzell, U., Sand Hansen, H. & Mutanen, P. (1983) Nasal and sinonasal cancer. Connection with occupational exposures in Denmark, Finland and Sweden. *Scand. J. Work Environ. Health, 9*, 315-326

[16]Newhouse, M.L., Oakes, D. & Woolley, A.J. (1985) Mortality of welders and other craftsmen at a shipyard in NE England. *Br. J. ind. Med., 42*, 406-410

[17]Cornell, R.G. & Landis, J.R. (1984) *Mortality patterns among nickel/chromium alloy foundry workers*. In: Sunderman, F.W., Jr, ed., *Nickel in the Human Environment (IARC Scientific Publications No. 53)*, Lyon, International Agency for Research on Cancer, pp. 87-93

[18]Langård, S. & Norseth, T. (1979) Cancer in the gastrointestinal tract in chromate pigment workers. *Arh. Hig. Rada. Toksikol., 30* (Suppl.), 301-304

[19]Abe, S., Ohsaki, Y., Kimura, K., Tsuneta, Y., Mikami, H. & Murao, M. (1982) Chromate lung cancer with special reference to its cell type and relation to the manufacturing process. *Cancer, 49*, 783-787

[20]Levy, L.S., Martin, P.A. & Bidstrup, P.L. (1986) Investigation of the potential carcinogenicity of a range of chromium containing materials on rat lung. *Br. J. ind. Med., 43*, 243-256

[21]*IARC Monographs, Suppl. 6*, 168-175, 1987

CHRYSOIDINE (Group 3)

A. Evidence for carcinogenicity to humans (*inadequate*)

A report of bladder cancer in three amateur anglers with exposure to chrysoidine-dyed maggots[1] stimulated reports of four further cases[2,3] and two case-control studies[4,5]. A study in Yorkshire, UK, used an existing large-scale bladder cancer case-control study (over 900 pairs) and made further enquiries regarding fishing, maggots and dyes used on or in the maggots. The relative risks were 0.7 (95% confidence interval, 0.2-2.3) based on five exposed cases for the use of bronze (surface-coloured) maggots, and 2.0 (0.6-6.2) based on nine exposed cases for yellow maggots (ready or self-coloured)[4]. A study in the West Midlands, UK, was smaller (202 pairs) but showed a higher percentage of use of dyed maggots (14% of cases, 8% of controls). A three-fold excess risk was noted for the use of bronze maggots for more than five years[5]. This study almost certainly included five cases from the previous case reports that stimulated the case-control studies, but this factor is unlikely to remove the statistically significant excess risk.

B. Evidence for carcinogenicity to animals (*limited*)

Chrysoidine was tested for carcinogenicity in single experiments in mice and rats by oral administration only. In mice, it produced liver-cell adenomas and carcinomas, leukaemia and reticulum-cell sarcomas. The experiment on rats was inadequately reported[6].

C. Other relevant data

No data were available on the genetic and related effects of chrysoidine in humans. It was mutagenic to bacteria[7].

References

[1]Searle, C.E. & Teale, J. (1982) Chrysoidine-based bait: a possible carcinogenic hazard to anglers? *Lancet*, *i*, 564

[2]Massey, J.A., Feneley, R.C.L. & Abrams, P.H. (1984) Maggots dyed with chrysoidine. *Br. med. J.*, *289*, 1451-1452

[3]Sole, G.M. (1984) Maggots dyed with chrysoidine: a possible risk to anglers. *Br. med. J.*, *289*, 1043-1044

[4]Cartwright, R.A., Robinson, M.R.G., Glashan, R.W., Gray, B.K., Hamilton-Stewart, P., Cartwright, S.C. & Barham-Hall, D. (1983) Does the use of stained maggots present a risk of bladder cancer to coarse fishermen? *Carcinogenesis*, *4*, 111-113

[5]Sole, G. & Sorahan, T. (1985) Coarse fishing and risk of urothelial cancer. *Lancet*, *i*, 1477-1479

[6]*IARC Monographs*, *8*, 91-96, 1975

[7]*IARC Monographs*, *Suppl. 6*, 176-177, 1987

CISPLATIN (Group 2A)

A. Evidence for carcinogenicity to humans (*inadequate*)

No epidemiological study of cisplatin as a single agent was available to the Working Group. Occasional case reports of exposure to cisplatin, especially in the presence of concurrent therapy with other putative carcinogens, such as ionizing radiation, alkylating agents and other potent oncotherapeutic drugs, do not constitute evidence of carcinogenesis[1-3].

B. Evidence for carcinogenicity to animals (*sufficient*)

Multiple intraperitoneal administrations of cisplatin to mice significantly increased the incidence and number of lung adenomas. Similar treatments caused a significant increase in the incidence of skin papillomas in mice given promoting treatment of croton oil applied to the skin. The incidences of epidermoid carcinomas and of both malignant and benign tumours in internal organs were increased by the same treatment, but were not significantly different from those in controls[1,4]. In two studies, multiple intraperitoneal injections of cisplatin to rats induced leukaemia[5,6].

C. Other relevant data

In one study, cisplatin-adriamycin combination chemotherapy induced sister chromatid exchanges in peripheral blood lymphocytes of patients treated with this agent. In another study, antigenicity against cisplatin-DNA adducts was demonstrated in blood cells of treated patients[7].

Cisplatin induced structural chromosomal aberrations and sister chromatid exchanges in cells of rodents treated *in vivo*, but it did not induce dominant lethal mutations in mice. It transformed Syrian hamster embryo cells; it induced chromosomal aberrations, micronuclei and sister chromatid exchanges in both human and rodent cells *in vitro*, and mutation and DNA damage (including DNA cross-links) in rodent cells *in vitro*. In *Drosophila*, cisplatin induced aneuploidy and dominant lethal and sex-linked recessive lethal mutations. It induced chromosomal aberrations and mutation in plants. Cisplatin induced mutation, gene conversion and DNA damage in fungi and mutation and DNA damage in bacteria[7].

References

[1]*IARC Monographs*, 26, 151-164, 1981

[2]Mead, G.M., Green, J.A., Macbeth, F.R., Williams, C.J., Whitehouse, J.M.A. & Buchanan, R. (1983) Second malignancy after cisplatin, vinblastin, and bleomycin (PVB) chemotherapy: a case report. *Cancer Treat. Rep.*, 67, 410

[3]Pedersen-Bjergaard, J., Rørth, M., Avnstrøm, S., Philip, P. & Hou-Jensen, K. (1985) Acute nonlymphocytic leukemia following treatment of testicular cancer and gastric cancer with combination chemotherapy not including alkylating agents: report of two cases. *Am. J. Hematol.*, 18, 425-429

[4]Leopold, W.R., Batzinger, R.P., Miller, E.C., Miller, J.A. & Earhart, R.H. (1981) Mutagenicity, tumorigenicity, and electrophilic reactivity of the stereoisomeric platinum (II) complexes of 1,2-diaminocyclohexane. *Cancer Res., 41*, 4368-4377

[5]Kempf, S.R. & Ivankovic, S. (1986) Chemotherapy-induced malignancies in rats after treatment with cisplatin as single agent and in combination: preliminary results. *Oncology, 43*, 187-191

[6]Kempf, S.R. & Ivankovic, S. (1986) Carcinogenic effect of *cis*platin(*cis*-diammine-dichloro-platinum(II), CDDP) in BD IX rats. *J. Cancer Res. clin. Oncol., 111*, 133-136

[7]*IARC Monographs, Suppl. 6*, 178-181, 1987

CLOFIBRATE (Group 3)

A. Evidence for carcinogenicity to humans (*inadequate*)

Results of a further four years of follow-up to the clofibrate trial of the World Health Organization[1] have become available[2]. On average, the total follow-up period was 13.2 years, 5.3 of which were during the actual treatment phase (range, four to eight years) and 7.9 thereafter. Three groups of men, divided according to their cholesterol levels, were studied, comprising 208 000 man-years of observation. The first two groups included subjects in the upper third of the serum cholesterol distribution, randomly allocated either to treatment by clofibrate (1.6 g daily) or an olive-oil placebo. The third group was composed of half of the men in the lowest third of the distribution, who received an olive-oil placebo. At the conclusion of follow-up, the age-standardized death rates from malignant neoplasms per 1000 per annum were 2.4, 2.4 and 2.3, respectively (based on 206, 197 and 173 deaths from neoplasms). However, the age-standardized death rates for malignant neoplasms during the treatment phase had been 1.9 (42 deaths), 1.2 (25 deaths) and 1.7 (30 deaths), respectively.

Reports of two of four other clofibrate trials did not include information on the occurrence of cancer[1]. Of those which did, one showed no excess of cancer in treated groups over the six-year period of the trial (eight cancer deaths in all)[3], and, in the other, covering a follow-up period of five to 8.5 years, the death rates for all cancers were 0.9% for the group receiving clofibrate, 0.8% for a group receiving niacin and 0.9% for the placebo group[4]. Two further trials of clofibrate showed no excess of cancer in treated groups[2].

In a single case report, a man who received clofibrate (among other drugs) for 15 years developed a jejunal adenocarcinoma[2].

B. Evidence for carcinogenicity to animals (*limited*)

Clofibrate was tested in two studies by oral administration to male rats; it produced hepatocellular carcinomas, and a few pancreatic exocrine acinar adenomas and carcinomas were observed[1]. Clofibrate decreased the incidence of 7,12-dimethylbenz[*a*]anthracene-induced mammary carcinomas in rats, but did not affect the carcinogenic action of

N-methyl-N-nitrosourea[5] or of dimethylhydrazine (isomer unspecified)[6]. In two studies, it enhanced N-nitrosodiethylamine-induced liver tumorigenesis[7,8], but, in a limited bioassay, when fed after the induction of liver foci by 2-acetylaminofluorene, it did not enhance liver carcinogenesis[9].

C. Other relevant data

No data were available on the genetic and related effects of clofibrate in humans. It did not induce chromosomal aberrations in Chinese hamster fibroblasts *in vitro* and was not mutagenic to bacteria[10].

References

[1]*IARC Monographs*, 24, 39-58, 1980

[2]Committee of Principal Investigators (1984) WHO cooperative trial on primary prevention of ischaemic heart disease with clofibrate to lower serum cholesterol: final mortality follow-up. *Lancet*, ii, 600-604

[3]Research Committee of the Scottish Society of Physicians (1971) Ischaemic heart disease: a secondary prevention trial using clofibrate. *Br. med. J.*, iv, 775-784

[4]The Coronary Drug Project Research Group (1975) Clofibrate and niacin in coronary heart disease. *J. Am. Med. Assoc.*, 231, 360-381

[5]Anisimov, V.N., Danetskaya, E.V., Miretsky, G.I., Troitskaya, M.N. & Dilman, V.M. (1981) Influence of miscleron (clofibrate) on carcinogenic effect of 7,12-dimethylbenz[a]anthracene and nitrosomethylurea in female rats (Russ.). *Vopr. Onkol.*, 27, 64-67

[6]Bershtein, L.M., Pozharisskii, K.M. & Dil'man, V.M. (1980) Effect of miscleron (clofibrate) on induction of intestinal tumours by dimethylhydrazine in rats (Russ.). *Bull. exp. Biol. Med.*, 90, 350-354

[7]Mochizuki, Y., Furukawa, K. & Sawada, N. (1982) Effects of various concentrations of ethyl-α-p-chlorophenoxyisobutyrate (clofibrate) on diethylnitrosamine-induced hepatic tumorigenesis in the rat. *Carcinogenesis*, 3, 1027-1029

[8]Mochizuki, Y., Furukawa, K. & Sawada, N. (1983) Effect of simultaneous administration of clofibrate with diethylnitrosamine on hepatic tumorigenesis in the rat. *Cancer Lett.*, 19, 99-105

[9]Numoto, S., Furukawa, K., Furuya, K. & Williams, G.M. (1984) Effects of the hepatocarcinogenic peroxisome-proliferating hypolipidemic agents clofibrate and nafenopin on the rat liver cell membrane enzymes γ-glutamyltranspeptidase and alkaline phosphatase and on the early stages of liver carcinogenesis. *Carcinogenesis*, 5, 1603-1611

[10]*IARC Monographs*, Suppl. 6, 182-183, 1987

CLOMIPHENE CITRATE (Group 3)

A. Evidence for carcinogenicity to humans (*inadequate*)

Only case reports of benign and malignant tumours occurring at various sites are available[1-5]. These include testicular tumours in three young men who had received clomiphene as part of hormonal treatment for oligospermia[2], a hepatoblastoma in a female infant whose mother had received clomiphene citrate as treatment for infertility[3], a liver-cell adenoma in a women who had received clomiphene citrate for oligomenorrhoea[4], and unilateral testicular neoplasms in two of 650 oligospermic men who had received monthly treatments with clomiphene citrate (daily for three weeks followed by a week of rest) for six to 12 months[5].

B. Evidence for carcinogenicity to animals (*inadequate*)

Clomiphene citrate was tested in an inadequate experiment in newborn rats by single subcutaneous injection; reproductive-tract abnormalities, including uterine and ovarian tumours, were reported[1].

C. Other relevant data

No data were available on the genetic and related effects of clomiphene citrate in humans. It did not induce chromosomal aberrations or micronuclei in bone-marrow cells of mice treated *in vivo*[6].

References

[1]*IARC Monographs, 21*, 551-561, 1979

[2]Neoptolemos, J.P., Locke, T.J. & Fossard, D.P. (1981) Testicular tumour associated with hormonal treatment for oligospermia. *Lancet, ii*, 754

[3]Melamed, I., Bujanover, Y., Hammer, J. & Spirer, Z. (1982) Hepatoblastoma in an infant born to a mother after hormonal treatment for sterility. *New Engl. J. Med., 307*, 820

[4]Carrasco, D., Barrachina, M., Prieto, M. & Berenguer, J. (1983) Clomiphene citrate and liver-cell adenoma. *New Engl. J. Med., 310*, 1120-1121

[5]Nilsson, A. & Nilsson, S. (1985) Testicular germ cell tumors after clomiphene therapy for subfertility. *J. Urol., 134*, 560-562

[6]*IARC Monographs, Suppl. 6*, 184-185, 1987

COAL GASIFICATION (Group 1)

A. Evidence for carcinogenicity to humans (*sufficient*)

Case reports of tumours of the skin (including the scrotum), bladder and respiratory tract in association with employment in industries involving the destructive distillation of coal suggested a link between work in that industry and human cancer. Descriptive epidemiological studies based on death certificates corroborated these early suggestions[1].

A series of detailed analytical epidemiological studies of the British gas industry add further weight to the hypothesis that work in such coal gasification plants carries a risk for tumours of the lung, bladder and scrotum. There appeared to be a relationship between elevated relative risk of tumours and work in retort houses, particularly when the job had entailed exposure to fumes emanating from the retorts[1].

B. Other relevant data

No relevant data were available to the Working Group.

References

[1]*IARC Monographs, 34*, 65-99, 1984

COAL-TAR PITCHES (Group 1)

A. Evidence for carcinogenicity to humans (*sufficient*)

A mortality analysis in the UK from 1946 showed a greatly increased risk for scrotal cancer among patent-fuel workers; furthermore, a large number of case reports describe the development of skin (including the scrotum) cancer in workers exposed to coal-tars (see p. 175) or coal-tar pitch[1]. Several epidemiological studies have shown excesses of lung and bladder cancer among workers exposed to pitch fumes in aluminium production plants[2]. A slight excess of lung cancer was found among furnace and maintenance workers exposed to coal-tar pitch fumes in a calcium carbide production plant[3]. A cohort study of US roofers indicated an increased risk for cancer of the lung and suggested increased risks for cancers of the oral cavity, larynx, oesophagus, stomach, skin and bladder and for leukaemia. Some support for excess risks of lung, laryngeal and oral-cavity cancer is provided by other studies of roofers. One study showed a small excess of bladder cancer in tar distillers and in patent-fuel workers. An elevated risk of cancer of the renal pelvis was seen in workers exposed to 'petroleum or tar or pitch'[1]. One study of millwrights and welders exposed to coal-tars and coal-tar pitch in a stamping plant showed significant excesses of leukaemia and of cancers of the lung and digestive organs[4].

B. Evidence for carcinogenicity to animals (*sufficient*)

Application of coal-tar pitches and extracts of coal-tar pitches to the skin of mice produced malignant skin tumours. Extracts of coal-tar pitches had both initiating and promoting activities in mouse skin[1,5,6].

C. Other relevant data

No data were available on the genetic and related effects of coal-tar pitches in humans.

Extracts of coal-tar pitches and 'coal-tar' paints (formulated with coal-tar pitches) were mutagenic to *Salmonella typhimurium* in the presence of an exogenous metabolic system. Extracts of emissions from a roofing-tar pot (coal-tar pitch-based tar) enhanced viral transformation in Syrian hamster embryo cells but did not cause DNA strand breaks. The same material induced sister chromatid exchanges and mutation in cultured rodent cells, both in the presence and absence of an exogenous metabolic system, and was mutagenic to *S. typhimurium* in the presence of an exogenous metabolic system[7].

References

[1]*IARC Monographs*, *35*, 83-159, 1985

[2]*IARC Monographs*, *34*, 37-64, 1984

[3]Kjuus, H., Andersen, A. & Langård, S. (1986) Incidence of cancer among workers producing calcium carbide. *Br. J. ind. Med.*, *43*, 237-242

[4]Silverstein, M., Maizlish, N., Park, R. & Mirer, F. (1985) Mortality among workers exposed to coal tar pitch volatiles and welding emissions: an exercise in epidemiologic triage. *Am. J. public Health*, *75*, 1283-1287

[5]Robinson, M., Bull, R.J., Munch, J. & Meier, J. (1984) Comparative carcinogenic and mutagenic activity of coal tar and petroleum asphalt paints used in potable water supply systems. *J. appl. Toxicol.*, *4*, 49-56

[6]Niemeier, R.W., Thayer, P.S., Menzies, K.T., von Thuna, P., Moss, C.E. & Burg, J. (1987) *A comparison of the skin carcinogenicity of condensed roofing asphalt and coal tar pitch fumes*. In: Cooke, M. & Dennis, A.J., eds, *Proceedings of the 10th International Symposium on Polynuclear Aromatic Hydrocarbons, Chemistry, Characterization and Carcinogenesis*, Columbus, OH, Battelle, pp. 609-647

[7]*IARC Monographs*, *Suppl. 6*, 186, 1987

COAL-TARS (Group 1)

A. Evidence for carcinogenicity to humans (*sufficient*)

There have been a number of case reports of skin cancer in patients who used tar ointments for a variety of skin diseases[1,2]. A mortality analysis in the UK from 1946 showed a greatly increased scrotal cancer risk for patent-fuel workers. Furthermore, a large number of case reports describe the development of skin (including the scrotum) cancer in workers exposed to coal-tars or coal-tar pitches (see p. 174)[1]. Several epidemiological studies have shown an excess of lung cancer among workers exposed to coal-tar fumes in coal gasification and coke production[3,4]. One study showed a small excess of bladder cancer in tar distillers and in patent-fuel workers. An elevated risk of cancer of the renal pelvis was seen in workers exposed to 'petroleum or tar or pitch'[1]. One study of millwrights and welders exposed to coal-tars and coal-tar pitch in a stamping plant showed significant excesses of leukaemia and of cancers of the lung and digestive organs[5].

B. Evidence for carcinogenicity to animals (*sufficient*)

Coal-tars from blast furnaces, coke ovens and coal gasification plants, as well as pharmaceutical coal-tars, were tested for carcinogenicity by skin application in mice, producing skin tumours. Pharmaceutical coal-tars and tars from coal gasification plants also produced skin tumours when applied to the ears of rabbits. Pharmaceutical coal-tars applied to the skin of rats produced lung tumours but not skin tumours. Inhalation of tar from coke ovens produced benign and malignant lung tumours in mice and rats and skin tumours in mice[1,3,4].

C. Other relevant data

An increased frequency of chromosomal aberrations was observed in peripheral lymphocytes of coal-tar workers, both smokers and nonsmokers. Extracts of urine from patients undergoing combined treatment with coal-tar preparations and ultraviolet light were mutagenic to *Salmonella typhimurium*[6].

Coal-tar induced transformation of Syrian hamster embryo cells. Samples of therapeutic coal-tar, extracts of coal-tar shampoos, an industrial coal-tar and vapours emitted from a coal-tar sample at 37°C were mutagenic to *S. typhimurium* in the presence of an exogenous metabolic system[6].

References

[1]*IARC Monographs, 35*, 83-159, 1985

[2]Stern, R.S., Scotto, J. & Fears, T.R. (1985) Psoriasis and susceptibility to nonmelanoma skin cancer. *J. Am. Acad. Dermatol., 12*, 67-73

[3]*IARC Monographs, 34*, 65-99, 1984

[4]*IARC Monographs, 34*, 101-131, 1984

[5]Silverstein, M., Maizlish, N., Park, R. & Mirer, F. (1985) Mortality among workers exposed to coal tar pitch volatiles and welding emissions: an exercise in epidemiologic triage. *Am. J. public Health, 75*, 1283-1287

[6]*IARC Monographs, Suppl. 6*, 186, 1987

COKE PRODUCTION (Group 1)

A. Evidence for carcinogenicity to humans (*sufficient*)

In the first half of the century, case reports of tumours of the skin (including the scrotum), bladder and respiratory tract, in association with employment in industries involving the destructive distillation of coal, suggested a link between that industry and human cancer. Despite their methodological shortcomings, descriptive epidemiological studies based on death certificates corroborated these early suggestions[1].

Later studies carried out in Japan, Sweden, the UK and the USA identified the lung as the site at which the excess cancer rates occurred most commonly among workers in coke production. All but two of the pertinent analytical epidemiological cohort studies provided evidence that work in coke production carries a significantly elevated risk of lung cancer. The two studies showing no lung cancer excess suffered from serious methodological limitations. The risk was evident in comparison with both the general population and non-coke production workers, and the extent of the increased relative risk estimates varied from three to seven fold. In those studies in which the relevant information was available, differences in smoking habits were shown not to have severely confounded the risk estimates[1].

Excess risk of kidney cancer has been repeatedly associated with work in coke plants. In one study in the USA, a seven-fold increase in risk was seen for workers employed for five years or more at coke ovens. In single studies, excess risks were reported for cancers of the large intestine and pancreas[1].

The largest study was conducted on a cohort of some 59 000 steel workers in the Pittsburgh area (USA)[1]. The study has recently been extended up to 1975 and the dose-response analysis of exposure to coal-tar pitch volatiles and lung cancer reviewed. Coke-oven workers (both white and nonwhite) exhibited a large, statistically significant increase in lung cancer mortality that was strongly associated with duration of exposure to coke-oven fumes and intensity of exposure, as documented by comparing topside- with side-oven experience. Significantly elevated mortality from prostatic and kidney cancer was also noted, but without clear evidence of an exposure-response relationship. Non-oven workers had no excess of lung cancer but a significantly increased mortality from cancer of the large intestine and pancreas. Cumulative exposure indices of exposure to coal-tar pitch volatiles were calculated and increasing lung cancer risk with increasing estimated exposure was found[2,3]. A possible causative agent is coal-tar fumes.

B. Other relevant data

An increase in the incidence of sister chromatid exchanges was observed in cultured peripheral blood lymphocytes from 12 nonsmoking coke-oven workers in a steel plant, when they were compared to a group of age-matched controls. Urine samples from nonsmoking coke-plant workers were mutagenic to *Salmonella typhimurium* in the presence of an exogenous metabolic system. In a second study of coke-plant workers, the mutagenic activity in *S. typhimurium* of extracts of urine samples collected after work was not statistically different from that of samples taken before work. Antigenicity against benzo[a]pyrene diol epoxide-DNA adducts has been demonstrated in peripheral blood lymphocytes of coke-oven workers[4].

References

[1]*IARC Monographs, 34*, 101-131, 1984

[2]Redmond, C.K. (1983) Cancer mortality among coke oven workers. *Environ. Health Perspect., 52*, 67-73

[3]Rockette, H.E. & Redmond, C.K. (1985) Selection, follow-up, and analysis in the coke oven study. *Natl Cancer Inst. Monogr., 67*, 89-94

[4]*IARC Monographs, Suppl. 6*, 187, 1987

CREOSOTES (Group 2A)

A. Evidence for carcinogenicity to humans (*limited*)

In a number of case reports, the development of skin cancer in workers exposed to creosotes is described. One study involved a review of 3753 cases of cutaneous epithelioma from 1920 to 1945 and showed that 35 cases (12 of which were of the scrotum) had had exposure to creosotes. Most cases occurred in workers handling creosotes or creosoted wood during timber treatment. A mortality analysis of workers in many occupations indicated an increased risk of scrotal cancer for creosote-exposed brickmakers[1].

B. Evidence for carcinogenicity to animals (*sufficient*)

Creosotes, creosote oils and anthracene oils were tested for carcinogenicity in mice by skin application, producing skin tumours, including carcinomas. One of the creosotes also produced lung tumours in mice after skin application[1].

C. Other relevant data

No occupationally related increase in mutagenicity was detected in the urine of creosote workers, but urine from rats administered creosote was mutagenic to *Salmonella typhimurium* in the presence of an exogenous metabolic system[2].

Creosote enhanced transformation of Syrian hamster embryo cells initiated with benzo[*a*]pyrene in a two-stage transformation assay, and creosote and a coal-tar/creosote mixture gave positive results in the mouse lymphoma L5178Y system. Creosote, vapour emitted from creosote at 37°C and a coal-tar/creosote mixture were mutagenic to *S. typhimurium* in the presence of an exogenous metabolic system[2].

References
[1]*IARC Monographs, 35*, 83-159, 1985
[2]*IARC Monographs, Suppl. 6*, 188, 1987

CYCLAMATES (Group 3)

A. Evidence for carcinogenicity to humans (*inadequate*)

The evidence that the risk of cancer is increased among users of artificial sweeteners is inconsistent[1]. Since the positive report of Howe *et al.*[2], reports have become available on six case-control studies and on one population study of bladder cancer.

The largest was a population-based study in ten areas of the USA, with 3010 bladder cases and 5783 controls. The relative risk for bladder cancer associated with use of artificial sweeteners was 1.0 (95% confidence interval, 0.89-1.1) among men and 1.1 (0.89-1.3) among women. Significant trends of increasing risk with increasing average daily consumption were found in certain subgroups examined *a priori* on the basis of the results of animal experiments; these subgroups were female nonsmokers and male heavy smokers[3]. Subsequent, independent re-analysis of the same data by a different statistical technique (multiple logistic regression) confirmed the original findings overall but cast doubt on the significance of the findings in the two subgroups because of inconsistent dose-response trends, especially among the male heavy smokers[4]. In response, the original investigators noted that the inconsistency derived from the development of risk scores which, in their opinion, were not correctly derived, as two relevant variables had been omitted[5]. In a subsequent report on data from one of the areas participating in this study, the use of hospital and population controls was compared. A higher proportion of hospital controls was found to have used artificial sweeteners than population controls[6]. This had been postulated earlier[2] as a possible reason for the negative findings of a hospital-based case-control study[7]. Bias resulting from use of prevalent rather than incident cases[8] has been suggested as a possible reason for the negative findings of another hospital-based case-control study[9].

Two other case-control studies have also shown increased risks among subgroups. In one, conducted simultaneously in Japan, the UK and the USA, the relative risks among women in the US component of the study associated with 'any' use of diet drinks and of sugar substitutes were 1.6 and 1.5, respectively, and 2.6 and 2.1, respectively, for non-smokers[10]. In the other two areas, however, a history of use of sugar substitutes, primarily saccharin, was not associated with an elevated bladder cancer risk[11]. In the other study, conducted in West Yorkshire, UK, although elevated risks were found for saccharin takers (see p. 334) who were nonsmokers, the risks associated with cyclamate use were not examined[12].

Two studies in Denmark[13,14], one in the USA[15] and a further case-control study in Canada[16], however, gave negative results. In one of the Danish studies, incidence of bladder cancer at ages 20-34 among people born 1941-1945 (when use of saccharin was high in Denmark) was compared with that among those born 1931-1940. The risk for men was 1.0 (0.7-1.6) and that for women, 0.3 (0.1-1.0)[13]. The other two studies were population-based case-control studies of bladder cancer. In Denmark, the relative risk for people of the two sexes combined was 0.78 (0.58-1.05)[14]. In a study in the USA of bladder cancer in women aged 20-49, the odds ratio for regular use of artificially sweetened beverages, table-top sweetener or both was 1.1 (0.7-1.7)[15]. In Canada, the odds ratio for use of cyclamate was 1.09 (0.60-1.97) in males and 0.92 (0.63-1.36) in females[16]. In neither study were the increased risks seen in subgroups in other studies replicated.

In the USA, in a study of 1862 patients hospitalized for cancer and of 10 874 control patients, a greater proportion of artificial sweetener users was found only among women with cancer of the stomach. Little information was available on urinary-tract cancer. No overall association was found between artificial sweetener use and cancer[17].

B. Evidence for carcinogenicity to animals (*limited*)

Sodium cyclamate was tested for carcinogenicity both alone and in combination with other chemicals in different animal species and by several routes of administration. Following its oral administration to two strains of mice, an increased incidence of lymphosarcomas was observed in female mice of one strain; a few bladder tumours were seen in rats exposed orally. Several other experiments in mice, rats, hamsters and monkeys were inadequate for evaluation. A 10:1 mixture of sodium cyclamate:sodium saccharin was given to mice in one multigeneration experiment and to rats in two single-generation experiments: transitional-cell carcinomas were induced in the bladders of male rats of one strain given the highest dose[1]. In a similar two-generation experiment in rats, no treatment-related tumour was observed[18]. Instillation of low doses of N-methyl-N-nitrosourea into the bladder of rats fed sodium cyclamate for long periods resulted in a dose-related induction of transitional-cell neoplasms of the bladder. After subcutaneous injection of rats with sodium cyclamate, no tumour was observed at the site of injection, the only site for which tumour incidence was reported. A significant increase in the incidence of bladder carcinomas was observed in mice given bladder implants of pellets containing sodium cyclamate[1]. Transplacental application of cyclamate to rats did not produce an increase in tumour incidence at any site[19].

Calcium cyclamate did not alter tumour incidence when tested by oral administration in a two-generation experiment in rats but produced local tumours in another experiment following its subcutaneous injection[1].

Cyclohexylamine was tested by oral administration at several dose levels in different strains of mice and rats, and in one multigeneration study in mice. No tumour related to treatment was observed[1].

C. Other relevant data

No data were available on the genetic and related effects of calcium cyclamate, dicyclohexylamine or cyclohexylamine in humans. In a single study, eight persons ingesting sodium cyclamate (70 mg/kg per day) did not exhibit chromosomal aberrations in their lymphocytes[20].

Calcium cyclamate induced chromosomal aberrations in bone-marrow cells of gerbils, but not in bone-marrow cells or spermatogonia of rats, treated in vivo. It did not induce dominant lethal mutations in rats or mice or micronuclei or sperm abnormalities in mice treated in vivo. It induced chromosomal aberrations in human lymphocytes but not in rat kangaroo cells in culture. It did not induce aneuploidy in Drosophila, but contradictory results were reported in assays for sex-linked recessive lethal mutations and heritable translocations. Calcium cyclamate was not mutagenic to bacteria[20].

Sodium cyclamate did not induce dominant lethal mutations or chromosomal aberrations in spermatogonia or spermatocytes of mice treated in vivo. It induced sister chromatid exchanges and chromosomal aberrations in cultured human lymphocytes and chromosomal aberrations in cultured Chinese hamster cells. It did not induce aneuploidy or sex-linked recessive lethal mutations in Drosophila or chromosomal aberrations in plants[20].

Cyclohexylamine did not induce dominant lethal mutations in one study in rats, but contradictory results were obtained in mice. It gave weakly positive results in the mouse spot test. Cyclohexylamine induced chromosomal aberrations in lymphocytes but not in bone-marrow cells of hamsters and lambs or in spermatogonia of hamsters and mice treated in vivo. In treated rats, chromosomal aberrations were induced in spermatogonia but not in leucocytes, and contradictory results were obtained for bone-marrow cells. Cyclohexylamine induced sister chromatid exchanges in cultured human lymphocytes, but, again, conflicting results were obtained concerning the induction of chromosomal aberrations. Cyclohexylamine enhanced virus-induced transformation of Syrian hamster embryo cells and induced chromosomal aberrations in cultured rat kangaroo cells. It did not induce somatic or sex-linked recessive lethal mutations, aneuploidy or heritable translocations in *Drosophila* and was not mutagenic and did not induce prophage in bacteria. In host-mediated assays, it did not induce mutation in bacteria or chromosomal aberrations in human leucocytes[20].

Dicyclohexylamine induced chromosomal aberrations in cultured human lymphocytes. It was not mutagenic to bacteria[20].

References

[1]*IARC Monographs*, 22, 55-109, 171-185, 1980

[2]Howe, G.R., Burch, J.D., Miller, A.B., Cook, G.M., Estève, J., Morrison, B., Gordon, P., Chambers, L.W., Fodor, G. & Winsor, G.M. (1980) Tobacco use, occupation, coffee, various nutrients, and bladder cancer. *J. natl Cancer Inst.*, 64, 701-713

[3]Hoover, R.M. & Strasser, P.H. (1980) Artificial sweeteners and human bladder cancer. Preliminary results. *Lancet*, i, 837-840

[4]Walker, A.M., Dreyer, N.A., Friedlander, E., Loughlin, J., Rothman, K.J. & Kohn, H.I. (1982) An independent analysis of the National Cancer Institute study on non-nutritive sweeteners and bladder cancer. *Am. J. public Health*, 72, 376-381

[5]Hoover, R. & Hartge, P. (1982) Non-nutritive sweeteners and bladder cancer. *Am. J. public Health*, 72, 382-383

[6]Silverman, D.T., Hoover, R.N. & Swanson, G.M. (1983) Artificial sweeteners and lower urinary tract cancer: hospital vs. population controls. *Am. J. Epidemiol.*, 117, 326-334

[7]Wynder, E.L. & Stellman, S.D. (1980) Artificial sweetener use and bladder cancer: a case-control study. *Science*, 207, 1214-1216

[8]Goldsmith, D.F. (1982) Calculation of potential bias in the odds ratio illustrated by a study of saccharin use and bladder cancer. *Environ. Res.*, 27, 298-306

[9]Kessler, I.I. & Clark, J.P. (1978) Saccharin, cyclamate, and human bladder cancer. No evidence of an association. *J. Am. med. Assoc.*, 240, 349-355

[10]Morrison, A.S. & Buring, J.E. (1980) Artificial sweeteners and cancer of the lower urinary tract. *New Engl. J. Med.*, 302, 537-541

[11]Morrison, A.S., Verhoek, W.G., Leck, I., Aoki, K., Ohno, Y. & Obata, K. (1982) Artificial sweeteners and bladder cancer in Manchester, UK, and Nagoya, Japan. *Br. J. Cancer*, 45, 332-336

[12]Cartwright, R.A., Adib, R., Glashan, R. & Gray, B.K. (1981) The epidemiology of bladder cancer in West Yorkshire. A preliminary report on non-occupational aetiologies. *Carcinogenesis*, 2, 343-347

[13]Jensen, O.M. & Kamby, C. (1982) Intra-uterine exposure to saccharine and risk of bladder cancer in man. *Int. J. Cancer*, 29, 507-509

[14]Møller-Jensen, O., Knudsen, J.B., Sørensen, B.L. & Clemmesen, J. (1983) Artificial sweeteners and absence of bladder cancer risk in Copenhagen. *Int. J. Cancer*, 32, 577-582

[15]Piper, J.M., Matanoski, G.M. & Tonascia, J. (1986) Bladder cancer in young women. *Am. J. Epidemiol.*, *123*, 1033-1042

[16]Risch, H.A., Burch, J.D., Miller, A.B., Hill, G.B., Steele, R. & Howe, G.R. (1987) Dietary factors and the incidence of cancer of the urinary bladder. *Am. J. Epidemiol.* (in press)

[17]Morrison, A.S. (1979) Use of artificial sweeteners by cancer patients. *J. natl Cancer Inst.*, *62*, 1397-1399

[18]Schmähl, D. & Habs, M. (1984) Investigations on the carcinogenicity of the artificial sweeteners sodium cyclamate and sodium saccharin in rats in a two-generation experiment. *Arzneimittel.-Forsch.*, *34*, 604-606

[19]Schmähl, D. & Habs, M. (1980) Absence of carcinogenic response to cyclamate and saccharin in Sprague-Dawley rats after transplacental application. *Arzneimittel.-Forsch.*, *30*, 1905-1906

[20]*IARC Monographs*, *Suppl. 6*, 188-195, 240-241, 1987

CYCLOPHOSPHAMIDE (Group 1)

A. Evidence for carcinogenicity to humans (*sufficient*)

Many cases of cancer have been reported following therapy with cyclophosphamide[1].

Excess frequencies of bladder cancer following therapy with cyclophosphamide for nonmalignant diseases have been clearly demonstrated in two epidemiological studies[1,2]. Three recent studies confirmed that cyclophosphamide is also a leukaemogen. Among 602 patients treated predominantly with cyclophosphamide for non-Hodgkin's lymphoma in Denmark, nine cases of acute nonlymphocytic leukaemia (ANLL) or preleukaemia were observed, compared to 0.12 expected on the basis of incidence rates in the general population[3]. In the USA, three cases of ANLL or preleukaemia were observed among 333 women treated only with cyclophosphamide for ovarian cancer; 1.2 were expected[4]. In the German Democratic Republic, a case-control study was carried out of leukaemia arising as a second primary malignancy following breast or ovarian cancer. Relative risks of 1.5, 3.3 and 7.3 were estimated in association with cumulative doses of <10 g, 10-29 g and >30 g of cyclophosphamide, respectively[5].

Cyclophosphamide is a far less potent leukaemogen than 1,4-butanediol dimethane-sulphonate (Myleran; see p. 137) when used following surgery for lung cancer[6]. Similarly, melphalan (see p. 239) produces a much higher incidence of leukaemia than cyclophosphamide when used in the therapy of multiple myeloma[7] and of ovarian cancer[4].

B. Evidence for carcinogenicity to animals (*sufficient*)

Cyclophosphamide has been tested for carcinogenicity by oral administration and by intravenous and intraperitoneal injection in rats and by subcutaneous and intraperitoneal injection in mice. It produced benign and malignant tumours at various sites, including the bladder, in rats after its oral or intravenous administration, and benign and malignant tumours at the site of injection and at distant sites in mice following its subcutaneous injection. There was some evidence of its carcinogenicity to mice and rats following intraperitoneal injection[1]. A study in which cyclophosphamide was given intraperitoneally to rats in combination with methotrexate (see p. 241) and 5-fluorouracil (see p. 210) resulted in induction of tumours in the nervous system, haematopoietic and lymphatic tissues, the urinary bladder and adrenal glands; however, because of lack of matched controls, it could not be concluded whether tumour induction was due to a combined effect of the three chemicals or of any one of them[8].

C. Other relevant data

Cyclophosphamide is metabolized to an alkylating intermediate. Increased incidences of chromosomal aberrations and sister chromatid exchanges were observed in peripheral blood lymphocytes and, in one study, in bone-marrow cells of patients treated with cyclophosphamide for a variety of malignant and nonmalignant diseases[9].

Cyclophosphamide has been tested extensively for genetic effects in a wide variety of tests *in vivo* and *in vitro*, giving consistently positive results. It bound to DNA in kidney, lung and liver of mice and induced dominant lethal mutations, chromosomal aberrations, micronuclei, sister chromatid exchanges, mutation and DNA damage in rodents treated *in vivo*. In human cells *in vitro*, it induced chromosomal aberrations, sister chromatid exchanges and DNA damage. In rodent cells *in vitro*, it induced transformation, chromosomal aberrations, sister chromatid exchanges, mutation and unscheduled DNA synthesis. In *Drosophila*, it induced aneuploidy, heritable translocations and somatic and sex-linked recessive lethal mutations. In fungi, it induced aneuploidy, mutation, recombination, gene conversion and DNA damage. In bacteria, it induced mutation and DNA damage. In bacteria, it induced mutation and DNA damage. In host-mediated assays, it induced chromosomal aberrations and sister chromatid exchanges in human lymphoid cells, mutation and sister chromatid exchanges in Chinese hamster cells, gene conversion in yeast, and mutation in bacteria. It was active in body-fluid assays of urine from humans and rodents exposed *in vivo*, and in one study using serum from rats[9].

References

[1]*IARC Monographs*, *26*, 165-202, 1981

[2]Kinlen, L.J. (1985) Incidence of cancer in rheumatoid arthritis and other disorders after immunosuppressive treatment. *Am. J. Med.*, *78 (Suppl. 1A)*, 44-49

[3]Pedersen-Bjergaard, J., Ersbøll, J., Sørensen, H.M., Keiding, N., Larsen, S.O., Philip, P., Larsen, M.S., Schultz, H. & Nissen, N.I. (1985) Risk of acute nonlymphocytic leukemia and preleukemia in patients treated with cyclophosphamide for non-Hodgkin's lymphomas. Comparison with results obtained in patients treated for Hodgkin's disease and ovarian carcinoma with other alkylating agents. *Ann. int. Med.*, *103*, 195-200

[4]Greene, M.H., Harris, E.L., Gershenson, D.M., Malkasian, G.D., Jr, Melton, L.J., III, Dembo, A.J., Bennett, J.M., Moloney, W.C. & Boice, J.D., Jr (1986) Melphalan may be a more potent leukemogen than cyclophosphamide. *Ann. int. Med.*, *105*, 360-367

[5]Haas, J.F., Kittelmann, B., Mehnert, W.H., Staneczek, W., Möhner, M., Kaldor, J.M. & Day, N.E. (1987) Risk of leukaemia in ovarian tumour and breast cancer patients following treatment by cyclophosphamide. *Br. J. Cancer*, *55*, 213-218

[6]Stott, H., Fox, W., Girling, D.J., Stephens, R.J. & Galton, D.A.G. (1977) Acute leukaemia after busulphan. *Br. med. J.*, *ii*, 1513-1517

[7]Cuzick, J., Erskine, S., Edelman, D. & Galton, D.A.G. (1987) A comparison of the incidence of myelodysplastic syndrome and acute myeloid leukaemia following melphalan and cyclophosphamide treatment for myelomatosis. A report to the Medical Research Council's Working Party on leukaemia in adults. *Br. J. Cancer*, *55*, 523-529

[8]Habs, M., Schmähl, D. & Lin, P.Z. (1981) Carcinogenic activity in rats of combined treatment with cyclophosphamide, methotrexate and 5-fluorouracil. *Int. J. Cancer*, *28*, 91-96

[9]*IARC Monographs, Suppl. 6*, 196-205, 1987

DACARBAZINE (Group 2B)

A. Evidence for carcinogenicity to humans (*inadequate*)

No epidemiological study of dacarbazine as a single agent was available to the Working Group. Occasional case reports of exposure to dacarbazine, especially in the presence of concurrent therapy with other putative carcinogens, such as ionizing radiation, alkylating agents and other potent oncotherapeutic drugs, do not constitute evidence of carcinogenesis[1].

In a large systematic follow-up of patients with Hogdkin's disease treated with an intensive chemotherapeutic combination including dacarbazine (plus adriamycin [see p. 82], vinblastine [see p. 371] and bleomycins [see p. 134]) but no alkylating agent, preliminary evidence suggested no excess of acute nonlymphocytic leukaemia in the first decade after therapy[2].

B. Evidence for carcinogenicity to animals (*sufficient*)

Following its oral or intraperitoneal administration to rats, dacarbazine produced tumours at various sites, including the mammary gland, thymus, spleen and brain, in as little as 18 weeks after initial exposure[1]. After its intraperitoneal administration to rats at the end of pregnancy, dacarbazine produced tumours, the majority of which were malignant neurinomas, in offspring[3]. Dacarbazine produced tumours at various sites, including lung, haematopoietic tissue and uterus, after intraperitoneal administration to mice[1].

C. Other relevant data

Dacarbazine did not induce sister chromatid exchanges in lymphocytes of treated patients in one study. It gave weakly positive results for induction of sister chromatid exchanges in Chinese hamster cells *in vitro* and was mutagenic to cultured rodent cells and to bacteria[4].

References

[1]*IARC Monographs*, 26, 203-212, 1981

[2]Valagussa, P., Santoro, A., Bellani, F.F., Franchi, F., Banfi, A. & Bonadonna, G. (1982) Absence of treatment-induced second neoplasms after ABVD in Hodgkin's disease. *Blood*, 59, 488-494

[3]Zeller, W.J. (1980) Prenatal carcinogenic action of 5-(3,3-dimethyl-1-triazeno)imidazole-4-carboxamide (DTIC) in the offspring of BD IX rats (Ger.). *Arch. Geschwulstforsch.*, 50, 306-308

[4]*IARC Monographs, Suppl.* 6, 208-209, 1987

DAPSONE (Group 3)

A. Evidence for carcinogenicity to humans (*inadequate*)

Cases of cancer have been reported in patients treated with dapsone for dermatitis herpetiformis[1] and leprosy[2]. Several follow-up studies have been undertaken of patients with leprosy, some of whom were treated with dapsone[1,3-6]. Increased mortality from cancer, restricted to males (standardized mortality ratio [SMR], 1.5; 95% confidence interval, 1.1-1.9), has been observed only in the most recent of them. The excess was most evident for cancers of the oral cavity and bladder and for lymphoma in males (SMRs, 4.5, 4.0 and 3.0, respectively) and for dapsone users. Possible confounding effects of tobacco and alcohol intake could not be addressed, but there was no substantial increase in mortality from lung cancer[6].

B. Evidence for carcinogenicity to animals (*limited*)

Dapsone has been tested by oral administration in mice and rats, by intraperitoneal administration in mice and by prenatal and lifetime oral exposure in mice and rats. In three different studies in rats, high doses of dapsone induced mesenchymal tumours of the spleen in males (and of the peritoneum in two studies). An increased incidence of tumours of the thyroid was found in rats of each sex in one study and in males in a further study. The experiment in mice involving intraperitoneal administration of dapsone could not be evaluated. The other two experiments in mice did not provide evidence of carcinogenicity[1].

C. Other relevant data

No data were available on the genetic and related effects of dapsone in humans. It was not mutagenic to bacteria[7].

References

[1]*IARC Monographs*, 24, 59-76, 1980

[2]Troy, J.L., Grossman, M.E. & Walther, R.R. (1980) Squamous-cell carcinoma arising in a leprous neurotrophic ulcer. Report of a case. *J. Dermatol. Surg. Oncol.*, 6, 659-661

[3]Oleinick, A. (1968) Survival among leprosy patients with special consideration of cancer as a cause of death. *Int. J. Lepr.*, *36*, 318-327

[4]Kolonel, L.N. & Hirohata, T. (1977) Leprosy and cancer: a retrospective cohort study in Hawaii. *J. natl Cancer Inst.*, *58*, 1577-1581

[5]Tokudome, S., Kono, S., Ikeda, M., Kuratsune, M. & Kumamaru, S. (1981) Cancer and other causes of death among leprosy patients. *J. natl Cancer Inst.*, *67*, 285-289

[6]Brinton, L.A., Hoover, R., Jacobson, R.R. & Fraumeni, J.F., Jr (1984) Cancer mortality among patients with Hansen's disease. *J. natl Cancer Inst.*, *72*, 109-114

[7]*IARC Monographs, Suppl. 6*, 210-211, 1987

DDT (Group 2B)

A. Evidence for carcinogenicity to humans (*inadequate*)

Alveolar-cell carcinoma of the lung has been reported in five patients with granulomatous disease of the lungs associated with the inhalation of DDT powder[1]. In four studies[2-5], tissue levels of DDT were reported to be higher in cancer patients than in subjects who died from other causes; no significant difference was found in four other studies[2,6-8], one of which was confined to cancer of the breast and included some living patients[7]. Serum DDT levels appeared to be elevated in another study of nine cancer patients[9], but the study is difficult to interpret. In two case-control studies of soft-tissue sarcoma[10,11] and in three of malignant lymphoma[12-14], relative risks for the association of these diseases with exposure to DDT were 1.2, 1.3, 1.6, 1.5 and 1.8, respectively. Some of the men in these studies had also been exposed to chlorophenoxy herbicides (see p. 156) and chlorophenols (see p. 154), for which there were higher relative risks. Excesses of leukaemia (particularly chronic lymphocytic leukaemia) were noted in two studies[15,16]. A case-control study of colon cancer[17] showed no increased relative risk for exposure to DDT. A small excess of deaths from cancer (3 observed, 1.0 expected) was found in forestry foremen exposed to DDT, 2,4-D and 2,4,5-T[18]. In two other cohort studies of men involved in the manufacture of DDT, there was no increase in mortality from cancer overall[19,20] (standardized mortality ratio [SMR], 68 and 95, respectively), although in one[20], mortality from respiratory cancer was increased slightly (SMR, 156; 95% confidence interval, 74-286). An increase in lung cancer mortality was also observed in agricultural workers who had used DDT and a variety of other pesticides and herbicides (180 [140-240])[21], but a small case-control study of lung cancer deaths in orchardists showed no excess[22]. Studies of pesticide applicators, who use DDT as well as a number of other pesticides, showed excesses of lung cancer[23,24]. In one of these studies, the risk for lung cancer increased with duration of holding a licence to nearly three fold among those licensed for 20 or more years[24]. Exposure to multiple pesticides in these studies prevents a clear evaluation of the cancer risk associated with DDT alone.

B. Evidence for carcinogenicity to animals (*sufficient*)

DDT has been tested for carcinogenicity by oral administration in mice, rats, hamsters, dogs and monkeys and by subcutaneous injection in mice. After oral administration to mice, it caused benign and malignant liver neoplasms, lymphomas and lung neoplasms[2,25]; oral administration to rats caused liver neoplasms[26,27]. Three feeding studies with hamsters gave negative results[2,28,29], and feeding studies with dogs and monkeys were inconclusive[2]. Following subcutaneous injection to mice, it produced liver tumours, lymphomas and lung tumours[25]. Oral administration of DDT enhanced the incidence of liver neoplasms induced in mice by oral administration of *N*-nitrosodiethylamine[30], and the incidences of liver preneoplastic lesions induced in rats by oral administration of 3'-methyl-4-(dimethylamino)-azobenzene[31] and of liver tumours induced in rats by oral administration of *N*-nitrosodiethylamine[32]. Feeding of DDT to rats also accelerated the development of mammary-gland tumours induced by 2-acetamidophenanthrene[33].

C. Other relevant data

In a single study, it was reported that workers exposed to DDT and other pesticides showed increases in chromatid-type aberrations, but not in chromosomal aberrations, in peripheral lymphocytes[34].

Conflicting results were obtained for the induction of dominant lethal mutations in mice and rats. DDT induced chromosomal aberrations in bone-marrow cells of mice, but not of rats, and chromosomal aberrations in spermatocytes of mice treated *in vivo*; it did not induce micronuclei in bone-marrow cells of treated mice. In human cells *in vitro*, it did not induce chromosomal aberrations, mutation or unscheduled DNA synthesis. It did not induce mutation, DNA strand breaks or unscheduled DNA synthesis in cultured rodent cells; conflicting results were obtained for chromosomal aberrations in Chinese hamster cells. DDT inhibited intercellular communication in human and rodent cell systems. It did not induce sex-linked recessive lethal mutations in *Drosophila*, but conflicting results were obtained with regard to aneuploidy; it caused dominant lethal mutations. It did not induce mutation in fungi, either after direct exposure or in a host-mediated assay. DDT was not mutagenic to bacteria and did not induce breakage of plasmid DNA[34].

References

[1]Pimentel, J.C. & Menezes, A.P. (1979) Granulomatous disease with alveolar cell carcinoma due to the inhalation of powdered DDT (Abstract). *Pathology*, *165*, 140

[2]*IARC Monographs*, *5*, 83-124, 1974

[3]Kasai, A., Asanuma, S. & Nakamura, S. (1972) Studies on organochlorine pesticide residues in human organs. Part III (Jpn.). *Nippon Noson Igakkai Zasshi*, *21*, 296-297

[4]Unger, M. & Olsen, J. (1980) Organochlorine compounds in the adipose tissue of deceased people with and without cancer. *Environ. Res.*, *23*, 257-263

[5]Unger, M., Olsen, J. & Clausen, J. (1982) Organochlorine compounds in the adipose tissue of deceased persons with and without cancer: a statistical survey of some potential confounders. *Environ. Res.*, *29*, 371-376

[6]Maier-Bode, H. (1960) DDT in human body fat (Ger.). *Med. exp. (Basel)*, *1*, 146-152

[7]Unger, M., Kiaer, H., Blichert-Toft, M., Olsen, J. & Clausen, J. (1984) Organochlorine compounds in human breast fat from deceased with and without breast cancer and in a biopsy material from newly diagnosed patients undergoing breast surgery. *Environ. Res., 34,* 24-28

[8]Davies, J.E., Barquet, A., Morgade, C. & Raffonelli, A. (1975) *Epidemiologic studies of DDT and dieldrin residues and their relationship to human carcinogenesis.* In: *Proceedings of the International Symposium on Recent Advances Assessing Health Effects of Environmental Pollution, 1974,* Vol. 2 (*EUR 5360*), Luxembourg, Commission of the European Communities, pp. 695-702

[9]Caldwell, G.G., Cannon, S.B., Pratt, C.B. & Arthur, R.D. (1981) Serum pesticide levels in patients with childhood colorectal carcinoma. *Cancer, 48,* 774-778

[10]Hardell, L. & Sandström, A. (1979) Case-control study: soft-tissue sarcomas and exposure to phenoxyacetic acids or chlorophenols. *Br. J. Cancer, 39,* 711-717

[11]Eriksson, M., Hardell, L., Berg, N.O., Möller, T. & Axelson, O. (1981) Soft-tissue sarcomas and exposure to chemical substances: a case-referent study. *Br. J. ind. Med., 38,* 27-33

[12]Hardell, L., Eriksson, M., Lenner, P. & Lundgren, E. (1981) Malignant lymphoma and exposure to chemicals, especially organic solvents, chlorophenols and phenoxy acids: a case-control study. *Br. J. Cancer, 43,* 169-176

[13]Cantor, K., Everett, G., Blair, A., Gibson, R., Schuman, L. & Isacson, P. (1984) Farming and non-Hodgkin's lymphoma (Abstract). *Am. J. Epidemiol., 122,* 535

[14]Woods, J.S., Polissar, L., Severson, R.K., Heuser, L.S. & Kulander, B.G. (1987) Soft-tissue sarcoma and non-Hodgkin's lymphoma in relation to phenoxy herbicide and chlorinated exposure in western Washington. *J. natl Cancer Inst., 78,* 899-910

[15]Blair, A., Everett, G., Cantor, K., Gibson, R., Schuman, L., Isacson, P., Blattner, W. & Van Lier, S. (1985) Leukemia and farm practices (Abstract). *Am. J. Epidemiol., 122,* 535

[16]Flodin, U., Fredriksson, M., Persson, B. & Axelson, O. (1987) Chronic lymphatic leukaemia and engine exhausts, fresh wood and DDT. A case-referent study. *Br. J. ind. Med.* (in press)

[17]Hardell, L. (1981) Relation of soft-tissue sarcoma, malignant lymphoma and colon cancer to phenoxy acids, chlorophenols and other agents. *Scand. J. Work Environ. Health, 7,* 119-130

[18]Hogstedt, C. & Westerlund, B. (1980) Cohort studies on causes of death of forestry workers with and without exposure to phenoxyacid preparations (Swed.). *Läkartidningen, 77,* 1828-1831

[19]Ditraglia, D., Brown, D.P., Namekata, T. & Iverson, N. (1981) Mortality study of workers employed at organochlorine pesticide manufacturing plants. *Scand. J. Work Environ. Health, 7 (Suppl. 4),* 140-146

[20]Wong, O., Brocker, W., Davis, H.V. & Nagle, G.S. (1984) Mortality of workers potentially exposed to organic and inorganic brominated chemicals, DBCP, Tris, PBB, and DDT. *Br. J. ind. Med., 41,* 15-24

[21]Bartel, E. (1981) Increased risk of lung cancer in pesticide-exposed male agricultural workers. *J. Toxicol. environ. Health, 8,* 1027-1040

[22]Wiklund, K.G.K. (1983) Respiratory cancer among orchardists in Washington State, 1968-1980 (Abstract). *Diss. Abstr. int., 44,* 128-B

[23]Wang, H.H. & MacMahon, B. (1979) Mortality of pesticide applicators. *J. occup. Med., 21,* 741-744

[24]Blair, A., Grauman, D.J., Lubin, J.H. & Fraumeni, J.F., Jr (1983) Lung cancer and other causes of death among licensed pesticide applicators. *J. natl Cancer Inst., 71,* 31-37

[25]Kashyap, S.K., Nigam, S.K., Karnik, A.B., Gupta, R.C. & Chatterjee, S.K. (1977) Carcinogenicity of DDT (dichlorodiphenyltrichloroethane) in pure inbred Swiss mice. *Int. J. Cancer*, *19*, 725-729

[26]Rossi, L., Ravera, M., Repetti, G. & Santi, L. (1977) Long-term administration of DDT or phenobarbital-Na in Wistar rats. *Int. J. Cancer*, *19*, 179-185

[27]Cabral, J.R.P., Hall, R.K., Rossi, L., Bronczyk, S.A. & Shubik, P. (1982a) Effects of long-term intake of DDT on rats. *Tumori*, *68*, 11-17

[28]Cabral, J.R.P., Hall, R.K., Rossi, L., Bronczyk, S.A. & Shubik, P. (1982b) Lack of carcinogenicity of DDT in hamsters. *Tumori*, *68*, 5-10

[29]Rossi, L., Barbieri, O., Sanguineti, M., Cabral, J.R.P., Bruzzi, P. & Santi, L. (1983) Carcinogenicity study with technical-grade dichlorodiphenyltrichloroethane and 1,1-dichloro-2,2-bis(*p*-chlorophenyl)ethylene in hamsters. *Cancer Res.*, *43*, 776-781

[30]Williams, G.M. & Numoto, S. (1984) Promotion of mouse liver neoplasms by the organochlorine pesticides chlordane and heptachlor in comparison to dichlorodiphenyltrichloroethane. *Carcinogenesis*, *5*, 1689-1696

[31]Kitagawa, T., Hino, O., Nomura, K. & Sugano, H. (1984) Dose-response studies on promoting and anticarcinogenic effects of phenobarbital and DDT in the rat hepatocarcinogenesis. *Carcinogenesis*, *5*, 1653-1656

[32]Nishizumi, M. (1979) Effect of phenobarbital, dichlorodiphenyltrichloroethane, and polychlorinated biphenyls on diethylnitrosamine-induced hepatocarcinogenesis. *Gann*, *70*, 835-837

[33]Scribner, J.D. & Mottet, N.K. (1981) DDT acceleration of mammary gland tumors induced in the male Sprague-Dawley rat by 2-acetamidophenanthrene. *Carcinogenesis*, *2*, 1235-1239

[34]*IARC Monographs, Suppl. 6*, 212-215, 1987

DIAZEPAM (Group 3)

A. Evidence for carcinogenicity to humans (*inadequate*)

A short-term screening study of 12 961 users of diazepam showed no evidence of excess of any cancer, and one negative association (lower risks of lymphoma and leukaemia than expected) was found over a four-year period. The morbidity ratio for all cancers was 1.0[1]. Subsequent studies have tended to concentrate on the suggestion that diazepam acts as a promoter in cancer[2], and most relate to breast cancer. No evidence of increased risk of breast cancer with diazepam use was found in a breast cancer screening study. The relative risk for 'ever' use of diazepam was 0.87 (95% confidence interval, 0.7-1.1). For use of diazepam 15 or more years earlier, the relative risk was 1.1 (0.5-2.4); for three or more years since last use of diazepam, the relative risk was 0.94 (0.7-1.3)[3]. Subsequent evaluation of the data from this study showed a negative association between diazepam use and extent of breast cancer and lymph node involvement[4]. These data suggest that diazepam does not act during the late stages of induction of breast cancer. The hypothesis was further evaluated in two case-control studies of breast cancer[5,6]. In one, 1236 cases of breast cancer and 728 controls with other malignancies were evaluated. The relative risk for women who had used diazepam four days a week for at least six months was 0.9 (0.5-1.6)[5]. In the second study, no increased risk from diazepam use was found in 151 breast cancer cases in comparison with 151 hospital controls (relative risk, 0.95)[6]. In a further study of women newly diagnosed with breast cancer, the age-adjusted risk ratio for diazepam use six months prior to diagnosis was 0.9 (0.7-1.3)[7]. Diazepam use was also studied in relation to malignant melanoma in a case-control study of 166 cases and 498 controls, using both medical records and questionnaires. Although 35% of the cases and 33% of the controls did not return questionnaires, neither data source suggested excess use of diazepam by the cases[8].

The evidence that diazepam is not a breast carcinogen could not be described as 'suggesting lack of carcinogenicity' for breast cancer, because of (1) the restricted statistical power to detect increases after long latent periods or to detect small increases (i.e., relative risks under 2.0), even though these might be expected under reasonable hypotheses, and (2) the special problems of studying a human cancer closely tied to life events in relation to usage of a drug given for poorly defined indications.

B. Evidence for carcinogenicity to animals (*inadequate*)

Oral administration of diazepam to mice resulted in an elevated incidence of liver tumours in males[9]. In rats, a study reported in detail[9] and one reported briefly[10] showed no increase in the incidence of tumours of any type compared to controls. In limited bioassays, oral administration of diazepam enhanced the occurrence of liver preneoplastic lesions and neoplasms induced in mice by N-nitrosodiethylamine[11], but not that induced in rats by 3'-methyl-4-(dimethylamino)azobenzene or 2-acetylaminofluorene[12,13].

C. Other relevant data

A metabolite of diazepam, oxazepam, produced liver tumours in mice after its oral administration[14].

Neither chromosomal aberrations nor sister chromatid exchanges (one study) were observed in the lymphocytes of patients receiving treatment with diazepam[15].

Diazepam did not induce chromosomal aberrations in bone-marrow cells of Chinese hamsters treated *in vivo*, or in human or Chinese hamster cells *in vitro*. It did not inhibit intercellular communication in cultured rat hepatocytes. It was not mutagenic to bacteria, but urine from mice treated with diazepam showed increased mutagenicity as compared to controls[15].

References

[1]Friedman, G.D. & Ury, H.K. (1980) Initial screening for carcinogenicity of commonly used drugs. *J. natl Cancer Inst.*, *65*, 723-733

[2]Horrobin, D.F. (1981) Diazepam as tumour promoter. *Lancet*, *i*, 277-278

[3]Kleinerman, R.A., Brinton, L.A., Hoover, R. & Fraumeni, J.F., Jr (1981) Diazepam and breast cancer. *Lancet*, *i*, 1153

[4]Kleinerman, R.A., Brinton, L.A., Hoover, R. & Fraumeni, J.F., Jr (1984) Diazepam use and progression of breast cancer. *Cancer Res.*, *44*, 1223-1225

[5]Kaufman, D.W., Shapiro, S., Slone, D., Rosenberg, L., Helmrich, S.P., Miettinen, O.S., Stolley, P.D., Levy, M. & Schottenfeld, D. (1982) Diazepam and the risk of breast cancer. *Lancet*, *i*, 537-539

[6]Wallace, R.B., Sherman, B.M. & Bean, J.A. (1982) A case-control study of breast cancer and psychotropic drug use. *Oncology*, *39*, 279-283

[7]Danielson, D.A., Jick, H., Hunter, J.R., Stergachis, A. & Madsen, S. (1982) Nonestrogenic drugs and breast cancer. *Am. J. Epidemiol.*, *116*, 329-332

[8]Adam, S. & Vessey, M. (1981) Diazepam and malignant melanoma. *Lancet*, *ii*, 1344

[9]de la Iglesia, F.A., Barsoum, N., Gough, A., Mitchell, L., Martin, R.A., Di Fonzo, C. & McGuire, E.J. (1981) Carcinogenesis bioassay of prazepam (Verstran) in rats and mice. *Toxicol. appl. Pharmacol.*, *57*, 39-54

[10]Jackson, M.R. & Harris, P.A. (1981) Absence of effect of diazepam on tumours. *Lancet*, *i*, 104

[11]Diwan, B.A., Rice, J.M. & Ward, J.M. (1986) Tumor-promoting activity of benzodiazepine tranquilizers, diazepam and oxazepam, in mouse liver. *Carcinogenesis*, *7*, 789-794

[12]Hino, O. & Kitagawa, T. (1982) Effect of diazepam on hepatocarcinogenesis in the rat. *Toxicol. Lett.*, *11*, 155-157

[13]Remandet, B., Gouy, D., Berthe, J., Mazue, G. & Williams, G.M. (1984) Lack of initiating or promoting activity of six benzodiazepine tranquilizers in rat liver limited bioassays monitored by histopathology and assay of liver and plasma enzymes. *Fundam. appl. Toxicol.*, *4*, 152-163

[14]*IARC Monographs*, *13*, 57-73, 1977

[15]*IARC Monographs*, *Suppl. 6*, 216-218, 1987

1,2-DIBROMO-3-CHLOROPROPANE (Group 2B)

A. Evidence for carcinogenicity to humans (*inadequate*)

Among a cohort of 550 chemical workers exposed to many compounds including 1,3-dibromo-3-chloropropane, a moderate, statistically nonsignificant increase in mortality from cancers at all sites was found (12 observed, 7.7 expected), due mainly to deaths from respiratory cancer. The slight excess was not removed after controlling for exposure to arsenicals[1].

A group of some 3500 workers classified as having had exposure on a 'routine' or 'nonroutine' basis to several brominated chemicals, including 1,2-dibromo-3-chloro-propane, was studied in four facilities in the USA. Among the 1034 workers ever exposed to 1,2-dibromo-3-chloropropane, a slightly increased, statistically nonsignificant mortality rate from cancer was observed. Nine respiratory cancers were observed, whereas 5.0 would have been expected; of these, seven were due to lung cancer (4.8 expected). Among 238 workers exposed on a 'routine' basis, no cancer death was observed[2].

In view of the numbers involved and the lack of control of confounding factors, the studies were considered to be inadequate.

B. Evidence for carcinogenicity to animals (*sufficient*)

1,2-Dibromo-3-chloropropane has been tested by oral administration and inhalation in mice and rats. After oral administration, it produced squamous-cell carcinomas of the forestomach in animals of each species and adenocarcinomas of the mammary gland in female rats[3]. After inhalation, it induced nasal cavity and lung tumours in mice, and nasal cavity and tongue tumours in rats of each sex and adrenal cortex adenomas in females[4].

C. Other relevant data

Several reports indicate that occupational exposure to 1,2-dibromo-3-chloropropane may result in azospermia[5].

1,2-Dibromo-3-chloropropane induced dominant lethal mutations in rats, but not in mice, and DNA strand breaks in rat testicular cells and unscheduled DNA synthesis in mouse testicular cells, but not abnormalities in sperm morphology in mice treated *in vivo*. In studies *in vitro*, it induced chromosomal aberrations and sister chromatid exchanges in Chinese hamster cells and DNA strand breaks in rat testicular cells. In *Drosophila*, it induced aneuploidy and sex-linked recessive lethal mutations; heritable translocation was seen in one study but not in another, although crossing-over was found in the latter. It was mutagenic to bacteria but did not cause DNA damage[5].

References

[1]Hearn, S., Ott, M.G., Kolesar, R.C. & Cook, R.R. (1984) Mortality experience of employees with occupational exposure to DBCP. *J. occup. Med., 39*, 49-55

[2]Wong, O., Brocker, W., Davis, H.V. & Nagle, G.S. (1984) Mortality of workers potentially exposed to organic and inorganic brominated chemicals, DBCP, Tris, PBB, and DDT. *Br. J. ind. Med., 41*, 15-24

[3]*IARC Monographs, 20*, 83-96, 1979

[4]National Toxicology Program (1982) *Carcinogenesis Bioassay of 1,2-Dibromo-3-chloropropane (CAS No. 96-12-8) in F344 Rats and B6C3F₁ Mice (Inhalation Studies) (NTP Technical Report 206; NIH Publ. No. 82-1762)*, Research Triangle Park, NC

[5]*IARC Monographs, Suppl. 6*, 219-221, 1987

ortho-DICHLOROBENZENE (Group 3) and *para*-DICHLOROBENZENE (Group 2B)

A. Evidence for carcinogenicity to humans (*inadequate*)

One report of a series of five cases has suggested an association between leukaemia and exposure to dichlorobenzenes[1].

B. Evidence for carcinogenicity to animals (*inadequate* for *ortho*-dichlorobenzene; *sufficient* for *para*-dichlorobenzene)

ortho-Dichlorobenzene was tested in mice and rats by gastric intubation; no evidence of carcinogenicity was observed[2]. A study by inhalation in several species was considered inadequate[1].

para-Dichlorobenzene was tested in mice and rats by gastric intubation; it caused renal tubular-cell adenocarcinomas in male rats and hepatocellular carcinomas in male and female mice[3]. It was also tested in mice and rats by inhalation; no increase in the incidence of tumours was noted, but the duration of exposure was limited[4].

C. Other relevant data

No data were available on the genetic and related effects of *ortho*- or *para*-dichlorobenzene in humans. *ortho*-Dichlorobenzene was not mutagenic to fungi or bacteria. *para*-Dichlorobenzene was mutagenic to fungi but not to bacteria[5].

References

[1]*IARC Monographs*, 29, 213-238, 1982

[2]National Toxicology Programme (1985) *Toxicology and Carcinogenesis Studies of 1,2-Dichlorobenzene (o-Dichlorobenzene) (CAS No. 95-50-1) in F344/N Rats and B6C3F$_1$ Mice (Gavage Studies) (NTP TR 255; NIH Publ. No. 86-2511)*, Research Triangle Park, NC

[3]National Toxicology Program (1987) *Toxicology and Carcinogenesis Studies of 1,4-Dichlorobenzene (CAS No. 106-46-7) in F344/N Rats and B6C3F$_1$ Mice (Gavage Studies) (NTP TR No. 319; NIH Publ. No. 87-2575)*, Research Triangle Park, NC

[4]Loeser, E. & Litchfield, M.H. (1983) Review of recent toxicology studies on *p*-dichlorobenzene. *Food chem. Toxicol., 21*, 825-832

[5]*IARC Monographs, Suppl. 6*, 222-225, 1987

3,3'-DICHLOROBENZIDINE (Group 2B)

A. Evidence for carcinogenicity to humans (*inadequate*)

Three retrospective epidemiological studies of workers exposed to 3,3'-dichlorobenzidine gave no evidence of carcinogenicity, but the studies were of insufficient quality or statistical power to permit confident exclusion of this possibility. Because 3,3'-dichlorobenzidine and benzidine (see p. 123) may be made in the same plant, 3,3'-dichlorobenzidine may have contributed to the incidence of bladder cancer attributed to benzidine[1].

B. Evidence for carcinogenicity to animals (*sufficient*)

3,3'-Dichlorobenzidine was tested for carcinogenicity in mice, rats, hamsters and dogs by oral administration, in rats by subcutaneous administration and in mice by transplacental exposure. Following its oral administration, it produced liver-cell tumours in mice, hepatocellular carcinomas in dogs, mammary and Zymbal-gland tumours in rats and carcinomas of the urinary bladder in hamsters and dogs. Increased incidences of leukaemias were observed in rats following oral administration and in mice following transplacental exposure[1].

C. Other relevant data

No data were available on the genetic and related effects of 3,3'-dichlorobenzidine in humans. It has been reported to induce unscheduled DNA synthesis in cultured human cells. It was mutagenic to bacteria[2].

References

[1]*IARC Monographs, 29*, 239-256, 1982
[2]*IARC Monographs, Suppl. 6*, 226-227, 1987

DICHLOROMETHANE (Group 2B)

A. Evidence for carcinogenicity to humans (*inadequate*)

No excess risk of death from malignancies was observed in one proportionate mortality study of 334 persons or in two cohort studies, one of which was a 13-year cohort mortality study of 751 employees exposed to dichloromethane, of whom 252 had had at least 20 years of work exposure, and the other a cohort study of 1271 workers in a fibre production plant in which dichloromethane was used as a solvent[1]. The first cohort study was later updated through to 1984 and expanded to comprise 1013 full-time, hourly employees. No statistically significant excess was observed for such hypothesized causes of mortality as lung cancer (14 observed, 21 expected) and liver cancer (none observed, 0.8 expected) or for cancer at any other site[2]. The proportionate mortality study and the first cohort mortality study concern partially overlapping populations. The studies had limited power to detect excess risk[1].

B. Evidence for carcinogenicity to animals (*sufficient*)

Dichloromethane was tested by oral administration in mice and rats, by inhalation exposure in mice, rats and hamsters, and by intraperitoneal injection in a lung-adenoma assay in mice. Exposure by inhalation increased the incidences of benign and malignant lung and liver tumours in mice of each sex, the incidence and multiplicity of benign mammary tumours in rats of each sex and the incidence of sarcomas located in the neck of male rats[1]. In another study in rats exposed by inhalation, an increase in the total number of malignant tumours was found in rats of each sex. After its oral administration, an increased incidence of lung tumours was seen in male mice and an increased incidence of malignant mammary tumours in female rats[3]. Other studies by oral administration in mice and in male rats and a study by inhalation in male hamsters gave negative results. Inconclusive results were obtained after oral administration to female rats and after exposure by inhalation of female hamsters. In a mouse-lung adenoma bioassay by intraperitoneal injection, negative results were obtained[1].

C. Other relevant data

No data were available on the genetic and related effects of dichloromethane in humans.

It did not induce chromosomal aberrations in bone-marrow cells of rats or micronuclei in mice treated *in vivo*. Unscheduled DNA synthesis was not induced in human cells *in vitro*. Dichloromethane induced transformation of virus-infected Fischer rat and Syrian hamster embryo cells. It induced chromosomal aberrations, but not mutation or DNA damage, in rodent cells *in vitro*; conflicting results were reported for the induction of sister chromatid exchanges in Chinese hamster cells. It induced sex-linked recessive lethal mutations in *Drosophila*. It was mutagenic to plants and induced mutation, mitotic recombination and gene conversion in *Saccharomyces cerevisiae* under conditions in which endogenous levels of cytochrome P450 were enhanced. It was mutagenic to bacteria[4].

References

[1]*IARC Monographs, 41*, 43-85, 1986

[2]Hearne, F.T., Grose, F., Pifer, J.W., Friedlander, B.R. & Raleigh, R.L. (1987) Methylene chloride mortality study: dose-response characterization and animal model comparison. *J. occup. Med., 29*, 217-228

[3]Maltoni, C., Cotti, G. & Perino, G. (1986) *Experimental research on methylene chloride carcinogenesis.* In: Maltoni, C. & Mehlman, M.A., eds, *Archives of Research on Industrial Carcinogenesis*, Vol. IV, Princeton, Princeton Scientific Publishing, pp. 1-244

[4]*IARC Monographs, Suppl. 6*, 228-230, 1987

1,3-DICHLOROPROPENE (TECHNICAL-GRADE) (Group 2B)

A. Evidence for carcinogenicity to humans (*inadequate*)

Two cases of malignant histiocytic lymphoma were reported among nine fireman accidentally exposed to 1,3-dichloropropene six years prior to diagnosis[1]. Because firemen are exposed to a large number of chemicals, the role of 1,3-dichloropropene cannot be evaluated.

B. Evidence for carcinogenicity to animals (*sufficient*)

Technical-grade 1,3-dichloropropene (containing 1.0% epichlorohydrin [see p. 202]), administered by gavage, produced tumours of the urinary bladder, lung and forestomach in mice and of the liver and forestomach in rats. After subcutaneous administration to mice, the purified *cis*-isomer produced malignant tumours at the site of injection[1].

C. Other relevant data

No data were available on the genetic and related effects of 1,3-dichloropropene in humans. It induced unscheduled DNA synthesis in human cells *in vitro* and sex-linked recessive lethal mutations but not reciprocal translocations in *Drosophila*. Both the individual *cis* and *trans* isomers and a mixture of the two were mutagenic to bacteria[2].

References

[1]*IARC Monographs, 41*, 113-130, 1986

[2]*IARC Monographs, Suppl. 6*, 237-239, 1987

DIELDRIN (Group 3)

A. Evidence for carcinogenicity to humans (*inadequate*)

Mean tissue levels of dieldrin were reported to be elevated in one necropsy study of 50 cancer patients compared to 42 control subjects[1]. Mean serum levels were also reported to be elevated in cancer patients compared with controls in one study[2], but not in another[3]. Follow-up for four to 29 years (mean, 24 years) of 233 workers employed for four to 27 years (mean, 11 years) in the manufacture of aldrin (see p. 88), dieldrin and endrin revealed nine deaths from cancer with 12 expected (standardized mortality ratio [SMR], 75; 95% confidence interval, 25-125)[4,5]. In a similar study, 90% of 1155 men employed in the manufacture of aldrin, dieldrin and endrin were followed for 13 years or more. Mortality from all cancers was not increased (82; 56-116), although there were apparent increases in mortality from cancers of the oesophagus, rectum and liver, based on very small numbers[6].

B. Evidence for carcinogenicity to animals (*limited*)

Dieldrin has been tested by oral administration in mice, rats, trout, hamsters, dogs and monkeys. In mice, it produced benign and malignant liver neoplasms[1,7-10]; no carcinogenic effect was observed in feeding studies using several strains of rats[1,8,11], trout[12] and hamsters[13], the latter having been given relatively high doses. Feeding studies in dogs and monkeys were inadequate for evaluation[1]. Dietary administration to trout of dieldrin enhanced the incidence of liver tumours induced by dietary administration of aflatoxin B_1[12].

C. Other relevant data

In one study, chromosomal aberrations were not found in peripheral blood lymphocytes of workers exposed to dieldrin[14].

Dieldrin did not induce dominant lethal mutations in mice or chromosomal aberrations in bone-marrow cells of Chinese hamsters treated *in vivo*. It induced unscheduled DNA synthesis in transformed human fibroblasts but not in rat hepatocytes; it did not induce single-strand breaks in Chinese hamster V79 cells. Dieldrin inhibited intercellular communication in human and rodent cell systems. It did not induce sex-linked recessive lethal mutations in *Drosophila*, was not mutagenic to bacteria and did not induce breakage of plasmid DNA[14].

References

[1]*IARC Monographs, 5*, 125-156, 1974

[2]Caldwell, G.G., Cannon, S.B., Pratt, C.B. & Arthur, R.D. (1981) Serum pesticide levels in patients with childhood colorectal carcinoma. *Cancer, 48*, 774-778

[3]Davies, J.E., Barquet, A., Morgade, C. & Raffonelli, A. (1975) *Epidemiologic studies of DDT and dieldrin residues and their relationship to human carcinogenesis.* In: *Proceedings of an International Symposition on Recent Advances in Assessing Health Effects of Environmental Pollution*, Vol. 2 (*EUR 5360*), Luxembourg, Commission of the European Communities, pp. 695-702

[4]van Raalte, H.G.S. (1977) Human experience with dieldrin in perspective. *Ecotoxicol. environ. Saf., 1*, 203-210

[5]Ribbens, P.H. (1985) Mortality study of industrial workers exposed to aldrin, dieldrin and endrin. *Int. Arch. occup. environ. Health, 56*, 75-79

[6]Ditraglia, D., Brown, D.P., Namekata, T. & Iverson, N. (1981) Mortality study of workers employed at organochlorine pesticide manufacturing plants. *Scand. J. Work Environ. Health, 7 (Suppl. 4)*, 140-146

[7]Tennekes, H.A., Wright, A.S., Dix, K.M. & Koeman, J.H. (1981) Effects of dieldrin, diet, and bedding on enzyme function and tumor incidence in livers of male CF-1 mice. *Cancer Res., 41*, 3615-3620

[8]National Cancer Institute (1978) *Bioassays of Aldrin and Dieldrin for Possible Carcinogenicity* (*Tech. Rep. Ser. No. 21; DHEW Publ. No. (NIH) 78-821*), Bethesda, MD, Carcinogenesis Testing Program, Division of Cancer Cause and Prevention

[9]Ruebner, B.H., Gershwin, M.E., Hsieh, L. & Dunn, P. (1980) Ultrastructure of spontaneous neoplasms induced by diethylnitrosamine and dieldrin in the C_3H mouse. *J. environ. Pathol. Toxicol., 4*, 237-254

[10]Meierhenry, E.F., Ruebner, B.H., Gershwin, M.E., Hsieh, L.S. & French, S.W. (1983) Dieldrin-induced Mallory bodies in hepatic tumors of mice of different strains. *Hepatology, 3*, 90-95

[11]National Cancer Institute (1978) *Bioassay of Dieldrin for Possible Carcinogenicity* (*Tech. Rep. Ser. No. 22; DHEW Publ. No. (NIH) 78-822*), Bethesda, MD, Carcinogenesis Testing Program, Division of Cancer Cause and Prevention

[12]Hendricks, J.D., Putnam, T.P. & Sinnhuber, R.O. (1979) Effect of dietary dieldrin on aflatoxin B_1 carcinogenesis in rainbow trout (*Salmo gairdneri*). *J. environ. Pathol. Toxicol., 2*, 719-728

[13]Cabral, J.R.P., Hall, R.K., Bronczyk, S.A. & Shubik, P. (1979) A carcinogenicity study of the pesticide dieldrin in hamsters. *Cancer Lett., 6*, 241-246

[14]*IARC Monographs, Suppl. 6*, 242-244, 1987

DIETHYL SULPHATE (Group 2A)

A. Evidence for carcinogenicity to humans (*limited*)

A historical cohort study of 335 process workers and 408 chemical mechanics and refinery workers at a plant manufacturing isopropyl alcohol (see p. 229) and ethanol in a petrochemical complex showed excess mortality (standardized mortality ratio, 504) from upper respiratory (laryngeal) cancers based on four cases. These persons had spent most of their time working in the strong acid-ethanol plant, which produced high concentrations of diethyl sulphate[1].

B. Evidence for carcinogenicity to animals (*sufficient*)

Diethyl sulphate produced local tumours in rats following its subcutaneous administration and produced tumours of the nervous system after prenatal exposure. A few tumours of the forestomach occurred in rats given diethyl sulphate by gavage[2].

C. Other relevant data

Diethyl sulphate is an alkylating agent[2]. No data were available on the genetic and related effects of this compound in humans.

Diethyl sulphate induced chromatid breaks in mouse embryos treated transplacentally and dominant lethal mutations in mice. It induced unscheduled DNA synthesis in human cells *in vitro* and chromosomal aberrations, micronuclei, sister chromatid exchanges, mutation, DNA strand breaks and DNA alkylation in rodent cells *in vitro*. In *Drosophila*, it induced sex-linked recessive lethal mutations, crossing-over and chromosomal aberrations. It induced chromosomal aberrations, mutation and DNA damage in plants and mutation in fungi. It was mutagenic to bacteria[3].

References

[1]Lynch, J., Hanis, N.M., Bird, M.G., Murray, K.J. & Walsh, J.P. (1979) An association of upper respiratory cancer with exposure to diethyl sulphate. *J. occup. Med.*, *21*, 333-341

[2]*IARC Monographs*, *4*, 277-281, 1974

[3]*IARC Monographs*, *Suppl. 6*, 257-259, 1987

3,3′-DIMETHOXYBENZIDINE (*ortho*-DIANISIDINE) (Group 2B)

A. Evidence for carcinogenicity to humans (*inadequate*)

3,3′-Dimethoxybenzidine (together with 3,3′-dichlorobenzidine [see p. 193] and *ortho*-toluidine [see p. 362]) has been prepared in the same plants as benzidine (see p. 123) and may therefore have contributed to the bladder cancer risk associated with benzidine[1]. No case is on record in the USSR of an occupational urinary bladder neoplasm produced solely by this compound[2].

B. Evidence for carcinogenicity to animals (*sufficient*)

Following its oral administration, 3,3′-dimethoxybenzidine produced tumours in rats at various sites, including the bladder, intestine, skin and Zymbal gland; it produced forestomach papillomas in hamsters[3].

C. Other relevant data

3,3′-Dimethoxybenzidine has been found in the urine of workers exposed to it[3].

No data were available on the genetic and related effects of 3,3′-dimethoxybenzidine in humans. It induced sister chromatid exchanges in Chinese hamster cells *in vitro* and unscheduled DNA synthesis in human cells and rat hepatocytes *in vitro*. It was mutagenic to bacteria[4].

References

[1]Clayson, D.B. (1976) Occupational bladder cancer. *Prev. Med., 5*, 228-244

[2]Genin, V.A. (1974) Hygienic assessment of dianisidine-sulphate production from standpoint of carcinogenous hazard for workers (Russ.). *Gig. Tr. prof. Zabol., 6*, 18-22

[3]*IARC Monographs, 4*, 41-47, 1974

[4]*IARC Monographs, Suppl. 6*, 262-263, 1987

DIMETHYLCARBAMOYL CHLORIDE (Group 2A)

A. Evidence for carcinogenicity to humans (*inadequate*)

No death from cancer was reported in an investigation of 39 dimethylcarbamoyl chloride production workers, 26 processing workers and 42 ex-workers aged 17-65 exposed for periods ranging from six months to 12 years[1].

B. Evidence for carcinogenicity to animals (*sufficient*)

Dimethylcarbamoyl chloride was tested for carcinogenicity by skin application and by subcutaneous and intraperitoneal injection in female mice of one strain; it induced local tumours[1]. In another experiment, exposure of rats and male hamsters to dimethyl-carbamoyl chloride by inhalation induced a high incidence of nasal-tract carcinomas[2].

C. Other relevant data

No data were available on the genetic and related effects of dimethylcarbamoyl chloride in humans.

Dimethylcarbamoyl chloride induced micronuclei but not sister chromatid exchanges in mice treated *in vivo*. It did not cause unscheduled DNA synthesis in human fibroblasts *in vitro*. It induced transformation of Syrian hamster embryo cells and chromosomal aberrations in Chinese hamster cells; conflicting results were obtained with regard to the induction of sister chromatid exchanges. It was mutagenic to mouse lymphoma cells; it did not induce unscheduled DNA synthesis in rat hepatocytes but did induce DNA strand breaks in Chinese hamster cells. Dimethylcarbamoyl chloride did not induce sex-linked recessive lethal mutations in *Drosophila*; it induced aneuploidy, mutation, gene conversion and DNA damage in yeast. It was mutagenic to bacteria and caused DNA damage[3].

References

[1]*IARC Monographs*, *12*, 77-84, 1976

[2]Sellakumar, A.R., Laskin, S., Kuschner, M., Rusch, G., Katz, G.V., Snyder, C.A. & Albert, R.E. (1980) Inhalation carcinogenesis by dimethylcarbamoyl chloride in Syrian golden hamsters. *J. environ. Pathol. Toxicol.*, *4*, 107-115

[3]*IARC Monographs*, *Suppl. 6*, 265-268, 1987

DIMETHYL SULPHATE (Group 2A)

A. Evidence for carcinogenicity to humans (*inadequate*)

Four cases of bronchial carcinoma were reported in men exposed occupationally to dimethyl sulphate[1]. Additional case reports have since appeared: a case of pulmonary carcinoma in a man exposed for seven years to 'small amounts' of dimethyl sulphate but to larger amounts of bis(chloromethyl)ether and chloromethyl methyl ether (see p. 131)[2], and a case of choroidal melanoma in a man exposed for six years to dimethyl sulphate[3].

B. Evidence for carcinogenicity to animals (*sufficient*)

Dimethyl sulphate produced mainly local tumours in rats following its inhalation or subcutaneous injection; it produced tumours of the nervous system after prenatal exposure[1].

C. Other relevant data

Dimethyl sulphate is an alkylating agent[4]. No data were available on the genetic and related effects of this compound in humans.

Dimethyl sulphate induced both structural and numerical chromosomal aberrations in bone-marrow cells of rats treated *in vivo* and chromatid breaks in mouse embryos treated transplacentally. It alkylated DNA in rats treated *in vivo* and in cultured rodent cells. It induced sister chromatid exchanges, unscheduled DNA synthesis and DNA strand breaks in human and rodent cells *in vitro*, and chromosomal aberrations and mutation in cultured rodent cells. It induced sex-linked recessive lethal mutations in *Drosophila* and mutation and mitotic recombination in yeast. Conflicting results were obtained for chromosomal aberrations and mutation in plants. It induced mutation and DNA damage in bacteria[4].

References

[1]*IARC Monographs*, 4, 271-276, 1974

[2]Bettendorf, U. (1977) Occupational lung cancer after inhalation of alkylating compounds. Dichlorodimethyl ether, monochlorodimethyl ether and dimethyl sulphate (Ger.). *Dtsch. med. Wochenschr.*, 102, 396-398

[3]Albert, D.M. & Puliafito, C.A. (1977) Choroidal melanoma: possible exposure to industrial toxins. *New Engl. J. Med.*, 296, 634-635

[4]*IARC Monographs, Suppl. 6*, 269-271, 1987

1,4-DIOXANE (Group 2B)

A. Evidence for carcinogenicity to humans (*inadequate*)

In a mortality study of 165 workers who had been exposed to low concentrations of 1,4-dioxane since 1954, seven deaths had occurred by 1975, two of which were from cancer[1].

B. Evidence for carcinogenicity to animals (*sufficient*)

Administration of 1,4-dioxane in drinking-water at several dose levels to rats and male guinea-pigs produced adenomas and carcinomas of the liver in rats of each sex, hepatomas in guinea-pigs, carcinomas of the nasal cavity in male and female rats and carcinomas of the gall-bladder in guinea-pigs. No increase in the incidence of tumours was observed in rats following its inhalation. It increased the incidence of skin tumours in mice when applied after 7,12-dimethylbenz[a]anthracene[2]. In a mouse-lung adenoma assay, 1,4-dioxane produced a statistically significant increase in the incidence of tumours in males given an intermediate intraperitoneal dose; no such increase was noted in males given a lower or higher intraperitoneal dose or in females given three intraperitoneal doses or in either males or females given 1,4-dioxane orally[3].

C. Other relevant data

No data were available on the genetic and related effects of 1,4-dioxane in humans. It induced DNA strand breaks in rat hepatocytes *in vitro*. It did not induce sex-linked recessive lethal mutations in *Drosophila* or aneuploidy in yeast. It induced chromosomal aberrations in plants. It was not mutagenic to bacteria[4].

References

[1]Buffler, P.A., Wood, S.M., Suarez, L. & Kilian, D.J. (1978) Mortality follow-up of workers exposed to 1,4-dioxane. *J. occup. Med.*, 20, 255-259

[2]*IARC Monographs*, 11, 247-256, 1976

[3]Stoner, G.D., Conran, P.B., Greisiger, E.A., Stober, J., Morgan, M. & Pereira, M.A. (1986) Comparison of two routes of chemical administration on the lung adenoma response in strain A/J mice. *Toxicol. appl. Pharmacol.*, 82, 19-31

[4]*IARC Monographs, Suppl. 6*, 272-274, 1987

EPICHLOROHYDRIN (Group 2A)

A. Evidence for carcinogenicity to humans (*inadequate*)

A cohort study of 474 and 389 workers exposed in 1948-1965 and 1955-1965 to epichlorohydrin in two factories in Texas and Louisiana, USA, showed slight excesses of lung cancer. In one of the factories, six cases were observed, with 4.2 expected; four of these workers had also been engaged in the manufacture of isopropyl alcohol (see p. 229). In the other, four cases were observed, with 3.1 expected. None of these excesses was statistically significant, even after pooling the data on lung cancer[1].

Another cohort study of 606 workers exposed to epichlorohydrin and other chemicals in four European factories was inconclusive due to small cohort size and short follow-up. The expected number of all cancers was 5.0; four cases were found[2].

B. Evidence for carcinogenicity to animals (*sufficient*)

Epichlorohydrin was tested in rats by oral administration, inducing papillomas and carcinomas of the forestomach[3,4], and by inhalation, inducing papillomas and carcinomas of the nasal cavity[5]. It was also tested in mice by skin application and by subcutaneous and intraperitoneal injection; it gave negative results after continuous skin painting but was active as an initiator on skin. It produced local sarcomas after subcutaneous injection[6] and was active in a mouse-lung tumour bioassay by intraperitoneal injection[7].

C. Other relevant data

Epichlorohydrin is a bifunctional alkylating agent. Chromosomal aberrations have been observed in workers exposed to this compound, although the studies are difficult to interpret[8].

Epichlorohydrin induced sister chromatid exchanges in bone-marrow cells but not micronuclei or dominant lethal mutations in mice treated *in vivo*; equivocal findings were found for chromosomal aberrations. It induced chromosomal aberrations, sister chromatid exchanges and unscheduled DNA synthesis in human cells *in vitro*. Weakly positive results were obtained in a cell transformation assay in C3H 10T1/2 cells. It induced chromosomal aberrations, sister chromatid exchanges, mutation and DNA strand breaks in rodent cells *in vitro*. Epichlorohydrin induced sex-linked recessive lethal mutations in *Drosophila*; aneuploidy, mutation, recombination, gene conversion and DNA damage in fungi; and mutation and DNA damage in bacteria[8].

References

[1]Enterline, P.E. (1982) Importance of sequential exposure in the production of epichlorohydrin and isopropanol. *Ann. N.Y. Acad. Sci., 381*, 344-349

[2]Tassignon, J.P., Bos, G.D., Craigen, A.A., Jacquet, B., Kueng, H.L., Lanouziere-Simon, C. & Pierre, C. (1983) Mortality in an European cohort occupationally exposed to epichlorohydrin (ECH). *Int. Arch. occup. environ. Health, 51*, 325-336

[3]Konishi, Y., Kawabata, A., Denda, A., Ikeda, T., Katada, H., Maruyama, H. & Higashiguchi, R. (1980) Forestomach tumors induced by orally administered epichlorohydrin in male Wistar rats. *Gann, 71*, 922-923

[4]Wester, P.W., van der Heijden, C.A., Bisschop, A. & van Esch, G.J. (1985) Carcinogenicity study with epichlorohydrin (CEP) by gavage in rats. *Toxicology, 36*, 325-339

[5]Laskin, S., Sellakumar, A.R., Kuschner, M., Nelson, N., La Mendola, S., Rusch, G.M., Katz, G.V., Dulak, N.C. & Albert, R.E. (1980) Inhalation carcinogenicity of epichlorohydrin in noninbred Sprague-Dawley rats. *J. natl Cancer Inst., 65*, 751-757

[6]*IARC Monographs, 11*, 131-139, 1976

[7]Stoner, G.D., Conran, P.B., Greisiger, E.A., Stober, J., Morgan, M. & Pereira, M.A. (1986) Comparison of two routes of chemical administration on the lung adenoma response in strain A/J mice. *Toxicol. appl. Pharmacol., 82*, 19-31

[8]*IARC Monographs, Suppl. 6*, 286-290, 1987

ERIONITE (Group 1)

A. Evidence for carcinogenicity to humans (*sufficient*)

Descriptive studies have demonstrated very high mortality from malignant mesothelioma, mainly of the pleura, in three Turkish villages where there was contamination from erionite and where exposure had occurred from birth[1].

B. Evidence for carcinogenicity to animals (*sufficient*)

Erionite has been tested in mice by intraperitoneal injection and in rats by inhalation, intrapleural and intraperitoneal administration, producing high incidences of mesotheliomas[1,2].

C. Other relevant data

Erionite fibres were identified in lung tissue samples in cases of pleural mesothelioma; ferruginous bodies were found in a much higher proportion of inhabitants in contaminated villages in Turkey than in those of two control villages[1].

No data were available on the genetic and related effects of erionite in humans. It induced unscheduled DNA synthesis in human cells *in vitro* and transformation and unscheduled DNA synthesis in mouse C3H 10T1/2 cells[3].

References

[1]*IARC Monographs, 42*, 225-239, 1987

[2]Pott, F. (1987) The fibre as a carcinogenic agent (Ger.). *Zbl. Bakt. Hyg. B, 184*, 1-23

[3]*IARC Monographs, Suppl. 6*, 291-292, 1987

ETHYLENE DIBROMIDE (Group 2A)

A. Evidence for carcinogenicity to humans (*inadequate*)

In one study, the mortality of 161 men exposed to ethylene dibromide in two factories since the mid-1920s and 1942, respectively, was investigated. By 1 January 1976, 36 workers had died, seven of them from cancer (5.8 expected)[1]. In another study, the mortality of 2510 male workers employed at a chemical plant was investigated. Ethylene dibromide was one of several chemicals used and was apparently a minor component of the mixed exposure. No statistically significant excess of cancer at any site was found[2]. An excess of lymphoma was detected n a mortality study of grain workers in the USA who may have had exposure to ethylene dibromide, among other compounds[3].

B. Evidence for carcinogenicity to animals (*sufficient*)

Ethylene dibromide has been tested for carcinogenicity by oral administration and by inhalation in mice and rats and by skin application in mice. Following its oral administration, it produced squamous-cell carcinomas of the forestomach in animals of each species, an increased incidence of alveolar/bronchiolar lung tumours in mice of each sex, liver carcinomas in female rats, haemangiosarcomas in male rats and oesophageal papillomas in female mice[4-6]. Following its inhalation, ethylene dibromide produced adenomas and carcinomas of the nasal cavity, haemangiosarcomas of the spleen, mammary tumours, subcutaneous mesenchymal tumours, an increased incidence of alveolar/bronchiolar lung tumours in animals of each species[7-9], and an increased incidence of peritoneal mesotheliomas in male rats[7]. Ethylene dibromide induced skin and lung tumours in mice after skin application[10].

C. Other relevant data

Ethylene dibromide did not induce chromosomal aberrations or sister chromatid exchanges in exposed pine-tree sprayers and fruit packers[11].

Ethylene dibromide did not induce dominant lethal mutations in mice or rats or chromosomal aberrations or micronuclei in bone-marrow cells of mice treated *in vivo*; however, a weak sister chromatid exchange response was observed. It bound covalently to DNA in rat hepatocytes and induced DNA strand breaks in mouse and rat hepatocytes and in rat testicular cells in studies of rodents treated *in vivo*. Sister chromatid exchanges, mutation and unscheduled DNA synthesis were induced in human cells *in vitro*, and chromosomal aberrations, sister chromatid exchanges, mutation, DNA strand breaks and unscheduled DNA synthesis in rodent cells *in vitro*. Ethylene dibromide induced sex-linked recessive lethal mutations in *Drosophila* and chromosomal aberrations and mutation in plants. It was mutagenic to fungi and bacteria and produced DNA damage in bacteria. Ethylene dibromide bound covalently to isolated DNA[11].

References

[1]Ott, M.G., Scharnweber, H.C. & Langner, R.R. (1980) Mortality experience of 161 employees exposed to ethylene dibromide in two production units. *Br. J. ind. Med.*, *37*, 163-168

[2]Sweeney, M.H., Beaumont, J.J., Waxweiler, R.J. & Halperin, W.E. (1986) An investigation of mortality from cancer and other causes of death among workers employed at an East Texas chemical plant. *Arch. environ. Health, 41*, 23-28

[3]Alavanja, M.C.R., Rush, G.A., Stewart, P. & Blair, A. (1987) Proportionate mortality study of workers in the grain industry. *J. natl Cancer Inst., 78*, 247-252

[4]*IARC Monographs, 15*, 195-209, 1977

[5]National Cancer Institute (1978) *Bioassay of 1,2-Dibromoethane for Possible Carcinogenicity (Tech. Rep. Ser. No. 86; DHEW Publ. No. (NIH) 78-1336)*, Bethesda, MD, US Department of Health, Education, and Welfare

[6]Van Duuren, B.L., Seidman, I., Melchionne, S. & Kline, S. A. (1985) Carcinogenicity bioassays of bromoacetaldehyde and bromoethanol — potential metabolites of dibromoethane. *Teratog. Carcinog. Mutagenesis, 5*, 393-403

[7]National Toxicology Program (1982) *Carcinogenesis Bioassay of 1,2-Dibromoethane (CAS No. 106-93-4) in F344 Rats and B6C3F$_1$ Mice (Inhalation Study) (Tech. Rep. Ser. No. 210; NIH Publ. No. 82-1766)*, Research Triangle Park, NC

[8]Stinson, S.F., Reznik, G. & Ward, J.M. (1981) Characteristics of proliferative lesions in the nasal cavities of mice following chronic inhalation of 1,2-dibromoethane. *Cancer Lett., 12*, 121-129

[9]Wong, L.C.K., Winston, J.M., Hong, C.B. & Plotnick, H. (1982) Carcinogenicity and toxicity of 1,2-dibromoethane in the rat. *Toxicol. appl. Pharmacol., 63*, 155-165

[10]Van Duuren, B.L., Goldschmidt, B.M., Loewengart, G., Smith, A.C., Melchionne, S., Seidman, I. & Rock, D. (1979) Carcinogenicity of halogenated olefinic and aliphatic hydrocarbons in mice. *J. natl Cancer Inst., 63*, 1433-1439

[11]*IARC Monographs, Suppl. 6*, 296-299, 1987

ETHYLENE OXIDE (Group 2A)

A. Evidence for carcinogenicity to humans (*limited*)

Five studies[1,2] have investigated the cancer mortality of workers exposed to ethylene oxide.

Case reports of two myeloid leukaemias and one morbus Waldenström (later reclassified as a non-Hodgkin's lymphoma) were initially found among persons on the work force of a small Swedish factory who had been exposed primarily to ethylene oxide during a sterilizing process. In a subsequent five-year follow-up, a further death from leukaemia (acute 'blastic') was reported. Hence, altogether, four deaths from malignancies of the lymphatic and haematopoietic system (three leukaemias) occurred among the workers, compared with 0.3 expected[1,2].

Another Swedish study comprising 89 ethylene oxide operators with all-day exposure and 86 intermittently exposed maintenance workers involved in the production of ethylene oxide by the chlorohydrin process showed a statistically significant excess of leukaemia, based on two deaths and two incident cases (two lymphocytic, two myelogenous). The expected number was 0.52. There was also a statistically significant excess of deaths from stomach cancer (5 observed, 0.6 expected; in addition, a sixth incident case was reported). These excesses were confined to the workers exposed all day[1,2]. It should be noted that these workers had been exposed to a mixture of chemical compounds, including dichloromethane (see p. 194), ethylene chlorohydrin and small amounts of bis(2-chloroethyl)ether[1].

A third Swedish cohort consisted of 355 workers exposed at a plant producing ethylene oxide through oxygenation of ethylene. Of these, 128 workers had had almost pure exposure to ethylene oxide. Eight deaths occurred compared with 11.6 expected. There was one case of myelogenous leukaemia (0.16 expected) and one of lung cancer among men with mixed exposure[2].

The total number of leukaemias observed in the three Swedish studies was thus eight, with 0.83 expected. Stomach cancer occurred in excess in one plant only (six cases in a group of 89 workers)[2].

In a cohort study of 767 ethylene oxide production workers in the USA, no case of leukaemia was found. However, there was only low potential exposure to ethylene oxide among the workforce and an unusually large deficit in total deaths compared to the number expected, indicating diluting errors in the design of the study[1].

A cohort study of 602 factory workers in the Federal Republic of Germany exposed to ethylene oxide, propylene oxide (see p. 328), benzene (see p. 120) and ethylene chlorohydrin showed a deficit of all deaths compared with four different expected figures. There were 14 deaths due to cancer (16.6 expected from national statistics), one of which was a myeloid leukaemia (0.15 expected) and four of which were stomach cancers (2.7 expected). The expected numbers used were not calendar period-specific over the whole observation period, however, and it is not clear whether they were computed on the basis of the 92% of identified workers or the full cohort[1].

In the light of these data, a causal relationship between exposure to ethylene oxide and leukaemia is possible, but the five small epidemiological studies so far available suffer from various disadvantages, especially confounding exposures, which make their interpretation difficult.

B. Evidence for carcinogenicity to animals (*sufficient*)

Ethylene oxide was tested by intragastric intubation in rats and produced local tumours, mainly squamous-cell carcinomas, of the forestomach. When rats were fed diets fumigated with ethylene oxide, no increased incidence of tumours was observed[1]. In two experiments in which rats of one strain were exposed by inhalation, ethylene oxide increased the incidences of mononuclear-cell leukaemia, brain tumours and proliferative lesions of the adrenal cortex in animals of each sex and of peritoneal mesotheliomas in males[1,3,4]. In mice, inhalation of ethylene oxide resulted in increased incidences of alveolar/bronchiolar lung tumours and tumours of the Harderian gland in animals of each sex and of uterine adenocarcinomas, mammary carcinomas and malignant lymphomas in females[5]. Ethylene oxide was also tested by subcutaneous injection in mice, producing local tumours, which were mainly fibrosarcomas[1].

C. Other relevant data

Significant increases in haemoglobin alkylation, in the incidences of chromosomal aberrations and sister chromatid exchanges in peripheral lymphocytes and, in a single study, micronuclei in erythrocytes have been observed in workers exposed occupationally to ethylene oxide[6].

Ethylene oxide induced chromosomal aberrations and sister chromatid exchanges in peripheral lymphocytes of monkeys exposed *in vivo*. It alkylated haemoglobin and DNA and induced chromosomal aberrations, micronuclei, dominant lethal mutations, heritable translocations and sister chromatid exchanges in rodents treated *in vivo*. In human cells *in vitro*, it induced sister chromatid exchanges, chromosomal aberrations and unscheduled DNA synthesis. It enhanced cell transformation in virus-infected Syrian hamster embryo cells and induced mutation in rodent cells *in vitro*. Ethylene oxide induced somatic and sex-linked recessive lethal mutations and heritable translocations in *Drosophila*. It induced mutation and chromosomal aberrations in plants. Ethylene oxide was mutagenic to fungi and bacteria and induced DNA damage in bacteria[6].

References

[1]*IARC Monographs*, *36*, 189-226, 1985

[2]Hogstedt, C., Aringer, L. & Gustavsson, A. (1986) Epidemiologic support for ethylene oxide as a cancer-causing agent. *J. Am. med. Assoc.*, *255*, 1575-1578

[3]Garman, R.H., Snellings, W.M. & Maronpot, R.R. (1985) Brain tumors in F344 rats associated with chronic inhalation exposure to ethylene oxide. *Neurotoxicology*, *6*, 117-138

[4]Garman, R.H., Snellings, W.M. & Maronpot, R.R. (1986) Frequency, size and location of brain tumours in F-344 rats chronically exposed to ethylene oxide. *Food chem. Toxicol.*, *24*, 145-153

[5]National Toxicology Program (1986) *Toxicology and Carcinogenesis Studies of Ethylene Oxide (CAS No. 75-21-8) in B6C3F$_1$ Mice (Inhalation Studies) (NTP TR 326; NIH Publ. No. 86-2582)*, Research Triangle Park, NC

[6]*IARC Monographs*, *Suppl. 6*, 300-303, 1987

ETHYLENE THIOUREA (Group 2B)

A. Evidence for carcinogenicity to humans (*inadequate*)

In one incidence study, 1929 workers were identified as having worked at some time with ethylene thiourea in one of several rubber manufacturing companies and in one firm producing ethylene thiourea. No case of thyroid cancer was reported in this group to the regional cancer registry between 1957 and 1971, although less than one case would have been expected[1].

B. Evidence for carcinogenicity to animals (*sufficient*)

In three studies, ethylene thiourea produced high incidences of follicular carcinomas of the thyroid in rats after its oral administration; animals of each sex were affected, although male rats had a higher incidence. Lower doses produced thyroid follicular hyperplasia[2-6]. In mice, oral administration of ethylene thiourea produced liver tumours; the thyroids of these animals were not examined[2]. In dosed rats, either shortened survival due to thyroid tumours or altered body weights may have obscured a potential carcinogenic effect on the liver due to administration of ethylene thiourea. A feeding study in hamsters showed no effect[6].

C. Other relevant data

No data were available on the genetic and related effects of ethylene thiourea in humans.

Ethylene thiourea did not induce dominant lethal mutations, micronuclei or sister chromatid exchanges in mice or chromosomal aberrations in rats treated *in vivo*. It did not induce unscheduled DNA synthesis in human fibroblasts *in vitro* or chromosomal aberrations, sister chromatid exchanges, mutation or unscheduled DNA synthesis in rodent cells *in vitro*. Ethylene thiourea did not induce sex-linked recessive lethal mutations in *Drosophila*, but it induced aneuploidy and mutation in yeast. Studies on gene conversion and DNA damage in yeast and on mutation in bacteria have given conflicting results[7].

References

[1]Smith, D. (1976) Ethylene thiourea — a study of possible teratogenicity and thyroid carcinogenicity. *J. Soc. occup. Med.*, *26*, 92-94

[2]*IARC Monographs*, *7*, 45-52, 1974

[3]Graham, S.L., Hansen, W.H., Davis, K.J. & Perry, C.H. (1973) Effects of one-year administration of ethylenethiourea upon the thyroid of the rat. *J. agric. Food Chem.*, *21*, 324-329

[4]Graham, S.L., Davis, K.J., Hansen, W.H. & Graham, C.H. (1975) Effects of prolonged ethylene thiourea ingestion on the thyroid of the rat. *Food Cosmet. Toxicol.*, *13*, 493-499

[5]Weisburger, E.K., Ulland, B.M., Nam, J.-M., Gart, J.J. & Weisburger, J.H. (1981) Carcinogenicity tests of certain environmental and industrial chemicals. *J. natl Cancer Inst.*, *67*, 75-88

[6]Gak, J.-C., Graillot, C. & Truhaut, R. (1976) Difference in sensitivity of the hamster and of the rat with regard to the effects of the long-term administration of ethylene thiourea (Fr.). *Eur. J. Toxicol.*, *9*, 303-312

[7]*IARC Monographs*, *Suppl. 6*, 304-307, 1987

FLUORIDES (INORGANIC, USED IN DRINKING-WATER) (Group 3)

A. Evidence for carcinogenicity to humans (*inadequate*)

Only studies on water fluoridation and cancer were reviewed. Comparisons have been made of mortality from cancers at all sites and from particular types of cancer between areas with high concentrations of inorganic fluoride in drinking-water (either occurring naturally or as a consequence of fluoridation) and areas with low concentrations, or before and after fluoridation; the areas or groups of areas most frequently studied are in Australia, Canada, China, England and Wales, New Zealand, Norway and the USA[1-6]. When possible, confounding of fluoride concentration with relevant variables such as age, sex, race and ethnic composition of the populations was taken into account. Fluoridation of drinking-water was introduced in the USA in 1950[1], and thus the studies in the USA encompass periods of observation of 20 years or more. Studies of areas with different levels of naturally fluoridation cover longer periods of exposure[1,6]. The studies have shown no consistent tendency for people living in areas with high concentrations of fluoride in the water to have higher cancer rates than those living in areas with low concentrations or for cancer mortality rates to increase following fluoridation.

In several studies, trends in cancer incidence or mortality in naturally or artificially fluoridated areas and in areas with low natural fluoride content and no artificially fluoridated water were evaluated according to individual cancer sites or groups of sites[1,3,4,6]. Since a large number of comparisons was made, some would be expected by chance alone to show differences. However, no consistent difference has been seen, and there have been as many significant negative associations between fluoridated water supplies and cancer incidence or mortality as there have been positive associations.

Many studies, therefore, cover the range of doses of fluoride in drinking-water to which humans are exposed, and these are mutually consistent in not showing a positive association between exposure to fluoride and overall cancer rates or rates of different cancers. The Working Group noted that the studies involved were of the ecological or correlation type. The Group was therefore unable to classify the evidence for inorganic fluorides used in drinking-water as 'suggesting lack of carcinogenicity'.

B. Evidence for carcinogenicity to animals (*inadequate*)

Sodium fluoride was tested in three experiments in three different strains of mice by oral administration. The available data are insufficient to allow an evaluation to be made[1].

C. Other relevant data

Epidemiological studies have shown no association between the presence of fluorides in drinking-water and the incidence of Down's syndrome[7].

Sodium fluoride did not induce DNA strand breaks in testicular cells of rats treated *in vivo* and did not cause chromosomal aberrations in bone-marrow or testicular cells or sister chromatid exchanges in bone-marrow cells of mice treated *in vivo*. It was reported to induce unscheduled DNA synthesis in cultured human cells, and conflicting results were obtained on the induction of chromosomal aberrations; it did not induce sister chromatid exchanges. It induced transformation, sister chromatid exchanges and chromosomal aberrations in Syrian hamster embryo cells *in vitro*. At high doses and low cell survival, sodium fluoride induced dose-related increases in mutations in cultured mouse lymphoma cells. It did not induce aneuploidy in *Drosophila*. It induced chromosomal aberrations in plants. It did not induce gene conversion in yeast and was not mutagenic to bacteria[7].

Stannous fluoride, sodium monofluorophosphate and sodium silicofluoride did not induce sex-linked recessive lethal mutations in *Drosophila*, and sodium monofluorophosphate did not induce dominant lethal mutations in *Drosophila*[7].

References

[1]*IARC Monographs*, 27, 237-303, 1982

[2]Wang, B. (1981) The relationship between malignancy and fluorine content in the drinking water in Xilinkuolemeng, Nei Menggu (Chin.). *Zhonghua Zhongliu Zazhi, 3*, 19-21

[3]Neuberger, J.S. (1982) Fluoridation and cancer: an epidemiologic appraisal. *J. Kansas med. Soc., 83*, 134-139

[4]Chilvers, C. (1982) Cancer mortality by site and fluoridation of water supplies. *J. Epidemiol. Commun. Health, 36*, 237-242

[5]Chilvers, C. (1983) Cancer mortality and fluoridation of water supplies in 35 US cities. *Int. J. Epidemiol., 12*, 397-404

[6]Chilvers, C. & Conway, D. (1985) Cancer mortality in England in relation to levels of naturally occurring fluoride in water supplies. *J. Epidemiol. Commun. Health, 39*, 44-47

[7]*IARC Monographs, Suppl. 6*, 312-315, 1987

5-FLUOROURACIL (Group 3)

A. Evidence for carcinogenicity to humans (*inadequate*)

No epidemiological study of 5-fluorouracil as a single agent was available to the Working Group. Occasional case reports of exposure to 5-fluorouracil, especially in the presence of concurrent therapy with other putative carcinogens, such as ionizing radiation, alkylating agents and other potent oncotherapeutic drugs, do not constitute evidence of carcinogenesis[1].

No increased risk of second malignancies was found among 276 patients with colorectal cancer randomized to low-dose (20 mg/kg bw) 5-fluoro-2′-deoxyuridine adjuvant therapy, followed for 1774 person-years (14 second noncolorectal cancers observed, 15 expected)[2].

B. Evidence for carcinogenicity to animals (*inadequate*)

5-Fluorouracil was tested by intravenous administration in mice and rats and by oral administration in rats. No evidence of carcinogenicity was found, but the studies suffered from limitations with regard to duration or dose[1]. It was reported that ingestion of 5-fluorouracil prevented or delayed the appearance of spontaneous mammary and pituitary tumours in old female rats; no histopathological evaluation was made of the tumours that developed[3]. A study in which 5-fluorouracil was given intraperitoneally to rats in combination with methotrexate (see p. 241) and cyclophosphamide (see p. 182) resulted in induction of tumours in the nervous system, haematopoietic and lymphatic tissue, the urinary bladder and the adrenal glands; however, because of the lack of matched controls, it could not be concluded whether tumour induction was due to a combined effect of the three chemicals or of any one of them[4].

C. Other relevant data

Neither chromosomal aberrations (in two patients) nor sister chromatid exchanges (in three patients) were induced following administration of 5-fluorouracil[5].

5-Fluorouracil induced micronuclei but not specific locus mutations in mice treated *in vivo*. It induced aneuploidy, chromosomal aberrations and sister chromatid exchanges in cultured Chinese hamster cells. It did not induce sex-linked recessive lethal mutations in *Drosophila*, but caused genetic crossing-over in fungi. Studies on mutation in bacteria were inconclusive[5].

References

[1]*IARC Monographs*, 26, 217-235, 1981

[2]Boice, J.D., Greene, M.H., Keehn, R.J., Higgins, G.A. & Fraumeni, J.F., Jr (1980) Late effects of low-dose adjuvant chemotherapy in colorectal cancer. *J. natl Cancer Inst.*, 64, 501-511

[3]Ferguson, T. (1980) Prevention and delay of spontaneous mammary and pituitary tumors by long- and short-term ingestion of 5-fluorouracil in Wistar-Furth rats. *Oncology*, 37, 353-356

[4]Habs, M., Schmähl, D. & Lin, P.Z. (1981) Carcinogenic activity in rats of combined treatment with cyclophosphamide, methotrexate and 5-fluorouracil. *Int. J. Cancer*, 28, 91-96

[5]*IARC Monographs*, Suppl. 6, 316-318, 1987

FORMALDEHYDE (Group 2A)

A. Evidence for carcinogenicity to humans (*limited*)

A number of epidemiological studies using different designs have been completed on persons in a variety of occupations with potential exposure to formaldehyde[1-24]. Cancers that occurred in excess in more than one study are: Hodgkin's disease, leukaemia, and cancers of the buccal cavity and pharynx (particularly nasopharynx), lung, nose, prostate, bladder, brain, colon, skin and kidney[1]. The studies reported are not entirely independent; the plant studied by Liebling *et al.*[2] and Marsh[1,3] is also included in the study by Blair *et al.*[4]; the case-control study of Fayerweather *et al.*[5] includes some subjects who were later studied by Blair *et al.*[4]. Detailed estimates of formaldehyde exposure levels were made in the studies of British chemical workers[6], US formaldehyde producers and users[4], Finnish wood workers[7] and US chemical workers[5], and for the case-control studies of Vaughan *et al.*[8,9] and Hayes *et al.*[10].

In the study of US producers and users of formaldehyde, 11% of the subjects were not exposed, 12% had an estimated time-weighted average (TWA) exposure of <0.1 ppm (<0.12 mg/m³), 34% a TWA of 0.1-<0.5 ppm (0.12-<0.6 mg/m³), 40% a TWA of 0.5-<2 ppm

$(0.6-<2.4$ mg/m³) and 4% a TWA of >2.0 ppm $(>2.4$ mg/m³)[4]. On the basis of the job held that incurred the highest level of exposure, the distribution among British chemical workers was: nil/background, <0.1 ppm $(<0.12$ mg/m³), 25%; 0.1-0.5 ppm (0.12-0.6 mg/m³), 24%; 0.6-2.0 ppm (0.7-2.4 mg/m³), 9%; >2.0 ppm $(>2.4$ mg/m³), 35%; and unknown, 6%[6].

Excesses of cancers of the buccal cavity and pharynx have been reported in five studies[2,8,11-13], with a statistically significant excess for cancer of the buccal cavity based on three deaths[11] in one study and statistically significant excesses for cancer at both sites in another study, based on two deaths[2]. Interpretation of the results of the last study is difficult because the deaths were not obtained systematically from the entire workforce, but rather were ascertained from worker reports and obituaries. The occurrence of cancer of the nasopharynx was elevated in a cohort study of industrial workers[4] and in case-control studies[8,9,14]. Among industrial workers exposed to formaldehyde-containing particulates, standardized mortality rates (SMRs) for nasopharyngeal cancer rose with cumulative exposure to formaldehyde: 192 (one death) for <0.5 ppm(<0.6 mg/m³)-years, 403 (two deaths) for $0.5-<5.5$ ppm($0.6-<6.7$ mg/m³)-years and 746 (two deaths) for >5.5 ppm(>6.7 mg/m³)-years. There was a similar trend with duration of exposure to formaldehyde, and all five cases held jobs in which hourly exposures exceeded 4.0 ppm formaldehyde[15]. A rising relative risk (RR) for nasopharyngeal cancer was seen by type of exposure to formaldehyde: 1.7 for occupation alone, 2.8 for living in mobile homes and 6.7 for both occupational and mobile-home exposures. These risks were unaffected by potentially confounding factors such as smoking, alcohol use and socioeconomic status[8,9]. An excess of nasopharyngeal cancer was reported in one study among women (RR, 2.6) exposed to formaldehyde, but not among men (RR, 0.7)[14]. Several other studies showed no excess[5,6,11,16], but no death from this tumour was reported in any of these studies.

Sinonasal cancer was associated with employment in jobs in which there is potential contact with formaldehyde in case-control studies in Denmark (RR, 2.8 in men and women)[14,17] and in the Netherlands (RR, 2.5 and 1.9 from two independent classifications of exposure)[10]. Risk for this tumour increased with level of exposure in the Netherlands[10] and with duration of exposure in Denmark[14]. Excess risks persisted in both studies when analyses were restricted to persons without exposure to wood dust (an established risk factor for this tumour, see p. 380), although they were no longer statistically significant. In one of the studies[10], the excess of sinonasal cancer from exposure to formaldehyde was found to be limited primarily to squamous-cell carcinoma, further differentiating the formaldehyde-associated excess from that caused by wood dust, with which adeno-carcinoma predominates. In another of the studies[17], however, the excess was not confined to squamous-cell carcinoma. No excess of sinonasal cancer was found in industrial workers (SMR, 91), but only two deaths occurred[4]. Sinonasal cancer was not associated with occupational or residential exposure to formaldehyde in another study[8,9]. None of the other studies reported any death from sinonasal cancer. The RRs for sinonasal cancer in the studies of Hayes[10] and Vaughan[8,9] were adjusted for smoking habits.

Slight excesses in the occurrence of lung cancer have been noted in several studies[2,4,7,12,18,19]. These excesses have shown no consistent pattern with increasing level or duration of exposure to formaldehyde. A statistically significant excess (SMR, 132) was reported among wage workers 20 or more years after first exposure. The risk of lung cancer did not increase among this, or any other group, with either level or duration of exposure[4]. In the UK, the risk of lung cancer rose with level of exposure in one factory from an SMR of 58 among those with low exposure to an SMR of 118 among those with high exposure[6]. No such pattern was seen, however, for the other factories[6], nor was risk associated with cumulative exposure[20]. In a case-control study of respiratory cancer among Finnish plywood and particle-board workers, an odds ratio of 1.6 (adjusted for smoking) was found after ten years of latency. RRs, however, decreased with level and duration of exposure to formaldehyde[7]. In a cohort mortality study of 1332 workers in a formaldehyde-resin plant in Italy, there was an overall excess of lung cancer (SMR, 186). The excess occurred among those not exposed to formaldehyde (SMR, 148) as well as among those exposed (SMR, 136), with the greatest excess among those with uncertain exposure (SMR, 358). Lung cancer mortality was not clearly associated with duration of exposure[19].

Studies of professional groups have shown rather consistent deficits of lung cancer. None of these studies, however, included information on smoking, and the lower prevalence of tobacco use in these groups would probably lead to such deficits. No excess occurrence of lung cancer was noted among Danish physicians[21] or among persons exposed to formaldehyde at a US chemical production facility[22].

Mortality from leukaemia and/or cancer of the brain has been found consistently to be elevated in studies of professional groups[1,12,13,16,23,24]. Except for a very slight excess of leukaemia reported in one study[5] (which was not statistically significant), excesses of these tumours have not been found among industrial workers exposed to formaldehyde. Among professionals, gliomas were the predominant cell type of brain cancer, and the leukaemias were predominantly of the myeloid type. The absence of excesses for these cancers among industrial workers, however, argues against a role of formaldehyde.

Mortality from prostatic cancer has been found to be elevated among professionals[13] and among industrial workers[4,5], but the excess was statistically significant only among embalmers[13]. This tumour has shown a dose-response gradient in both studies of industrial workers, although the test for trend in the study of Blair[4] was not statistically significant.

Slight excesses of mortality from bladder cancer have been reported among professionals[13,23] and among industrial workers[5]. No such excess occurred, however, in the other large industrial cohorts, and none of the excesses was statistically significant. Significant excesses of colon cancer were noted among professionals[12,13] and among industrial workers[2]; nonsignificant elevations have also been reported[11,16]. A significant excess mortality from cancer of the skin was reported among New York embalmers (proportionate mortality ratio, 221)[12], and a slight excess was noted among industrial workers (based on two deaths)[11]. Excesses of Hodgkin's disease were seen among white industrial workers in two studies, based on 14 deaths (SMR, 142)[4] and on one death[11]. The risk of Hodgkin's disease rose with level of formaldehyde exposure among wage and salaried workers alike, although each stratum had small numbers[4].

Although excess occurrence of a number of cancers has been reported, the evidence for a possible involvement of formaldehyde is strongest for nasal and nasopharyngeal cancer. The occurrence of these cancers showed an exposure-response gradient in more than one study, but the numbers of exposed cases were often small and some studies did not show excesses. The nose and nasopharynx could come into direct contact with formaldehyde through inhalation. Excess mortality from leukaemia and cancer of the brain was generally not seen among industrial workers, which suggests that the excesses for these cancers among professionals is due to factors other than formaldehyde. The slight excesses of cancer of the lung noted in several studies generally did not display the patterns of increasing risk with various measures of exposure (i.e., latency, duration, level or cumulative) usually seen for occupational carcinogens. No other cancer showed a consistent excess across the various studies.

B. Evidence for carcinogenicity to animals (*sufficient*)

Formaldehyde was tested for carcinogenicity by inhalation in two strains of rats and in one strain of mice. Significant increases in the incidence of squamous-cell carcinomas of the nasal cavity were induced in both strains of rats but not in mice[1,25]. A slight increase in the incidence of nasal cavity polypoid adenomas was also observed in male rats[25]. The tumours in the nasal cavity of rats were localized precisely: in the anterior portion of the lateral aspect of the nasoturbinate and adjacent lateral wall[26]. Experiments in which rats were exposed to both hydrogen chloride and formaldehyde showed that the carcinogenic response to formaldehyde does not result from the presence of bis(chloromethyl)ether (see p. 131), which is formed from the mixture of gases[27]. Another study in mice and one in hamsters by inhalation, one in rats by subcutaneous administration and one in rabbits by exposure in oral tanks were considered inadequate for evaluation[1,28].

C. Other relevant data

In single studies of persons exposed to formaldehyde, increases in the frequencies of chromosomal aberrations and sister chromatid exchanges in peripheral lymphocytes have been reported, but negative results have also been published. The interpretation of both the positive and negative studies is difficult due to the small number of subjects studied and inconsistencies in the findings[29].

No increase in the frequency of micronuclei or chromosomal aberrations was observed in rodents treated with formaldehyde *in vivo*; assays for dominant lethal mutations and DNA damage gave inconclusive results. Formaldehyde induced sperm-head anomalies in rats It induced DNA-protein cross-links, unscheduled DNA synthesis, chromosomal aberrations, sister chromatid exchanges and mutation in human cells *in vitro*. It induced transformation of mouse C3H 10T1/2 cells and chromosomal aberrations, sister chromatid exchanges, DNA strand breaks and DNA-protein cross-links in rodent cells *in vitro*. In *Drosophila*, administration of formaldehyde in the diet induced lethal and visible mutations, deficiencies, duplications, inversions and translocations and crossing-over in spermatogonia. It induced mutation, gene conversion, DNA strand breaks and DNA-protein cross-links in fungi and mutation and DNA damage in bacteria[29].

References

[1]*IARC Monographs*, *29*, 345-389, 1982

[2]Liebling, T., Rosenman, K.D., Pastides, H., Griffith, R.G. & Lemeshow, S. (1984) Cancer mortality among workers exposed to formaldehyde. *Am. J. ind. Med.*, *5*, 423-428

[3]Marsh, G.M. (1982) Proportional mortality patterns among chemical plant workers exposed to formaldehyde. *Br. J. ind. Med.*, *39*, 313-322

[4]Blair, A., Stewart, P., O'Berg, M., Gaffey, W., Walrath, J., Ward, J., Bales, R., Kaplan, S. & Cubit, D. (1986) Mortality among industrial workers exposed to formaldehyde. *J. natl Cancer Inst.*, *76*, 1071-1084

[5]Fayerweather, W.E., Pell, S. & Bender, J.R. (1983) *Case-control study of cancer deaths in DuPont workers with potential exposure to formaldehyde*. In: Clary, J.J., Gibson, J.E. & Waritz, R.S., eds, *Formaldehyde: Toxicology, Epidemiology, Mechanisms*, New York, Marcel Dekker, pp. 47-125

[6]Acheson, E.D., Gardner, M.J., Pannett, B., Barnes, H.R., Osmond, C. & Taylor, C.P. (1984) Formaldehyde in the British chemical industry. *Lancet*, *i*, 611-616

[7]Partanen, T., Kauppinen, T., Nurminen, M., Nickels, J., Hernberg, S., Hakulinen, T., Pukkala, E. & Savonen, E. (1985) Formaldehyde exposure and respiratory and related cancers: a case-referent study among Finnish woodworkers. *Scand. J. Work Environ. Health*, *11*, 409-415

[8]Vaughan, T.L., Strader, C., Davis, S. & Daling, J.R. (1986) Formaldehyde and cancers of the pharynx, sinus and nasal cavity: I. Occupational exposures. *Int. J. Cancer*, *38*, 677-683

[9]Vaughan, T.L., Strader, C., Davis, S. & Daling, J.R. (1986) Formaldehyde and cancers of the pharynx, sinul and nasal cavity. II. Residential exposures. *Int. J. Cancer*, *38*, 685-688

[10]Hayes, R.B., Raatgever, J.W., De Bruyn, A. & Gérin, M. (1986) Cancer of the nasal cavity and paranasal sinuses, and formaldehyde exposure. *Int. J. Cancer*, *37*, 487-492

[11]Stayner, L., Smith, A.B., Reeve, G., Blade, L., Elliott, L., Keenlyside, R. & Halperin, W. (1985) Proportionate mortality study of workers in the garment industry exposed to formaldehyde. *Am. J. ind. Med.*, *7*, 229-240

[12]Walrath, J. & Fraumeni, J.F., Jr (1983) Mortality patterns among embalmers. *Int. J. Cancer*, *31*, 407-411

[13]Walrath, J. & Fraumeni, J.F., Jr (1984) Cancer and other causes of death among embalmers. *Cancer Res.*, *44*, 4638-4641

[14]Olsen, J.H., Jensen, S.P., Hink, M., Faurbo, K., Breum, N.O. & Jensen, O.M. (1984) Occupational formaldehyde exposure and increased nasal cancer risk in man. *Int. J. Cancer*, *34*, 639-644

[15]Blair, A., Stewart, P.A., Hoover, R.N., Fraumeni, J.F., Jr, Walrath, J., O'Berg, M. & Gaffey, W. (1987) Cancers of the nasopharynx and oropharynx and formaldehyde exposure. *J. natl Cancer Inst.*, *78*, 191-192

[16]Stroup, N.E., Blair, A. & Erikson, G.E. (1986) Brain cancer and other causes of death in anatomists. *J. natl Cancer Inst.*, *77*, 1217-1224

[17]Olsen, J.H. & Asnaes, S. (1986) Formaldehyde and the risk of squamous cell carcinoma of the sinonasal cavities. *Br. J. ind. Med.*, *43*, 769-774

[18]Coggon, D., Pannett, B. & Acheson, E.D. (1984) Use of job-exposure matrix in an occupational analysis of lung and bladder cancers on the basis of death certificates. *J. natl Cancer Inst.*, *72*, 61-65

[19]Bertazzi, P.A., Pesatori, A.C., Radice, L., Zocchetti, C. & Vai, T. (1986) Exposure to formaldehyde and cancer mortality in a cohort of workers producing resins. *Scand. J. Work Environ. Health*, *12*, 461-468

[20]Acheson, E.D., Barnes, H.R., Gardner, M.J., Osmond, C., Pannett, B. & Taylor, C.P. (1984) Formaldehyde process workers and lung cancer. *Lancet*, *i*, 1066-1067

[21]Jensen, O.M. & Andersen, S.K. (1982) Lung cancer risk from formaldehyde. *Lancet*, *i*, 913

[22]Bond, G.G., Flores, G.H., Shellenberger, R.J., Cartmill, J.B., Fishbeck, W.A. & Cook, R.R. (1986) Nested case-control study of lung cancer among chemical workers. *Am. J. Epidemiol.*, *124*, 53-66

[23]Harrington, J.M. & Oakes, D. (1984) Mortality study of British pathologists 1974-80. *Br. J. ind. Med.*. *41*, 188-191

[24]Levine, R.J., Andjelkovich, D.A. & Shaw, L.K. (1984) The mortality of Ontario undertakers and a review of formaldehyde-related mortality studies. *J. occup. Med.*, *26*, 740-746

[25]Kerns, W.D., Pavkov, K.L., Donofrio, D.J., Gralla, E.J. & Swenberg, J.A. (1983) Carcinogenicity of formaldehyde in rats and mice after long-term inhalation exposure. *Cancer Res.*, *43*, 4382-4392

[26]Morgan, K.T., Jiang, X.-Z., Starr, T.B. & Kerns, W.D. (1986) More precise localization of nasal tumors associated with chronic exposure of F-344 rats to formaldehyde gas. *Toxicol. appl. Pharmacol.*, *82*, 264-271

[27]Sellakumar, A.R., Snyder, C.A., Solomon, J.J. & Albert, R.E. (1985) Carcinogenicity of formaldehyde and hydrogen chloride in rats. *Toxicol. appl. Pharmacol.*, *81*, 401-406

[28]Dalbey, W.E. (1982) Formaldehyde and tumors in hamster respiratory tract. *Toxicology*, *24*, 9-14

[29]*IARC Monographs, Suppl. 6*, 321-324, 1987

HAEMATITE AND FERRIC OXIDE:
FERRIC OXIDE (Group 3)
HAEMATITE (Group 3)
UNDERGROUND HAEMATITE MINING WITH EXPOSURE TO RADON (Group 1)

A. Evidence for carcinogenicity to humans (*inadequate* for haematite and ferric oxide; *sufficient* for underground haematite mining with exposure to radon)

Underground haematite miners have a higher incidence of lung cancer in the presence of exposure to radon daughters (although other agents might also contribute to the risk) than surface haematite miners[1-11]. Haematite mining with low-grade exposure to radon daughters and silica dust was not associated with excess lung cancer in a relatively large cohort[12]. The importance of exposure to radon daughters in the occurrence of lung cancer in haematite miners is also suggested by the time trend of lung cancer rates in a mining population[4]. One mining population with an increased lung cancer risk but with current low exposure to radon daughters might have had higher exposures in the past due to poorer ventilation[13,14].

Some studies of metal workers exposed to ferric oxide dusts have shown an increased incidence of lung cancer[1,15], but the influence of factors in the workplace other than ferric oxide, i.e., soots (see p. 343), silica (see p. 341) and asbestos (see p. 106) in foundry work, cannot be discounted. In other studies of metal and chemical workers exposed to ferric oxide, the incidence of lung cancer has generally not been increased[1,16].

B. Evidence for carcinogenicity to animals (*inadequate* for haematite; *evidence suggesting lack of carcinogenicity* for ferric oxide)

No conclusive carcinogenic effect was observed in mice, hamsters or guinea-pigs given ferric oxide intratracheally or by inhalation[1]. Repeated intratracheal instillation to hamsters of benzo[a]pyrene bound to fine ferric oxide dust particles induced squamous-cell and anaplastic carcinomas[17]. There was no increase in tumour yield in hamsters administered a constant dose of benzo[a]pyrene and increasing amounts of ferric oxide intratracheally, indicating that, beyond a certain ratio of benzo[a]pyrene to ferric oxide, the latter does not affect tumour yield[18]. Administration of ferric oxide particles alone occasionally induced interstitial fibrosis, indicating that ferrous oxide particles act as cofactors in this system, mainly as carriers[19]. In one study, intrapleural inoculation of the respirable fraction of iron ore mine dust to female BALB/c mice resulted in an increased incidence of lung adenomas; in a second study, an increased incidence of lymphoma/leukaemia was observed in female C57BL/6J mice exposed chronically to the same dust. In neither study was the number of animals specified, nor whether the mice were killed serially or died; in the second study, the type of exposure was not specified[20]. In several studies in hamsters, ferric oxide was not carcinogenic when given alone but enhanced lung and nasal-cavity carcinogenesis induced by N-nitrosodiethylamïne and N-nitrosodimethylamine, respectively[21-23].

C. Other relevant data

No data were available on the genetic and related effects of ferric oxide in humans. It did not induce transformation of Syrian hamster embryo cells[24].

References

[1]*IARC Monographs, 1*, 29-39, 1972

[2]Damber, L. & Larsson, L.-G. (1985) Underground mining, smoking, and lung cancer: a case-control study in the iron ore municipalities in northern Sweden. *J. natl Cancer Inst., 74*, 1207-1213

[3]Edling, C. (1982) Lung cancer and smoking in a group of iron ore miners. *Am. J. ind. Med., 3,* 191-199

[4]Edling, C. & Axelson, O. (1983) Quantitative aspects of radon daughter exposure and lung cancer in underground miners. *Br. J. ind. Med., 40,* 182-187

[5]Ĺsó, J. & Szöllösová, M. (1984) The incidence of lung cancer in the miners of iron-ore mines (Czech). *Pracov. Lék., 36,* 294-298

[6]Jorgensen, H.S. (1973) A study of mortality from lung cancer among miners in Kiruna 1950-1970. *Work Environ. Health, 10,* 126-133

[7]Jorgensen, H.S. (1984) Lung cancer among underground workers in the iron ore mine of Kiruna based on thirty years of observation. *Ann. Acad. Med., 13 (Suppl.),* 371-377

[8]Larsson, L.-G. & Damber, L. (1982) Interaction between underground mining and smoking in the causation of lung cancer: a study of nonuranium miners in northern Sweden. *Cancer Detect. Prev., 5,* 385-389

[9]Radford, E.P. (1981) *Radon daughters in the induction of lung cancer in underground miners.* In: Peto, R. & Schneiderman, M., eds, *Quantification of Occupational Exposure (Banbury Report 9),* Cold Spring Harbor, NY, CSH Press, pp. 151-163

[10]Radford, E.P. & St Clair Renard, K.G. (1984) Lung cancer in Swedish iron miners exposed to low doses of radon daughters. *New Engl. J. Med., 310,* 1485-1494

[11]St Clair Renard, K.G. (1974) Respiratory cancer mortality in an iron ore mine in northern Sweden. *Ambio, 3,* 67-69

[12]Lawler, A.B., Mandel, J.S., Schuman, L.M. & Lubin, J.H. (1985) A retrospective cohort mortality study of iron ore (hematite) miners in Minnesota. *J. occup. Med., 27,* 507-517

[13]Anthoine, D., Braun, P., Cervoni, P., Schwartz, P. & Lamy, P. (1979) Should the lung cancer of iron miners in the Lorraine be considered an occupational disease? 270 new cases observed from 1964-1978 (Fr.). *Rev. fr. Mal. respir., 7,* 63-65

[14]Pham, Q.T., Gaertner, M., Mur, J.M., Braun, P., Gabiano, M. & Sadoul, P. (1983) Incidence of lung cancer among iron miners. *Eur. J. respir. Dis., 64,* 534-540

[15]Tola, S., Koskela, R.-S., Hernberg, S. & Järvinen, E. (1979) Lung cancer mortality among iron foundry workers. *J. occup. Med., 21,* 753-760

[16]Axelson, O. & Sjöberg, A. (1979) Cancer incidence and exposure to iron oxide dust. *J. occup. Med., 21,* 419-422

[17]Saffiotti, U. (1969) Experimental respiratory tract carcinogenesis. *Prog. exp. Tumor Res., 11,* 302-333

[18]Sellakumar, A.R., Montesano, R., Saffiotti, U. & Kaufman, D.G. (1973) Hamster respiratory carcinogenesis induced by benzo[a]pyrene and different dose levels of ferric oxide. *J. natl Cancer Inst., 50,* 507-510

[19]Stenbäck, F., Rowland, J. & Sellakumar, A. (1976) Carcinogenicity of benzo[a]pyrene and dusts in the hamster lung (instilled intratracheally with titanium oxide, aluminum oxide, carbon and ferric oxide). *Oncology, 33,* 29-34

[20]Keast, D., Tam, N., Sheppard, N. & Papadimitriou, J.M. (1985) The role of tobacco smoke, iron ore mine dusts, viruses, and chemicals in experimental cancer. *Arch. environ. Health, 40,* 296-300

[21]Stenbäck, F., Ferrero, A., Montesano, R. & Shubik, P. (1973) Synergistic effect of ferric oxide on dimethylnitrosamine carcinogenesis in the Syrian golden hamster. *Z. Krebsforsch., 79,* 31-38

[22]Nettesheim, P., Creasia, D.A. & Mitchell, T.J. (1975) Carcinogenic and cocarcinogenic effects of inhaled synthetic smog and ferric oxide particles. *J. natl Cancer Inst., 55*, 159-169

[23]Feron, V.J., Emmelot, P. & Vossenaar, T. (1972) Lower respiratory tract tumours in Syrian golden hamsters after intratracheal instillations of diethylnitrosamine alone and with ferric oxide. *Eur. J. Cancer, 8*, 445-449

[24]*IARC Monographs, Suppl. 6*, 310-311, 1987

HEXACHLOROBENZENE (Group 2B)

A. Evidence for carcinogenicity to humans (*inadequate*)

No report of a direct association between hexachlorobenzene and human cancer is available. Hepatocellular carcinoma has been associated with porphyria[1-5]. However, although abnormal porphyrin metabolism persisted at least 20 years after an epidemic of porphyria cutanea tarda in Turkey, caused by consumption of grain treated with hexachlorobenzene[6], no excess cancer occurrence has been reported in this population 25 years after the accident[7].

B. Evidence for carcinogenicity to animals (*sufficient*)

Hexachlorobenzene was tested by oral administration in one experiment in mice and in one in hamsters. In mice, it produced liver-cell tumours in animals of each sex; in hamsters of each sex, it produced hepatomas, liver haemangioendotheliomas and thyroid adenomas. An experiment involving intraperitoneal administration in mice was considered to be inadequate[6]. In a study in rats fed hexachlorobenzene in the diet, hepatomas, hepatocellular carcinomas, bile-duct adenomas and renal-cell adenomas were observed[8]. In a two-generation feeding study in rats with lower dose levels, increased incidences of parathyroid adenomas and adrenal phaeochromocytomas were observed in animals of each sex and liver neoplastic nodules in females of the F_1 generation[9]. After 90 weeks' feeding of hexachlorobenzene to rats, 100% of surviving females and only 16% of males had developed liver tumours[10].

C. Other relevant data

No data were available on the genetic and related effects of hexachlorobenzene in humans. It did not induce dominant lethal mutations in rats treated *in vivo*. It did not induce chromosomal aberrations in cultured Chinese hamster cells or mutation in bacteria[11].

References

[1]Kordač, V. (1972) Frequency of occurrence of hepatocellular carcinoma in patients with porphyria cutanea tarda in long-term follow-up. *Neoplasma, 19*, 135-139

[2]Solis, J.A., Betancor, P., Campos, R., Enriquez de Salamanca, R., Rojo, P., Marin, I. & Schüller, A. (1982) Association of porphyria cutanea tarda and primary liver cancer: report of ten cases. *J. Dermatol.*, *9*, 131-137

[3]Lithner, F. & Wetterberg, L. (1984) Hepatocellular carcinoma in patients with acute intermittent porphyria. *Acta med. scand.*, *215*, 271-274

[4]Hardell, L., Bengtsson, N.O., Jonsson, U., Eriksson, S. & Larsson, L.G. (1984) Aetiological aspects on primary liver cancer with special regard to alcohol, organic solvents and acute intermittent porphyria — an epidemiological investigation. *Br. J. Cancer*, *50*, 389-397

[5]Axelson, O. (1986) *A review of porphyria and cancer and the missing link with human exposure to hexachlorobenzene*. In: Morris, C.R. & Cabral, J.R.P., eds, *Hexachlorobenzene: Proceedings of an International Symposium (IARC Scientific Publications No. 77*), Lyon, International Agency for Research on Cancer, pp. 585-589

[6]*IARC Monographs*, *20*, 155-178, 1979

[7]Peters, H.A., Gocmen, A., Cripps, D.J., Bryan, G.T. & Dogramaci, I. (1982) Epidemiology of hexachlorobenzene-induced porphyria in Turkey. Clinical and laboratory follow-up after 25 years. *Arch. Neurol.*, *39*, 744-749

[8]Ertürk, E., Lambrecht, R.W., Peters, H.A., Cripps, D.J., Gocmen, A., Morris, C.R. & Bryan, G.T. (1986) *Oncogenicity of hexachlorobenzene*. In: Morris, C.R. & Cabral, J.R.P., eds, *Hexachlorobenzene: Proceedings of an International Symposium (IARC Scientific Publications No. 77*), Lyon, International Agency for Research on Cancer, pp. 417-423

[9]Arnold, D.L., Moodie, C.A., Charbonneau, S.M., Grice, H.C., McGuire, P.F., Bryce, F.R., Collins, B.T., Zawidzka, Z.Z., Krewski, D.R., Nera, E.A. & Munro, I.C. (1985) Long-term toxicity of hexachlorobenzene in the rat and the effect of dietary vitamin A. *Food chem. Toxicol.*, *23*, 779-793

[10]Smith, A.G., Francis, J.E., Dinsdale, D., Manson, M.M. & Cabral, J.R.P. (1985) Hepatocarcinogenicity of hexachlorobenzene in rats and the sex difference in hepatic iron status and development of porphyria. *Carcinogenesis*, *6*, 631-636

[11]*IARC Monographs, Suppl. 6*, 331-332, 1987

HEXACHLOROCYCLOHEXANES (Group 2B)

A. Evidence for carcinogenicity to humans (*inadequate*)

Four cases of leukaemia were reported in men exposed to γ-hexachlorocyclohexane (lindane) with or without other chemicals[1,2]. Cases of aplastic anaemia have also been associated with exposure to this compound[1]. Mean tissue levels of hexachlorocyclohexanes were reported to be elevated in two of three studies of autopsy patients; in one of these, in four liver cancer patients, the level of the β-isomer was abnormally high[3-5]. Mean serum levels of β-hexachlorocyclohexane were not appreciably higher in four cancer patients than in three controls[6]. Exposure to γ-hexachlorocyclohexane was recorded in case-control studies of soft-tissue sarcomas and of lymphomas[7,8] but was insufficiently frequent for any conclusion to be drawn. An increase in lung cancer mortality was observed in agricultural workers who had used hexachlorocyclohexane (unspecified) and a variety of other pesticides and herbicides (standardized mortality ratio, 180 [95% confidence interval, 140-240])[9].

B. Evidence for carcinogenicity to animals (*sufficient* for technical-grade and the α isomer; *limited* for the β and γ isomers)

Technical-grade, α- and β-hexachlorocyclohexane and the γ isomer (lindane) produced liver tumours in mice when administered orally[1,10,11]; the technical grade also produced lymphoreticular neoplasms[10]. In two studies in rats, an increased incidence of liver tumours was observed with the α isomer[1,12], and in one study in rats a few thyroid tumours were observed with the γ isomer[1]; other studies in rats[11,13-15] were considered to be inadequate. Studies in hamsters[11] and dogs[16] were also inadequate. Technical-grade hexachlorocyclohexane and the γ isomer were tested inadequately by skin application in mice[1,10]. α-Hexachlorocyclohexane enhanced the incidence of liver neoplasms induced in rats by *N*-nitrosodiethylamine[12].

C. Other relevant data

In a single study, chromosomal aberrations were not found in workers involved in the production of γ-hexachlorocyclohexane (lindane)[17].

Technical-grade hexachlorocyclohexane, but not γ-hexachlorocyclohexane, induced dominant lethal mutations in mice; chromosomal aberrations were not found in bone-marrow cells of mice exposed to technical-grade or γ-hexachlorocyclohexane *in vivo*. γ-Hexachlorocyclohexane did not induce unscheduled DNA synthesis in human cells *in vitro* and did not induce micronuclei or chromosomal aberrations in cultured rodent cells; it induced DNA strand breaks but not unscheduled DNA synthesis. It inhibited intercellular communication in Chinese hamster V79 cells. It did not induce sex-linked recessive lethal mutations in *Drosophila*. α-Hexachlorocyclohexane was not mutagenic to yeast, but the γ isomer induced gene conversion. Neither γ- nor β-hexachlorocyclohexane was mutagenic to bacteria, and α- and β-hexachlorocyclohexane did not cause DNA damage in bacteria[17].

References

[1]*IARC Monographs, 20*, 195-239, 1979

[2]Sidi, Y., Kiltchevsky, E., Shaklai, M. & Pinkhas, J. (1983) Acute myeloblastic leukemia and insecticide. *N.Y. State J. Med., 83*, 161

[3]Hoffman, W.S., Adler, H., Fishbein, W.I. & Bauer, F.C. (1967) Relation of pesticide concentrations in fat to pathological changes in tissues. *Arch. environ. Health, 15*, 758-765

[4]Radomski, J.L., Deichmann, W.B., Clizer, E.E. & Rey, A. (1968) Pesticide concentrations in the liver, brain and adipose tissue of terminal hospital patients. *Food Cosmet. Toxicol., 6*, 209-220

[5]Kasai, A., Asanuma, S. & Nakamura, S. (1972) Studies on organochlorine pesticide residues in human organs. Part III (Jpn.). *Nippon Noson Igakkai Zasshi, 21*, 296-297

[6]Caldwell, G.G., Cannon, S.B., Pratt, C.B. & Arthur, R.D. (1981) Serum pesticide levels in patients with childhood colorectal carcinoma. *Cancer, 48*, 774-778

[7]Eriksson, M., Hardell, L., Berg, N.O., Möller, T. & Axelson, O. (1981) Soft-tissue sarcomas and exposure to chemical substances: a case-referent study. *Br. J. ind. Med.*, *38*, 27-33

[8]Hardell, L., Eriksson, M., Lenner, P. & Lundgren, E. (1981) Malignant lymphoma and exposure to chemicals, especially organic solvents, chlorophenols and phenoxy acids: a case-control study. *Br. J. Cancer*, *43*, 169-176

[9]Barthel, E. (1981) Increased risk of lung cancer in pesticide-exposed male agricultural workers. *J. Toxicol. environ. Health*, *8*, 1027-1040

[10]Kashyap, S.K., Nigam, S.K., Gupta, R.C., Karnik, A.B. & Chatterjee, S.K. (1979) Carcinogenicity of hexachlorocyclohexane (BHC) in pure inbred Swiss mice. *J. environ. Sci. Health*, *B14*, 305-318

[11]Munir, K.M., Soman, C.S. & Bhide, S.V. (1983) Hexachlorocyclohexane-induced tumorigenicity in mice under different experimental conditions. *Tumori*, *69*, 383-386

[12]Schulte-Hermann, R. & Parzefall, W. (1981) Failure to discriminate initiation from promotion of liver tumors in a long-term study with the phenobarbital-type inducer *alpha*-hexachlorocyclohexane and the role of sustained stimulation of hepatic growth and monooxygenases. *Cancer Res.*, *41*, 4140-4146

[13]Angsubhakorn, S., Bhamarapravati, N., Romruen, K., Sahaphong, S. & Thamavit, W. (1977) Alpha benzene hexachloride inhibition of aflatoxin B_1-induced hepatocellular carcinoma. A preliminary report. *Experientia*, *34*, 1069-1970

[14]Hiasa, Y., Ohshima, M., Ohmori, T. & Murata, Y. (1978) Effect of *alpha*-benzene hexachloride on 2-fluorenylacetamide carcinogenesis in rats. *Gann*, *69*, 423-426

[15]Angsubhakorn, S., Bhamarapravati, N., Romruen, K., Sahaphong, S., Thamavit, W. & Miyamoto, M. (1981) Further study of *alpha* benzene hexachloride inhibition of aflatoxin B_1 hepatocarcinogenesis in rats. *Br. J. Cancer*, *43*, 881-883

[16]Rivett, K.F., Chesterman, H., Kellett, D.N., Newman, A.J. & Worden, A.N. (1978) Effects of feeding lindane to dogs for periods of up to 2 years. *Toxicology*, *9*, 273-289

[17]*IARC Monographs*, *Suppl. 6*, 333-335, 1987

HYDRALAZINE (Group 3)

A. Evidence for carcinogenicity to humans (*inadequate*)

Two studies suggest an association between exposure to hydralazine and cancer. One was confined to patients with and without signs of toxicity due to hydralazine, and potential confounding factors were not controlled for. The other involved a small number of subjects exposed to hydralazine, but the possibility of selection bias could not be excluded[1]. However, a study of 3988 participants in a hypertensive detection and follow-up programme suggested no increased risk for cancers at all sites from use of hydralazine. A logistic regression estimate of cancer risk after controlling for age, sex, race, smoking behaviour and concomitant drug therapy was 0.89 (95% confidence interval, 0.45-1.8). It was noted that this estimate of no excess risk was restricted to a hypertensive population over 40 years of age, exposed to hydralazine for various periods (none longer than five years)[2]. Another study involving women with breast cancer also showed no increased risk with use of hydralazine (relative risk, 0.9; 0.5-1.7)[3].

B. Evidence for carcinogenicity to animals (*limited*)

Hydralazine hydrochloride was tested in one experiment in mice by oral administration. A significant increase in the incidence of lung tumours was reported[1].

C. Other relevant data

No data were available on the genetic and related effects of hydralazine in humans.

In a single, limited study, hydralazine did not induce DNA damage in animals treated *in vivo*. It induced sister chromatid exchanges in human lymphocytes *in vitro*, whereas assays for chromosomal aberrations in rodent cells *in vitro* were inconclusive. Hydralazine induced unscheduled DNA synthesis in rat and rabbit hepatocytes *in vitro* and induced mutation and DNA damage in bacteria[4].

References

[1]*IARC Monographs*, *24*, 85-100, 1980

[2]Rogers, A.S. (1984) Hydralazine: an estimate of cancer risk in a hypertensive program (Abstract). *Diss. Abstr. int.*, *44*, 2123

[3]Kaufman, D.W., Kelly, J.P., Rosenberg, L., Stolley, P.D., Schottenfeld, D. & Shapiro, S. (1987) Hydralazine and breast cancer. *J. natl Cancer Inst.*, *78*, 243-246

[4]*IARC Monographs*, *Suppl. 6*, 338-340, 1987

HYDRAZINE (Group 2B)

A. Evidence for carcinogenicity to humans (*inadequate*)

Two reports of cancer mortality in workers exposed to hydrazine have appeared in recent years. Choroidal melanoma was observed in one man who had been exosed to hydrazine for six years[1]. A preliminary report of an epidemiological study of men engaged in hydrazine manufacture revealed no unusual excess of cancer. This study comprised 423 men, with a 64% vital status ascertainment. None of the five cancers reported (three of the stomach, one prostatic and one neurogenic) occurred in the group with the highest exposure[2]. A follow-up study of this cohort[3] has extended it to 1982. Mortality from all causes was not elevated (49 observed, 61.5 expected), and the only excess entailed two lung cancer cases within the highest exposure category, with a relative risk of 1.2 (95% confidence interval, 0.2-4.5).

B. Evidence for carcinogenicity to animals (*sufficient*)

Hydrazine has been tested in mice by oral administration, producing liver and mammary tumours and lung tumours in both P and F_1 generations; after intraperitoneal administration to mice, it produced lung tumours, leukaemias and sarcomas[4,5]. After oral administration to rats, it produced lung and liver tumours[4]. When tested by inhalation, it produced benign and malignant nasal tumours in rats, benign nasal polyps, a few colon tumours and thyroid adenomas in hamsters, and a slight increase in the incidence of lung adenomas in mice[6].

C. Other relevant data

No data were available on the genetic and related effects of hydrazine in humans.

Hydrazine did not induce dominant lethal mutation or micronuclei in bone-marrow cells of mice treated *in vivo*. It induced unscheduled DNA synthesis in human cells *in vitro*. It did not induce chromosomal aberrations in rat cells *in vitro* but induced sister chromatid exchanges in Chinese hamster cells; conflicting results were obtained for the induction of mutation in mouse lymphoma cells. It induced DNA strand breaks in rat hepatocytes *in vitro*. Hydrazine induced somatic mutation in *Drosophila* and chromosomal aberrations and mutation in plants. It was mutagenic to yeast and bacteria and induced DNA damage in bacteria[7].

References

[1]Albert, D.M. & Puliafito, C.A. (1977) Choroidal melanoma: possible exposure to industrial toxins. *New Engl. J. Med.*, *296*, 634-635

[2]Roe, F.J.C. (1978) Hydrazine. *Ann. occup. Hyg.*, *21*, 323-326

[3]Wald, N., Boreham, J., Doll, R. & Bonsall, J. (1984) Occupational exposure to hydrazine and subsequent risk of cancer. *Br. J. ind. Med.*, *41*, 31-34

[4]*IARC Monographs*, *4*, 127-136, 1974

[5]Menon, M.M. & Bhide, S.V. (1983) Perinatal carcinogenicity of izoniazid (INH) in Swiss mice. *J. Cancer Res. clin. Oncol.*, *105*, 258-261

[6]Vernot, E.H., MacEwen, J.D., Bruner, R.H., Haun, C.C., Kinkead, E.R., Prentice, D.E., Hall, A., Schmidt, R.E., Eason, R.L., Hubbard, G.B. & Young, J.T. (1985) Long-term inhalation toxicity of hydrazine. *Fundam. appl. Toxicol.*, *5*, 1050-1064

[7]*IARC Monographs*, *Suppl. 6*, 341-343, 198

IRON AND STEEL FOUNDING (Group 1)

A. Evidence for carcinogenicity to humans (*sufficient*)

Analytical cohort epidemiological studies of foundry workers conducted in a number of countries have typically noted risks of lung cancer elevated between 1.5 and 2.5 fold[1,2]. Proportionate mortality studies have also shown the proportion of deaths from lung cancer to be 1.5- to 1.8-fold greater than that in the general population. Associations between foundry work and lung cancer have similarly been observed in studies of mortality statistics[1].

In two studies in which site-specific cancer deaths among iron and steel foundry workers were compared with corresponding rates for the general population, significantly increased risks for cancer of the digestive system were observed; in one, the elevated risk was for cancers in the 'digestive system', in the other, it was for 'stomach cancer'[1].

Results of studies of a single cohort of steel foundry workers in the USA showed a significantly elevated risk of cancer of the genito-urinary system when compared with the entire steel worker population under study, the risk being significantly elevated also for some specific sites (prostate and kidney)[1].

Elevated lung cancer risks have also been reported in a grey-iron foundry[2], in steel foundries[3], in iron and steel foundries[2] and among persons living near steel foundries[4]. No consistent excess of lung cancer, however, was reported among foundrymen employed in a nickel-chromium alloy foundry[5]. Other cancer excesses reported have included leukaemia, stomach cancer and urogenital cancer[2]. Despite the absence of information to specify definitely the carcinogenic substances in the work environment (e.g., polynuclear aromatic hydrocarbons, silica [see p. 341], metal fumes, formaldehyde [see p. 211]), the consistency of the excess in studies from around the world shows that certain exposures in iron and steel founding can cause lung cancer in humans. Most studies lacked information on smoking, but, when it was available, it did not appear that tobacco use could explain the lung cancer excess.

B. Other relevant data

Antigenicity against benzo[a]pyrene diol epoxide-DNA adducts has been demonstrated in peripheral lymphocytes of foundry workers[5].

References

[1]IARC Monographs, 34, 133-190, 1984

[2]IARC Monographs, 42, 39-143, 1987

[3]Fletcher, A.C. & Ades, A. (1984) Lung cancer mortality in a cohort of English foundry workers. Scand. J. Work Environ. Health, 10, 7-16

[4]Lloyd, O.L., Smith, G., Lloyd, M.M., Holland, Y. & Gailey, F. (1985) Raised mortality from lung cancer and high sex ratios of births associated with industrial pollution. Br. J. ind. Med., 42, 475-480

[5]Cornell, R.G. & Landris, J.R. (1984) Mortality patterns among nickel/chromium alloy foundry workers. In: Sunderman, F.W., Jr, ed., Nickel in the Human Environment (IARC Scientific Publications No. 53), Lyon, International Agency for Research on Cancer, pp. 87-93

[6]IARC Monographs, Suppl. 6, 344, 1987

IRON-DEXTRAN COMPLEX (Group 2B)

A. Evidence for carcinogenicity to humans (*inadequate*)

An early report was made of a woman who had developed an undifferentiated soft-tissue sarcoma following multiple injections of iron-dextran complex[1]. In a report on 196 cases of sarcoma of the buttock, four of 90 for whom records on drug use were still available had been given intramuscular injections of iron. In three of the cases, an interval of at least two years had elapsed[2]. A selective tendency to report receiving iron injections may have introduced bias. A review of reports during the period 1960-1977 indicated that nine malignancies had been described in five reports. Two were thought to have been foreign-body reactions to fat necrosis; one was a metastatic carcinoma at the site of an iron-dextran injection; and one was a reticulum-cell sarcoma with fractures of the pelvis possibly only coincidentally related to iron injections six years before. Several of the remainder were of different histological type[3]. Only one, a poorly differentiated spindle-cell fibrosarcoma, was believed likely to be related to iron-dextran injections given 14 years previously[4]. No further case report or epidemiological study is known to the Working Group. It seems probable that the considerable publicity given to the initial case report[1] and the tendency to give parenteral iron therapy intravenously may have considerably reduced human exposure to intra-muscularly administered iron-dextran complex.

B. Evidence for carcinogenicity to animals (*sufficient*)

Iron-dextran complex has been tested in mice, rabbits and rats by repeated sub-cutaneous or intramuscular injections, producing local tumours at the injection site[1,5]. The Working Group noted that iron-dextran complex accumulates at the site of injection in rodents, in contrast to its rapid dispersal after injection in human beings.

C. Other relevant data

No adequate data were available to the Working Group.

References

[1]*IARC Monographs*, 2, 161-178, 1973

[2]Greenberg, G. (1976) Sarcoma after intramuscular iron injection. *Br. med. J.*, *ii*, 1508-1509

[3]Fielding, J. (1977) Does sarcoma occur in man after intramuscular iron? *Scand. J. Haematol.*, *Suppl. 32*, 100-104

[4]Robertson, A.G. & Dick, W.C. (1977) Intramuscular iron and local oncogenesis. *Br. med. J.*, *i*, 946

[5]Hrubý, M. & Damková, E. (1985) Induction and transplantability of ferridextran tumours in inbred strains of *Rattus norvegicus* (Czech.). *Sbornik Lék.*, *87*, 114-120

ISONICOTINIC ACID HYDRAZIDE (ISONIAZID) (Group 3)

A. Evidence for carcinogenicity to humans (*inadequate*)

Several early studies showed no significant excess of cancer among patients treated with isoniazid[1]. A study of 3842 tuberculosis patients followed for 16-24 years showed slight excesses of deaths from malignant neoplasms of the bronchus, lung and pleura in 2041 patients treated with isoniazid during 1953-1957 and followed through to 1973 (relative risk, 1.6; 95% confidence interval, 1.2-2.1), but none in 655 treated for tuberculosis in 1950-1952 when isoniazid was not generally available (0.7; 0.1-1.5). An excess of all malignant neoplasms was seen in patients treated in 1953-1957 (1.4; 1.2-1.7), but also in 145 patients not treated with isoniazid over the same period (1.8; 0.7-2.9). Again, no excess was observed in those treated for tuberculosis in 1950-1952. No dose-response effect was seen either for total consumption or for maximum daily dose of isoniazid[2]. Additional studies of cancer incidence and mortality among patients treated with isoniazid have shown no excess of lung cancer, or of cancer as a whole, that could be attributed to treatment[3-6]. A cancer incidence study in patients with tuberculosis, involving heavy smokers, showed an excess of lung cancer among men exposed to isoniazid (3.4, based on 88 cases observed, 26.2 expected) but also among those not exposed (2.6, based on 18 cases observed, 7.0 expected). The difference between the two ratios was not statistically significant. The corresponding figures for women were 4.6, based on 14 cases exposed, and 0.5, based on one case not exposed[7]. In a preliminary analysis of one-year case records, 72 (4.9%) cancer patients had healed tuberculosis compared with 26 (2%) noncancer patients[8]. Four case-control studies concerning bladder and kidney cancers[9], bladder cancer[10,11] and cancer in children[12] have provided no conclusive evidence of a risk associated with isoniazid therapy. A single case of mesothelioma has been reported in a nine-year-old child whose mother was treated with isoniazid for a positive tuberculin skin test in the second and third trimesters of pregnancy[13].

B. Evidence for carcinogenicity to animals (*limited*)

Isoniazid produced lung tumours in mice after its oral, intraperitoneal or subcutaneous administration[1,8,14-16]. Studies in rats were considered inadequate for evaluation. No tumour was produced in hamsters after oral administration of isoniazid[1].

C. Other relevant data

In the one available study, isoniazid did not induce chromosomal aberrations in lymphocytes of treated patients[17].

Isoniazid did not induce dominant lethal mutations in mice, or chromosomal aberrations, sister chromatid exchanges or DNA damage in rodents treated *in vivo*. Results for chromosomal aberrations and sister chromatid exchanges in human cells *in vitro* were inconclusive; it did not induce unscheduled DNA synthesis. In cultured rodent cells, it induced chromosomal aberrations and sister chromatid exchanges, but not DNA damage. It did not induce transformation of Syrian hamster embryo cells. It did not induce gene conversion in yeast. Isoniazid was mutagenic to *Salmonella typhimurium* but not, in a single study, to *Escherichia coli*[17].

References

[1]*IARC Monographs*, *4*, 159-172, 1974

[2]Stott, H., Peto, J., Stephens, R., Fox, W., Sutherland, I., Foster-Carter, A.F., Teare, H.D. & Fenning, J. (1976) An assessment of the carcinogenicity of isoniazid in patients with pulmonary tuberculosis. *Tubercle*, *57*, 1-15

[3]Glassroth, J.L., White, M.C. & Snider, D.E., Jr (1977) An assessment of the possible association of isoniazid with human cancer deaths. *Am. Rev. respir. Dis.*, *116*, 1065-1074

[4]Howe, G.R., Lindsay, J., Coppock, E. & Miller, A.B. (1979) Isoniazid exposure in relation to cancer incidence and mortality in a cohort of tuberculosis patients. *Int. J. Epidemiol.*, *8*, 305-312

[5]Boice, J.D. & Fraumeni, J.F., Jr (1980) Late effects following isoniazid therapy. *Am. J. public Health*, *70*, 987-989

[6]Costello, H.D. & Snider, D.E., Jr (1980) The incidence of cancer among participants in a controlled, randomized isoniazid preventive therapy trial. *Am. J. Epidemiol.*, *111*, 67-74

[7]Clemmesen, J. & Hjalgrim-Jensen, S. (1979) Is isonicotinic acid hydrazide (INH) carcinogenic to man? A 24-year follow-up of 3371 tuberculosis cases. *Ecotoxicol. environ. Saf.*, *3*, 439-450

[8]Bhide, S.V., Maru, G.B., Mate, N.B., Menon, M. & Gangadharan, P. (1981) Metabolic studies on the possible mode of action of isoniazid tumorigenicity. *J. Cancer Res. clin. Oncol.*, *99*, 153-166

[9]Glassroth, J.L., Snider, D.E. & Comstock, G.W. (1977) Urinary tract cancer and isoniazid. *Am. Rev. respir. Dis.*, *116*, 331-333

[10]Miller, C.T., Neutel, C.I., Nair, R.C., Marrett, L.D., Last, J.M. & Collins, W.E. (1978) Relative importance of risk factors in bladder carcinogenesis. *J. chron. Dis.*, *31*, 51-56

[11]Kantor, A.F., Hartge, P., Hoover, R.N. & Fraumeni, J.F., Jr (1985) Tuberculosis chemotherapy and risk of bladder cancer. *Int. J. Epidemiol.*, *14*, 182-184

[12]Sanders, B.M. & Draper, G.J. (1979) Childhood cancer and drugs in pregnancy. *Br. med. J.*, *i*, 717-718

[13]Tuman, K.J., Chilcote, R.R., Berkow, R.I. & Moohr, J.W. (1980) Mesothelioma in child with prenatal exposure to isoniazid. *Lancet*, *ii*, 362

[14]Maru, G.B., Sawai, M.M. & Bhide, S.V. (1980) Prevention of isoniazid tumorigenicity by antitoxicants of isoniazid in Swiss mice. *J. Cancer Res. clin. Oncol.*, *97*, 145-151

[15]Maru, G.B. & Bhide, S.V. (1982) Effect of antioxidants and antitoxicants of isoniazid on the formation of lung tumours in mice by isoniazid and hydrazine sulphate. *Cancer Lett.*, *17*, 75-80

[16]Menon, M.M. & Bhide, S.V. (1983) Perinatal carcinogenicity of isoniazid (INH) in Swiss mice. *J. Cancer Res. clin. Oncol.*, *105*, 258-261

[17]*IARC Monographs*, *Suppl. 6*, 347-350, 1987

ISOPROPYL ALCOHOL MANUFACTURE (STRONG-ACID PROCESS) (Group 1),

ISOPROPYL ALCOHOL (Group 3) and

ISOPROPYL OILS (Group 3)

A. Evidence for carcinogenicity to humans (*sufficient* for the manufacture of isopropyl alcohol by the strong-acid process; *inadequate* for isopropyl alcohol and isopropyl oils)

An increased incidence of cancer of the paranasal sinuses was observed in workers at factories where isopropyl alcohol was manufactured by the strong-acid process[1,2]. The risk for laryngeal cancer may also have been elevated in these workers[1]. It is unclear whether the cancer risk is due to the presence of diisopropyl sulphate, which is an intermediate in the process, to isopropyl oils, which are formed as by-products, or to other factors, such as sulphuric acid. Epidemiological data concerning the manufacture of isopropyl alcohol by the weak-acid process are insufficient for an evaluation of carcinogenicity[3]. (See also the summary of data for diethyl sulphate, p. 198.)

B. Evidence for carcinogenicity to animals (*inadequate* for isopropyl alcohol and isopropyl oils)

Isopropyl oils, formed during the manufacture of isopropyl alcohol by both the strong-acid and weak-acid processes, were tested inadequately in mice by inhalation, skin application and subcutaneous administration. Isopropyl oils formed during the strong-acid process were also tested inadequately in dogs by inhalation and instillation into the sinuses[1].

The available data on isopropyl alcohol were inadequate for evaluation[1].

C. Other relevant data

No data were available to the Working Group.

References

[1]*IARC Monographs*, *15*, 223-243, 1977

[2]Alderson, M.R. & Rattan, N.S. (1980) Mortality of workers on an isopropyl alcohol plant and two MEK dewaxing plants. *Br. J. ind. Med.*, *37*, 85-89

[3]Wright, U. (1979) *The hidden carcinogen in the manufacture of isopropyl alcohol.* In: Deichmann, W.B., ed., *Toxicology and Occupational Medicine*, New York, Elsevier, pp. 93-97

LEAD AND LEAD COMPOUNDS:
LEAD AND INORGANIC LEAD COMPOUNDS (Group 2B)
ORGANOLEAD COMPOUNDS (Group 3)

A. Evidence for carcinogenicity to humans (*inadequate*)

Three epidemiological studies of workers exposed to lead and lead compounds were reviewed previously[1]: one on smelters and battery workers in the USA, one on workers exposed to tetraethyllead in the USA, and one on copper smelters in the USA; data on the first of these populations have been updated[2]. A study on battery workers in the UK[3] is now available, and studies of a US lead smelter[4] and of a Swedish copper smelter[5] have also been reported. A statistically significant excess of cancers of the digestive system (21 observed, 12.6 expected) was found in the study of battery workers in the UK, spanning 1925-1976, although the excess was confined to the years 1963-1966[3]. Significant excesses of stomach cancer (34 observed, 20.2 expected) and of respiratory cancers (116 observed, 93.5 expected) were seen in the study of US battery plant workers[2], although there was a downward trend in standardized mortality ratio by number of years of employment; in the lead production facilities, the excesses noted for stomach and respiratory cancers were not significant[2]. A nonsignificant excess of respiratory cancer (41 observed, 36.9 expected) was reported in one of the studies of smelters[4], with 28 observed and 25.7 expected in the group with high exposure to lead. Excesses were also noted in this study for kidney cancer (6 observed, 2.9 expected) and bladder cancer (6 observed, 4.2 expected)[4]. A small study of workers at a Swedish smelter[5] with long-term exposure to lead demonstrated a nonsignificant excess of lung cancers (8 observed, 5 expected). Two cases of kidney cancer in lead smelter workers have also been reported[6,7].

The excesses of respiratory cancer in these studies were relatively small, showed no clear-cut trend with length or degree of exposure, and could have been confounded by factors such as smoking or exposure to arsenic (see p. 100).

A study of workers manufacturing tetraethyllead revealed excesses of respiratory cancer (15 observed, 11.2 expected) and brain cancer (3 observed, 1.6 expected)[8].

B. Evidence for carcinogenicity to animals (*sufficient* for inorganic lead compounds; *inadequate* for organolead compounds)

Lead acetate and lead subacetate were tested for carcinogenicity by oral, subcutaneous and intraperitoneal administration in rats, lead phosphate was tested by subcutaneous and intraperitoneal administration in rats, and lead subacetate was tested by oral administration in mice. Renal tumours were produced in animals of each species by each route of administration. Rats given lead acetate or lead subacetate orally developed gliomas. Lead subacetate also produced an increased incidence of lung adenomas in mice after its intraperitoneal administration[1]. Oral administration of lead dimethyldithiocarbamate (ledate) increased the incidence of reticulum-cell sarcomas in male mice of one strain[9] but was not carcinogenic to mice or rats in another experiment[10].

Synergistic effects were reported[1,11-14] in the kidneys of rats given lead acetate and
N-nitroso-N-(hydroxyethyl)ethylamine, N-(4'-fluoro-4-biphenyl)acetamide or 2-(nitroso-
ethylamine)ethanol orally and in the lungs of hamsters given lead oxide with benzo-
[a]pyrene intratracheally. Lead subacetate given in the diet enhanced the incidences of liver
and kidney tumours induced in rats by 2-acetylaminofluorene given in the diet[1].

The lead compounds tested for carcinogenicity in animals are almost all soluble salts
that were selected on the basis of ease of administration. Metallic lead, lead oxide and lead
tetraalkyls have not been tested adequately.

C. Other relevant data

Studies of chromosomal aberrations in people exposed to lead have given conflicting
results: positive reports have been published concerning workers in lead-battery industries
and lead smelters, but other studies of workers under comparable conditions have given
negative results. Increased incidences of sister chromatid exchanges have been reported in
the peripheral blood lymphocytes of workers exposed to lead but not in those of children
exposed to high levels of lead in the environment. An increased incidence of sperm
abnormalities was seen in men exposed occupationally to lead[15].

Although a few studies in rodents treated with lead salts in vivo have shown small (but
significant) increases in the frequency of chromosomal aberrations and micronuclei in
bone-marrow cells, most studies showed no increase. Lead salts caused morphological
sperm abnormalities in mice but not in rabbits. Sister chromatid exchanges and unscheduled DNA synthesis were not induced in cells of animals treated with lead salts in vivo.
Lead salts did not induce chromosomal aberrations in human lymphocytes in vitro.
Conflicting results have been obtained in assays for transformation in cultured rodent cells.
Lead salts did not cause aneuploidy in Drosophila, mutation or gene conversion in yeast or
mutation or DNA damage in bacteria[15].

Tetraethyl- and tetramethyllead did not induce mutation in bacteria[15].

References

[1]IARC Monographs, 23, 39-141, 325-415, 1980

[2]Cooper, W.C., Wong, O. & Kheifets, L. (1985) Mortality among employees of lead battery plants and
lead-producing plants, 1947-1980. Scand. J. Work Environ. Health, 11, 331-345

[3]Malcolm, D. & Barnett, H.A.R. (1982) A mortality study of lead workers 1925-76. Br. J. ind. Med.,
39, 404-410

[4]Selevan, S.G., Landrigan, P.J., Stern, F.B. & Jones, J.H. (1985) Mortality of lead smelter workers.
Am. J. Epidemiol., 122, 673-783

[5]Gerhardsson, L., Lundström, N.-G., Nordberg, G. & Wall, S. (1986) Mortality and lead exposures: a
retrospective cohort study of Swedish smelter workers. Br. J. ind. Med., 43, 707-712

[6]Baker, E.L., Jr, Goyer, R.A., Fowler, B.A., Khettry, U., Bernard, D.B., Adler, S., White, R. deV.,
Babayan, R. & Feldman, R.G. (1980) Occupational lead exposure, nephropathy, and renal
cancer. Am. J. ind. Med., 1, 139-148

[7]Lilis, R. (1981) Long-term occupational lead exposure, chronic nephropathy, and renal cancer: a case report. *Am. J. ind. Med.*, *2*, 293-297

[8]Sweeney, M.H., Beaumont, J.J., Waxweiler, R.J. & Halperin, W.E. (1986) An investigation of mortality from cancer and other causes of death among workers employed at an East Texas chemical plant. *Arch. environ. Health*, *41*, 23-28

[9]*IARC Monographs*, *12*, 131-135, 1976

[10]National Cancer Institute (1979) *Bioassay of Lead Dimethyldithiocarbamate for Possible Carcinogenicity (Tech. Rep. Ser. No. 151; DHEW Publ. No. (NIH) 79-1707)*, Washington DC, US Department of Health, Education and Welfare

[11]Hinton, D.E., Lipsky, M.M., Heatfield, B.M. & Trump, B.F. (1979) Opposite effects of lead on chemical carcinogenesis in kidney and liver of rats. *Bull. environ. Contam. Toxicol.*, *23*, 464-469

[12]Tanner, D.C. & Lipsky, M.M. (1984) Effect of lead acetate on *N*-(4'-fluoro-4-biphenyl)acetamide-induced renal carcinogenesis in the rat. *Carcinogenesis*, *5*, 1109-1113

[13]Shirai, T., Ohshima, M., Masuda, A., Tamano, S. & Ito, N. (1984) Promotion of 2-(ethyl-nitrosamino)ethanol-induced renal carcinogenesis in rats by nephrotoxic compounds: positive responses with folic acid, basic lead acetate, and *N*-(3,5-dichlorophenyl)succinimide but not with 2,3-dibromo-1-propanol phosphate. *J. natl Cancer Inst.*, *72*, 477-482

[14]Hiasa, Y., Ohshima, M., Kitahori, Y., Fujita, T., Yuasa, T. & Miyashiro, A. (1983) Basic lead acetate: promoting effect on the development of renal tubular cell tumors in rats treated with *N*-ethyl-*N*-hydroxyethylnitrosamine. *J. natl Cancer Inst.*, *70*, 761-765

[15]*IARC Monographs*, *Suppl. 6*, 351-354, 1987

LEATHER INDUSTRIES:
BOOT AND SHOE MANUFACTURE AND REPAIR (Group 1)

Evidence for carcinogenicity to humans (*sufficient*)

Nasal adenocarcinoma has been caused by employment in boot and shoe manufacture and repair. Relative risks well in excess of ten fold have been reported from studies in the boot and shoe manufacturing industry in England and in Italy. There is also evidence that an increased risk exists for other types of nasal cancer[1-3]. A far higher risk of nasal cancer was found for people who worked in the dustiest operations, and for those classified into the category of 'heavy' exposure to leather dust, strongly suggesting a role for exposure to leather dust[2,3]. Thus, in comparison with the 'nonexposed' category, the sex-adjusted standardized odds ratio for the 'uncertain or light exposure' category was 7.5, and for the 'heavy exposure' category, 121.0. A similar, highly significant pattern was noted when only adenocarcinomas were considered. Exposure to solvents or to tobacco smoking could not account for the noted increased risk[3]. A mortality study of over 5000 men known to have been employed in the boot and shoe manufacturing industry in three towns in the UK in 1939 showed a large, significant excess of deaths from nasal cancer (10 observed, 1.9 expected). An observed:expected ratio of 14 was found among workers in the finishing room[4]. The elevated nasal cancer risk was almost totally confined to employees in the preparation and finishing rooms, where most of the dusty operations occurred. It was estimated that the risk to those men was 4.5 relative to that in other operations, and 9.8 relative to that of men resident in the area who had never been employed in the footwear industry[2].

Case reports have also suggested an association between exposure to leather, including during shoe manufacture, and mucinous adenocarcinoma of the nose and ethmoidal cancer in Switzerland and France, respectively[5,6].

One mortality study conducted in London, UK, showed no association between nasal cancer deaths occurring between 1968 and 1978 and occupation in the boot and shoe industry, as recorded on death certificates[7]. A proportionate mortality analysis of 3754 deaths among US shoeworkers revealed no death from nasal cancer, whereas 2.2 were expected on the basis of data for the general population[8]. Similar results were obtained from a study of 2798 deaths between 1954 and 1974 in a shoe and leather industry area in Massachusetts, USA; detailed occupational information was available, however, for only 289 of the deceased[9].

Early death certificate surveys showed an increased risk of bladder cancer among shoemakers and repairers. Later studies provided evidence of an increased risk associated with employment in the leather industry. Although boot and shoemakers were included in these studies, it was not possible to determine whether the risk was related to them in particular[1]. A nonsignificant increased risk for bladder cancer was reported in association with work in the boot and shoe industry in a case-control study based on deaths of male residents in certain London boroughs from 1968-1978. When data for these workers were combined with those for leather workers, the estimated risk became significant[7]. A significant association of leather work (leather or tanning industry, manufacture of leather goods, or shoemaking) with cancer of the lower urinary tract was found in a collaborative case-control study in the USA and the UK, but not in Japan[10]. A statistically significant increase was found among female shoe workers (7 deaths observed and 2.8 expected) in another, independent study in the USA. Male shoeworkers and leather workers showed no excess of bladder cancer in this study[9]. In Sweden, an increase in the incidence of bladder cancer (22 cases observed, 14.5 expected) was reported among shoe factory workers[11]. An elevated risk that was not statistically significant was also found among boot and shoe repairers in a British county. Smoking did not appear to account for the increase[12]. In another study in the UK, in a cohort of 5108 boot and shoe workers, 32 deaths from bladder cancer were observed, with 39.2 expected[13].

A possible increase in risk for kidney cancer among shoe workers was suggested by a study in Sweden[11]. However, a large cohort study among boot and shoe workers in the UK did not support this hypothesis[13]. Three cases of mesothelioma were reported among 3806 deaths in shoe workers[14]; it has further been reported that a female shoemaker (whose husband was also a shoemaker) died of mesothelioma[15].

The occurrence of leukaemia among shoemakers exposed to benzene (see p. 120) has been well documented[1,16], and this association has been supported further by a recent mortality study in one town in the UK[4].

Surveys conducted in the The Netherlands, the UK and the USA have suggested positive associations between boot and shoe manufacture/repair and cancers of the lung, oral cavity and pharynx and stomach[1]. These suggestions were later confirmed by a mortality survey in the USA, which also showed a significant increase in the proportion of deaths due to cancers of the rectum and of the liver and gall-bladder, in people of each sex[8]. Excess mortality from rectal cancer was also found among boot and shoemakers in two towns in the UK; the excess was significant for workers in the lasting and making room, who were probably exposed to solvents, glues and leather dust[4]. Exposure to solvents, dyes or metallic compounds in the footwear industry, among nonfactory shoemakers and repairers and among operatives making leather and leather products, was deemed to be associated with the increased risk of bowel cancer noted in a US study[17]. An increased proportion of cancer of the digestive tract among male shoeworkers was found in another US study; however, it was suggested that factors other than their occupation could have been responsible for the excess noted[9]. In a study of gall-bladder cancer occurring in Sweden between 1961 and 1969, in which information on occupation was drawn from 1960 census data, the incidences of cancers of the gall-bladder and of the biliary tract were found to be significantly elevated among men employed in shoemaking and repair[18]. In view of the exploratory nature and design of these studies, the findings were considered to be inadequate for a definite evaluation.

No indication of a link between Hodgkin's disease and work in 'textile, shoes, leather' industries emerged from investigations in Italy[19].

References

[1]*IARC Monographs*, *25*, 249-277, 1981

[2]Acheson, E.D., Pippard, E.C. & Winter, P.D. (1982) Nasal cancer in the Northamptonshire boot and shoe industry: is it declining? *Br. J. Cancer*, *46*, 940-946

[3]Merler, E., Baldasseroni, A., Laria, R., Faravelli, P., Agostini, R., Pisa, R. & Berrino, F. (1986) On the causal association between exposure to leather dust and nasal cancer: further evidence from a case-control study. *Br. J. ind. Med.*, *43*, 91-95

[4]Pippard, E.C. & Acheson, E.D. (1985) The mortality of boot and shoe makers, with special reference to cancer. *Scand. J. Work Environ. Health*, *11*, 249-255

[5]Penneau, D., Pineau, B., Dubin, J., Géraut, C., Penneau, M. & Proteau, J. (1984) Pilot retrospective study of relative risk of ethmoidal cancer in leather work and shoe manufacture (Fr.). *Arch. Mal. prof.*, *45*, 633-638

[6]Rüttner, J.R. & Makek, M. (1985) Mucinous adenocarcinoma of the nose and paranasal sinuses, an occupational disease? (Ger.). *Schweiz. med. Wochenschr.*, *115*, 1838-1842

[7]Baxter, P.J. & McDowall, M.E. (1986) Occupation and cancer in London: an investigation into nasal and bladder cancer using the Cancer Atlas. *Br. J. ind. Med.*, *43*, 44-49

[8]Decouflé, P. & Walrath, J. (1983) Proportionate mortality among US shoeworkers, 1966-1977. *Am. J. ind. Med.*, *4*, 523-532

[9]Garabrant, D.H. & Wegman, D.H. (1984) Cancer mortality among shoe and leather workers in Massachusetts. *Am. J. ind. Med.*, *5*, 303-314

[10]Morrison, A.S., Ahlbom, A., Verhoek, W.G., Aoki, K., Leck, I., Ohno, Y. & Obata, K. (1985) Occupation and bladder cancer in Boston, USA, Manchester, UK, and Nagoya, Japan. *J. Epidemiol. Commun. Health*, *39*, 294-300

[11]Malker, H.R., Malker, B.K., McLaughlin, J.K. & Blot, W.J. (1984) Kidney cancer among leather workers. *Lancet, i*, 56

[12]Cartwright, R.A. & Boyko, R.W. (1984) Kidney cancer among leather workers. *Lancet, i*, 850-851

[13]Acheson, E.D. & Pippard, E.C. (1984) Kidney cancer among leather workers. *Lancet, i*, 563

[14]Decouflé, P. (1980) Mesothelioma among shoeworkers. *Lancet, i*, 259

[15]Vianna, N.J. & Polan, A.K. (1978) Non-occupational exposure to asbestos and malignant mesothelioma in females. *Lancet, i*, 1061-1063

[16]*IARC Monographs, 29*, 93-148, 391-397, 1982

[17]Berg, J.W. & Howell, M.A. (1975) Occupation and bowel cancer. *J. Toxicol. environ. Health, 1*, 75-89

[18]Malker, H.R.S., McLaughlin, J.K., Malker, B.K., Stone, B.J., Weiner, J.A., Ericsson, J.L.E. & Blot, W.J. (1986) Biliary tract cancer and occupation in Sweden. *Br. J. ind. Med., 43*, 257-262

[19]Fonte, R., Grigis, L., Grigis, P. & Franco, G. (1982) Chemicals and Hodgkin's disease. *Lancet, ii*, 5

LEATHER GOODS MANUFACTURE (Group 3)

Evidence for carcinogenicity to humans (*inadequate*)

A few cases of leukaemia have been reported following exposure to benzene (a known human carcinogen[1]; see p. 120) during the manufacture of leather goods other than boots and shoes. The number of cases of nasal cancer reported is insufficient to make an association with employment in the manufacture of leather goods (other than boots and shoes)[2]. A positive association between bladder cancer and employment in the leather products industry is suggested by a number of studies. A case-control study in West Yorkshire, UK, showed a statistically nonsignificant risk of bladder cancer associated with employment in leather goods production (as well as tanning, and boot and shoe repairing)[3]. Indications of an association with dusty leather occupations (not only shoemaking) came from a similar study in London[4]. In two of three areas in which a collaborative study of environmental risk factors for bladder cancer was conducted, a significant association with employment in 'leather' was found; the term 'leather' comprised the manufacture of leather goods, the leather and tanning industries and shoemaking[5]. Leather goods manufacture was most probably included in the leather exposure found to be statistically significantly associated with bladder cancer in another study in the USA[6]. None of the studies provides sufficient grounds to evaluate the specific role of the production of leather goods in the established association of leather work and cancer risk to humans.

References

[1]*IARC Monographs, 29*, 93-148, 391-397, 1982

[2]*IARC Monographs, 25*, 279-292, 1981

[3]Cartwright, R.A. & Boyko, R.W. (1984) Kidney cancer among leather workers. *Lancet, i*, 850-851

[4]Baxter, P.J. & McDowall, M.E. (1986) Occupation and cancer in London: an investigation into nasal and bladder cancer using the Cancer Atlas. *Br. J. ind. Med., 43*, 44-49

[5]Morrison, A.S., Ahlbom, A., Verhoek, W.G., Aoki, K., Leck, I., Ohno, Y. & Obata, K. (1985) Occupation and bladder cancer in Boston, USA, Manchester, UK, and Nagoya, Japan. *J. Epidemiol. Commun. Health, 39*, 294-300

[6]Marrett, L.D., Hartge, P. & Meigs, J.W. (1986) Bladder cancer and occupational exposure to leather. *Br. J. ind. Med., 43*, 96-100

LEATHER TANNING AND PROCESSING (Group 3)

Evidence for carcinogenicity to humans (*inadequate*)

Early studies of cancer risks possibly associated with leather industries provide little information specifically related to workers in tanneries. There was no evidence to suggest an association between leather tanning and nasal cancer[1]. Following the observation of an increased risk of nasal cancer among boot and shoe manufacturers, possibly associated with exposure to dust from leather tanned by a particular process[2], a study was designed to examine the possible cancer risk carried by different methods of leather tanning. The mortality experience of two groups of men working in tanneries in 1939 was compared to that of the population of England and Wales, and for no cause of death was a statistically significant increase above expectation found. Among the 573 men employed in tanneries using a process with vegetable extracts, one death from nasal cancer was observed (0.21 expected); among 260 employees using a tanning process with chromium salts (tri- and hexavalent; see p. 165), one death from soft-tissue tumour (0.07 expected) was reported[3].

In a Swedish study, a slight increase in mortality from stomach cancer and a three-fold, significantly increased risk for cancer of the pancreas were found to be associated with the occupational titles 'tanners' and 'tannery workers' as recorded in the registry of deaths and burials of a parish where a tannery had been in operation from 1873 to 1960. Tannery work involved exposure to chromium and, probably, to chlorophenols (see p. 154); smoking was an unlikely explanation for the findings, but the contribution of various dietary habits could not be ruled out[4]. Suggestions of increased risks for intestinal cancer and lung cancer and for cancer of the tonsils were imputed by a mortality study of workers employed in a tannery plant using chromium salts and synthetic tannins[5]. An association between lung cancer and tanning was also suggested by a study of incident cases in the UK[6] and by a study of cancer deaths among shoe and leather workers in the USA, in which the estimated risk for tannery workers relative to a group of workers classified as nonexposed was 4.2, which was statistically significant. Chromium and arsenicals (see p. 100) were mentioned as possibly contributing to the excess of lung cancer[7]. Significantly increased lung cancer mortality was also found among a group of fur tanners in the USA, who had probably been exposed to chrome (hexavalent) tanning agents[8].

In a study of bladder cancer and occupation, a relative risk of 1.5 was found for leather tanners, which is not statistically significant[1]. No significant excess of bladder cancer was found in another study of tanners in the UK[9]. In two of three areas in which a collaborative study of environmental risk factors for bladder cancer was conducted, a significant association with employment in 'leather' was found; the term 'leather' comprised the leather and tanning industries, the manufacture of leather goods and shoemaking[10].

In a cohort of 1629 leather tanners in Sweden, eight cases of kidney cancer were observed, while 3.4 would have been expected from regional rates[11]. The hypothesis of this association was not supported by another study[12].

References

[1]*IARC Monographs*, *25*, 201-247, 1981

[2]Acheson, E.D., Pippard, E.C. & Winter, P.D. (1982) Nasal cancer in the Northamptonshire boot and shoe industry: is it declining ? *Br. J. Cancer*, *46*, 940-946

[3]Pippard, E.C., Acheson, E.D. & Winter, P.D. (1985) Mortality of tanners. *Br. J. ind. Med.*, *42*, 285-287

[4]Edling, C., Kling, H., Flodin, U. & Axelson, O. (1986) Cancer mortality among leather tanners. *Br. J. ind. Med.*, *43*, 494-496

[5]Puntoni, R., Valerio, A., Cresta, E., Filiberti, R., Bonassi, S. & Vercelli, M. (1984) Mortality study in a tannery (Ital.). *Med. Lav.*, *75*, 471-477

[6]Coggon, D., Pannett, B., Osmond, C. & Acheson, E.D. (1986) A survey of cancer and occupation in young and middle aged men. I. Cancers of the respiratory tract. *Br. J. ind Med.*, *43*, 332-338

[7]Garabrant, D.H. & Wegman, D.H. (1984) Cancer mortality among shoe and leather workers in Massachusetts. *Am. J. ind. Med.*, *5*, 303-314

[8]Sweeney, M.H., Walrath, J. & Waxweiler, R.J. (1985) Mortality among retired fur workers. Dyers, dressers (tanners) and service workers. *Scand. J. Work Environ. Health*, *11*, 257-264

[9]Cartwright, R.A. & Boyko, R.W. (1984) Kidney cancer among leather workers. *Lancet*, *i*, 850-851

[10]Morrison, A.S., Ahlbom, A., Verhoek, W.G., Aoki, K., Leck, I., Ohno, Y. & Obata, K. (1985) Occupation and bladder cancer in Boston, USA, Manchester, UK, and Nagoya, Japan. *J. Epidemiol. Commun. Health*, *39*, 294-300

[11]Malker, H.R., Malker, B.K., McLaughlin, J.K. & Blot, W.J. (1984) Kidney cancer among leather workers. *Lancet*, *i*, 56

[12]Acheson, E.D. & Pippard, E.C. (1984) Kidney cancer among leather workers. *Lancet*, *i*, 563

MAGENTA (Group 3) and
MANUFACTURE OF MAGENTA (Group 1)

A. Evidence for carcinogenicity to humans (*inadequate* for magenta; *sufficient* for the manufacture of magenta)

The manufacture of magenta* was first reported to be associated with bladder tumours in 1895. One study in the UK in 1954 showed an association between magenta production and an increased incidence of bladder cancer, with three deaths (0.13 expected)[1]. An excess of bladder tumours was also noted in one Italian plant manufacturing new fuchsin ('new' magenta) and safranine T (5 observed deaths, 0.08 expected). In addition to magenta, the suspected agents include the precursors *ortho*-toluidine (see p. 362), 4,4'-methylene bis(2-methylaniline) (see p. 246) and *ortho*-nitrotoluene[2].

B. Evidence for carcinogenicity to animals (*inadequate* for magenta)

Magenta products were tested for carcinogenicity in mice, rats and hamsters by subcutaneous and oral administration. Subcutaneous administration of *para*-magenta, a component of commercial magenta, induced local sarcomas in rats[1]. Oral administration of magenta or *para*-magenta to rats and hamsters for life at the maximum tolerated dose produce no treatment-related tumour[3,4]. In one limited study in mice, there was no increase in tumour incidence following oral administration of commercial magenta[1].

C. Other relevant data

No data were available on the genetic and related effects of magenta in humans[5].

Technical-grade magenta consists of a mixture of magenta I, *para*-magenta and related compounds. In the studies considered below, one of these isomers was assayed rather than the complete mixture[5]. *para*-Magenta did not induce transformation of Syrian hamster embryo cells or unscheduled DNA synthesis in rat hepatocytes *in vitro*. It did not induce recombination in yeast. *para*-Magenta and magenta I were mutagenic to bacteria. *para*-Magenta did not induce prophage[5].

References

[1]*IARC Monographs, 4*, 57-64, 1974

[2]Rubino, G.F., Scansetti, G., Piolatto, G. & Pira, E. (1982) The carcinogenic effect of aromatic amines: an epidemiological study on the role of *o*-toluidine and 4,4'-methylene bis(2-methyl-aniline) in inducing bladder cancer in man. *Environ. Res., 27*, 241-254

---

*Included in the term 'magenta' are *para*-magenta and ring-methylated derivatives.

[3]Green, U., Holste, J. & Spikermann, A.R. (1979) A comparative study of the chronic effects of magenta, paramagenta and phenyl-β-naphthylamine in Syrian golden hamsters. *J. Cancer Res. clin. Oncol.*, *95*, 51-55

[4]Ketkar, M.B. & Mohr, U. (1982) The chronic effects of magenta, paramagenta and phenyl-β-naphthylamine in rats after intragastric administration. *Cancer Lett.*, *16*, 203-206

[5]*IARC Monographs*, *Suppl. 6*, 356-358, 1987

MELPHALAN (Group 1)

A. Evidence for carcinogenicity to humans (*sufficient*)

Epidemiological studies of patients with ovarian carcinoma[1-3], multiple myeloma[4,5] or breast cancer[6] have consistently shown very large excesses of acute nonlymphocytic leukaemia in the decade following therapy with melphalan. The relative risk was consistently estimated to be in excess of 100, to increase with increasing dose, and to be roughly the same with and without radiotherapy[7].

B. Evidence for carcinogenicity to animals (*sufficient*)

Melphalan has been tested in mice and rats by intraperitoneal injection, producing lymphosarcomas and a dose-related increase in the incidence of lung tumours in mice and peritoneal sarcomas in rats[8].

C. Other relevant data

Melphalan is a bifunctional alkylating agent. Patients treated therapeutically with melphalan had increased frequencies of chromosomal aberrations and sister chromatid exchanges in their peripheral lymphocytes[9].

Melphalan induced chromosomal aberrations in bone-marrow cells of rats treated *in vivo*. The compound induced chromosomal aberrations, sister chromatid exchanges and DNA damage in human cells *in vitro*. It induced transformation of C3H 10T1/2 cells. In cultured rodent cells, it induced chromosomal aberrations, sister chromatid exchanges, mutation and DNA damage. It induced aneuploidy and sex-linked recessive lethal mutations in *Drosophila* and mutation in bacteria[9].

References

[1]Einhorn, N., Eklund, G., Franzén, S., Lambert, B., Lindsten, J. & Söderhäll, S. (1982) Late side effects of chemotherapy in ovarian carcinoma. A cytogenetic, hematologic, and statistical study. *Cancer*, *49*, 2234-2241

[2]Reimer, R.R., Hoover, R., Fraumeni, J.F., Jr & Young, R.C. (1977) Acute leukemia after alkylating-agent therapy of ovarian cancer. *New Engl. J. Med.*, *297*, 177-181

[3]Greene, M.H., Boice, J.D., Jr, Greer, B.E., Blessing, J.A. & Dembo, A.J. (1982) Acute nonlymphocytic leukemia after therapy with alkylating agents for ovarian cancer. A study of five randomized clinical trials. *New Engl. J. Med.*, *307*, 1416-1421

[4]Law, I.P. & Blom, J. (1977) Second malignancies in patients with multiple myeloma. *Oncology*, *34*, 20-24

[5]Gonzalez, F., Trujillo, J.M. & Alexanian, R. (1977) Acute leukemia in multiple myeloma. *Ann. intern. Med.*, *86*, 440-443

[6]Greene, M.H., Harris, E.L., Gershenson, D.M., Malkasian, G.D., Jr, Melton, L.J., III, Dembo, A.J., Bennett, J.M., Moloney, W.C. & Boice, J.D., Jr (1986) Melphalan may be a more potent leukemogen than cyclophosphamide. *Ann. intern. Med.*, *105*, 360-367

[7]Fisher, B., Rockette, H., Fisher, E.R., Wickerham, D.L., Redmond, C. & Brown, A. (1985) Leukemia in breast cancer patients following adjuvant chemotherapy or postoperative radiotherapy: the NSABP experience. *J. clin. Oncol.*, *3*, 1640-1658

[8]*IARC Monographs*, *9*, 167-180, 1975

[9]*IARC Monographs*, *Suppl. 6*, 363-365, 1987

6-MERCAPTOPURINE (Group 3)

A. Evidence for carcinogenicity to humans (*inadequate*)

No epidemiological study of 6-mercaptopurine as a single agent was available to the Working Group. Occasional case reports of exposure to 6-mercaptopurine, especially in the presence of concurrent therapy with other putative carcinogens, such as ionizing radiation, alkylating agents and other potent oncotherapeutic drugs, do not constitute evidence of carcinogenesis[1].

B. Evidence for carcinogenicity to animals (*inadequate*)

6-Mercaptopurine was tested by intraperitoneal administration and by skin painting (followed by croton oil) in mice and by intraperitoneal, subcutaneous and intravenous injection in rats. Limitations to the data in all the reports precluded evaluation of the possible carcinogenicity of this compound[1].

C. Other relevant data

6-Mercaptopurine induced chromosomal aberrations and sister chromatid exchanges in lymphocytes of treated patients in single studies[2].

In rodents treated *in vivo*, 6-mercaptopurine induced dominant lethal mutations, chromosomal aberrations and micronuclei, but not aneuploidy. The compound induced chromosomal aberrations in human lymphocytes *in vitro*. It induced mutation in cultured rodent cells and chromosomal aberrations and sister chromatid exchanges but not aneuploidy in Chinese hamster cells *in vitro*. It did not transform mouse C3H 10T1/2 cells. 6-Mercaptopurine was mutagenic to and caused DNA damage in bacteria[2].

References

[1] *IARC Monographs*, 26, 249-266, 1981

[2] *IARC Monographs*, Suppl. 6, 366-368, 1987

METHOTREXATE (Group 3)

A. Evidence for carcinogenicity to humans (*inadequate*)

The relationship between methotrexate treatment and subsequent malignancy has been investigated in one cohort of 457 patients (3522 person-years) treated for trophoblastic tumours (2 observed, 3.5 expected)[1] and in a cohort of 248 patients treated for psoriasis (10 observed, 22 expected)[2]. A case-control study of treatment for psoriasis has also been performed, in which 26 cases of noncutaneous cancer (104 matched controls) and 80 cases of nonmelanoma skin cancer (297 matched controls) were studied; relative risks were 1.0 and 1.2, respectively[3]. In each comparison, no excess (significant or otherwise) or subsequent malignancy was observed.

B. Evidence for carcinogenicity to animals (*inadequate*)

Methotrexate was tested by oral administration in mice and hamsters, by intraperitoneal injection in mice and rats, and by intravenous injection in rats. One study in mice by oral administration showed a high incidence of lung carcinomas, but the study design did not include matched controls. No other study revealed a carcinogenic effect, but the significance of several was limited because of deficiencies in experimental design or reporting of data[4]. A study in which methotrexate was given intraperitoneally in combination with cyclophosphamide (see p. 182) and 5-fluorouracil (see p. 210) to rats resulted in induction of tumours in the nervous system, haematopoietic and lymphatic tissues, the urinary bladder and adrenal glands; however, because of lack of matched controls, it could not be concluded whether tumour induction was due to a combined effect of the three chemicals or to any one of them[5].

C. Other relevant data

In patients treated with methotrexate, chromosomal aberrations were observed in bone-marrow cells, and, in one of two studies, sister chromatid exchanges were induced in lymphocytes[6].

Methotrexate induced micronuclei in mice, but neither aneuploidy in mouse oocytes nor DNA strand breaks in granuloma cells of rats treated *in vivo*. It induced chromosomal aberrations in human and rodent cells *in vitro* and sister chromatid exchanges in rodent but not in human cells *in vitro*. It did not induce unscheduled DNA synthesis in human cells *in vitro*. It caused transformation of C3H 10T1/2 cells but not of Syrian hamster embryo cells and was mutagenic to mouse lymphoma cells but not to Chinese hamster cells *in vitro*. Methotrexate induced genetic crossing-over but not sex-linked recessive lethal mutations in *Drosophila*. It was not mutagenic to *Salmonella typhimurium* but gave conflicting results in *Escherichia coli* and was mutagenic to *Bacillus subtilis*. It did not induce DNA damage in bacteria[6].

References

[1]Rustin, G.J.S., Rustin, F., Dent, J., Booth, M., Salt, S. & Bagshawe, K.D. (1983) No increase in second tumors after cytotoxic chemotheraphy for gestational trophoblastic tumors. *New Engl. J. Med., 308*, 473-476

[2]Nyfors, A. & Jensen, H. (1983) Frequency of malignant neoplasms in 248 long-term methotrexate-treated psoriatics. A preliminary study. *Dermatologica, 167*, 260-261

[3]Stern, R.S., Zierler, S. & Parrish, J.A. (1982) Methotrexate used for psoriasis and the risk of noncutaneous or cutaneous malignancy. *Cancer, 50*, 869-872

[4]*IARC Monographs, 26*, 267-292, 1981

[5]Habs, M., Schmähl, D. & Lin, P.Z. (1981) Carcinogenic activity in rats of combined treatment with cyclophosphamide, methotrexate and 5-fluorouracil. *Int. J. Cancer, 28*, 91-96

[6]*IARC Monographs, Suppl. 6*, 372-374, 1987

5-METHOXYPSORALEN (Group 2A)

A. Evidence for carcinogenicity to humans (*inadequate*)

In a survey of 87 persons employed in the production of bergamot oil (of which 5-methoxypsoralen is a constituent), 19% of 79 exposed workers and 16% of a comparison group of 31 people resident in the same area were observed to have 'keratomas' or 'epitheliomas' of the skin. Possible confounding effects of age, sex and outdoor employment were not considered in this analysis[1].

B. Evidence for carcinogenicity to animals (*sufficient*)

5-Methoxypsoralen was tested in mice by skin application in combination with ultraviolet A radiation or solar-simulated radiation, producing skin papillomas and carcinomas; in these studies, no or few skin tumours were observed with ultraviolet A radiation or solar-simulated radiation alone. The studies were inadequate to evaluate the local and systemic carcinogenic effects of the compound itself[1].

C. Other relevant data

No data were available on the genetic and related effects of 5-methoxypsoralen in humans.

In the presence of ultraviolet A radiation, 5-methoxypsoralen induced chromosomal aberrations, sister chromatid exchanges and unscheduled DNA synthesis in human cells *in vitro*; sister chromatid exchanges, mutation and DNA cross-links in rodent cells *in vitro*; mutation, gene conversion and DNA cross-links in yeast; and mutation and prophage in bacteria[2].

5-Methoxypsoralen, tested in the absence of ultraviolet A radiation, was reported to be weakly mutagenic to bacteria[2].

References

[1] *IARC Monographs*, *40*, 327-347, 1986

[2] *IARC Monographs*, *Suppl. 6*, 377-379, 1987

8-METHOXYPSORALEN (METHOXSALEN) PLUS ULTRAVIOLET RADIATION (Group 1)

A. Evidence for carcinogenicity to humans (*sufficient*)

The development of nonmelanocytic skin cancer (basal- and squamous-cell skin cancers) has been reported in patients treated with 8-methoxypsoralen and long-wave ultraviolet light (UVA) (PUVA) for psoriasis or mycosis fungoides[1-5]. Three cases of malignant melanoma of the skin have been reported in patients with psoriasis treated with PUVA[6,7]. The strongest evidence for a causal association between PUVA treatment and nonmelanocytic skin cancer comes from the follow-up of 1380 psoriatic patients treated in the USA. The standardized incidence ratio (SIR) for squamous-cell carcinoma increased from 4.1 (95% confidence interval, 2.3-6.8) at low doses to 22.3 (13.5-34.1) at medium doses and 56.8 (42.7-74.2) at high doses; this effect was independent of possible confounding effects of therapy with ionizing radiation and topical tar. The effect on basal-cell cancer incidence was much weaker (high doses: SIR, 4.5; 2.8-6.9)[8]. One cohort study of 525 psoriatic patients treated with PUVA did not suggest an increase in the incidence of skin cancer (mean follow-up period, 2.1 years)[9]. This 'negative' result could have been due to lack of statistical power and to the low doses used in the study. Another study with a five-year follow up showed no skin tumour in 94 patients treated with PUVA for psoriasis or mycosis fungoides[10].

8-Methoxypsoralen alone did not alter the incidence of new skin cancer over two years in two small controlled trials of its use as a prophylactic for skin cancer[1].

B. Evidence for carcinogenicity to animals (*sufficient*)

8-Methoxypsoralen was tested by oral and intraperitoneal administration and by skin application in combination with ultraviolet A radiation in mice, producing epidermal and dermal tumours[1,11-15]. When it was tested alone in mice by intraperitoneal administration[13] or by skin application[12,13], it did not induce skin tumours. The studies were inadequate to evaluate the systemic carcinogenicity of 8-methoxypsoralen.

C. Other relevant data

In patients treated with PUVA, neither chromosomal aberrations (one study) nor sister chromatid exchanges were observed[16].

8-Methoxypsoralen in combination with ultraviolet A radiation induced sister chromatid exchanges in epithelial cells of cheek pouches of hamsters treated *in vivo*. In a large number of studies, it induced chromosomal aberrations, sister chromatid exchanges, mutation, DNA damage and DNA cross-links in human cells *in vitro*. It transformed mouse C3H 10T1/2 cells. In rodent cells in culture, it induced chromosomal aberrations, micronuclei, sister chromatid exchanges, mutation, unscheduled DNA synthesis and DNA cross-links. It induced mitotic recombination and mutation in fungi and mutation and DNA damage in bacteria[16].

8-Methoxypsoralen in the absence of ultraviolet A radiation induced mutation in bacteria, but inconclusive results were obtained with respect to chromosomal aberrations and sister chromatid exchanges in human cells *in vitro*, gene mutation and DNA damage in rodent cells *in vitro* and mutation in yeast[16].

References

[1]*IARC Monographs*, 24, 101-124, 1980

[2]Roenigk, H.H., Jr & Caro, W.A. (1981) Skin cancer in the PUVA-48 cooperative study. *J. Am. Acad. Dermatol.*, 4, 319-324

[3]Stüttgen, G., Kentsch, V., Schalla, W. & Schneider, L. (1981) The risks of photochemotherapy (Ger.). *Z. Hautkr.*, 56, 1379-1399

[4]Abel, E.A., Deneau, D.G., Farber, E.M., Price, N.M. & Hoppe, R.T. (1981) PUVA treatment of erythrodermic and plaque type mycosis fungoides. *J. Am. Acad. Dermatol.*, 4, 423-429

[5]Stern, R., Zierler, S. & Parrish, J.A. (1982) Psoriasis and the risk of cancer. *J. invest. Dermatol.*, 78, 147-149

[6]Frenk, E. (1983) Malignant melanoma in a patient with severe psoriasis treated by oral methoxsalen photochemotherapy. *Dermatologica*, 167, 152-154

[7]Marx, J.L., Auerbach, R., Possick, P., Myrow, R., Gladstein, A.H. & Kopf, A.W. (1983) Malignant melanoma *in situ* in two patients treated with psoralens and ultraviolet A. *J. Am. Acad. Dermatol.*, 9, 904-911

[8]Stern, R.S., Laird, N., Melski, J., Parrish, J.A., Fitzpatrick, T.B. & Bleich, H.L. (1984) Cutaneous squamous-cell carcinoma in patients treated with PUVA. *New Engl. J. Med.*, 310, 1156-1161

[9]Lassus, A., Reunala, T., Idänpää-Heikkilä, J., Juvakoski, T. & Salo, O. (1981) PUVA treatment and skin cancer: a follow-up study. *Acta dermatol. venereol.*, 61, 141-145

[10]Fitzsimons, C.P., Long, J. & MacKie, R.M. (1983) Synergistic carcinogenic potential of methotrexate and PUVA in psoriasis. *Lancet, i*, 235-236

[11]Kripke, M.L., Morison, W.L. & Parrish, J.A. (1982) Induction and transplantation of murine skin cancers induced by methoxsalen plus ultraviolet (320-400 nm) radiation. *J. natl Cancer Inst., 68*, 685-690

[12]Nagayo, K., Way, B.H., Tran, R.M. & Song, P.S. (1983) Photocarcinogenicity of 8-methoxypsoralen and aflatoxin B$_1$ with longwave ultraviolet light. *Cancer Lett., 18*, 191-198

[13]Young, A.R., Magnus, I.A., Davies, A.C. & Smith, N.P. (1983) A comparison of the photo-tumorigenic potential of 8-MOP and 5-MOP in hairless albino mice exposed to solar simulated radiation. *Br. J. Dermatol., 108*, 507-518

[14]Gibbs, N.K., Young, A.R. & Magnus, I.A. (1985) A strain of hairless mouse susceptible to tumorigenesis by TPA alone: studies with 8-methoxypsoralen and solar simulated radiation. *Carcinogenesis, 6*, 797-799

[15]Hannuksela, M., Stenbäck, F. & Lahti, A. (1986) The carcinogenic properties of topical PUVA. A lifelong study in mice. *Arch. dermatol. Res., 278*, 347-351

[16]*IARC Monographs, Suppl. 6*, 380-385, 1987

METHYL BROMIDE (Group 3)

A. Evidence for carcinogenicity to humans (*inadequate*)

Two cohort studies mention exposure to methyl bromide. In both study populations, exposure to a great number of other chemical compounds occurred, and, therefore, the slight excesses of some cancers found cannot be interpreted in terms of exposure to methyl bromide[1].

B. Evidence for carcinogenicity to animals (*limited*)

In one 90-day study by oral administration in rats, methyl bromide was reported to produce squamous-cell carcinomas of the forestomach[1]. In a second, 25-week study, it was found that early hyperplastic lesions of the forestomach regressed after discontinuation of treatment; one early carcinoma (1/11) developed after 25 weeks of continuous treatment by gavage[2].

C. Other relevant data

No data were available on the genetic and related effects of methyl bromide in humans.

Micronuclei were induced in the bone-marrow and peripheral blood cells of rats and mice following exposure to methyl bromide by inhalation. After treatment of mice with methyl bromide by different routes, DNA methylation of liver and spleen was observed. Methyl bromide induced sister chromatid exchanges in human lymphocytes *in vitro* and mutation in mouse lymphoma cells *in vitro*. It did not induce unscheduled DNA synthesis in rat hepatocytes. Methyl bromide induced sex-linked recessive lethal mutations in *Drosophila* and was mutagenic to plants and bacteria[3].

References

[1] *IARC Monographs*, *41*, 187-212, 1987

[2] Boorman, G.A., Hong, H.L., Jameson, C.W., Yoshitomi, K. & Maronpot, R.R. (1986) Regression of methyl bromide-induced forestomach lesions in the rat. *Toxicol. appl. Pharmacol.*, *86*, 131-139

[3] *IARC Monographs*, *Suppl. 6*, 386-388, 1987

METHYL CHLORIDE (Group 3)

A. Evidence for carcinogenicity to humans (*inadequate*)

In a small study of 852 butyl rubber manufacturing workers exposed to methyl chloride, there was a total of 30 deaths from cancer, which was fewer than expected on the basis of US mortality data. The study is uninformative for assessing the carcinogenicity of methyl chloride[1].

B. Evidence for carcinogenicity to animals (*inadequate*)

A study in which methyl chloride was tested for carcinogenicity in mice and rats by inhalation was reported only in an abstract and could not be evaluated[1].

C. Other relevant data

No data were available on the genetic and related effects of methyl chloride in humans.

Methyl chloride induced sister chromatid exchanges and mutation but not DNA strand breaks in human lymphocytes *in vitro*. It enhanced transformation of virus-infected Syrian hamster embryo cells. It induced chromosomal aberrations in plants and was mutagenic to bacteria[2].

References

[1] *IARC Monographs*, *41*, 161-186, 1987

[2] *IARC Monographs*, *Suppl. 6*, 389-390, 1987

4,4′-METHYLENE BIS(2-CHLOROANILINE) (MOCA) (Group 2A)

A. Evidence for carcinogenicity to humans (*inadequate*)

In a review, a higher than expected incidence of bladder cancer was reported among workers in a UK plant manufacturing MOCA[1]. An earlier study of workers manufacturing this compound in the USA, who were followed up for less than 16 years, failed to reveal any bladder tumour[2].

B. Evidence for carcinogenicity to animals (*sufficient*)

After oral administration of MOCA, mice developed haemangiosarcomas and hepatomas[2,3]; rats developed lung, liver, mammary gland and Zymbal gland tumours and haemangiosarcomas[2-5]; and dogs developed urinary bladder tumours[6]. Tumours of the lung and liver were produced after subcutaneous injection of rats[2].

C. Other relevant data

MOCA is an aromatic amine with structural similarities to benzidine, which is causally associated with cancer in humans (see p. 123).

No data were available on the genetic and related effects of MOCA in humans.

MOCA induced micronuclei in bone-marrow cells of mice treated *in vivo*. Conflicting results were obtained for the induction of sister chromatid exchanges in Chinese hamster cells *in vitro*; it induced unscheduled DNA synthesis in rodent hepatocytes. In yeast, MOCA induced aneuploidy, gave equivocal results in assays for gene conversion and did not cause mutation. It was mutagenic and induced prophage in bacteria[7].

References

[1]Cartwright, R.A. (1983) Historical and modern epidemiological studies on populations exposed to *N*-substituted aryl compounds. *Environ. Health Perspect.*, *49*, 13-19

[2]*IARC Monographs*, *4*, 65-71, 1974

[3]Russfield, A.B., Homburger, F., Boger, E., van Dongen, C.G., Weisburger, E.K. & Weisburger, J.H. (1975) The carcinogenic effect of 4,4′-methylene-bis-(2-chloroaniline) in mice and rats. *Toxicol. appl. Pharmacol.*, *31*, 47-54

[4]Kommineni, C., Groth, D.H., Frockt, I.J., Voelker, R.W. & Stanovick, R.P. (1978) Determination of the tumorigenic potential of methylene-bis-orthochloroaniline. *J. environ. Pathol. Toxicol.*, *2*, 149-171

[5]Stula, E.F., Sherman, H., Zapp, J.A., Jr & Clayton, J.W., Jr (1975) Experimental neoplasia in rats from oral administration of 3,3′-dichlorobenzidine, 4,4′-methylene-bis(2-chloroaniline), and 4,4′-methylene-bis(2-methylaniline). *Toxicol. appl. Pharmacol.*, *31*, 159-176

[6]Stula, E.F., Barnes, J.R., Sherman, H., Reinhardt, C.F. & Zapp, J.A., Jr (1977) Urinary bladder tumors in dogs from 4,4′-methylene-bis-(2-chloroaniline) (MOCA®). *J. environ. Pathol. Toxicol.*, *1*, 31-50

[7]*IARC Monographs*, *Suppl. 6*, 391-393, 1987

4,4'-METHYLENE BIS(2-METHYLANILINE) (Group 2B)

A Evidence for carcinogenicity to humans (*inadequate*)

A study of an Italian cohort of 906 dyestuffs workers employed between 1922 and 1970 revealed an impressive excess of deaths from bladder cancer (36 observed, 1.2 expected). Workers were classified into ten exposure categories. Among 53 workers employed in the manufacture of new fuchsin ('new' magenta [see p. 238]) and safranine T, five died from bladder cancer, whereas 0.08 would have been expected. Their minimum length of employment was 12 years. Three of the five deaths occurred among workers engaged in the synthesis of *ortho*-toluidine (see p. 362) and 4,4'-methylenebis(2-methylaniline), used as precursors in the production of new fuchsin and safranine T, which was carried out in a separate building within the plant[1].

B. Evidence for carcinogenicity to animals (*sufficient*)

4,4'-Methylene bis(2-methylaniline) was tested for carcinogenicity by oral administration in rats and dogs, inducing high incidences of hepatocellular carcinomas in animals of each species; neoplasms of the lung, mammary gland and skin in rats and of the lung in dogs were also reported[2-4].

C. Other relevant data

No data were available to the Working Group.

References

[1]Rubino, G.F., Scansetti, G., Piolatto, G. & Pira, E. (1982) The carcinogenic effect of aromatic amines: an epidemiological study on the role of *o*-toluidine and 4,4'-methylene bis(2-methylaniline) in inducing bladder cancer in man. *Environ. Res., 27,* 241-254

[2]*IARC Monographs, 4,* 73-77, 1974

[3]Stula, E.F., Sherman, H., Zapp, J.A., Jr & Clayton, J.W., Jr (1975) Experimental neoplasia in rats from oral administration of 3,3'-dichlorobenzidine, 4,4'-methylene-bis(2-chloroaniline), and 4,4'-methylene-bis(2-methylaniline). *Toxicol. appl. Pharmacol., 31,* 159-176

[4]Stula, E.F., Barnes, J.R., Sherman, H., Reinhardt, C.F. & Zapp, J.A., Jr (1978) Liver and lung tumors in dogs from 4,4'-methylene-bis(2-methylaniline). *J. environ. Pathol. Toxicol., 1,* 339-356

N-METHYL-*N*'-NITRO-*N*-NITROSOGUANIDINE (MNNG) (Group 2A)

A. Evidence for carcinogenicity to humans (*inadequate*)

Three cases of brain tumour (gliomas) and one of colon cancer have been reported from a genetics laboratory over a 13-year period. All the subjects were likely to have been exposed to MNNG for at least six to 15 years prior to death, but other carcinogens had been used in the laboratory[1,2].

B. Evidence for carcinogenicity to animals (*sufficient*)

MNNG has been tested for carcinogenicity in mice, rats, hamsters, rabbits and dogs, producing tumours at many sites. It has a predominantly local carcinogenic effect and is carcinogenic in single-dose experiments. Following its oral administration, papillomas and squamous-cell carcinomas of the oesophagus and forestomach, adenocarcinomas of the stomach, small intestine and large bowel, and sarcomas of the gastrointestinal tract were reported[3]. These findings have been extended in more recent studies after oral administration to rats[4-7], hamsters[8,9] and dogs[10,11]. After subcutaneous injection of mice, it produced lung and liver tumours and haemangioendotheliomas[12]; after intrarectal instillation in rats and guinea-pigs[13-15] and after intrauterine and intravaginal application to rats, it produced local tumours[16].

C. Other relevant data

MNNG is an alkylating agent[17]. No data were available to evaluate the genetic and related effects of this compound in humans.

MNNG induced DNA strand breaks in various organs of rats treated *in vivo*. It did not cause dominant lethal mutations in mice, but it gave positive results for mutation in the mouse spot test; it induced chromosomal aberrations and micronuclei in bone-marrow cells of mice and sister chromatid exchanges in bone-marrow cells of mice and Chinese hamsters treated *in vivo*. It induced chromosomal aberrations, sister chromatid exchanges, DNA strand breaks and unscheduled DNA synthesis in human and rodent cells *in vitro* and induced mutation in cultured rodent cells. It gave positive results in several assays for cell transformation. MNNG induced somatic and sex-linked recessive lethal mutations in *Drosophila*. It caused chromosomal aberrations, sister chromatid exchanges and mutation in plants and recombination and mutation in fungi. It was mutagenic to and caused DNA damage in bacteria, and gave positive results in host-mediated assays using bacteria or yeast as indicators and mice as hosts[17].

References

[1]Pleven, C., Audran, R., Falcy, M., Efthymiou, M.-L. & Philbert, M. (1983) Glioblastomas and chemical mutagenesis in biology laboratories. Report of 3 deaths in the same institute (Fr.). *Arch. Mal. prof.*, *44*, 411-418

[2]Pleven, C., Falcy, M., Audran, R., Philbert, M. & Efthymiou, M.L. (1984) Occurrence of glioblastomas in people working in research laboratories using nitroso compounds (Fr.). *J. Toxicol. méd.*, *4*, 249-257

[3]*IARC Monographs*, *4*, 183-195, 1974

[4]Martin, M.S., Martin, F., Justrabo, E., Michiels, R., Bastien, H. & Knobel, S. (1974) Susceptibility of inbred rats to gastric and duodenal carcinomas induced by *N*-methyl-*N'*-nitro-*N*-nitroso-guanidine. *J. natl Cancer Inst.*, *53*, 837-840

[5]Kartasheva, L.A. & Bykorez, A.I. (1975) Induction of adenocarcinomas of the stomach in rats by *N*-methyl-*N'*-nitro-*N*-nitrosoguanidine (Russ.). *Vopr. Onkol.*, *21*, 50-55

[6]Habs, M., Deutsch-Wenzel, R., Preussmann, R. & Schmähl, D. (1978) Induction of gastric tumors in BD-IV rats by single application of N-methyl-N'-nitro-N-nitrosoguanidine. *Z. Krebsforsch.*, *91*, 183-188

[7]Sherenesheva, N.I. (1979) Induction of gastrointestinal tumours in rats by N-methyl-N'-nitro-N-nitrosoguanidine (MNNG) (Russ.). *Vopr. Onkol.*, *25*, 72-74

[8]Kogure, K., Sasadaira, H., Kawachi, T., Shimosato, Y., Tokunaga, A., Fujimura, S. & Sugimura, T. (1974) Further studies on induction of stomach cancer in hamsters by N-methyl-N'-nitro-N-nitrosoguanidine. *Br. J. Cancer*, *29*, 132-142

[9]Ketkar, M., Reznik, G. & Green, U. (1978) Carcinogenic effect of N-methyl-N'-nitro-N-nitroso-guanidine (MNNG) in European hamsters. *Cancer Lett.*, *4*, 241-244

[10]Fujita, M., Taguchi, T., Takami, M., Usugane, M., Takahashi, A. & Shiba, S. (1974) Carcinoma and related lesion in dog stomach induced by oral administration of N-methyl-N'-nitro-N-nitroso-guanidine. *Gann*, *65*, 207-214

[11]Koyama, Y., Omori, K., Hirota, T., Sano, R. & Ishihara, K. (1976) Leiomyosarcomas of the small intestine induced in dogs by N-methyl-N'-nitro-N-nitrosoguanidine. *Gann*, *67*, 241-251

[12]Fujii, K. & Nakadate, M. (1977) Tumor induction by a single subcutaneous injection of N-methyl-N'-nitro-N-nitrosoguanidine and its derivatives in newborn mice. *Z. Krebsforsch.*, *90*, 313-319

[13]Nakano, H. (1973) Histopathological studies on rat colo-rectal carcinoma induced by N-methyl-N'-nitro-N-nitrosoguanidine. *Tohoku J. exp. Med.*, *110*, 7-21

[14]Chłap, Z. & Przewłocki, F. (1979) A study of colon cancer in rats after rectal administration of N-methyl-N'-nitro-N-nitrosoguanidine (Pol.). *Pat. Pol.*, *30*, 475-488

[15]Narisawa, T., Wong, C.Q. & Weisburger, J.H. (1976) Large bowel carcinoma in strain-2 guinea pigs by intrarectal instillation of N-methyl-N'-nitro-N-nitrosoguanidine. *Gann*, *67*, 41-46

[16]Tanaka, T. & Mori, H. (1983) Experimental induction of uterine cancer in rats by N-methyl-N'-nitro-N-nitrosoguanidine. *Pathol. Res. Pract.*, *178*, 20-26

[17]*IARC Monographs, Suppl. 6*, 394-398, 1987

METRONIDAZOLE (Group 2B)

A. Evidence for carcinogenicity to humans (*inadequate*)

Two epidemiological studies[1,2] of women treated with metronidazole showed some excesses of cancers of the uterine cervix, a neoplasm that has risk factors in common with vaginal trichomoniasis, the main indication in women for treatment with this drug. In one study[1], a greater excess of cervical cancer was observed in women with trichomoniasis who were not exposed to metronidazole than in those who were (relative risk, 2.1 *versus* 1.7). An excess of lung cancer (4 observed, 0.6 expected) seen in one of these studies[1] was not found in the other (2 observed, 2.6 expected)[3]. In the former, the excess was mainly of adeno-carcinoma (3/4 cases) and was concentrated after at least ten years from first use of metronidazole (3 observed, 0.3 expected)[4]. Further follow-up and analysis of these data have suggested that the excess could be explained entirely by confounding with smoking[5].

Another study in which 12 280 users of metronidazole were followed up for two and one-half years gave a relative risk of 0.9 (95% confidence interval, 0.5-1.9) for all cancers[6].

B. Evidence for carcinogenicity to animals (*sufficient*)

Metronidazole has been tested for carcinogenicity by oral administration to mice and rats. It significantly increased the incidences of lung tumours in mice of each sex, of lymphomas in female mice[7,8] and of mammary, pituitary, testicular and liver tumours in rats[7,9,10]. It increased the incidence of colonic tumours induced in rats by subcutaneous administration of 1,2-dimethylhydrazine[11,12].

C. Other relevant data

Studies on bone-marrow cells and lymphocytes from a series of patients treated with metronidazole showed no increase in the incidence of chromosomal damage. Metronidazole was active in body fluid assays using sweat, faeces and urine from humans exposed *in vivo* and urine from rodents exposed *in vivo*[13].

Metronidazole did not induce micronuclei in bone-marrow cells of mice or rats, sister chromatid exchanges in bone-marrow cells of Chinese hamsters or unscheduled DNA synthesis in germ cells of male rabbits treated *in vivo*. Human cells exposed to metronidazole *in vitro* did not show increased incidences of chromosomal aberrations, whereas results with respect to sister chromatid exchanges were inconclusive. Metronidazole did not induce sister chromatid exchanges in cultured hamster cells; conflicting results were reported for the induction of mutation and DNA damage in rodent cells *in vitro*. It did not induce sex-linked recessive lethal mutations in *Drosophila* or recombination in yeast. It induced mutation in fungi and bacteria and induced prophage in bacteria[13].

References

[1]Beard, C.M., Noller, K.L., O'Fallon, W.M., Kurland, L.T. & Dockerty, M.B. (1979) Lack of evidence for cancer due to use of metronidazole. *New Engl. J. Med., 301*, 519-522

[2]Friedman, G.D. & Ury, H.K. (1980) Initial screening for carcinogenicity of commonly used drugs. *J. natl Cancer Inst., 65*, 723-733

[3]Friedman, G.D. (1980) Cancer after metronidazole. *New Engl. J. Med., 302*, 519

[4]Beard, C.M. (1980) Cancer after metronidazole. *New Engl. J. Med., 302*, 520

[5]Beard, C., Noller, K. & O'Fallon, W.M. (1985) Metronidazole and subsequent malignant neoplasms (Abstract). *Am. J. Epidemiol., 122*, 529

[6]Danielson, D.A., Hannan, M.T. & Jick, H. (1982) Metronidazole and cancer. *J. Am. med. Assoc., 247*, 2498-2499

[7]*IARC Monographs, 13*, 113-122, 1977

[8]Cavaliere, A., Bacci, M., Amorosi, A., Del Gaudio, M. & Vitali, R. (1983) Induction of lung tumors and lymphomas in BALB/c mice by metronidazole. *Tumori, 69*, 379-382

[9]Rustia, M. & Shubik, P. (1979) Experimental induction of hepatomas, mammary tumors, and other tumors with metronidazole in noninbred Sas:MRC(WI)BR rats. *J. natl Cancer Inst., 63*, 863-868

[10]Cavaliere, A., Bacci, M. & Vitali, R. (1984) Induction of mammary tumors with metronidazole in female Sprague-Dawley rats. *Tumori, 70*, 307-311

[11]Sloan, D.A., Fleiszer, D.M., Richards, G.K., Murray, D. & Brown, R.A. (1983) Increased incidence of experimental colon cancer associated with long-term metronidazole therapy. *Am. J. Surg., 145*, 66-70

[12]A-Kareem, A.M., Fleiszer, D.M., Richards, G.K., Senterman, M.K. & Brown, R.A. (1984) Effect of long-term metronidazole (MTZ) therapy on experimental colon cancer in rats. *J. surg. Res., 36*, 547-552

[13]*IARC Monographs, Suppl. 6*, 399-402, 1987

MINERAL OILS:
UNTREATED AND MILDLY-TREATED OILS (Group 1)
HIGHLY-REFINED OILS (Group 3)

A. Evidence for carcinogenicity to humans (*sufficient* for untreated and mildly-treated oils; *inadequate* for highly-refined oils)

Exposure to mineral oils that have been used in a variety of occupations, including mulespinning, metal machining and jute processing, has been associated strongly and consistently with the occurrence of squamous-cell cancers of the skin, and especially of the scrotum[1]. Production processes for these oils have changed over time, and with more recent manufacturing methods highly-refined products are produced that contain smaller amounts of contaminants, such as polycyclic aromatic hydrocarbons.

Excess mortality or morbidity from gastrointestinal malignancies was seen in two out of three cohort studies of metal workers (stomach cancer in two studies, large-bowel cancer in one); however, the only significant excess was for the sum of stomach cancer plus large-bowel cancer in one study. Four cases of scrotal cancer were detected in one relatively small cohort study of metal industry workers[1]. Among 682 turners with five or more years of exposure to mineral oils, five cases of squamous-cell carcinoma of the skin (four of the scrotum) occurred, with 0.3 expected[2]. In a case-control study, a relative risk of 4.9 was reported for the association of scrotal cancer with potential exposure of metal workers to mineral oils. Neither the actual levels of exposure nor the classification of the mineral oil to which the machine workers were potentially exposed was available in the reports of the epidemiological studies[1].

In a case-control study, an excess of sinonasal cancers was seen in toolsetters, set-up men and toolmakers[1]. In a series of 344 cases of scrotal cancer from 1936 to 1976, 62% had held occupations in which exposure to mineral oils was likely to have occurred. The median latent period was 34 years[3].

An examination of the incidence of second primary cancers among men with scrotal cancer demonstrated excesses of respiratory, upper alimentary tract and skin cancers; when the occupations were grouped, the excess was largely confined to those with exposure to oil[1].

Excesses of bladder cancer have been reported in case-control studies in several countries among machinists and engineers, who were possibly exposed to cutting oils containing aromatic amines as additives[1].

With regard to printing pressmen, one of two cohort studies addressing lung cancer showed an excess and one of two proportionate mortality studies showed a small, statistically nonsignificant excess of lung cancer among newspaper pressmen but no excess among non-newspaper pressmen; the other study did not address lung cancer. One of three proportionate mortality studies on manual workers in the printing industry, not specifically addressing printing pressmen, did not show an increased lung cancer risk, whereas the other two studies found a statistically significant excess. One of two proportionate mortality studies of printing pressmen indicated a statistically significant increase of deaths from rectal cancer, and the other showed a statistically nonsignificant increase of deaths from colon cancer; the cohort study considering colorectal cancers did not show an increased occurrence. One proportionate mortality study among newspaper and other commercial printing pressmen showed a statistically significant excess of mortality from cancers of the buccal cavity and pharynx, whereas no such excess was observed in a cohort study. One case-control study indicated a statistically significant excess of cancers of the buccal cavity and pharynx. The findings regarding other malignancies were inconsistent; scrotal cancers were not mentioned. The type and amount of exposure were usually not described; exposure to both mineral oils and carbon blacks (see p. 142) would probably have been involved[1].

In mortality statistics from the UK and from Washington State, USA, excesses of lung and skin cancer have been registered for jobs entailing exposure to mineral oils[1].

B. Evidence for carcinogenicity to animals (*sufficient* for untreated and mildly-treated oils; *inadequate* for highly-refined oils)

Vacuum-distillate fractions, acid-treated oils, mildly-treated solvent-refined oils, mildly-treated hydrotreated oils, solvent extracts (aromatic oils) and some cutting oils produced skin tumours after repeated skin applications to mice. Similar treatment with high-boiling, catalytically-cracked oils produced skin tumours in rabbits and rhesus monkeys. Some severely solvent-refined oils did not produce skin tumours in mice. Highly-refined food-grade mineral oils did not produce skin tumours when applied to the skin of mice, although after intraperitoneal injection they produced plasma-cell neoplasms and reticulum-cell sarcomas in certain strains of mice[1]. It was agreed that, in accordance with the previous evaluation, 'the significant latter finding is difficult to interpret'[1].

C. Other relevant data

An increase in the frequency of chromosomal aberrations was observed in the peripheral blood lymphocytes of glass workers exposed to mineral oil mists. Urine from workers in a cold-rolling steel plant exposed to oil mists of solvent-refined oils was mutagenic to *Salmonella typhimurium* in the presence of an exogenous metabolic system[4].

Special test protocols may be necessary to evaluate mineral oils adequately in short-term tests. Vacuum distillates from oil refining were reported to be mutagenic to *S. typhimurium* in the presence of an exogenous metabolic system. Positive findings were also obtained when the concentration of the exogenous metabolic system was five to ten fold that used generally. Acid-treated oils were not mutagenic to *S. typhimurium* in the presence of an exogenous metabolic system; solvent-refined oils were reported to be mutagenic in the presence of an exogenous metabolic system. Hydrotreated oil was reported to be mutagenic to *S. typhimurium* in the presence of an exogenous metabolic system, while white oils, highly-refined steel-hardening oil and solvent-refined steel-rolling oils were not. Unused crankcase oil was mutagenic to *S. typhimurium* in the presence of an exogenous metabolic system, while in other studies no mutagenic activity was found. Used crankcase oil from both gasoline and diesel engines was mutagenic to *S. typhimurium* both in the presence and absence of a metabolic system[4].

Two insulation oils from highly-refined mineral-base oils induced transformation of Syrian hamster embryo cells and enhanced transformation of mouse C3H 10T1/2 cells. Unused new, re-refined and used crankcase oils induced transformation in Syrian hamster embryo cells[4].

References

[1]*IARC Monographs*, *33*, 87-168, 1984

[2]Järvholm, B., Fast, K., Lavenius, B. & Tomsic, P. (1985) Exposure to cutting oils and its relation to skin tumors and premalignant skin lesions on the hands and forearms. *Scand. J. Work Environ. Health*, *11*, 365-369

[3]Waldron, H.A., Waterhouse, J.A.H. & Tessema, N. (1984) Scrotal cancer in the West Midlands, 1936-76. *Br. J. ind. Med.*, *41*, 437-444

[4]*IARC Monographs*, *Suppl. 6*, 403, 1987

MOPP AND OTHER COMBINED CHEMOTHERAPY INCLUDING ALKYLATING AGENTS (Group 1)

A. Evidence for carcinogenicity to humans (*sufficient*)

In 1972, roughly five years after the introduction of intensive combined chemotherapy for Hodgkin's disease, the first report of subsequent acute nonlymphocytic leukaemia (ANLL) appeared[1]. Since then, investigators in more than 15 clinical centres and collaborative treatment groups in Europe and North America have performed a series of studies leading to the conclusion that the association is probably causal.

These studies are not easily compared with one another. The groups and subgroups of study subjects differ in distribution by age, stage at diagnosis, timing of initial therapy (both radiological and chemotherapeutic), interval between diagnosis and intensive chemotherapy, composition of the chemotherapeutic regimen and length of follow-up. Further, the methods of counting and allocating patients or person-years at risk, the criteria for diagnosis, the method of validating the separate identity of a second malignancy, the 'unexposed' group used as a reference standard, the method of statistical analysis, and the index used to summarize risk differences vary greatly from study to study. Finally, the extent to which such specific details are clearly described in the published reports is also variable.

Nonetheless, these reports are consistent in describing a strongly increased risk of ANLL after intensive treatment with combined chemotherapeutic regimens, particularly those containing alkylating agents. The most recent reports[2-18] describe a total of over 11 000 patients, reported roughly a decade after diagnosis, among whom more than 170 cases of ANLL have thus far occurred. About one-quarter of these patients had received no intensive combined chemotherapy, yet all but a few leukaemia cases have occurred among those patients who did. Summary estimates of the relative risk of ANLL after intensive chemotherapy (relative to reasonably appropriate healthy populations) have been calculated to vary from 9[11] through 40[4,10] to well over 100[6,9,16], precluding meaningful comparisons between studies, and estimates of the absolute (actuarial) risk observed in the first ten years range from 2-3%[3,4,10,14] through 5-6%[5,7-9,12] to 9-10%[2,13], again precluding direct comparisons between estimates. Observed variations in both relative risk and actuarial risk are probably due to differences in both methodology and exposure.

Although cases of leukaemia have been observed after radiotherapy in the absence of chemotherapy for Hodgkin's disease, the magnitude of the risk ratio is much lower, and may not even be elevated[6,19]. In contrast, the risk for ANLL is consistently high after chemotherapy even in the absence of radiation[7-9]. Although few untreated patient-years have been analysed recently, the relative absence of ANLL as an observed sequel of Hodgkin's disease prior to the era of intensive combined regimens[20,21], the absence of any relationship to histological subtype[13], and the appearance of ANLL during complete remission[5] emphasize the etiological role of chemotherapy, although interactions with stage of disease, with radiation or with factors important in the pathogenesis of Hodgkin's disease itself cannot be ruled out completely.

The only specific drug combination that has been used with sufficient frequency that it can be clearly linked to ANLL is MOPP (nitrogen mustard [see p. 269], vincristine [see p. 372], procarbazine [see p. 327] and prednisone [see p. 326]), although several reports describe excess cases not attributable to MOPP[9,11,14,16], and excesses of ANLL have appeared after treatment with other alkylating agent-containing combinations. The predominance of combined chemotherapy also precludes the identification of risk from individual constituents. Preliminary experience does indicate that risk for ANLL may be lower with some specific combinations, such as ABVD (adriamycin, bleomycin, vinblastine and dacarbazine)[14,22,23].

Solid tumours, especially non-Hodgkin's lymphomas[10,24-27] and lung cancer[3,6,12,28,29], but including sarcomas, melanoma, malignancies of the central nervous system and carcinomas of the thyroid and gastrointestinal system, have also been reported in abundance after combined chemotherapy for Hodgkin's disease[3,6,7,10,12,29-32], but comparisons of observed to expected frequencies have not yielded consistent results. In contrast to leukaemia, solid tumours are more common in the general population, increase rapidly in frequency with age (and therefore the passage of time after treatment), are more diverse in known etiology, and are considered to appear with greater frequency after intensive radiotherapy[6]. Moreover, they are observed to appear with increasing frequency only after longer average duration of follow-up[32]. Some reports have shown increased risk after intensive chemotherapy[10], and the plausibility of a relationship is further suggested by multiple case reports of second malignancies that are unusual because of their rarity, either at an age[33] or on an absolute basis[9,24,31]. At present, it would appear that solid tumours occur among survivors of Hodgkin's disease in excess of the expected frequency; but, because too few patients have been followed into the second decade after treatment, it is too early to determine whether the increase can be better attributed to chance or to factors other than chemotherapy[32].

Combined chemotherapy containing alkylating agents for non-Hodgkin's lymphoma may also lead to ANLL[34-37], although the reports are not consistent and the documentation is less complete.

Treatment of nonhaematological malignancies may also cause second tumours, but most reported cases have occurred after the use of single agents[38], and combination regimens are less commonly used. Intensive combination therapy including alkylating agents for small-cell carcinoma of the lung[39,40], and possibly for cancer of the testis[41], may increase the risk for ANLL.

B. Evidence for carcinogenicity to animals (*inadequate*)

No data on MOPP were available to the Working Group. Combined treatment with cyclophosphamide (see p. 182), methotrexate (see p. 241) and 5-fluorouracil (see p. 210) induced carcinogenic responses in several organs in rats[42]. See also the summaries of data on individual compounds: adriamycin (see p. 81), bleomycins (see p. 134), chlorambucil (see p. 144), cyclophosphamide, 5-fluorouracil, methotrexate, nitrogen mustard (see p. 269), prednisone (see p. 326), procarbazine hydrochloride (see p. 327), vinblastine sulphate (see p. 371) and vincristine sulphate (see p. 372).

C. Other relevant data

For data on genetic and related effects, see the summaries on individual compounds, listed above.

References

[1] Arseneau, J.C., Sponzo, R.W., Levin, D.L., Schnipper, L.E., Bonner, H., Young, R.C., Canellos, G.P., Johnson, R.E. & DeVita, V.T. (1972) Nonlymphomatous malignant tumours complicating Hodgkin's disease. Possible association with intensive therapy. *New Engl. J. Med., 287*, 1119-1122

[2] Aisenberg, A.C. (1983) Acute nonlymphocytic leukemia after treatment for Hodgkin's disease. *Am. J. Med., 75*, 449-454

[3] Baccarani, M., Bosi, A. & Papa, G. (1980) Second malignancy in patients treated for Hodgkin's disease. *Cancer, 46*, 1735-1740

[4]Bergsagel, D.E., Alison, R.E., Bean, H.A., Brown, T.C., Bush, R.S., Clark, R.M., Chua, T., Dalley, D., DeBoer, G., Gospodarowicz, M., Hasselback, R., Perrault, D. & Rideout, D.F. (1982) Results of treating Hodgkin's disease without a policy of laparotomy staging. *Cancer Treat. Rep.*, *66*, 717-731

[5]Brusamolino, E., Lazzarino, M., Salvaneschi, L., Canevari, A., Morra, E., Castelli, G., Pagnucco, G., Isernia, P. & Bernasconi, C. (1982) Risk of leukemia in patients treated for Hodgkin's disease. *Eur. J. Cancer clin. Oncol.*, *18*, 237-242

[6]Boivin, J.F., Hutchison, G.B., Lyden, M., Godbold, J., Chorosh, J. & Schottenfeld, D. (1984) Second primary cancers following treatment of Hodgkin's disease. *J. natl Cancer Inst.*, *72*, 233-241

[7]Coleman, C.N., Kaplan, H.S., Cox, R., Varghese, A., Butterfield, P. & Rosenburg, S.A. (1982) Leukaemias, non-Hodgkin's lymphomas and solid tumours in patients treated for Hodgkin's disease. *Cancer Surv.*, *1*, 733-744

[8]Coltman, C.A., Jr & Dixon, D.O. (1982) Second malignancies complicating Hodgkin's disease. A Southwest Oncology Group 10-year follow-up. *Cancer Treat. Rep.*, *66*, 1023-1033

[9]Glicksman, A.S., Pajak, T.F., Gottlieb, A., Nissen, N., Stutzman, L. & Cooper, M.R. (1982) Second malignant neoplasms in patients successfully treated for Hodgkin's disease: a Cancer and Leukemia Group B study. *Cancer Treat. Rep.*, *66*, 1035-1044

[10]Henry-Amar, M. (1983) Second cancers after radiotherapy and chemotherapy for early stages of Hodgkin's disease. *J. natl Cancer Inst.*, *71*, 911-916

[11]Jacquillat, C., Auclerc, G., Weil, M., Auclerc, M.F. & Maral, J. (1983) Acute leukaemias and solid tumours in the course of Hodgkin's disease (Fr.). *Bull. Cancer*, *70*, 61-66

[12]Tester, W.J., Kinsella, T.J., Waller, B., Makuch, R.W., Kelley, P.A., Glatstein, E. & DeVita, V.T. (1984) Second malignant neoplasms complicating Hodgkin's disease: the National Cancer Institute experience. *J. clin. Oncol.*, *2*, 762-769

[13]Pedersen-Bjergaard, J. & Larsen, S.O. (1982) Incidence of acute nonlymphocytic leukemia, preleukemia, and acute myeloproliferative syndrome up to 10 years after treatment of Hodgkin's disease. *New Engl. J. Med.*, *307*, 965-971

[14]Valagussa, P., Santoro, A., Fossati Bellani, F., Franchi, F., Banfi, A. & Bonadonna, G. (1982) Absence of treatment-induced second neoplasms after ABVD in Hodgkin's disease. *Blood*, *59*, 488-494

[15]Prosnitz, L.R., Farber, L.R., Kapp, D.S., Bertino, J.R., Nordlund, M. & Lawrence, R. (1982) Combined modality therapy for advanced Hodgkin's disease: long-term follow-up data. *Cancer Treat. Rep.*, *66*, 871-879

[16]Bartolucci, A.A., Liu, C., Durant, J.R. & Gams, R.A. (1983) Acute myelogenous leukemia as a second malignant neoplasm following the successful treatment of advanced Hodgkin's disease. *Cancer*, *52*, 2209-2213

[17]Andrieu, J.M., Montagnon, B., Asselain, B., Bayle-Weisgerber, C., Chastang, C., Teillet, F. & Bernard, J. (1980) Chemotherapy-radiotherapy association in Hodgkin's disease, clinical stages IA, II$_2$A: results of a prospective clinical trial with 166 patients. *Cancer*, *46*, 2126-2130

[18]Shishkin, I.P. (1984) Secondary tumours in patients with Hodgkin's disease following treatment (Russ.). *Med. Radiol. (Moscow)*, *29*, 24-28

[19]Selby, P. & Horwich, A. (1986) Secondary leukaemia in Hodgkin's disease. *Lancet*, *i*, 1027-1028

[20]Berg, J.W. (1967) The incidence of multiple primary cancers. 1. Development of further cancers in patients with lymphomas, leukemias, and myeloma. *J. natl Cancer Inst.*, *38*, 741-752

[21]Newman, D.R., Maldonado, J.E., Harrison, E.G., Jr, Kiely, J.M. & Linman, J.W. (1970) Myelomonocytic leukemia in Hodgkin's disease. *Cancer*, *25*, 128-134

[22]Amadori, S., Papa, G., Anselmo, A.P., Fidani, P. & Mandelli, F. (1983) Acute promyelocytic leukemia following ABVD (doxorubicin, bleomycin, vinblastine, and dacarbazine) and radiotherapy for Hodgkin's disease. *Cancer Treat. Rep.*, *67*, 603-604

[23]Valagussa, P., Santoro, A., Fossati-Bellani, F., Banfi, A., Bonadonna, G. & Veronesi, U. (1985) Second neoplasms in Hodgkin's disease (HD): progress report (Abstract No. 720). *Proc. Am. Assoc. Cancer Res.*, *26*, 182

[24]Armitage, J.O., Dick, F.R., Goeken, J.A., Foucar, M.K. & Gingrich, R.D. (1983) Second lymphoid malignant neoplasms occurring in patients treated for Hodgkin's disease. *Arch. intern. Med.*, *143*, 445-450

[25]Krikorian, J.G., Burke, J.S., Rosenberg, S.A. & Kaplan, H.S. (1979) Occurrence of non-Hodgkin's lymphoma after therapy for Hodgkin's disease. *New Engl. J. Med.*, *300*, 452-458

[26]Jacquillat, C., Khayat, D., Desprez-Curely, J.P., Weil, M., Brocheriou, C., Auclerc, G., Chamseddine, N. & Bernard, J. (1984) Non-Hodgkin's lymphoma occurring after Hodgkin's disease. Four new cases and a review of the literature. *Cancer*, *53*, 459-462

[27]Miettinen, M., Franssila, K.O. & Saxén, E. (1983) Hodgkin's disease, lymphocytic predominance nodular. Increased risk for subsequent non-Hodgkin's lymphomas. *Cancer*, *51*, 2293-2300

[28]Kaldor, J.M., Day, N.E., Band, P., Choi, N.W., Clarke, E.A., Coleman, M.P., Hakama, M., Koch, M., Langmark, F., Neal, F.E., Pettersson, F., Pompe-Kirn, V., Prior, P. & Storm, H.H. (1987) Second malignancies following testicular cancer, ovarian cancer and Hodgkin's disease: an international collaborative study among cancer registries. *Int. J. Cancer*, *39*, 571-585

[29]Valagussa, P., Santora, A., Kenda, R., Bellani, F.F., Franchi, F., Banfi, A., Rilke, F. & Bonadonna, G. (1980) Second malignancies in Hodgkin's disease: a complication of certain forms of treatment. *Br. med. J.*, *i*, 216-219

[30]Nelson, D.F., Cooper, S., Weston, M.G. & Rubin, P. (1981) Second malignant neoplasms in patients treated for Hodgkin's disease with radiotherapy or radiotherapy and chemotherapy. *Cancer*, *48*, 2386-2393

[31]Tucker, M.A., Misfeldt, D., Coleman, C.N., Clark, W.H., Jr & Rosenberg, S.A. (1985) Cutaneous malignant melanoma after Hodgkin's disease. *Ann. intern. Med.*, *102*, 37-41

[32]Boivin, J.-F. & O'Brien, K. (1987) Solid cancer risk after treatment of Hodgkin's disease. *Cancer* (in press)

[33]Brumbach, R.A., Gerber, J.E., Hicks, D.G. & Strauchen, J.A. (1984) Adenocarcinoma of the stomach following irradiation and chemotherapy for lymphoma in young patients. *Cancer*, *54*, 994-998

[34]Greene, M.H., Young, R.C., Merrill, J.M. & DeVita, V.T. (1983) Evidence of a treatment dose response in acute nonlymphocytic leukemias which occur after therapy of non-Hodgkin's lymphoma. *Cancer Res.*, *43*, 1891-1898

[35]Gomez, G.A., Aggarwal, K.K. & Han, T. (1982) Post-therapeutic acute malignant myeloproliferative syndrome and acute nonlymphocytic leukemia in non-Hodgkin's lymphoma. Correlation with intensity of treatment. *Cancer*, *50*, 2285-2288

[36]Harousseau, J.L., Andrieu, J.M., Dumont, J., Montagnon, B. Asselain, B., Daniel, M.T. & Flandrin, G. (1980) Acute myeloblastic leukaemia during the course of malignant non-Hodgkin's lymphomas (Fr.). *Nouv. Presse méd., 9*, 3513-3516

[37]Pedersen-Bjergaard, J., Ersbøll, J., Sørensen, H.M., Keiding, N., Larsen, S.O., Philip, P., Larsen, M.S., Schultz, H. & Nissen, N.I. (1985) Risk of acute nonlymphocytic leukemia and preleukemia in patients treated with cyclophosphamide for non-Hodgkin's lymphoma. Comparison with results obtained in patients treated for Hodgkin's disease and ovarian carcinoma with other alkylating agents. *Ann. intern. Med., 103*, 195-200

[38]Kyle, R.A. (1982) Second malignancies associated with chemotherapeutic agents. *Semin. Oncol., 9*, 131-142

[39]Markman, M., Pavy, M.D. & Abeloff, M.D. (1982) Acute leukemia following intensive therapy for small-cell carcinoma of the lung. *Cancer, 50*, 672-675

[40]May, J.T., Hsu, S.D. & Costanzi, J.J. (1981) Acute leukemia following combination chemotherapy for cancer of the lung. *Oncology, 38*, 134-137

[41]van Imhoff, G.W., Steijfer, D.T., Breuning, M.H., Anders, G.J.P.A., Mulder, N.H. & Halie, M.R. (1986) Acute nonlymphocytic leukemia 5 years after treatment with cisplatin, vinblastine, and bleomycin for disseminated testicular cancer. *Cancer, 57*, 984-987

[42]Habs, M., Schmähl, D. & Lin, P.Z. (1981) Carcinogenic activity in rats of combined treatment with cyclophosphamide, methotrexate and 5-fluorouracil. *Int. J. Cancer, 28*, 91-96

MUSTARD GAS (SULPHUR MUSTARD) (Group 1)

A. Evidence for carcinogenicity to humans (*sufficient*)

The mortality of British and American veterans who were exposed to mustard gas during the First World War has been compared with that of other veterans who experienced respiratory infections; the effect of smoking could not be directly controlled for in either group. Cumulative lung cancer risk was not affected in UK veterans and was only modestly elevated (relative risk, 1.5, compared with the effect of cigarette smoking, roughly 10) in US veterans[1].

In contrast, mustard gas production workers in Japan during the Second World War have been found to have experienced an increase in the proportion of deaths attributed to lung cancer (three fold) compared to the local population[1,2], and especially in respiratory cancer (40 fold) in comparison with the general population[1]. Although sophisticated analytical methods were not used, the prevalence of smoking appeared to be comparable in the exposed and unexposed groups, and there was increased risk with increased duration of exposure[3]. British workers engaged in mustard gas production during the Second World War have also been followed up. Among 511 individuals, 11 cases of cancer (nine of the larynx and two of the pharynx) were identified, whereas one would have been expected[4].

B. Evidence for carcinogenicity to animals (*limited*)

Mustard gas was tested for carcinogenicity in mice, producing lung tumours after its inhalation or intravenous injection and local sarcomas after its subcutaneous injection[1].

C. Other relevant data

Mustard gas is a bifunctional alkylating agent[5]. No data were available on its genetic and related effects in humans.

Evidence of covalent binding to cellular DNA, RNA and protein *in vivo* was obtained in mice injected intraperitoneally with ^{35}S-labelled mustard gas. It induced chromosomal aberrations and DNA damage in rodent cells *in vitro* and mutation in mouse lymphoma cells *in vitro* and in a host-mediated assay. It induced aneuploidy, heritable translocations, dominant lethal mutations and sex-linked recessive lethal mutations in *Drosophila*. It was mutagenic to fungi and induced DNA damage in bacteria[5].

References

[1]*IARC Monographs*, 9, 181-192, 1975

[2]Shigenobu, T. (1980) Occupational cancer of the lungs — cancer of the respiratory tract among workers manufacturing poisonous gases (Jpn.). *Jpn. J. thorac. Dis.*, 18, 880-885

[3]Nishimoto, Y., Yamakido, M., Shigenobu, T., Onari, K. & Yukutake, M. (1983) Long term observation of poison gas workers with special reference to respiratory cancers. *J. Univ. occup. environ. Health*, 5 (*Suppl.*), 89-94

[4]Manning, K.P., Skegg, D.C.G., Stell, P.M. & Doll, R. (1981) Cancer of the larynx and other occupational hazards of mustard gas workers. *Clin. Otolaryngol.*, 6, 165-170

[5]*IARC Monographs*, *Suppl.* 6, 403-405, 1987

1-NAPHTHYLAMINE (Group 3)

A. Evidence for carcinogenicity to humans (*inadequate*)

An excess occurrence of bladder cancer was observed in workers who had been exposed to commercial 1-naphthylamine for five or more years who had not also been engaged in the production of 2-naphthylamine or benzidine. However, commercial 1-naphthylamine made at that time may have contained 4-10% 2-naphthylamine (see p. 261)[1]. Among a cohort of 906 men employed for at least one year between 1922 and 1970 in a dyestuffs plant in Italy, a considerable excess of bladder cancer deaths (27 observed, 0.19 expected) was observed among 151 workers involved in the manufacture of 1- and 2-naphthylamine and benzidine (see p. 123)[2]. A case-control study of bladder cancer in the UK showed a significant, exposure-related increased risk for dyestuffs workers. 1-Naphthylamine was plausibly concerned, but it was not possible to single out any compound from the combined exposure to arylamines[3].

In view of the contamination of the commercial product and the mixed nature of the exposures investigated, it is not possible to assess the carcinogenicity of 1-naphthylamine alone.

B. Evidence for carcinogenicity to animals (*inadequate*)

1-Naphthylamine was tested for carcinogenicity in mice, hamsters and dogs by oral administration and in newborn mice by subcutaneous injection. No carcinogenic effect was observed following oral administration to hamsters[1] or dogs[1,4,5] or in a lung adenoma bioassay in mice[6]. Inconclusive results were obtained after oral administration to adult mice and after subcutaneous injection of newborn mice[1].

C. Other relevant data

No data were available on the genetic and related effects of 1-naphthylamine in humans.

1-Naphthylamine did not induce micronuclei in bone-marrow cells of mice treated *in vivo*; it induced DNA strand breaks in mice, but not in rats. 1-Naphthylamine increased the incidence of chromosomal aberrations in cultured rodent cells, but the results for sister chromatid exchanges, mutation and DNA damage were inconclusive; no cell transformation was induced in Syrian hamster embryo cells. It did not induce sex-linked recessive lethal mutations in *Drosophila*. It induced aneuploidy but not mutation in yeast; results for mitotic recombination were conflicting. It was mutagenic to bacteria[7].

References

[1]*IARC Monographs*, 4, 87-96, 1974

[2]Decarli, A., Peto, J., Piolatto, G. & La Vecchia, C. (1985) Bladder cancer mortality of workers exposed to aromatic amines: analysis of models of carcinogenesis. *Br. J. Cancer*, *51*, 707-712

[3]Boyko, R.W., Cartwright, R.A. & Glashan, R.W. (1985) Bladder cancer in dye manufacturing workers. *J. occup. Med.*, *27*, 799-803

[4]Radomski, J.L., Deichmann, W.B., Altman, N.H. & Radmonski, T. (1980) Failure of pure 1-naphthylamine to induce bladder tumors in dogs. *Cancer Res.*, *40*, 3537-3539

[5]Purchase, I.F.H., Kalinowski, A.E., Ishmael, J., Wilson, J., Gore, C.W. & Chart, I.S. (1981) Lifetime carcinogenicity study of 1- and 2-naphthylamine in dogs. *Br. J. Cancer*, *44*, 892-901

[6]Theiss, J.C., Shimkin, M.B. & Weisburger, E.K. (1981) Pulmonary adenoma response of strain A mice to sulfonic acid derivatives of 1- and 2-naphthylamines. *J. natl Cancer Inst.*, *67*, 1299-1302

[7]*IARC Monographs*, *Suppl. 6*, 406-409, 1987

2-NAPHTHYLAMINE (Group 1)

A. Evidence for carcinogenicity to humans (*sufficient*)

Case reports and epidemiological studies conducted independently in the 1950s and 1960s showed that occupational exposure to 2-naphthylamine, either alone or as an impurity in other compounds, is causally associated with the occurrence of bladder cancer[1].

Two studies in the USA examined cancer incidence and mortality in a group of chemical workers exposed mainly to 2-naphthylamine. In one, a remarkable and significantly increased incidence of bladder cancer was found (13 observed, 3.3 expected), which was not explained by smoking habits[2]. Investigation of mortality failed to pinpoint this increased risk and suggested an excess of oesophageal cancer, which, however, was not considered to be associated with the occupational exposure[3]. Two reports on one occupational population at a dyestuffs plant in Italy documented a very high bladder cancer risk linked specifically to 2-naphthylamine production (6 deaths observed, 0.04 expected) and a clear exposure-response relationship of the risk to exposures in the plant[4,5]. Incidence studies from Japan dealing with exposure to both 2-naphthylamine and benzidine (see p. 123) showed apparently increased risks of cancer of the urinary tract and bladder and, possibly, an increased occurrence of second primary cancers at several sites, including the liver[6-8]. Case reports and ecological studies also documented the relationship between exposure to 2-naphthylamine, as well as to benzidine, and bladder cancer risk[9,10]. 2-Naphthylamine was most probably involved in the exposure to aryl amines reported in a UK study as producing a significantly increased bladder cancer risk, which was not accounted for by smoking habits[11].

B. Evidence for carcinogenicity to animals (*sufficient*)

2-Naphthylamine was tested for carcinogenicity by oral administration in many animal species and by the mouse-lung adenoma bioassay. Following its oral administration, it induced bladder neoplasms in hamsters[1], dogs[1,12-14] and nonhuman primates[1], and liver tumours in mice[1]. A low incidence of bladder carcinomas was observed in rats after its oral administration[15]. In a lung-adenoma bioassay in mice by intraperitoneal injection, 2-naphthylamine produced positive results[16].

C. Other relevant data

No data were available on the genetic and related effects of 2-naphthylamine in humans.

Mice and rabbits treated with 2-naphthylamine had increased incidences of sister chromatid exchanges; micronuclei were not induced in bone-marrow cells of mice treated *in vivo*. 2-Naphthylamine was mutagenic in the mouse spot test and induced DNA strand breaks in hepatocytes of treated rats. It formed DNA adducts in bladder and liver cells of dogs *in vivo*. It induced unscheduled DNA synthesis in human cells *in vitro* and chromosomal aberrations, sister chromatid exchanges, DNA strand breaks and unscheduled DNA synthesis in rodent cells *in vitro*. Equivocal results were obtained for mutation, but it caused morphological transformation in Syrian hamster embryo and virus-infected rat cells. 2-Naphthylamine induced aneuploidy in *Drosophila*, but equivocal results were found for sex-linked recessive lethal mutations. It caused aneuploidy, mutation and mitotic recombination in yeast and was mutagenic to plants and bacteria[17].

References

[1] *IARC Monographs, 4*, 97-111, 1974

[2]Schulte, P.A., Ringen, K., Hemstreet, G.P., Altekruse, E.B., Gullen, W.H., Patton, M.G., Allsbrook, W.C., Jr, Crosby, J.H., West, S.S., Witherington, R., Koss, L., Bales, C.E., Tillet, S., Rooks, S.C.F., Stern, F., Stringer, W., Schmidt, V.A. & Brubaker, M.M. (1985) Risk assessment of a cohort exposed to aromatic amines. Initial results. *J. occup. Med.*, *27*, 115-121

[3]Stern, F.B., Murthy, L.I., Beaumont, J.J., Schulte, P.A. & Halperin, W.E. (1985) Notification and risk assessment for bladder cancer of a cohort exposed to aromatic amines. III. Mortality among workers exposed to aromatic amines in the last beta-naphthylamine manufacturing facility in the United States. *J. occup. Med.*, *27*, 495-500

[4]Rubino, G.F., Scansetti, G., Piolatto, G. & Pira, E. (1982) The carcinogenic effect of aromatic amines: an epidemiological study on the role of *o*-toluidine and 4,4'-methylene bis(2-methyl-aniline) in inducing bladder cancer in man. *Environ. Res.*, *27*, 241-254

[5]Decarli, A., Peto, J., Piolatto, G. & La Vecchia, C. (1985) Bladder cancer mortality of workers exposed to aromatic amines: analysis of models of carcinogenesis. *Br. J. Cancer*, *51*, 707-712

[6]Tsuchiya, K., Okubo, T. & Ishizu, S. (1975) An epidemiological study of occupational bladder tumours in the dye industry of Japan. *Br. J. ind. Med.*, *32*, 203-209

[7]Nakamura, J., Takamatsu, M., Doi, J., Ohkawa, T., Fujinaga, T., Ebisuno, S. & Sone, M. (1980) Clinical study on the occupational urinary tract tumor in Wakayama. *Jpn. J. Urol.*, *71*, 945-951

[8]Morinaga, K., Oshima, A. & Hara, I. (1982) Multiple primary cancers following exposure to benzidine and beta-naphthylamine. *Am. J. ind. Med.*, *3*, 243-246

[9]Budnick, L.D., Sokal, D.C., Falk, H., Logue, J.N. & Fox, J.M. (1984) Cancer and birth defects near the Drake Superfund site, Pennsylvania. *Arch. environ. Health*, *39*, 409-413

[10]Segnan, N. & Tanturri, G. (1976) A study on the geographical pathology of laryngeal, bladder and children cancer in the Province of Turin (Ital.). *Tumori*, *62*, 377-386

[11]Boyko, R.W., Cartwright, R.A. & Glashan, R.W. (1985) Bladder cancer in dye manufacturing workers. *J. occup. Med.*, *27*, 799-803

[12]Romanenko, A.M. & Martynenko, A.G. (1972) Morphological peculiarities of vesical tumours induced by beta-naphthylamine in dogs (Russ.). *Vopr. Onkol.*, *18*, 70-75

[13]Radomski, J.L., Krischer, C. & Krischer, K.N. (1978) Histologic and histochemical preneoplastic changes in the bladder mucosae of dogs given 2-naphthylamine. *J. natl Cancer Inst.*, *60*, 327-333

[14]Purchase, I.F.H., Kalinowski, A.E., Ishmael, J., Wilson, J., Gore, C.W. & Chart, I.S. (1981) Lifetime carcinogenicity study of 1- and 2-naphthylamine in dogs. *Br. J. Cancer*, *44*, 892-901

[15]Hicks, R.M., Wright, R. & Wakefield, J.St J. (1982) The induction of rat bladder cancer by 2-naphthylamine. *Br. J. Cancer*, *46*, 646-661

[16]Theiss, J.C., Shimkin, M.B. & Weisburger, E.K. (1981) Pulmonary adenoma response of strain A mice to sulfonic acid derivaties of 1- and 2-naphthylamines. *J. natl Cancer Inst.*, *67*, 1299-1302

[17]*IARC Monographs, Suppl. 6*, 410-414, 1987

1-NAPHTHYLTHIOUREA (ANTU) (Group 3)

A. Evidence for carcinogenicity to humans (*inadequate*)

Cases of bladder tumours have been reported among rat catchers exposed to ANTU (containing up to 0.2% 2-naphthylamine [see p. 261])[1].

B. Evidence for carcinogenicity to animals (*inadequate*)

ANTU was tested for carcinogenicity in mice and rats by administration in the diet. The studies were considered to be inadequate for evaluation[2].

C. Other relevant data

No data were available on the genetic and related effects of ANTU in humans. It did not induce unscheduled DNA synthesis in rat hepatocytes *in vitro*. It was mutagenic to bacteria[3].

References

[1]Davies, J.M., Thomas, H.F. & Manson, D. (1982) Bladder tumours among rodent operatives handling ANTU. *Br. med. J., 285*, 927-931

[2]*IARC Monographs, 30*, 347-357, 1983

[3]*IARC Monographs, Suppl. 6*, 415-416, 1987

NICKEL AND NICKEL COMPOUNDS (Group 1*)

A. Evidence for carcinogenicity to humans (*sufficient*)

Early epidemiological studies of populations of workers in nickel refineries in different countries clearly demonstrate excess incidences of cancers of the nasal cavity and lung and, possibly, excesses of cancer of the larynx. Although the carcinogen(s) could not be specified, the cancer hazards seemed to be associated primarily with the early stage of nickel refining. Nickel carbonyl was considered unlikely to be involved, while nickel subsulphide and nickel oxide emerged as the strongest candidates[1].

Later reports from Canada and the USA confirmed the increased risks for lung and sinonasal cancers carried by exposure during nickel refining operations, where the primary exposure was to nickel sulphides (including subsulphide) and nickel oxides[2-4]. The early studies of nickel refinery workers in Wales (UK) and Norway were extended and updated. Among workers in South Wales, the elevated risks for cancers of the lung and nasal sinuses persisted until 1930[5]. For both lung cancer (137 cases before 1925) and nasal cancer (56 cases before 1925), the increased risk was significantly associated with employment in calcining and at furnaces and with copper sulphate and nickel sulphate production[6,7]. In Norway, the highest incidence rates for cancers of the respiratory organs occurred among workers employed in roasting, smelting and electrolysis departments. The increased incidence of nasal cancers (21 cases; relative risk, 26.3) exhibited a very steep decrease with more recent

---

*This evaluation applies to the group of chemicals as a whole and not necessarily to all individual chemicals within the group (see also Methods, p. 38). After the meeting of the Working Group, the Secretariat became aware of epidemiological and experimental studies in progress on the carcinogenicity of nickel and nickel compounds.

year of first employment; the incidence of lung cancer (82 cases; relative risk, 3.7) gave no indication of a consistent decrease during the period 1916-1959. A slight, statistically nonsignificant excess of laryngeal cancer (5 cases observed, 2.4 expected) was also reported[8,9].

Reports of an increased occurrence of lung cancer among nickel smelting workers have also come from New Caledonia, Slovakia and the USSR[10-16].

There have been three case reports of cancers of the respiratory tract in workers who were involved in nickel plating and grinding operations[1].

Three investigations that examined the possible cancer risk associated with exposure to nickel and nickel compounds in nickel alloy plants showed no significant increase in mortality from cancer[17-19]. In one of these, excess mortality from lung cancer was noted in maintenance workers; however, it was unclear whether the risk was directly associated with nickel exposures[18]. Workers at a gaseous diffusion plant who were exposed to high-purity metallic nickel powder did not exhibit any increase in mortality from respiratory-tract cancers[20,21]. An incidence study at a hydrometallurgical nickel refining plant in Canada did not indicate an increased risk of cancer. Exposure was to metallic nickel and nickel concentrate dust[22].

Other investigations have addressed more complex and mixed exposure conditions and thus provide little evidence to evaluate the specific role of nickel and nickel compounds[23-30].

The association of specific types of cancer with nickel exposure has also been examined by means of case-control investigations. One study of cancer of the larynx supported an association with nickel exposure[31], but another did not[32]. Studies of sinonasal cancer and lung cancer yielded contradictory results; all suffered from inadequate description of the exposure to nickel[33-36]. In one of these[35], the risk was high in welders with nickel exposure (relative risk, 3.3, 95% confidence interval, 1.2-9.2); however, exposure to nickel compounds was so highly correlated with the presence of chromium that the observed exposure to nickel could have reflected a confounding effect of chromium (see p. 165). A study at an aircraft-engine factory showed no association between lung cancer deaths and exposure to nickel oxides, sulphate, chloride or alloys[37].

It is still not possible to state with certainty which specific nickel compounds are human carcinogens, and which are not. A large amount of evidence has accrued that nickel refining carries a carcinogenic risk to workers. The risk is particularly high in those exposed during certain processes, mainly entailing exposure to nickel (sub)sulphides and oxides. The lung and nasal sinuses are the most clearly established target organs.

B. Evidence for carcinogenicity to animals (*sufficient*)

Nickel subsulphide produced malignant tumours in rats after its inhalation[1] or intramuscular[1,38,39], intrarenal[40,41], intratesticular[42] or intraocular[43] administration and after its insertion into heterotransplanted tracheas[44]; it also produced local sarcomas in mice and rabbits after intramuscular administration[1,45-47]. Nickel powder, nickel oxide, hydroxide and carbonate, nickelocene and nickel-iron sulphide matte produced local sarcomas in mice, rats, hamsters and rabbits when given intramuscularly[1,38,48]. Intravenous administration of nickel carbonyl increased the incidences of various tumours in rats[1], and inhalation of nickel carbonyl produced a low incidence of lung tumours in rats[1]. Nickelous acetate administered intraperitoneally to mice produced an excess of lung adenomas and carcinomas[49]. Nickel sulphide produced renal tumours in rats when injected intrarenally[50].

With few exceptions, the nickel compounds tested produced sarcomas and/or carcinomas at the tissue sites where they were deposited. Bioavailability and persistence in the tissues appear to be important in nickel carcinogenesis.

C. Other relevant data

Studies of the uptake, content and release of nickel in nasal mucosa indicate that workers exposed to water-insoluble nickel salts (e.g., roasting and smelting workers) retain more nickel than those exposed to soluble compounds (e.g., electrolysis workers). Nickel accumulated during active work is retained in the mucous membrane for years after retirement[51-53].

Workers exposed to nickel in one refinery had slight excesses of chromosomal aberrations (mainly gaps) in their peripheral lymphocytes, but no increase in the incidence of sister chromatid exchanges was seen[54].

Nickel compounds did not induce dominant lethal mutations in mice. Soluble nickel compounds caused DNA strand breaks and cross-links in rats treated *in vivo*, and particles of crystalline nickel sulphide bound to DNA in Chinese hamster cells *in vitro*. Nickel compounds were weakly active in inducing chromosomal aberrations and sister chromatid exchanges in human lymphocytes and rodent cells *in vitro*. They induced transformation in several rodent cell systems *in vitro*. Particles of crystalline nickel sulphides induced mutation in a protozoan. In general, negative results were obtained in bacterial mutation assays; nickel compounds induced prophage in bacteria. Insoluble nickel compounds bound to isolated DNA[54].

References

[1]*IARC Monographs, 11,* 75-112, 1976

[2]Chovil, A., Sutherland, R.B. & Halliday, M. (1981) Respiratory cancer in a cohort of nickel sinter plant workers. *Br. J. ind. Med., 38,* 327-333

[3]Roberts, R.S., Julian, J.A., Muir, D.C.F. & Shannon, H.S. (1984) *Cancer mortality associated with the high-temperature oxidation of nickel subsulfide.* In: Sunderman, F.W., Jr, ed., *Nickel in the Human Environment (IARC Scientific Publications No. 53),* Lyon, International Agency for Research on Cancer, pp. 23-35

[4]Enterline, P.E. & Marsh, G.M. (1982) Mortality among workers in a nickel refinery and alloy manufacturing plant in West Virginia. *J. natl Cancer Inst., 68,* 925-933

[5]Doll, R., Mathews, J.D. & Morgan, L.G. (1977) Cancers of the lung and nasal sinuses in nickel workers: a reassessment of the period of risk. *Br. J. ind. Med., 34,* 102-105

[6]Peto, J., Cuckle, H., Doll, R., Hermon, C. & Morgan, L.G. (1984) *Respiratory cancer mortality of Welsh nickel refinery workers*. In: Sunderman, F.W., Jr, ed., *Nickel in the Human Environment (IARC Scientific Publications No. 53)*, Lyon, International Agency for Research on Cancer, pp. 37-46

[7]Kaldor, J., Peto, J., Easton, D., Doll, R., Hermon, C. & Morgan, L. (1986) Models for respiratory cancer in nickel refinery workers. *J. natl. Cancer Inst.*, *77*, 841-848

[8]Pedersen, E., Andersen, A. & Høgetveit, A. (1978) Second study of the incidence and mortality of cancer of respiratory organs among workers at a nickel refinery (Abstract). *Ann. clin. Lab. Sci.*, *8*, 503-504

[9]Magnus, K., Andersen, A. & Høgetveit, A.C. (1982) Cancer of respiratory organs among workers at a nickel refinery in Norway. Second report. *Int. J. Cancer*, *30*, 681-685

[10]Lessard, R., Reed, D., Maheux, B. & Lambert, J. (1978) Lung cancer in New Caledonia, a nickel smelting island. *J. occup. Med.*, *20*, 815-817

[11]Olejár, Š., Olejárová, E. & Vrábel, K. (1982) Neoplasia of the lungs in the workers of the nickel smelting plant (Czech.). *Pracov. Lék.*, *34*, 280-282

[12]Langer, A.M., Rohl, A.N., Selikoff, I.J., Harlow, G.E. & Prinz, M. (1980) Asbestos as a cofactor in carcinogenesis among nickel-processing workers. *Science*, *209*, 420-422

[13]Meininger, J., Raffinot, P. & Troly, G. (1982) Cancer in nickel-processing workers in New Caledonia. *Science*, *215*, 424-425

[14]Langer, A.M., Rohl, A.N., Fischbein, A. & Selikoff, I.J. (1982) Cancer in nickel-processing workers in New Caledonia. *Science*, *215*, 425-426

[15]Saknyn, A.V. & Shabynina, N.K. (1970) Some statistical data on the carcinogenous hazards for workers engaged in the production of nickel from oxidized ores (Russ.). *Gig. Tr. prof. Zabol.*, *14*, 10-13

[16]Saknyn, A.V. & Shabynina, N.K. (1973) Epidemiology of malignant new growths at nickel smelters (Russ.). *Gig. Tr. prof. Zabol.*, *17*, 25-29

[17]Cox, J.E., Doll, R., Scott, W.A. & Smith, S. (1981) Mortality of nickel workers: experience of men working with metallic nickel. *Br. J. ind. Med.*, *38*, 235-239

[18]Redmond, C.K. (1984) *Site-specific cancer mortality among workers involved in the production of high nickel alloys*. In: Sunderman, F.W., Jr, ed., *Nickel in the Human Environment (IARC Scientific Publications No. 53)*, Lyon, International Agency for Research on Cancer, pp. 73-86

[19]Cornell, R.G. (1984) *Mortality patterns among stainless-steel workers*. In: Sunderman, F.W., Jr, ed., *Nickel in the Human Environment (IARC Scientific Publications No. 53)*, Lyon, International Agency for Research on Cancer, pp. 65-71

[20]Goldbold, J.H., Jr & Tompkins, E.A. (1979) A long-term mortality study of workers occupationally exposed to metallic nickel at the Oak Ridge gaseous diffusion plant. *J. occup. Med.*, *21*, 799-806

[21]Cragle, D.L., Hollis, D.R., Newport, T.H. & Shy, C.M. (1984) *A retrospective cohort mortality study among workers occupationally exposed to metallic nickel powder at the Oak Ridge gaseous diffusion plant*. In: Sunderman, F.W., Jr, ed., *Nickel in the Human Environment (IARC Scientific Publications No. 53)*, Lyon, International Agency for Research on Cancer, pp. 57-63

[22]Egedahl, R. & Rice, E. (1984) *Cancer incidence at a hydrometallurgical nickel refinery*. In: Sunderman, F.W., Jr, ed., *Nickel in the Human Environment (IARC Scientific Publications No. 53)*, Lyon, International Agency for Research on Cancer, pp. 47-55

[23]Shannon, H.S., Julian, J.A. & Roberts, R.S. (1984) A mortality study of 11,500 nickel workers. *J. natl Cancer Inst.*, *74*, 1251-1258

[24]Cornell, R.G. & Landis, J.R. (1984) *Mortality patterns among nickel/chromium alloy foundry workers*. In: Sunderman, F.W., Jr, ed., *Nickel in the Human Environment (IARC Scientific Publications No. 53)*, Lyon, International Agency for Research on Cancer, pp. 87-93

[25]Becker, N., Claude, J. & Frentzel-Beyme, R. (1985) Cancer risk of arc welders exposed to fumes containing chromium and nickel. *Scand. J. Work Environ. Health*, *11*, 75-82

[26]Polednak, A.P. (1981) Mortality among welders, including a group exposed to nickel oxides. *Arch. environ. Health*, *36*, 235-242

[27]Newhouse, M.L., Oakes, D. & Woolley, A.J. (1985) Mortality of welders and other craftsmen at a shipyard in NE England. *Br. J. ind. Med.*, *42*, 406-410

[28]Sorahan, T. & Waterhouse, J.A.H. (1983) Mortality study of nickel-cadmium battery workers by the method of regression models in life tables. *Br. J. ind. Med.*, *40*, 293-300

[29]Sorahan, T. & Waterhouse, J.A.H. (1985) Cancer of prostate among nickel-cadmium battery workers. *Lancet*, *i*, 459

[30]Andersson, K., Elinder, C.G., Hogstedt, C., Kjellström, T. & Spång, G. (1984) Mortality among cadmium and nickel-exposed workers in a Swedish battery factory. *Toxicol. environ. Chem.*, *9*, 53-62

[31]Olsen, J. & Sabroe, S. (1984) Occupational causes of laryngeal cancer. *J. Epidemiol. Commun. Health*, *38*, 117-121

[32]Burch, J.D., Howe, G.R., Miller, A.B. & Semenciw, R. (1981) Tobacco, alcohol, asbestos, and nickel in the etiology of cancer of the larynx: a case-control study. *J. natl Cancer Inst.*, *67*, 1219-1224

[33]Roush, G.C., Meigs, J.W., Kelly, J., Flannery, J.T. & Burdo, H. (1980) Sinonasal cancer and occupation: a case-control study. *Am. J. Epidemiol.*, *111*, 183-193

[34]Acheson, E.D., Cowdell, R.H. & Rang, E.H. (1981) Nasal cancer in England and Wales: an occupational survey. *Br. J. ind. Med.*, *38*, 218-224

[35]Gérin, M., Siemiatycki, J., Richardson, L., Pellerin, J., Lakhani, R. & Dewar, R. (1984) *Nickel and cancer associations from a multicancer occupation exposure case-referent study: preliminary findings*. In: Sunderman, F.W., Jr, ed., *Nickel in the Human Environment (IARC Scientific Publications No. 53)*, Lyon, International Agency for Research on Cancer, pp. 105-115

[36]Hernberg, S., Collan, Y., Degerth, R., Englund, A., Engzell, U., Kuosma, E., Mutanen, P., Nordlinder, H., Sand Hansen, H., Schultz-Larsen, K., Søgaard, H. & Westerholm, P. (1983) Nasal cancer and occupational exposures. Preliminary report of a joint Nordic case-referent study. *Scand. J. Work Environ. Health*, *9*, 208-213

[37]Bernacki, E.J., Parsons, G.E. & Sunderman, F.W., Jr (1978) Investigation of exposure to nickel and lung cancer mortality. Case control study at aircraft engine factory. *Ann. clin. Lab. Sci.*, *8*, 190-194

[38]Sunderman, F.W., Jr & Maenza, R.M. (1976) Comparisons of carcinogenicities of nickel compounds in rats. *Res. Commun. chem. Pathol. Pharmacol.*, *14*, 319-330

[39]Yamashiro, S., Gilman, J.P.W., Hulland, T.J. & Abandowitz, H.M. (1980) Nickel sulphide-induced rhabdomyosarcomata in rats. *Acta pathol. jpn.*, *30*, 9-22

[40]Jasmin, G. & Riopelle, J.L. (1976) Renal carcinomas and erythrocytosis in rats following intrarenal injection of nickel subsulfide. *Lab. Invest.*, *35*, 71-78

[41]Sunderman, F.W., Jr, Maenza, R.M., Hopfer, S.M., Mitchell, J.M., Allpass, P.R. & Damjanov, I. (1979) Induction of renal cancers in rats by intrarenal injection of nickel subsulfide. *J. environ. Pathol. Toxicol., 21*, 1511-1527

[42]Damjanov, I., Sunderman, F.W., Jr, Mitchell, J.M. & Allpass, P.R. (1978) Induction of testicular sarcomas in Fischer rats by intratesticular injection of nickel subsulfide. *Cancer Res., 38*, 268-276

[43]Albert, D.M., Gonder, J.R., Papale, J., Craft, J.L., Dohlman, H.G., Reid, M.C. & Sunderman, F.W., Jr (1980) *Induction of ocular neoplasms in Fischer rats by intraocular injection of nickel subsulfide.* In: Brown, S.S. & Sunderman, F.W., Jr, eds, *Nickel Toxicology*, New York, Academic Press, pp. 55-58

[44]Yarita, T. & Nettesheim, P. (1978) Carcinogenicity of nickel subsulfide for respiratory tract mucosa. *Cancer Res., 38*, 3140-3145

[45]Hildebrand, H.F. & Biserte, G. (1979) Cylindrical laminated bodies in nickel-subsulphide-induced rhabdomyosarcoma in rabbits. *Eur. J. Cell Biol., 19*, 276-280

[46]Hildebrand, H.F. & Biserte, G. (1979) Nickel sub-sulphide-induced leiomyosarcoma in rabbit white skeletal muscle. A light microscopical and ultrastructural study. *Cancer, 43*, 1358-1374

[47]Hildebrand, H.F. & Tetaert, D. (1981) Ni_3S_2-induced leiomyosarcomas in rabbit skeletal muscle: analysis of the tumoral myosin and its significance in the retrodifferentiation concept. *Oncodev. Biol. Med., 2*, 101-108

[48]Kasprzak, K.S., Gabryel, P. & Jarczewska, K. (1983) Carcinogenicity of nickel(II)hydroxides and nickel(II)sulfate in Wistar rats and its relation to the *in vitro* dissolution rates. *Carcinogenesis, 4*, 275-279

[49]Stoner, G.D., Shimkin, M.B., Troxell, M.C., Thompson, T.L. & Terry, L.S. (1976) Test for carcinogenicity of metallic compounds by the pulmonary tumor response in strain A mice. *Cancer Res., 36*, 1744-1747

[50]Sunderman, F.W., Jr, McCully, K.S. & Hopfer, S.M. (1984) Association between erythrocytosis and renal cancers in rats following intrarenal injection of nickel compounds. *Carcinogenesis, 5*, 1511-1517

[51]Torjussen, W. (1979) Nickel as carcinogenic factor in nasal carcinoma. *Acta otolaryngol., Suppl. 360*, 125

[52]Barton, R.T. & Høgetveit, A.C. (1980) Nickel-related cancers of the respiratory tract. *Cancer, 45*, 3061-3064

[53]Torjussen, W. (1985) Occupational nasal cancer caused by nickel and nickel compounds. *Rhinology, 23*, 101-105

[54]*IARC Monographs, Suppl. 6*, 417-420, 1987

NITROGEN MUSTARD (Group 2A)

A. Evidence for carcinogenicity to humans (*limited*)

No epidemiological study of nitrogen mustard as a single agent was available to the Working Group. However, it is the principal alkylating agent in leukaemogenic combination chemotherapy given for Hodgkin's disease, and other alkylating agents are clearly leukaemogenic (see p. 254). The many case reports of cancer following topical application of nitrogen mustard cannot be interpreted with certainty because concurrent treatment with radiation and other potent drugs has been the rule rather than the exception, and occasionally such associations would be expected by chance.

Squamous-cell carcinomas of the skin following long-term topical application of nitrogen mustard alone or in combination with systemic therapy for mycosis fungoides[1-4] and psoriasis[5-7] have been observed to appear on skin surfaces not exposed to the sun.

B. Evidence for carcinogenicity to animals (*sufficient*)

Nitrogen mustard, administered mainly as the hydrochloride, has been tested for carcinogenicity in mice and rats by subcutaneous, intravenous and intraperitoneal administration and by skin painting. It produced mainly lung tumours and lymphomas in mice after subcutaneous, intravenous and intraperitoneal administration. Intravenous injection of nitrogen mustard to rats induced tumours in different organs[8]. Application by skin painting produced local tumours in mice in a dose-dependent manner[9,10].

C. Other relevant data

Nitrogen mustard is a bifunctional alkylating agent. In one study, it induced chromosomal aberrations in lymphocytes of treated patients[11].

Nitrogen mustard induced dominant lethal mutations and induced micronuclei in bone-marrow cells of mice exposed *in vivo* and alkylated DNA of ascites cells in experimental animals treated *in vivo*. It induced chromosomal aberrations, sister chromatid exchanges and unscheduled DNA synthesis in human cells *in vitro*. In rodent cells *in vitro*, it induced sister chromatid exchanges, chromosomal aberrations and DNA damage; studies on the induction of mutation were inconclusive. It transformed mouse C3H 10T1/2 cells. Nitrogen mustard induced aneuploidy and somatic mutation and recombination in *Drosophila*, chromosomal aberrations in plants, mitotic recombination and mutation in fungi, and mutation and DNA damage in bacteria[11].

References

[1]Du Vivier, A., Vonderheid, E.C., Van Scott, E.J. & Urbach, F. (1978) Mycosis fungoides, nitrogen mustard and skin cancer. *Br. J. Dermatol.*, *99*, 61-63

[2]Kravitz, P.H. & McDonald, C.J. (1978) Topical nitrogen mustard induced carcinogenesis. *Acta dermatol. venereol.*, *58*, 421-425

[3]Lee, L.A., Fritz, K.A., Golitz, L., Fritz, T.J. & Weston, W.L. (1982) Second cutaneous malignancies in patients with mycosis fungoides treated with topical nitrogen mustard. *J. Am. Acad. Dermatol.*, *7*, 590-598

[4]Abel, E.A., Sendagorta, E. & Hoppe, R.T. (1986) Cutaneous malignancies and metastatic squamous cell carcinoma following topical therapies for mycosis fungoides. *J. Am. Acad. Dermatol.*, *14*, 1029-1038

[5]Halprin, K.M., Comerford, M. & Taylor, J.R. (1982) Cancer in patients with psoriasis. *J. Am. Acad. Dermatol*, *7*, 633-638

[6]Ganor, S. (1983) Skin cancer in psoriatics treated with nitrogen mustard. *J. Am. Acad. Dermatol.*, *9*, 164

[7]Halprin, K.M., Comerford, M. & Taylor, J.R. (1982) Skin cancer in psoriatics treated with nitrogen mustard. *J. Am. Acad. Dermatol.*, *8*, 164-165

[8]*IARC Monographs*, *9*, 193-207, 1975

[9]Zackheim, H.S. & Smuckler, E.A. (1980) Tumorigenic effect of topical mechlorethamine, BCNU and CCNU in mice. *Experientia*, *36*, 1211-1212

[10]Epstein, J.H. (1984) Nitrogen mustard (mechlorethamine) and UVB photocarcinogenesis: a dose response effect. *J. invest. Dermatol.*, *83*, 320-322

[11]*IARC Monographs*, *Suppl. 6*, 421-424, 1987

OCHRATOXIN A (Group 3)

A. Evidence for carcinogenicity to humans (*inadequate*)

Incidence of and mortality from urothelial urinary-tract tumours have been correlated with the geographical distribution of Balkan endemic nephropathy in Bulgaria and Yugoslavia. A relatively high frequency of contamination of cereals and bread with ochratoxin A has been reported in an area of Yugoslavia where Balkan endemic nephropathy is present. No report of a direct association between ochratoxin A and human cancer is available[1].

B. Evidence for carcinogenicity to animals (*limited*)

When ochratoxin A was administered in the diet of mice for 24 months, renal adenomas and carcinomas were observed in males and some hepatocellular carcinomas were observed in females in one study[2] and hepatomas and renal-cell tumours in male mice in another study[3]. Other studies by oral administration and studies by subcutaneous injection to mice and rats were inadequate in terms of the numbers of animals used and survival rates[1].

C. Other relevant data

No data were available on the genetic and related effects of ochratoxin A in humans.

Ochratoxin A did not induce sister chromatid exchanges in bone-marrow cells of Chinese hamsters treated *in vivo* or mutation in rodent cells treated *in vitro*; conflicting results were obtained for induction of unscheduled DNA synthesis in rodent hepatocytes. Ochratoxin A did not induce mutation in yeast or bacteria[4].

References

[1]*IARC Monographs*, *31*, 191-206, 1983

[2]Bendele, A.M., Carlton, W.W., Krogh, P.A. & Lillehoj, E.B. (1985) Ochratoxin A carcinogenesis in the (C57BL/6J × C3H)F$_1$ mouse. *J. natl Cancer Inst.*, *75*, 733-742

[3]Kanisawa, M. (1984) Synergistic effect of citrinin on hepatorenal carcinogenesis of ochratoxin A in mice. *Dev. Food Sci.*, *7*, 245-254

[4]*IARC Monographs*, *Suppl. 6*, 434-436, 1987

OESTROGENS, PROGESTINS AND COMBINATIONS

I. INTRODUCTORY REMARKS

IARC Monographs Volume 21[1] should be consulted for a general discussion of sex hormones and cancer. The principles considered in that volume remain applicable. Attention is drawn to specific points previously noted therein as 'General Conclusions on Sex Hormones':

'Steroid hormones are essential for the growth, differentiation and function of many tissues in both animals and humans. It has been established by animal experimentation that modification of the hormonal environment by surgical removal of endocrine glands, by pregnancy or by exogenous administration of steroids can increase or decrease the spontaneous occurrence of tumours or the induction of tumours by applied carcinogenic agents.... The incidence of tumours in humans could be altered by exposure to various exogenous hormones, singly or in combination.'

These statements make explicit the facts that oestrogens and progestins occur naturally, and that the hormonal milieu and dose-effect relationships are generally inextricably involved in the carcinogenic effects of oestrogens and progestins.

In this section, we describe the human epidemiology, carcinogenicity studies in animals, and other relevant data for oestrogens and progestins alone and in combination. The human epidemiological data reflect the patterns of use of oestrogens and progestins and their combinations in medical practice, i.e., the available information concerns specific products used for particular indications. Although many of the products have the same constituents (or a similar class of constituents), doses vary among products and the compounds and doses have changed over time. The operating principle is to determine the ability of the chemical to produce cancer or other genetic and related effects without the strictures of mode of human use or the magnitude of the doses. Thus, there is a basic incongruity between the human data and the animal carcinogenicity data. As noted earlier, however, the effects of these chemicals in humans appear, at least in most cases, to be linked to the hormonal milieu.

In this section, the current status of 'evidence for carcinogenicity to humans' is described only for diethylstilboestrol, oestrogen replacement therapy, medroxyprogesterone acetate, sequential oral contraceptives, combined oral contraceptives and oestrogen-progestin replacement therapy. There is little evidence that various oestrogens and progestins differ in their effects on cancer risk when the effect is an oestrogenic/progestinic effect, and the reader should therefore consult the descriptions of other oestrogens and progestins.

The reader should also be aware that diethylstilboestrol, dienoestrol, hexoestrol and chlorotrianisene are nonsteroidal oestrogens, and their carcinogenic effects may not be due solely to their oestrogenic action.

Reference

[1]*IARC Monographs, 21*, 131-134, 1979

II. OESTROGENS

NONSTEROIDAL OESTROGENS (Group 1*)

Evidence for carcinogenicity to humans (*sufficient*)

Diethylstilboestrol (Group 1)

A. Evidence for carcinogenicity to humans (*sufficient*)

Diethylstilboestrol (DES) causes clear-cell adenocarcinoma of the vagina and cervix in women exposed *in utero*. There is sufficient evidence that administration of oestrogens for the control of symptoms of the climacteric is causally related to an increased incidence of endometrial carcinoma; DES is no different from other oestrogens in this respect[1].

There is also clear evidence that administration of DES in large doses during pregnancy increases the subsequent risk of breast cancer and that DES increases the risk of testicular cancer in males exposed *in utero*.

In four follow-up studies[2-5] of exposed and nonexposed groups of women, the possible effects of DES exposure during pregnancy on subsequent breast cancer risk have been evaluated. All have shown an increased risk in exposed women. Two were randomized trials[2,3]. In one[2], there were 32 (4.6%) breast cancers among 693 women exposed to an average total dose of 12 g DES, and 21 (3.1%) breast cancers among 668 control (placebo) women. In the other[3], there were four (5.0%) breast cancers among 80 women exposed to an average total dose of DES of 16 g (plus ethisterone, average total dose, 14 g), compared to none of 76 controls; all 156 women were diabetic. In two studies, an exposed group and a 'matched' unexposed group were followed up[4,5]. One[4] showed 118 (4.4%) breast cancer cases in 2680 women exposed to a mean DES dose of 5 g, and 80 (3.1%) among 2566 control women. The other[5] similarly showed 38 (2.5%) breast cancer cases among 1531 women exposed to a mean DES dose of 2 g, and 24 (1.7%) cases among the 1404 control women. The overall relative risk from these four studies is 1.5 ($p = 0.001$).

A further group of 408 DES-exposed women (median dose, 1.5 g) was followed up, and the eight breast cancer cases found were contrasted to the 8.1 cases expected on the basis of

---

*This evaluation applies to the group of chemicals as a whole and not necessarily to all individual chemicals within the group (see also Methods, p. 38).

local breast cancer incidence rates[6]. If this study is considered together with the four studies described above, the overall relative risk is 1.4 ($p = 0.0016$).

In all five papers[2-6], the possibility is discussed that there may be a long (15-20 years) 'latent' period before the first 'DES-induced' breast cancer would be seen. Clear evidence was found in a study[4] in which there was no difference in the breast cancer rates of exposed and nonexposed women until 22 years after exposure, but an increasing difference thereafter. Similarly, in another study[3], there was no case in the exposed group in the first 18 years after exposure. In a further study[5], the relative risk was 1.3 before age 50 and 1.7 thereafter; and, in another[6], three cases were reported with 5.1 expected before age 50 and five cases *versus* 3.0 expected thereafter. In contrast, however, a randomized study[2] showed 11 exposed cases and five nonexposed cases during the first 15 years of follow-up, compared to 21 exposed cases and 16 nonexposed cases thereafter. Further data are required to settle this issue.

The four follow-up studies[2-5] of exposed and nonexposed women also included information on other possibly 'hormone-related' cancers. The occurrence of endometrial cancer was not increased in any study. The study[2] of 693 women exposed to DES and 668 controls showed increases in the occurrence of cancer of the ovary (4 exposed, 1 nonexposed), cancer of the cervix (7 exposed, 3 nonexposed) and cancer of the colon-rectum (2 exposed, 1 nonexposed); there was also a risk for cancer at these sites in the study of 1531 women exposed to DES and 1404 controls[5] (6 exposed, 2 nonexposed; 9 exposed, 6 nonexposed; 11 exposed, 7 nonexposed for the three sites, respectively). A third study[4] showed, in contrast, no elevation of rates for cancer at any other site, and there were seven deaths from cervical cancer in the control group and none in the exposed group, suggesting that matching in the control group was 'inadequate'; the authors could not identify the matching problem, and, in particular, they found that the two groups were well matched on educational level. The data are too few to draw any firm conclusions.

A greater frequency of abnormalities of the reproductive tract has been found in males exposed prenatally to DES in comparison with nonexposed controls, although the data are few. Cryptorchidism, a major risk factor for testicular cancer, is one of the associated lesions[1]. Cancer of the testis has been investigated in five case-control studies of fetal exposure to DES[7-11]. One[7] showed that 5.1% (4/78) of cases and 1% of controls had been exposed to hormones (in all likelihood DES) for bleeding; the second[8] similarly found that 5.8% (11/190) *versus* 2.3% (7/304) had had such exposure; the third[9] found 1.9% (2/108) *versus* 0 (0/108) exposed to DES; the fourth[10] found 1.0% (2/202) *versus* 1.0% (2/206) exposed to DES; and the fifth[11] found 1.9% (4/211) *versus* 0.9% (2/214) exposed to DES. The combined relative risk is 2.5 ($p = 0.014$).

A number of unusual tumours have been reported in women exposed to DES *in utero*: a fatal adenocarcinoma of the endometrium at age 26[12]; a pituitary adenoma at age 18[13]; an invasive squamous-cell carcinoma of the cervix at age 21[14]; an invasive adenosquamous-cell carcinoma of the cervix at age 27[15]; and an ovarian teratoma at age 12[16].

There has been no further report to add to the six cases of primary breast cancer in males with prostatic cancer treated with DES[1]. A case has been reported of a Leydig-cell tumour developing in a man treated with DES at 1 mg per day for 2.5 years[17]. There has been a case report of hepatic angiosarcoma in a man treated over a long period with DES for prostatic cancer[1,18], and a second case report of a hepatoma in a prostatic cancer patient treated with DES at 3 mg per day for 4.5 years (to diagnosis of hepatoma)[1,19]. Three renal carcinomas have been reported after exposure to DES for prostatic cancer[20,21].

B. Evidence for carcinogenicity to animals (*sufficient*)

DES has been tested in mice, rats, hamsters, frogs and squirrel monkeys, producing tumours principally in oestrogen-responsive tissues[1]. Female newborn mice injected with DES developed epidermoid carcinomas and granular-cell myoblastomas of the cervix and squamous carcinomas of the vagina[22]. Mice treated prenatally with DES developed adenocarcinomas of the uterus, cervix and vagina, epidermoid carcinomas of the uterine cervix and vagina and ovarian and mammary tumours[23-28]. Female mice fed diets containing DES developed cervical and endometrial adenocarcinomas, mammary adeno-carcinomas, osteosarcomas and mesotheliomas[29-33]. Mice treated subcutaneously with DES had a slightly increased incidence of lymphomas and subcutaneous fibrosarcomas[34,35]. Prenatal exposure to DES potentiated mammary tumorigenesis in rats given 7,12-di-methylbenz[a]anthracene at about 50 days of age[36]. Rats given DES by subcutaneous pellet developed mammary and pituitary tumours. When these animals were also treated with X-rays or neutrons, they developed a higher incidence of mammary tumours[37-39]. In other studies (subcutaneous, transplacental, oral), rats treated with DES developed mammary, hepatic and pituitary tumours[40-44]. When hamsters were treated prenatally with DES, females developed endometrial adenocarcinoma, squamous-cell papillomas of the cervix and vagina, and a mixed Mullerian tumour of the cervix (myosarcoma); in males, a leiomysarcoma of the seminal vesicles and a Cowper's gland adenoma were found[45]. Male hamsters castrated as adults and given DES subcutaneously developed renal tumours[46,47].

C. Other relevant data

No data were available on the genetic and related effects of DES in humans.

DES induced chromosomal aberrations in bone-marrow cells of mice treated *in vivo*, but data on induction of sister chromatid exchanges and micronuclei were equivocal; it induced sister chromatid exchanges in one study in rats. Unusual nucleotides were found in kidney DNA following chronic treatment of hamsters with DES. Aneuploidy was induced in human cells *in vitro*, but data on induction of sister chromatid exchanges, chromosomal aberrations and mutation were inconclusive; it induced DNA strand breaks, but not unscheduled DNA synthesis, except in a single study. Tests for transformation in rat and Syrian hamster embryo cells gave positive results, while results for mouse cells were negative. Aneuploidy and DNA strand breaks were induced in rodent cells *in vitro*, but results for chromosomal aberrations, micronuclei and sister chromatid exchanges were equivocal; DES did not induce mutation or unscheduled DNA synthesis, except in a single study in Syrian hamster embryo cells. It did not inhibit intercellular communication of Chinese hamster V79 cells. It induced aneuploidy in fungi, but, in most studies, it did not induce mutation, recombination or gene conversion. It did not induce mutation in a variety of bacterial and insect systems, but it was mutagenic in plants. DNA damage was not induced in fungi or bacteria. DES induced single-strand breaks in bacteriophage DNA in the presence of a horseradish peroxidase activation system[48].

References

[1]*IARC Monographs, 21,* 131-134, 173-231, 1979

[2]Bibbo, M., Haenszel, W.M., Wied, G.L., Hubby, M. & Herbst, A.L. (1978) A twenty-five-year follow-up of women exposed to diethylstilbestrol during pregnancy. *New Engl. J. Med., 298,* 763-767

[3]Beral, V. & Colwell, L. (1980) Randomised trial of high doses of stilboestrol and ethisterone in pregnancy: long-term follow-up of mothers. *Br. med. J., 281,* 1098-1101

[4]Greenberg, E.R., Barnes, A.B., Resseguie, L., Barrett, J.A., Burnside, S., Lanza, L.L., Neff, R.K., Stevens, M., Young, R.H. & Colton, T. (1984) Breast cancer in mothers given diethylstilbestrol in pregnancy. *New Engl. J. Med., 311,* 1393-1398

[5]Hadjimichael, O.C., Meigs, J.W., Falcier, F.W., Thompson, W.D. & Flannery, J.T. (1984) Cancer risk among women exposed to exogenous estrogens during pregnancy. *J. natl Cancer Inst., 73,* 831-834

[6]Brian, D.D., Tilley, B.C., Labarthe, D.R., O'Fallon, W.M., Noller, K.L. & Kurland, L.T. (1980) Breast cancer in DES-exposed mothers. Absence of association. *Mayo Clin. Proc., 55,* 89-93

[7]Henderson, B.E., Benton, B., Jing, J., Yu, M.C. & Pike, M.C. (1979) Risk factors for cancer of the testis in young men. *Int. J. Cancer, 23,* 598-602

[8]Schottenfeld, D., Warshauer, M.E., Sherlock, S., Zauber, A.G., Leder, M. & Payne, R. (1980) The epidemiology of testicular cancer in young adults. *Am. J. Epidemiol., 112,* 232-246

[9]Depue, R.H., Pike, M.C. & Henderson, B.E. (1983) Estrogen exposure during gestation and risk of testicular cancer. *J. natl Cancer Inst., 71,* 1151-1155

[10]Brown, L.M., Pottern, L.M. & Hoover, R.N. (1986) Prenatal and perinatal risk factors for testicular cancer. *Cancer Res., 46,* 4812-4816

[11]Moss, A.R., Osmond, D., Bacchetti, P., Torti, F.M. & Gurgin, V. (1986) Hormonal risk factors in testicular cancer. A case-control study. *Am. J. Epidemiol., 124,* 39-52

[12]Barter, J.F., Austin, J.M., Jr & Shingleton, H.M. (1986) Endometrial adenocarcinoma after in utero diethylstilbestrol exposure. *Obstet. Gynecol., 67 (Suppl.),* 84S-85S

[13]Cunningham, J.R., Gidwani, G.P., Gupta, M.S., Duchesneau, P.M. & Schumacher, O.P. (1982) Prolactin-secreting pituitary adenoma: occurrence following prenatal exposure to diethyl-stilbestrol. *Cleveland Clin. Q., 49,* 249-254

[14]Lamb, E.J. (1977) Invasive squamous cell carcinoma of the cervix in a diethylstilbestrol-exposed offspring. *Am. J. Obstet. Gynecol., 129,* 924-925

[15]Vandrie, D.M., Puri, S., Upton, R.T. & Demeester, L.J. (1983) Adenosquamous carcinoma of the cervix in a woman exposed to diethylstilbestrol *in utero. Obstet. Gynecol., 61 (Suppl.),* 84S-87S

[16]Lazarus, K.H. (1984) Maternal diethylstilboestrol and ovarian malignancy in offspring. *Lancet, i,* 53

[17]Deshmukh, A.S. & Hartung, W.H. (1983) Leydig cell tumor in patient on estrogen therapy. *Urology, 21,* 538-539

[18]Ham, J.M., Pirola, R.C. & Crouch, R.L. (1980) Hemangioendothelial sarcoma of the liver associated with long-term estrogen therapy in a man. *Dig. Dis. Sci., 25,* 879-883

[19]Brooks, J.J. (1982) Hepatoma associated with diethylstilbestrol therapy for prostatic carcinoma. *J. Urol.*, *128*, 1044-1045

[20]Bellet, R.E. & Squitieri, A.P. (1974) Estrogen-induced hypernephroma. *J. Urol.*, *112*, 160-161

[21]Nissenkorn, I., Servadio, C. & Avidor, I. (1979) Oestrogen-induced renal carcinoma. *Br. J. Urol.*, *51*, 6-9

[22]Dunn, T.B. (1979) Cancer and other lesions in mice receiving estrogens. *Recent Results Cancer Res.*, *66*, 175-192

[23]McLachlan, J.A. (1979) Transplacental effects of diethylstilbestrol in mice. *Natl Cancer Inst. Monogr.*, *51*, 67-72

[24]McLachlan, J.A., Newbold, R.R. & Bullock, B.C. (1980) Long-term effects on the female mouse genital tract associated with prenatal exposure to diethylstilbestrol. *Cancer Res.*, *40*, 3988-3999

[25]Lamb, J.C., IV, Newbold, R.R. & McLachlan, J.A. (1981) Visualization by light and scanning electron microscopy of reproductive tract lesions in female mice treated transplacentally with diethylstilbestrol. *Cancer Res.*, *41*, 4057-4062

[26]Newbold, R.R. & MacLachlan, J.A. (1982) Vaginal adenosis and adenocarcinoma in mice exposed prenatally or neonatally to diethylstilbestrol. *Cancer Res.*, *42*, 2003-2011

[27]Walker, B.E. (1983) Uterine tumors in old female mice exposed prenatally to diethylstilbestrol. *J. natl Cancer Inst.*, *70*, 477-484

[28]Nagasawa, H., Mori, T. & Nakajima, Y. (1980) Long-term effects of progesterone or diethylstilbestrol with or without estrogen after maturity on mammary tumorigenesis in mice. *Eur. J. Cancer*, *16*, 1583-1589

[29]Highman, B., Greenman, D.L., Norvell, M.J., Farmer, J. & Shellenberger, T.E. (1980) Neoplastic and preneoplastic lesions induced in female C3H mice by diets containing diethylstilbestrol or 17β-estradiol. *J. environ. Pathol. Toxicol.*, *4*, 81-95

[30]Highman, B., Roth, S.I. & Greenman, D.L. (1981) Osseous changes and oesteosarcomas in mice continuously fed diets containing diethylstilbestrol or 17β-estradiol. *J. natl Cancer Inst.*, *67*, 653-662

[31]Greenman, D.L., Highman, B., Kodell, R.L., Morgan, K.T. & and Norvell, M. (1984) Neoplastic and nonneoplastic responses to chronic feeding of diethylstilbestrol in C3H mice. *J. Toxicol. environ. Health*, *14*, 551-567

[32]Greenman, D.L., Kodell, R.L., Highman, B., Schieferstein, G.J. & Norvell, M. (1984) Influence of strain and age on the induction of mammary tumours by diethylstilboestrol in C3H mice. *Food chem. Toxicol.*, *22*, 871-874

[33]Greenman, D.L., Highman, B., Chen, J.J., Schieferstein, G.J. & Norvell, M.J. (1986) Influence of age on induction of mammary tumors by diethylstilbestrol in C3H/HeN mice with low murine mammary tumor virus titer. *J. natl Cancer Inst.*, *77*, 891-898

[34]Boján, F., Rédai, I. & Gomba, S. (1979) Induction of lymphomas by urethane in combination with diethylstilboestrol in CFLP mice. *Experientia*, *35*, 378-379

[35]Ways, S. (1982) Local induction of fibrosarcomas by diethylstilbestrol. *Int. Res. Commun. System med. Sci.*, *10*, 796-797

[36]Boylan, E.S. & Calhoon, R.E. (1979) Mammary tumorigenesis in the rat following prenatal exposure to diethylstilbestrol and postnatal treatment with 7,12-dimethylbenz(a)anthracene. *J. Toxicol. environ. Health*, *5*, 1059-1071

[37]Holtzman, S., Stone, J.P. & Shellabarger, C.J. (1979) Synergism of diethylstilbestrol and radiation in mammary carcinogenesis in female F344 rats. *J. natl Cancer Inst.*, *63*, 1071-1074

[38]Holtzman, S., Stone, J.P. & Shellabarger, C.J. (1981) Synergism of estrogens and X-rays in mammary carcinogenesis in female ACI rats. *J. natl Cancer Inst.*, *67*, 455-459

[39]Shellabarger, C.J., Chmelevsky, D., Kellerer, A.M., Stone, J.P. & Holtzman, S. (1982) Induction of mammary neoplasms in the ACI rat by 430-keV neutrons, X-rays, and diethylstilbestrol. *J. natl Cancer Inst.*, *69*, 1135-1146

[40]Sumi, C., Yokoro, K. & Matsushima, R. (1983) Induction of hepatic tumors by diethylstilbestrol alone or in synergism with N-nitrosobutylurea in castrated male WF rats. *J. natl Cancer Inst.*, *70*, 937-942

[41]Phelps, C. & Hymer, W.C. (1983) Characterization of estrogen-induced adenohypophyseal tumors in the Fischer 344 rat. *Neuroendocrinology*, *37*, 23-31

[42]Rothschild, T.C., Calhoon, R.E. & Boylan, E.S. (1985) Transplacental carcinogenicity of diethylstilbestrol (DES) in female ACI rats (Abstract No. 770). *Proc. Am. Assoc. Cancer Res.*, *26*, 195

[43]Inoh, A., Kamiya, K., Fujii, Y. & Yokoro, K. (1985) Protective effects of progesterone and tamoxifen in estrogen-induced mammary carcinogenesis in ovariectomized W/FU rats. *Jpn. J. Cancer Res. (Gann)*, *76*, 699-704

[44]Wanless, I.R. & Medline, A. (1982) Role of estrogens as promoters of hepatic neoplasia. *Lab. Invest.*, *46*, 313-320

[45]Rustia, M. (1979) Role of hormone imbalance in transplacental carcinogenesis induced in Syrian golden hamsters by sex hormones. *Natl Cancer Inst. Monogr.*, *51*, 77-87

[46]Li, J.J., Li, S.A., Klicka, J.K., Parsons, J.A. & Lam, L.K.T. (1983) Relative carcinogenic activity of various synthetic and natural estrogens in the Syrian hamster kidney. *Cancer Res.*, *43*, 5200-5204

[47]Li, J.J. & Li, S.A. (1984) Estrogen-induced tumorigenesis in hamsters: roles for hormonal and carcinogenic activities. *Arch. Toxicol.*, *55*, 110-118

[48]*IARC Monographs*, Suppl. *6*, 250-256, 1987

Dienoestrol

A. Evidence for carcinogenicity to animals (*limited*)

Dienoestrol was tested in female guinea-pigs by subcutaneous injection and in female mice by intravaginal administration. Although these experiments indicated induction of 'uterine tumours' in guinea-pigs and of ovarian tumours in mice, they were regarded as inadequate[1]. Renal tumours were produced by administration of α-dienoestrol in male hamsters castrated as adults[2,3]. In noninbred rats, dienoestrol given prenatally and neonatally did not increase tumour incidence[4].

B. Other relevant data

No data were available on the genetic and related effects of dienoestrol in humans.

There are two stable stereoisomers of dienoestrol — Z,Z-dienoestrol (*cis,cis*-dienoestrol, β-dienoestrol) and E,E-dienoestrol (*trans,trans*-dienoestrol, α-dienoestrol). E,E-Dienoestrol is the principal constituent of dienoestrol-containing medications, whereas Z,Z-dienoestrol is a metabolite of diethylstilboestrol. Z,Z-Dienoestrol induced sister chromatid exchanges in human fibroblasts *in vitro*. Z,Z-Dienoestrol, but not E,E-dienoestrol, transformed cultured hamster cells. Z,Z-Dienoestrol produced single-strand breaks in hamster cells in the absence of an exogenous metabolic system, whereas both Z,Z- and E,E-dienoestrol gave weakly positive results in tests for unscheduled DNA synthesis in hamster cells, only in the presence of a metabolic system. Z,Z-Dienoestrol did not induce single-strand breaks in bacteriophage DNA in the presence of a horseradish peroxidase activation system. Z,Z-Dienoestrol and E,E-dienoestrol were not mutagenic to bacteria[5].

References

[1]*IARC Monographs*, *21*, 161-171, 1979

[2]Li, J.J., Li, S.A., Klicka, J.K., Parsons, J.A. & Lam, L.K.T. (1983) Relative carcinogenic activity of various synthetic and natural estrogens in the Syrian hamster kidney. *Cancer Res.*, *43*, 5200-5204

[3]Li, J.J. & Li, S.A. (1984) Estrogen-induced tumorigenesis in hamsters: roles for hormonal and carcinogenic activities. *Arch. Toxicol.*, *55*, 110-118

[4]Ird, Y.A. (1983) Blastomogenesis induced in rats by transplacental treatment with estrogens (Russ.). *Vopr. Onkol.*, *29*, 61-66

[5]*IARC Monographs*, *Suppl. 6*, 245-247, 1987

Hexoestrol

A. Evidence for carcinogenicity to animals (*sufficient*)

Hexoestrol was tested for carcinogenicity in intact male hamsters and in males castrated as adults by subcutaneous implantation as a pellet, producing renal tumours, some of which were described as renal carcinomas, in 85-100% of tested animals[1-3].

B. Other relevant data

No data were available on the genetic and related effects of hexoestrol in humans. Unusual nucleotides were found in kidney DNA of hamsters treated with hexoestrol *in vivo*. The compound was not mutagenic to bacteria[4].

References

[1]Li, J.J., Li, S.A., Klicka, J.K., Parsons, J.A. & Lam, L.K.T. (1983) Relative carcinogenic activity of various synthetic and natural estrogens in the Syrian hamster kidney. *Cancer Res.*, *43*, 5200-5204

[2]Li, J.J. & Li, S.A. (1984) Estrogen-induced tumorigenesis in hamsters: roles for hormonal and carcinogenic activities. *Arch. Toxicol.*, *55*, 110-118

[3]Liehr, J.G., Ballatore, A.M., Dague, B.B. & Ulubelen, A.A. (1985) Carcinogenicity and metabolic activation of hexestrol. *Chem.-biol. Interactions, 55*, 157-176

[4]*IARC Monographs, Suppl. 6*, 336-337, 1987

Chlorotrianisene

A. Evidence for carcinogenicity to animals (*inadequate*)

Chlorotrianisene was tested in only one experiment in rats by oral administration. The data were insufficient to evaluate the carcinogenicity of this compound[1].

B. Other relevant data

No data were available to the Working Group.

Reference

[1]*IARC Monographs, 21*, 139-146, 1979

STEROIDAL OESTROGENS (Group 1*)

Evidence for carcinogenicity to humans (*sufficient*)

Oestrogen replacement therapy (Group 1)

A. Evidence for carcinogenicity to humans (*sufficient*)

A number of studies, utilizing a variety of designs, have shown a consistent, strongly positive association between exposure to a number of oestrogenic substances and risk of endometrial cancer, with evidence of positive dose-response relationships both for strength of medication and duration of use[1]. Consistent findings have also been seen in more recent studies[2-16]. The rise and fall of incidence of endometrial cancer in several areas of the USA was compatible with trends in oestrogen use[1,15].

Of the 20 epidemiological studies of oestrogen replacement therapy and breast cancer risk[16-35], nine show a positive relation between oestrogen use and breast cancer[17-20,22-24,28,33]. The increased risks tend to be small; for example, a 50% increase was found with 20 years of menopausal oestrogen replacement therapy use[24]. All except one[33] of the positive studies involved use of population controls (eight of the nine studies with population controls gave positive results), and most showed increased risk after prolonged use or after ten or more years since initial exposure. One study showed a positive association with current oestrogen use[23].

---

*This evaluation applies to the group of chemicals as a whole and not necessarily to all individual chemicals within the group (see also Methods, p. 38).

One possible reason that studies with hospital controls gave negative results and those with population controls positive results is that oestrogen replacement therapy may be used more frequently in hospitalized women than in the general population. However, in two studies involving use of both hospital and population control groups, one giving positive[29] and the other largely negative[25] results, similar results were obtained when hospital and population controls were used to estimate the relative risk. Three of the studies with negative results[26,27,34] probably did not permit the authors to address satisfactorily the question of long-term use of oestrogen replacement therapy. The large hospital-based study that showed a positive finding used as controls subjects with a large spectrum of acute conditions unrelated to any of the known or suspected risk factors for breast cancer[33].

One cohort study of 1439 women initially treated for benign breast disease showed increased risk for women who took exogenous oestrogens after biopsy, but not for those who had taken them before biopsy. The increased risk in the former group appeared to be associated with epithelial hyperplasia or calcification in the initial lesion[35].

References

[1]*IARC Monographs*, *21*, 95-102, 147-159, 1979

[2]Buring, J.E., Bain, C.J. & Ehrmann, R.L. (1986) Conjugated estrogen use and risk of endometrial cancer. *Am. J. Epidemiol.*, *124*, 434-441

[3]Ewertz, M., Machado, S.G., Boice, J.D., Jr & Jensen, O.M. (1984) Endometrial cancer following treatment for breast cancer: a case-control study in Denmark. *Br. J. Cancer*, *50*, 687-692

[4]Henderson, B.E., Casagrande, J.T., Pike, M.C., Mack, T., Rosario, I. & Duke, A. (1983) The epidemiology of endometrial cancer in young women. *Br. J. Cancer*, *47*, 749-756

[5]Hulka, B.S., Fowler, W.C., Jr, Kaufman, D.G., Grimson, R.C., Greenberg, B.G., Hogue, C.J.R., Berger, G.S. & Pulliam, C.C. (1980) Estrogen and endometrial cancer: cases and two control groups from North Carolina. *Am. J. Obstet. Gynecol.*, *137*, 92-101

[6]Kelsey, J.L., LiVolsi, V.A., Holford, T.R., Fischer, D.B., Mostow, E.D., Schwartz, P.E., O'Connor, T. & White, C. (1982) A case-control study of cancer of the endometrium. *Am. J. Epidemiol.*, *116*, 333-342

[7]La Vecchia, C., Franceschi, S., Gallus, G., DeCarli, A., Colombo, E., Mangioni, C. & Tognoni, G. (1982) Oestrogens and obesity as risk factors for endometrial cancer in Italy. *Int. J. Epidemiol.*, *11*, 120-126

[8]La Vecchia, C., Franceschi, S., DeCarli, A., Gallus, G. & Tognoni, G. (1984) Risk factors for endometrial cancer at different ages. *J. natl Cancer Inst.*, *73*, 667-671

[9]Öbrink, A., Bunne, G., Collén, J. & Tjernberg, B. (1981) Estrogen regimen of women with endometrial carcinoma. A retrospective case-control study at Radiumhemmet. *Acta obstet. gynecol. scand.*, *60*, 191-197

[10]Shapiro, S., Kaufman, D.W., Slone, D., Rosenberg, L., Miettinen, O.S., Stolley, P.D., Rosenshein, N.B., Watring, W.G., Leavitt, T., Jr & Knapp, R.C. (1980) Recent and past use of conjugated estrogens in relation to adenocarcinoma of the endometrium. *New Engl. J. Med.*, *303*, 485-489

[11]Shapiro, S., Kelly, J.P., Rosenberg, L., Kaufman, D.W., Helmrich, S.P., Rosenshein, N.B., Lewis, J.L., Jr, Knapp, R.C., Stolley, P.D. & Schottenfeld, D. (1985) Risk of localized and widespread endometrial cancer in relation to recent and discontinued use of conjugated estrogens. *New Engl. J. Med., 313*, 969-972

[12]Spengler, R.F., Clarke, E.A., Woolever, C.A., Newman, A.M. & Osborn, R.W. (1981) Exogenous estrogens and endometrial cancer: a case-control study and assessment of potential biases. *Am. J. Epidemiol., 114*, 497-506

[13]Stavraky, K.M., Collins, J.A., Donner, A. & Wells, G.A. (1981) A comparison of estrogen use by women with endometrial cancer, gynecologic disorders, and other illnesses. *Am. J. Obstet. Gynecol., 141*, 547-555

[14]Weiss, N.S., Farewell, V.T., Szekely, D.R., English, D.R. & Kiviat, N. (1980) Oestrogens and endometrial cancer: effect of other risk factors on the association. *Maturitas, 2*, 185-190

[15]Marrett, L.D., Meigs, J.W. & Flannery, J.T. (1982) Trends in the incidence of cancer of the corpus uteri in Connecticut, 1964-1969, in relation to consumption of exogenous estrogens. *Am. J. Epidemiol., 116*, 57-67

[16]Vakil, D.V., Morgan, R.W. & Halliday, M. (1983) Exogenous estrogens and development of breast and endometrial cancer. *Cancer Detect. Prev., 6*, 415-424

[17]Hoover, R., Gray, L.A., Sr, Cole, P. & MacMahon, B. (1976) Menopausal estrogens and breast cancer. *New Engl. J. Med., 295*, 401-405

[18]Ross, R.K., Paganini-Hill, A., Gerkins, V.R., Mack, T.M., Pfeffer, R., Arthur, M. & Henderson, B.E. (1980) A case-control study of menopausal estrogen therapy and breast cancer. *J. Am. med. Assoc., 243*, 1635-1639

[19]Hoover, R., Glass, A., Finkle, W.D., Azevedo, D. & Milne, K. (1981) Conjugated estrogens and breast cancer risk in women. *J. natl Cancer Inst., 67*, 815-820

[20]Hulka, B.S., Chambless, L.E., Deubner, D.C. & Wilkinson, W.E. (1982) Breast cancer and estrogen replacement therapy. *Am. J. Obstet. Gynecol., 143*, 638-644

[21]Gambrell, R.D., Jr, Maier, R.C. & Sanders, B.I. (1983) Decreased incidence of breast cancer in postmenopausal estrogen-progestogen users. *Obstet. Gynecol., 62*, 435-443

[22]Hiatt, R.A., Bawol, R., Friedman, G.D. & Hoover, R. (1984) Exogenous estrogen and breast cancer after bilateral oophorectomy. *Cancer, 54*, 139-144

[23]McDonald, J.A., Weiss, N.S., Daling, J.R., Francis, A.M. & Polissar, L. (1986) Menopausal estrogen use and the risk of breast cancer. *Breast Cancer Res. Treat., 7*, 193-199

[24]Brinton, L.A., Hoover, R. & Fraumeni, J.F., Jr (1986) Menopausal oestrogens and breast cancer risk: an expanded case-control study. *Br. J. Cancer, 54*, 825-832

[25]Nomura, A.M.Y., Kolonel, L.N., Hirohata, T. & Lee, J. (1986) The association of replacement estrogens with breast cancer. *Int. J. Cancer, 37*, 49-53

[26]Sartwell, P.E., Arthes, F.G. & Tonascia, J.A. (1977) Exogenous hormones, reproductive history, and breast cancer. *J. natl Cancer Inst., 59*, 1589-1592

[27]Ravnihar, B., Seigel, D.G. & Lindtner, J. (1979) An epidemiologic study of breast cancer and benign breast neoplasias in relation to the oral contraceptive and estrogen use. *Eur. J. Cancer, 15*, 395-405

[28]Jick, H., Walker, A.M., Watkins, R.N., D'Ewart, D.C., Hunter, J.R., Danford, A., Madsen, S., Dinan, B.J. & Rothman, K.J. (1980) Replacement estrogens and breast cancer. *Am. J. Epidemiol.*, *112*, 586-594

[29]Kelsey, J.L., Fischer, D.B., Holford, T.R., LiVolsi, V.A., Mostow, E.D., Goldenberg, I.S. & White, C. (1981) Exogenous estrogens and other factors in the epidemiology of breast cancer. *J. natl Cancer Inst.*, *67*, 327-333

[30]Sherman, B., Wallace, R. & Bean, J. (1983) Estrogen use and breast cancer. Interaction with body mass. *Cancer*, *51*, 1527-1531

[31]Kaufman, D.W., Miller, D.R., Rosenberg, L., Helmrich, S.P., Stolley, P., Schottenfeld, D. & Shapiro, S. (1984) Noncontraceptive estrogen use and the risk of breast cancer. *J. Am. med. Assoc.*, *252*, 63-67

[32]Horwitz, R.I. & Stewart, K.R. (1984) Effect of clinical features on the association of estrogens and breast cancer. *Am. J. Med.*, *76*, 192-198

[33]La Vecchia, C., Decarli, A., Parazzini, F., Gentile, A., Liberati, C. & Franceschi, S. (1986) Non-contraceptive oestrogens and the risk of breast cancer in women. *Int. J. Cancer*, *38*, 853-858

[34]Wingo, P.A., Layde, P.M., Lee, N.C., Rubin, G. & Ory, H.W. (1987) The risk of breast cancer in postmenopausal women who have used estrogen replacement therapy. *J. Am. med. Assoc.*, *257*, 209-215

[35]Thomas, D.B., Persing, J.P. & Hutchison, W.B. (1982) Exogenous estrogens and other risk factors for breast cancer in women with benign breast diseases. *J. natl Cancer Inst.*, *69*, 1017-1025

Conjugated oestrogens

A. Evidence for carcinogenicity to animals (*limited*)

Conjugated oestrogens were tested inadequately in rats by oral administration in one study[1]. In male hamsters castrated as adults, equilin administered as a subcutaneously implanted pellet produced renal tumours in 6/8 treated animals. In contrast, *d*-equilenin administered similarly did not induce renal tumours[2,3].

B. Other relevant data

No data were available on the genetic and related effects of conjugated oestrogens in humans.

A commercial preparation of conjugated oestrogens did not induce chromosomal aberrations in human lymphoblastoid cells *in vitro* or in Chinese hamster V79 cells exposed in diffusion chambers implanted into mice after oestrogen treatment. It was not mutagenic to bacteria[4].

References

[1]*IARC Monographs*, *21*, 147-159, 1979

[2]Li, J.J., Li, S.A., Klicka, J.K., Parsons, J.A. & Lam, L.K.T. (1983) Relative carcinogenic activity of various synthetic and natural estrogens in the Syrian hamster kidney. *Cancer Res.*, *43*, 5200-5204

[3]Li, J.J. & Li, S.A. (1984) Estrogen-induced tumorigenesis in hamsters: roles for hormonal and carcinogenic activities. *Arch. Toxicol.*, *55*, 110-118

[4]*IARC Monographs, Suppl. 6*, 187, 1987

Oestradiol-17β and esters

A. Evidence for carcinogenicity to animals (*sufficient*)

Oestradiol-17β and its esters were tested in mice, rats, hamsters and guinea-pigs by oral and subcutaneous administration. Administration to mice increased the incidences of mammary, pituitary, uterine, cervical, vaginal, testicular, lymphoid and bone tumours[1-5]. In rats, there was an increased incidence of mammary and/or pituitary tumours[1,6]. Oestradiol-17β produced a nonstatistically significant increase in the incidence of foci of altered hepatocytes and hepatic nodules induced by partial hepatectomy and administration of *N*-nitrosodiethylamine in rats[7]. In hamsters, a high incidence of malignant kidney tumours occurred in intact and castrated males[1,8-10] and in ovariectomized females, but not in intact females[1]. In guinea-pigs, diffuse fibromyomatous uterine and abdominal lesions were observed[1].

B. Other relevant data

No data were available on the genetic and related effects of oestradiol-17β in humans.

Oestradiol-17β did not induce chromosomal aberrations in bone-marrow cells of mice treated *in vivo*. Unusual nucleotides were found in kidney DNA of treated hamsters. It induced micronuclei but not aneuploidy, chromosomal aberrations or sister chromatid exchanges in human cells *in vitro*. In rodent cells *in vitro*, it induced aneuploidy and unscheduled DNA synthesis but was not mutagenic and did not induce DNA strand breaks or sister chromatid exchanges. Oestradiol-17β was not mutagenic to bacteria[11].

References

[1]*IARC Monographs*, *21*, 279-326, 1979

[2]Huseby, R.A. (1980) Demonstration of a direct carcinogenic effect of estradiol on Leydig cells of the mouse. *Cancer Res.*, *40*, 1006-1013

[3]Highman, B., Roth, S.I. & Greenman, D.L. (1981) Osseous changes and osteosarcomas in mice continuously fed diets containing diethylstilbestrol or 17β-estradiol. *J. natl Cancer Inst.*, *67*, 653-662

[4]Highman, B., Greenman, D.L., Norvell, M.J., Farmer, J. & Shellenberger, T.E. (1980) Neoplastic and preneoplastic lesions induced in female C3H mice by diets containing diethylstilbestrol or 17β-estradiol. *J. environ. Pathol. Toxicol.*, *4*, 81-95

[5]Nagasawa, H., Mori, T. & Nakajima, Y. (1980) Long-term effects of progesterone or diethylstilbestrol with or without estrogen after maturity on mammary tumorigenesis in mice. *Eur. J. Cancer*, *16*, 1583-1589

[6]Inoh, A., Kamiya, K., Fujii, Y. & Yokoro, K. (1985) Protective effects of progesterone and tamoxifen in estrogen-induced mammary carcinogenesis in ovariectomized W/FU rats. *Jpn. J. Cancer Res. (Gann)*, *76*, 699-704

[7]Yager, J.D., Campbell, H.A., Longnecker, D.S., Roebuck, B.D. & Benoit, M.C. (1984) Enhancement of hepatocarcinogenesis in female rats by ethinyl estradiol and mestranol but not estradiol. *Cancer Res.*, *44*, 3862-3869

[8]Li, J.J., Li, S.A., Klicka, J.K., Parsons, J.A. & Lam, L.K.T. (1983) Relative carcinogenic activity of various synthetic and natural estrogens in the Syrian hamster kidney. *Cancer Res.*, *43*, 5200-5204

[9]Li, J.J. & Li, S.A. (1984) Estrogen-induced tumorigenesis in hamsters: roles for hormonal and carcinogenic activities. *Arch. Toxicol.*, *55*, 110-118

[10]Liehr, J.G., Stancel, G.M., Chorich, L.P., Bousfield, G.R. & Ulubelen, A.A. (1986) Hormonal carcinogenesis: separation of estrogenicity from carcinogenicity. *Chem.-biol. Interactions*, *59*, 173-184

[11]*IARC Monographs, Suppl. 6*, 437-439, 1987

Oestriol

A. Evidence for carcinogenicity to animals (*limited*)

Oestriol was tested by subcutaneous implantation in castrated mice and in rats and hamsters. It increased the incidence and accelerated the appearance of mammary tumours in both male and female mice and produced kidney tumours in hamsters[1].

B. Other relevant data

No data were available on the genetic and related effects of oestriol in humans. It did not induce aneuploidy in cultured lymphocytes from one pregnant woman; results for induction of sister chromatid exchanges were inconclusive. No effect was seen in lymphocytes from one man[2].

References

[1]*IARC Monographs*, *21*, 327-341, 1979

[2]*IARC Monographs, Suppl. 6*, 440-441, 1987

Oestrone

A. Evidence for carcinogenicity to animals (*sufficient*)

Oestrone was tested in mice by oral administration, in mice, rats and hamsters by subcutaneous injection and implantation, and in mice by skin painting. Its administration resulted in an increased incidence of mammary tumours in mice, in pituitary, adrenal and mammary tumours in rats, and in renal tumours in both castrated and intact male hamsters[1]. Oestrone implanted subcutaneously as a pellet produced renal tumours in 80% of treated male hamsters castrated as adults[2,3].

B. Other relevant data

No data were available on the genetic and related effects of oestrone in humans. It was not mutagenic to Chinese hamster cells *in vitro*[4].

References

[1] *IARC Monographs*, *21*, 343-362, 1979

[2] Li, J.J., Li, S.A., Klicka, J.K., Parsons, J.A. & Lam, L.K.T. (1983) Relative carcinogenic activity of various synthetic and natural estrogens in the Syrian hamster kidney. *Cancer Res., 43*, 5200-5204

[3] Li, J.J. & Li, S.A. (1984) Estrogen-induced tumorigenesis in hamsters: roles for hormonal and carcinogenic activities. *Arch. Toxicol., 55*, 110-118

[4] *IARC Monographs*, *Suppl. 6*, 442-443, 1987

Ethinyloestradiol

A. Evidence for carcinogenicity to animals (*sufficient*)

Ethinyloestradiol was tested in mice, rats, dogs and monkeys by oral administration and in rats by subcutaneous injection. In mice, it increased the incidences of pituitary tumours and of malignant mammary tumours in both males and females and produced malignant tumours of the uterus and cervix in females[1]. In rats, it increased the incidence of liver-cell tumours[1,2], pituitary chromophobe adenomas[2] and mammary adenocarcinomas[2,3]. Ethinyloestradiol administered as a subcutaneous injection of pellets produced a low but increased incidence of renal tumours in hamsters castrated as adults[4,5]. In rats, it induced foci of altered hepatocytes, a presumed preneoplastic lesion; when administered following initiation of hepatocarcinogenesis with *N*-nitrosodiethylamine, ethinyloestradiol enhanced the development of foci of altered hepatocytes and of hepatic nodules[6]. In female rats given partial hepatectomy and treated with *N*-nitrosodiethylamine, ethinyloestradiol potentiated the development of foci of altered hepatocytes and of hepatocellular carcinomas[7]. In *N*-nitrosodiethylamine-initiated rats, ethinyloestradiol increased the number of γ-glutamyl transpeptidase-positive hepatic foci[8]. Dietary administration of ethinyloestradiol combined with subcutaneous injections of 3,2'-dimethyl-4-aminobiphenyl caused a high incidence of prostatic carcinomas in male rats[9]. In rats, ethinyloestradiol significantly enhanced the development of tumours of the liver and kidneys induced by several agents[10].

B. Other relevant data

No data were available on the genetic and related effects of ethinyloestradiol alone in humans. See, however, the summary of data for combined oral contraceptives (p. 297).

Ethinyloestradiol did not induce chromosomal aberrations in human lymphocytes, chromosomal aberrations or mutation in Chinese hamster cells or unscheduled DNA synthesis in rat hepatocytes *in vitro*. Studies on cell transformation were inconclusive. It was weakly active in an assay for inhibition of intercellular communication in Chinese hamster V79 cells. It did not induce sex-linked recessive lethal mutations in *Drosophila* or mutation in yeast and did not induce mutation or DNA damage in bacteria[11].

References

[1] *IARC Monographs, 21*, 233-255, 1979

[2] Schardein, J.L. (1980) Studies of the components of an oral contraceptive agent in albino rats. I. Estrogenic component. *J. Toxicol. environ. Health, 6*, 885-894

[3] Holtzman, S., Stone, J.P. & Shellabarger, C.J. (1981) Synergism of estrogens and X-rays in mammary carcinogenesis in female ACI rats. *J. natl Cancer Inst., 67*, 455-459

[4] Li, J.J., Li, S.A., Klicka, J.K., Parsons, J.A. & Lam, L.K.T. (1983) Relative carcinogenic activity of various synthetic and natural estrogens in the Syrian hamster kidney. *Cancer Res., 43*, 5200-5204

[5] Li, J.J. & Li, S.A. (1984) Estrogen-induced tumorigenesis in hamsters: roles for hormonal and carcinogenic activities. *Arch. Toxicol., 55*, 110-118

[6] Wanless, I.R. & Medline, A. (1982) Role of estrogens as promoters of hepatic neoplasia. *Lab. Invest., 46*, 313-320

[7] Yager, J.D., Campbell, H.A., Longnecker, D.S., Roebuck, B.D. & Benoit, M.C. (1984) Enhancement of hepatocarcinogenesis in female rats by ethinyl estradiol and mestranol but not estradiol. *Cancer Res., 44*, 3862-3869

[8] Yager, J.D., Roebuck, B.D., Paluszcyk, T.L. & Memoli, V.A. (1986) Effects of ethinyl estradiol and tamoxifen on liver DNA turnover and new synthesis and appearance of gamma glutamyl transpeptidase-positive foci in female rats. *Carcinogenesis, 12*, 2007-2014

[9] Shirai, T., Fukushima, S., Ikawa, E., Tagawa, Y. & Ito, N. (1986) Induction of prostate carcinoma *in situ* at high incidence in F344 rats by a combination of 3,2'-dimethyl-4-aminobiphenyl and ethinyl estradiol. *Cancer Res., 46*, 6423-6426

[10] Shirai, T., Tsuda, H., Ogiso, T., Hirose, M. & Ito, N. (1987) Organ specific modifying potential of ethinyl estradiol on carcinogenesis initiated with different carcinogens. *Carcinogenesis, 8*, 115-119

[11] *IARC Monographs, Suppl. 6*, 293-295, 1987

Mestranol

A. Evidence for carcinogenicity to animals (*sufficient*)

Mestranol was tested in mice, rats, dogs and monkeys by oral administration. It increased the incidence of pituitary tumours and malignant mammary tumours in mice[1,2] and increased the incidence of malignant mammary tumours in female rats. Studies in monkeys were still in progress; although no tumour had been observed after seven years, no conclusive evaluation could be made[1]. Feeding of mestranol to rats following partial hepatectomy and treatment with *N*-nitrosodiethylamine enhanced the development of foci of altered hepatocytes and of hepatocellular carcinomas[3,4]. No significant increase in mammary tumour occurrence was seen in dogs treated with mestranol[5,6].

B. Other relevant data

No data were available on the genetic and related effects of mestranol alone in humans. See, however, the summary of data for combined oral contraceptives (p. 297).

Mestranol did not induce DNA strand breaks in hepatocytes of rats or chromosomal aberrations in bone-marrow cells of mice treated *in vivo*. It did not induce chromosomal aberrations in human lymphocytes *in vitro*. It was weakly active in an assay for inhibition of intercellular communication in Chinese hamster V79 cells. It did not induce unscheduled DNA synthesis in cultured rat hepatocytes or sex-linked recessive lethal mutations in *Drosophila*. It was not mutagenic to bacteria[7].

References

[1]*IARC Monographs*, *21*, 257-278, 1979

[2]El Etreby, M.F. & Neumann, F. (1980) *Influence of sex steroids and steroid antagonists on hormone-dependent tumors in experimental animals.* In: Iacobelli, S., King, R.J.B., Lindner, H.R. & Lippman, M.E., eds, *Hormones and Cancer*, New York, Raven Press, pp. 321-336

[3]Yager, J.D., Jr & Yager, R. (1980) Oral contraceptive steroids as promoters of hepatocarcinogenesis in female Sprague-Dawley rats. *Cancer Res.*, *40*, 3680-3695

[4]Yager, J.D., Campbell, H.A., Longnecker, D.S., Roebuck, B.D. & Benoit, M.C. (1984) Enhancement of hepatocarcinogenesis in female rats by ethinylestradiol and mestranol but not estradiol. *Cancer Res.*, *44*, 3862-3869

[5]El Etreby, M.F. & Gräf, K.-J. (1979) Effect of contraceptive steroids on mammary gland of beagle dog and its relevance to human carcinogenicity. *Pharmacol. Ther.*, *5*, 369-402

[6]Kwapien, R.P., Giles, R.C., Geil, R.G. & Casey, H.W. (1980) Malignant mammary tumors in beagle dogs dosed with investigational oral contraceptive steroids. *J. natl Cancer Inst.*, *65*, 137-144

[7]*IARC Monographs*, *Suppl. 6*, 369-371, 1987

III. PROGESTINS (Group 2B)

Evidence for carcinogenicity to humans (*inadequate*)

Medroxyprogesterone acetate (Group 2B)

A. Evidence for carcinogenicity to humans (*inadequate*)

The results of one cross-sectional study of the development of breast nodules in women given medroxyprogesterone acetate was difficult to interpret because of methodological considerations[1]. Two small cohort studies in the USA showed relative risks (and 95% confidence limits) of breast cancer in women exposed to medroxyprogesterone acetate of 0.69 (0.3-1.4)[2] and 1.1 (0.5-2.4)[3], but both included only women with short-term exposure and limited duration of follow-up. A case-control study of 30 women with breast cancer and 179 controls[4] yielded a relative risk of 1.0 (no confidence limits given) for use of medroxy-progesterone acetate at some time. Preliminary analyses of a collaborative case-control study in Thailand, Kenya and Mexico sponsored by the World Health Organization[5], based on 427 cases (39 'ever' users) and 5951 controls (557 'ever' users), provided estimates of relative risk (and 95% confidence limits) for breast cancer of 1.0 (0.7-1.5) in women who 'ever' used medroxyprogesterone acetate, 1.1 (0.7-1.9) for users for 1-12 months, 1.2 (0.7-2.2) for users for 13-36 months and 0.8 (0.4-1.7) for users for $\geqslant$37 months.

Medroxyprogesterone acetate causes reversible changes in the endometrium, from proliferative to secretory or suppressed[4]. In one small cohort study, one case of uterine leiomyosarcoma was found, with 0.83 cancers of the uterine corpus expected, giving a relative risk of 1.2 [0.03-6.7][2]. In the collaborative study[5], the estimated relative risk for endometrial cancer in 'ever' users of medroxyprogesterone acetate was 0.3 (0.04-2.4), based on 57 cases, only one of which was exposed, and 316 matched controls (30 exposed).

In one small cohort study[2], one ovarian cancer case occurred in a medroxyprogesterone acetate user, with 1.16 expected, giving a relative risk of 0.86 [0.02-4.6]. Preliminary analysis of data from the collaborative study[5], based on 105 cases (seven exposed) and 637 matched controls (74 exposed) yielded a relative risk for ovarian cancer of 0.7 (0.3-1.7) in 'ever' users of medroxyprogesterone acetate.

The results of two cohort studies of dysplasia and of carcinoma *in situ* of the uterine cervix in women given medroxyprogesterone acetate were conflicting and difficult to interpret because of methodological problems[1]. Preliminary results from the collaborative study[5], based on 920 cases of invasive cervical carcinoma (126 exposed to medroxy-progesterone acetate) and 5833 controls (545 exposed) yielded estimated relative risks of 1.2 (0.9-1.5) in 'ever' users, after controlling for parity, history of vaginal discharge, age at first sexual relationship, number of sexual partners, number of prior Pap smears and use of an intrauterine device and oral contraceptives. Relative risks in users for 1-12, 13-24, 25-60 and $\geqslant$61 months were estimated to be 1.4 (1.0-2.0), 1.2 (0.7-2.0), 0.6 (0.4-1.1) and 1.4 (0.9-2.2), respectively.

Preliminary analyses of data from the collaborative study[5] showed the relative risk for primary liver cancer (all histological types combined) in women who had ever used medroxyprogesterone acetate to be 1.0 (0.4-2.8), based on 57 cases (seven exposed) and 290 controls (34 exposed).

B. Evidence for carcinogenicity to animals (*sufficient*)

Medroxyprogesterone acetate was tested by intramuscular injection in dogs and by subcutaneous implantation in mice. It induced adenocarcinomas of the mammary gland in one study in female mice[6], and produced malignant mammary tumours in dogs[1]. After four years of intramuscular treatment of dogs with a human contraceptive dose, a dose-related increase in the incidence of mammary nodules was seen; the incidence of mammary-gland nodules at that time was comparable with that seen in dogs given progesterone at 25 times the canine luteal level[7]. Female dogs treated with medroxyprogesterone acetate for at least one year had a significant increase in the incidence of large and small mammary nodules as compared with control animals in one study[8], and a dose-related increase in the incidence of large mammary nodules was found in another after intramuscular administration[9].

C. Other relevant data

No data were available on the genetic and related effects of medroxyprogesterone acetate alone in humans. See, however, the summary of data for combined oral contraceptives (p. 297). Medroxyprogesterone acetate induced sister chromatid exchanges in mouse cells *in vitro*[10].

References

[1]*IARC Monographs*, *21*, 417-429, 1979

[2]Liang, A.P., Levenson, A.G., Layde, P.M., Shelton, J.D., Hatcher, R.A., Potts, M. & Michelson, M.J. (1983) Risk of breast, uterine corpus, and ovarian cancer in women receiving medroxy-progesterone injections. *J. Am. med. Assoc.*, *249*, 2909-2912

[3]Danielson, D.A., Jick, H., Hunter, J.R., Stergachis, A. & Madsen, S. (1982) Nonestrogenic drugs and breast cancer. *Am. J. Epidemiol.*, *116*, 329-332

[4]Greenspan, A.R., Hatcher, R.A., Moore, A., Rosenberg, M.J. & Ory, H.W. (1980) The association of depo-medroxyprogesterone acetate and breast cancer. *Contraception*, *21*, 563-569

[5]Special Programme of Research, Development and Research Training in Human Reproduction (1986) Depot-medroxyprogesterone acetate (DMPA) and cancer. Memorandum from a WHO meeting. *WHO Bull.*, *64*, 375-382

[6]Lanari, C., Molinolo, A.A. & Pasqualini, C.D. (1986) Induction of mammary adenocarcinomas by medroxyprogesterone acetate in BALB/c female mice. *Cancer Lett.*, *33*, 215-223

[7]Frank, D.W., Kirton, K.T., Murchison, T.E., Quinlan, W.J., Coleman, M.E., Gilbertson, T.J., Feenstra, E.S. & Kimball, F.A. (1979) Mammary tumors and serum hormones in the bitch treated with medroxyprogesterone acetate or progesterone for four years. *Fertil. Steril.*, *31*, 340-346

[8]van Os, J.L., van Laar, P.H., Oldenkamp, E.P. & Verschoor, J.S.C. (1981) Oestrus control and the incidence of mammary nodules in bitches, a clinical study with two progestogens. *Vet. Q.*, *3*, 46-56

[9]Concannon, P.W., Spraker, T.R., Casey, H.W. & Hansel, W. (1981) Gross and histopathologic effects of medroxyprogesterone acetate and progesterone on the mammary glands of adult beagle bitches. *Fertil. Steril.*, *36*, 373-387

[10]*IARC Monographs, Suppl. 6*, 359-360, 1987

Chlormadinone acetate

A. Evidence for carcinogenicity to animals (*limited*)

Chlormadinone acetate was tested in mice, rats and dogs by oral administration. In dogs, it produced mammary tumours in one study[1] and increased the incidence of mammary-gland hyperplasia and mammary nodules in another[2].

B. Other relevant data

No data were available on the genetic and related effects of chlormadinone acetate alone in humans. See, however, the summary of data for combined oral contraceptives (p. 297). Chlormadinone acetate did not induce chromosomal aberrations in cultured human lymphocytes and was not mutagenic to bacteria[3].

References

[1]*IARC Monographs*, *21*, 365-375, 1979

[2]El Etreby, M.F. & Gräf, K.-J. (1979) Effect of contraceptive steroids on mammary gland of beagle dog and its relevance to human carcinogenicity. *Pharmacol. Ther.*, *5*, 369-402

[3]*IARC Monographs, Suppl. 6*, 148-149, 1987

Dimethisterone

A. Evidence for carcinogenicity to animals (*inadequate*)

Dimethisterone was reported to have been tested in monkeys in one study. No increase in tumour incidence was found[1].

B. Other relevant data

No data were available on the genetic and related effects of dimethisterone in humans. It did not induce chromosomal aberrations in cultured human lymphocytes[2].

References

[1]Weikel, J.H., Jr & Nelson, L.W. (1977) Problems in evaluating chronic toxicity of contraceptive steroids in dogs. *J. Toxicol. environ. Health, 3*, 167-177

[2]*IARC Monographs, Suppl. 6*, 260-261, 1987

Ethynodiol diacetate

A. Evidence for carcinogenicity to animals (*limited*)

Ethynodiol diacetate was tested in mice and rats by oral administration. It increased the incidence of benign liver tumours in male mice and of mammary tumours in castrated male mice, and produced benign mammary tumours in male rats[1].

B. Other relevant data

No data were available on the genetic and related effects of ethynodiol diacetate alone in humans. See, however, the summary of data for combined oral contraceptives (p. 297). Ethynodiol diacetate did not induce sex-linked recessive lethal mutations in *Drosophila*[2].

References

[1]*IARC Monographs, 21*, 387-398, 1979

[2]*IARC Monographs, Suppl. 6*, 308-309, 1987

17α-Hydroxyprogesterone caproate

A. Evidence for carcinogenicity to animals (*inadequate*)

17α-Hydroxyprogesterone caproate was tested in rabbits by repeated intramuscular injection, giving inconclusive results[1]. It was reported to have accelerated the growth of a transplantable cervical tumour line in mice[2].

B. Other relevant data

No data were available to the Working Group.

References

[1]*IARC Monographs, 21*, 399-406, 1979

[2]Umancheeva, A.F., Novikova, A.I. & Anisomov, V.N. (1981) Stimulating effect of pregnancy on the growth of cervical cancer (Russ.). *Akush. Ginekol., 1*, 53-55

Lynoestrenol

A. Evidence for carcinogenicity to animals (*inadequate*)

Lynoestrenol was tested by oral administration in mice and rats. It induced a slight increase in the incidence of benign liver-cell tumours in male mice and of malignant mammary tumours in female mice. In female rats, a slight but nonsignificant increase in the incidence of malignant mammary tumours was observed after administration of lynoestrenol[1].

B. Other relevant data

No data were available to the Working Group.

References

[1]*IARC Monographs*, *21*, 407–415, 1979

Megestrol acetate

A. Evidence for carcinogenicity to animals (*limited*)

Megestrol acetate was tested by oral administration in mice, rats, dogs and monkeys. It produced nodular hyperplasia, and benign and malignant mammary tumours in dogs[1]. No tumour was reported in monkeys[2].

B. Other relevant data

No data were available on the genetic and related effects of megestrol acetate alone in humans. See, however, the summary of data for combined oral contraceptives (p. 297). Megestrol acetate did not induce chromosomal aberrations in cultured human lymphocytes[3].

References

[1]*IARC Monographs*, *21*, 431–439, 1979

[2]Weikel, J.H., Jr & Nelson, L.W. (1977) Problems in evaluating chronic toxicity of contraceptive steroids in dogs. *J. Toxicol. environ. Health*, *3*, 361–362, 1987

[3]*IARC Monographs*, *Suppl. 6*, 361–362, 1987

Norethisterone

A. Evidence for carcinogenicity to animals (*sufficient*)

Norethisterone and its acetate were tested by oral administration in mice and rats, and by subcutaneous implantation in mice. In mice, norethisterone and its acetate increased the incidence of benign liver-cell tumours in males; norethisterone increased the incidence of pituitary tumours in females and produced granulosa-cell tumours in the ovaries of females. Norethisterone increased the incidence of benign liver-cell tumours and benign and malignant mammary tumours in male rats[1]. Rats fed 3-4 mg/kg bw per day norethisterone acetate (about 100 times the daily human dose) for two years had an increased incidence of neoplastic nodules of the liver; an increase in the incidence of uterine polyps was seen in females[2]. In rats given weekly intramuscular injections for 104 weeks of norethisterone enanthate at doses of 10, 30 and 100 mg/kg bw (20, 60 and 200 times the daily human contraceptive dose), there was a dose-related increase in pituitary-gland tumours in males, whereas in females no effect on pituitary glands was observed with the lowest dose and a reduction in pituitary tumours was observed with the highest dose. Benign mammary tumours were observed in males at all doses, but there was little effect in females; the incidence of malignant mammary tumours was greatly increased in both males and females given the two higher dose levels and was dose-related. A dose-related increase in the incidence of liver tumours was also seen in animals of each sex[3].

B. Other relevant data

No data were available on the genetic and related effects of norethisterone alone in humans. See, however, the summary of data for combined oral contraceptives (p. 297).

Aneuploidy was observed in oocytes of mice treated with high doses of norethisterone acetate. In a test for dominant lethal mutations in which female mice were exposed orally to norethisterone acetate, no increase was seen in one strain of mice, and a second strain showed an increase only when females were mated within two weeks after treatment. The compound did not induce aneuploidy or chromosomal aberrations in cultured human lymphocytes. Neither norethisterone nor its acetate was mutagenic to bacteria[4].

References

[1]*IARC Monographs*, *21*, 441-460, 1979

[2]Schardein, J.L. (1980) Studies on the components of an oral contraceptive agent in albino rats. II. Progestogenic component and comparison of effects of the components and the combined agent. *J. Toxicol. environ. Health*, *6*, 895-906

[3]El Etreby, M.F. & Neumann, F. (1980) *Influence of sex steroids and steroid antagonists on hormone-dependent tumors in experimental animals.* In: Iacobelli, S., King, R.J.B., Lindner, H.R. & Lippman, M.E., eds, *Hormones and Cancer*, New York, Raven Press, pp. 321-336

[4]*IARC Monographs*, *Suppl. 6*, 427-429, 1987

Norethynodrel

A. Evidence for carcinogenicity to animals (*limited*)

Norethynodrel was tested by oral administration in mice and rats and by subcutaneous implantation in mice. It increased the incidence of pituitary tumours in mice of each sex and that of mammary tumours in castrated males of one strain. It also increased the incidence of benign and malignant liver-cell, pituitary and mammary (benign and malignant) tumours in male rats[1]. Feeding of norethynodrel to rats following partial hepatectomy and treatment with *N*-nitrosodiethylamine increased the number of γ-glutamyl transpeptidase-positive hepatic foci at four months, but there was no significant difference by nine months[2].

B. Other relevant data

No data were available on the genetic and related effects of norethynodrel alone in humans. See, however, the summary of data for combined oral contraceptives (p. 297). Norethynodrel did not induce aneuploidy in human cells in culture or unscheduled DNA synthesis in rat hepatocytes *in vitro*. It inhibited intercellular communication in Chinese hamster V79 cells. The compound was not mutagenic to bacteria[3].

References

[1]*IARC Monographs*, *21*, 461-477, 1979

[2]Yager, J.D., Jr & Yager, R. (1980) Oral contraceptive steroids as promoters of hepatocarcinogenesis in female Sprague-Dawley rats. *Cancer Res.*, *40*, 3680-3685

[3]*IARC Monographs*, *Suppl. 6*, 430-431, 1987

Norgestrel

A. Evidence for carcinogenicity to animals (*inadequate*)

Norgestrel was tested by oral administration in mice and rats. No increase in the incidence of tumours was observed in either species[1].

B. Other relevant data

No data were available on the genetic and related effects of norgestrel alone in humans. See, however, the summary of data for combined oral contraceptives (p. 297). Norgestrel gave inconclusive results in tests for sex-linked recessive lethal mutations in *Drosophila*. It was not mutagenic to bacteria[2].

References

[1]*IARC Monographs*, *21*, 479-490, 1979

[2]*IARC Monographs*, *Suppl. 6*, 432-433, 1987

Progesterone

A. Evidence for carcinogenicity to animals (*sufficient*)

Progesterone was tested by subcutaneous and by intramuscular injection in mice, rabbits and dogs, and by subcutaneous implantation in mice. It increased the incidences of ovarian, uterine and mammary tumours in mice. Neonatal treatment with progesterone enhanced the occurrence of precancerous and cancerous lesions of the genital tract and increased mammary tumorigenesis in female mice[1]. Dogs treated with progesterone for four years at one to 25 times the luteal-phase levels for that species developed a dose-related incidence of mammary-gland nodules[2].

B. Other relevant data

No data were available on the genetic and related effects of progesterone in humans.

Progesterone did not induce dominant lethal mutations in mice or chromosomal aberrations in rats treated *in vivo*. It did not induce chromosomal aberrations or sister chromatid exchanges in cultured human cells, nor chromosomal aberrations or DNA strand breaks in rodent cells. Studies on transformation of rodent cells *in vitro* were inconclusive: a clearly positive result was obtained for rat embryo cells, a weakly positive result for mouse cells and a negative result for Syrian hamster embryo cells. Progesterone was not mutagenic to bacteria[3].

References

[1]*IARC Monographs*, *21*, 491-515, 1979

[2]Frank, D.W., Kirton, K.T., Murchison, T.E., Quinlan, W.J., Coleman, M.E., Gilbertson, T.J., Feenstra, E.S. & Kimball, F.A. (1979) Mammary tumors and serum hormones in the bitch treated with medroxyprogesterone acetate or progesterone for four years. *Fertil. Steril.*, *31*, 340-346

[3]*IARC Monographs*, *Suppl. 6*, 479-481, 1987

IV. OESTROGEN-PROGESTIN COMBINATIONS

SEQUENTIAL ORAL CONTRACEPTIVES (Group 1)

A. Evidence for carcinogenicity to humans (*sufficient*)

Case reports of endometrial cancer occurring at an unusually young age in users of sequential oral contraceptives provide evidence that these preparations can cause endometrial cancer[1]. Three case-control studies have provided the following estimates of the relative risk (and 95% confidence intervals) for endometrial cancer in women who had used sequential oral contraceptives: 2.2 (0.6-7.3)[2], 2.1 (0.8-5.8)[3] and [1.9 (0.7-5.3)][4]. One study[2] showed a relative risk of 7.3 (1.4-38.8) in users of a preparation that contained a relatively large amount of a potent oestrogen (0.1 mg ethinyloestradiol) and only a weak progestin (25 mg dimethisterone); another[4] showed a relative risk of 4.6 in users of more than two years' duration. The finding of an increased risk for endometrial cancer in relation to sequential oral contraceptives is in contrast with a reduction in risk for endometrial cancer found in association with the use of combined oral contraceptives (see below).

B. Evidence for carcinogenicity to animals (*inadequate* for dimethisterone in combination with ethinyloestradiol)

Dimethisterone and oestrogen

When dimethisterone and ethinyloestradiol were given sequentially to female dogs by oral administration, a few palpable mammary nodules were reported to have occurred in treated (4/16) and in untreated animals (2/16)[5].

C. Other relevant data

No adequate data were available on the genetic and related effects of sequential oral contraceptives in humans. See, however, the summaries of data on individual compounds commonly found in sequential oral contraceptives: chlormadinone acetate (p. 291), dimethisterone (p. 291), ethinyloestradiol (p. 286) and mestranol (p. 288).

References

[1] *IARC Monographs, 21*, 111-112, 133, 1979

[2] Weiss, N.S. & Sayvetz, T.A. (1980) Incidence of endometrial cancer in relation to the use of oral contraceptives. *New Engl. J. Med., 302*, 551-554

[3] Centers for Disease Control Cancer and Steroid Hormone Study (1983) Oral contraceptive use and the risk of endometrial cancer. *J. Am. med. Assoc., 249*, 1600-1604

[4] Henderson, B.E., Casagrande, J.T., Pike, M.C., Mack, T., Rosario, I. & Duke, A. (1983) The epidemiology of endometrial cancer in young women. *Br. J. Cancer, 47*, 749-756

[5] *IARC Monographs, 21*, 233-255, 377-385, 1979

COMBINED ORAL CONTRACEPTIVES (Group 1)

A. Evidence for carcinogenicity to humans (*sufficient*)

There is sufficient evidence that combined oral contraceptives cause benign and malignant liver tumours. There is also conclusive evidence that these agents protect against cancers of the ovary and endometrium.

Liver cancer

Numerous case reports and series of hepatic-cell adenomas occurring almost exclusively in women who had used combined oral contraceptives strongly suggest that such benign tumours may result from exposure to these products[1]. Two case-control studies[1] have shown that risk of hepatic-cell adenomas increases strongly with duration of use and have provided estimates of the relative risk in users for more than seven and nine years duration of 500[2] and 25[3], respectively. The many reports of focal nodular hyperplasia occurring in users of oral contraceptives could also represent a causal relationship, but these lesions also occur in men and older women, and no case-control study on these populations has been conducted.

Reports of hepatocellular carcinomas occurring in conjunction with liver-cell adenomas in users of oral contraceptives have been published[1]. In addition, three case-control studies of hepatocellular carcinomas, one in the USA[4] and two in the UK[5,6], have shown strong trends of increasing risk with duration of use. Relative risks (95% confidence limits) in the three studies in users of more than five, eight and eight years' duration, respectively, were estimated to be [13.5 (1.2-152.2)][4], 7.2 (2.0-25.7)[5] and 20.1 (2.3-175.7)[4], respectively. When data for all three studies are combined, relative risks of 2.5 (1.1-5.5) and 10.0 (3.7-27.2) in 'ever' users and users for more than five to eight years (depending on the study) were derived by the Working Group. Although all three case-control studies of liver cancers and oral contraceptives are small and have methodological deficiencies that could have resulted in biased results, the magnitude of the relative risks and the consistency of the results provide strong evidence that the results are not spurious. Case reports of cholangiocarcinoma in users of oral contraceptives have also been published, but one case-control study of 11 cases[6] showed no association with use of oral contraceptives [(relative risk, 0.3 in women who ever used oral contraceptives; 0.9 in users of four or more years)].

Ovarian cancer

Ten case-control studies have provided the following estimates of the relative risk (95% confidence limits) for ovarian cancer in women who had ever used combined oral contraceptives: 0.6 [0.3-1.1][7], [0.7 (0.4-1.1)][8], 0.8 (0.4-1.5)[9], 0.5 (0.2-1.5)[10], 0.6 [0.4-1.0][11], 0.7 (0.4-1.1)[12], 0.4 (0.2-1.0)[13], 0.6 (0.4-0.9)[14], 0.6 (0.4-0.9)[15] and 0.6 (0.4-1.0)[16]. Six of these studies assessed risk in relation to duration of use, and five provide at least some evidence that the risk declines with years of exposure, although this trend is less striking than that for endometrial cancer (see below). Relative risks in women who had used combined oral contraceptives for up to or more than five, five, seven and nine years were found in four different studies to be 0.3 (0.1-0.8)[14], 0.4 (0.2-0.6)[15], 0.6 [0.3-1.4][8] and 0.4 (0.2-1.3)[11].

Endometrial cancer

Five case-control studies have provided the following estimates of the relative risk (95% confidence limits) for endometrial cancer in women who had ever used combined oral contraceptives: 0.5 (0.1-1.0)[17], 0.4 (0.2-0.8)[18], 0.4 [0.2-1.2][19], 0.5 (0.3-0.8)[20] and 0.6 (0.2-1.3)[16]. Three of these[18-20], and two others[21,22], assessed risk in relation to duration of use, and all showed a decline in risk with duration of exposure. Relative risks in users of five or more years' duration were estimated in two studies to be 0.3 (0.1-1.3)[19] and 0.6 (0.4-0.9)[20], and one study showed a relative risk of 0.1[22] in women with six or more years of use.

Cervical cancer

Four case-control studies[23-26] of cervical squamous dysplasia provide estimates of relative risk in women who had ever used combined oral contraceptives ranging from 1.2 to 3, and the lower limit of the 95% confidence limits of two of the estimates was greater than 1.0. Relative risks (95% confidence limits) from three cohort studies were [5.0 (1.2-20.8)][1], 1.5 [(0.8-2.6)][27] and 1.1 [(0.8-1.7)][28]. Relative risks for squamous dysplasia were found to increase with duration of use in two[24,26] of three case-control studies in which risk in relation to length of exposure was considered, and those for women who had used oral contraceptives for more than four years were found in two cohort studies to be [4.9 (1.1-21.8)[1]] and 2.0 [(1.1-3.6)][27].

Four case-control studies of cervical carcinoma *in situ*[1,23-25] provide estimates of relative risk in women who had ever used combined oral contraceptives ranging from 0.6 to 1.1[25], with 95% confidence limits that include 1.0; but one additional such study yielded an estimated relative risk of [1.6 (1.2-2.0)][1], and estimates from three cohort studies were [3.7 (1.5-9.0)][1], 1.6 [(0.8-3.0)][27] and 1.2 (0.8-1.7)[28]. One case-control study showed a strong increase in risk for carcinoma *in situ* with duration of use[24], but two others did not[1,25]. Relative risks in users of more than four years' duration were estimated in two cohort studies to be [5.4 (2.1-13.7)][1] and 1.7 [(0.9-3.2)][27]. Another cohort study[1] showed the risk of progression from dysplasia to carcinoma *in situ* to be six times greater in users than in nonusers of oral contraceptives.

Three case-control studies of invasive cervical cancer yielded relative risks in women who had ever used combined oral contraceptives of 1.2 (1.0-1.4)[29], 1.5 (1.1-2.1)[30] and 1.7 (0.8-3.6)[16]; and three cohort studies gave incidence rates of invasive cervical cancer per 1000 women years in users and nonusers of oral contraceptives of 0.20 and 0[27], 0.15 and 0.07[31] and 0.12 and 0[28]. All three case-control studies also showed that risk increased with duration of use; and the two in which relative risks were assessed in women who had used oral contraceptives for more than five years gave values of 1.5 (1.1-2.1)[29] and [1.9 (1.3-2.7)][30].

There is evidence that one or more sexually transmitted, infective agents play an important role in the development of cervical cancer. Since this agent(s) has not been unequivocally identified, and, in particular, was not considered in the studies under review, surrogate measures were used to reflect degree of sexual activity and to adjust for this. Any observed effect of oral contraceptives on risk of cervical cancer may therefore be confounded by an association of oral contraceptive use with exposure to the putative infective agent. Since the specific factor by which the analysis should be adjusted is not known, the Working Group considered that adjusting for age at first intercourse and number of sexual partners may not be sufficient to remove the confounding and, therefore, that they could not regard a causal association of oral contraceptives and cervical cancer as proven.

Breast cancer

Relative risks for breast cancer in women who had ever used combined oral contraceptives have been assessed in 18 case-control studies[1,16,32-43] and in seven cohort studies[1,44-47]. All provide point estimates of relative risk close to unity, with 95% confidence intervals that include 1.0. Six case-control studies have provided estimates of the relative risk in women who had used combined oral contraceptives for more than a decade: four[36,39,40,43] yield relative risks between 0.7 and 1.1 with 95% confidence limits that included 1.0 in users of ten or more years' duration; another[48] provides a relative risk estimate of 2.2 (1.2-4.0) in users of 12 or more years' duration; and one[42] gives a relative risk of 0.6 (0.4-0.9) in women who had used oral contraceptives for 15 or more years. Eight case-control studies[16,36-38,40,42,43,48] and two cohort studies[44,45] give estimated relative risks for breast cancer ten or more to 20 or more years after initial exposure to combined oral contraceptives, and all are close to 1.0, with 95% confidence intervals that include unity. Eleven case-control studies have assessed risk for breast cancer among women who had used combined oral contraceptives before their first full-term pregnancy. The results are inconsistent, six studies[39,40,43,47,49,50] showing no significant elevation in risk, three[34,37,51] showing a significant trend of increasing risk with duration of use, and two[48,52] showing an increased risk without a significant trend. The reasons for these discrepant findings have not been identified. Five case-control studies have assessed risk in women who had used combined oral contraceptives before 25 years of age. The initial study of this issue showed a strong trend of increasing risk with years of use before age 25[53]. A subsequent study from Sweden[54] showed a relative risk of 3.3 in women who had ever used oral contraceptives at age 20-24, but ascertainment of prior use was not comparable for cases and controls, rendering this finding suspect. Another study from Norway and Sweden[48] gave a relative risk of 2.7 in women who had used oral contraceptives for eight or more years before the age of 25, but the confidence limits for this included 1.0 (0.7-11.0), and no consistent trend of increasing risk with duration of use was observed. The fourth study, from New Zealand[43], showed a nonsignificant ($p = 0.4$) trend of declining risk with duration of use before age 25 and estimated the relative risk in users of six or more years to be 0.6. The fifth study[50] gave relative risks of 1.0 to 1.3 in six categories of duration of use (<12, 13-48 and >48 months in women less than 20 and in women 20-24 years of age) but no trend of increasing risk with duration of use. Risk was also initially reported to be particularly enhanced by use before age 25[53] of oral contraceptives with a high progestogen potency, but the authors' classification has been disputed; and results from a large collaborative study in the USA do not confirm their findings[50].

Other tumours

The relative risk for malignant melanoma in women who had ever taken oral contraceptives has been estimated in eight case-control[1,55-61] and three cohort[55,62,63] studies. Values from all the case-control studies were close to unity, with 95% confidence limits that included 1.0. Values from the three cohort studies were 0.3 [0.1-0.8][55], 1.5 (0.7-2.9)[62] and 3.5 (1.4-9.0)[63]. The reasons for these widely discrepant results are unknown. Trends of increasing risk with duration of use have been observed in some investigations but not in others. The two case-control studies in which analyses were performed to estimate the relative risk in users of more than two[56] and five[59] years' duration, ten or more years after initial exposure, showed elevated risks of 2.3 (0.8-6.9) and 1.5 (1.0-2.1), respectively. Two case-control studies showed trends of increasing risk specifically for superficial spreading melanoma with increasing duration of use[57,60], although a third did not[63]. Also, two studies have shown relative risks for superficial spreading-type melanoma to be increased in users of five or more years' duration after latent periods of over ten[59] and 12[57] years: [1.6 (1.0-2.6)] and 4.4 (2.0-9.7), respectively.

Two case-control studies and two prospective studies have shown no increase in risk for pituitary adenomas[1,64,65].

Women who took oral contraceptives after evacuation of a hydatidiform mole were reported in one study[1] subsequently to have developed trophoblastic tumours more frequently than women who had used other methods of contraception after a molar evacuation, but this was not confirmed in another investigation[66].

A single case-control study showed a reduction in risk for carcinomas of the colon and rectum with duration of use of combined oral contraceptives[67], but two cohort studies showed no alteration in risk for these neoplasms in users[63,68].

A protective effect of combined oral contraceptives against both fibroadenoma and fibrocystic disease of the breast has been found in many investigations[1,63,69-72], although a single recent study found an increase in risk for the latter condition in postmenopausal women[73]. One study showed no protective effect of oral contraceptives against fibrocystic disease with atypical histological features[1], but one subsequent investigation did[70].

A reduction in risk for retention cysts of the ovary has been documented in two cohort studies and in one case-control study[1]. A reduction in risk for uterine leiomyoma has been documented in one case-control study[74].

B. Evidence for carcinogenicity to animals (*sufficient* for norethynodrel in combination with mestranol; *limited* for chlormadinone acetate in combination with mestranol or ethinyloestradiol, for ethynodiol acetate in combination with mestranol or ethinyl-oestradiol, for megestrol acetate in combination with ethinyloestradiol, for norethisterone in combination with mestranol or ethinyloestradiol, for progesterone in combination with oestradiol-17β, and for investigational contraceptives; *inadequate* for lynoestrenol in combination with mestranol and for norgestrel in combination with ethinyloestradiol)

Chlormadinone acetate and oestrogens

Chlormadinone acetate, in combination with mestranol, was tested for carcinogenicity by oral administration to mice; an increased incidence of pituitary tumours was observed in animals of each sex. Oral administration of chlormadinone acetate in combination with ethinyloestradiol to mice resulted in an increased incidence of mammary tumours in intact and castrated males[75].

Ethynodiol diacetate and oestrogens

Following oral administration of ethynodiol diacetate plus mestranol to mice, increased incidences of pituitary tumours were observed in animals of each sex. Ethynodiol diacetate plus ethinyloestradiol was tested for carcinogenicity by oral administration to mice and rats.

In mice, it induced increased incidences of pituitary tumours in animals of each sex and of malignant tumours of connective tissues of the uterus. In rats, malignant mammary tumours were produced in animals of each sex[76].

Lynoestrenol and oestrogens

Lynoestrenol, in combination with mestranol, was tested in mice and female rats by oral administration. A slight, nonsignificant increase in the incidence of malignant mammary tumours was observed in female mice[77].

Megestrol acetate and oestrogens

Megestrol acetate plus ethinyloestradiol was tested for carcinogenicity by oral administration to mice and rats. In mice, increased incidences of malignant mammary tumours were observed in animals of each sex. No increase in tumour incidence was observed in rats[78].

Norethisterone and oestrogens

Norethisterone acetate plus ethinyloestradiol was tested for carcinogenicity by oral administration to mice, rats and monkeys. In mice, pituitary tumours were observed in animals of each sex. In rats, increased incidences of benign mammary tumours were found in males in one study and of benign liver-cell and mammary tumours in animals of each sex in the other[79]. Norethisterone acetate plus ethinyloestradiol administered orally to rats induced endometrial carcinomas[80]. Oral administration of norethisterone acetate plus ethinyloestradiol to female rats for 12 months resulted in hyperplastic nodules of the liver in all animals and a hepatocellular carcinoma in one (preliminary results)[81]. Norethisterone acetate and ethinyloestradiol given orally to monkeys for ten years did not produce malignant tumours[82].

Norethisterone plus mestranol was tested for carcinogenicity in mice and rats by oral administration. In mice, pituitary tumours developed in animals of each sex. In rats, an increased incidence of malignant mammary tumours was found in females. Norethisterone plus ethinyloestradiol, tested in mice by oral administration, induced an increased incidence of pituitary tumours in females[79].

Norethynodrel and oestrogens

Norethynodrel in combination with mestranol was tested for carcinogenicity in mice, rats, hamsters and monkeys orally and by subcutaneous implantation. Increased incidences of pituitary, mammary, vaginal and cervical tumours were found in female mice and of pituitary tumours in male mice. In castrated male mice, the combined treatment resulted in an increase in the incidence of mammary tumours. In rats, benign liver-cell tumours were observed in males and pituitary tumours and malignant mammary tumours in animals of each sex. A study of hamsters was of too short a duration to be considered for evaluation.

The combined treatment given to *Macaca mulatta* monkeys for five years did not increase the incidence of mammary tumours[83].

Norgestrel and oestrogens

Norgestrel plus ethinyloestradiol was tested for carcinogenicity in mice and rats by oral administration. No increase in the incidence of tumours was observed in either species[84].

Progesterone and oestrogen

Neonatal exposure of mice to progesterone plus oestradiol-17β resulted in an increased incidence of mammary tumours[85].

Investigational oral contraceptives

Three investigational oral contraceptives (ethynerone, chloroethynyl norgestrel or anagestone acetate plus mestranol) were tested for carcinogenicity by oral administration to dogs. An increased incidence of malignant mammary tumours was observed after treatment with chloroethynyl norgestrel plus mestranol or with anagestone acetate plus mestranol; no difference in the total number of mammary-gland nodules was observed with these two contraceptives. One dog given ethynerone plus mestranol had 14 malignant mammary fibrosarcomas[86].

C. Other relevant data

The results reported in the available studies relate to a variety of different oral contraceptives.

Several studies showed no increase in the incidence of structural chromosomal changes in lymphocytes taken from women after oral contraceptive use (norethisterone with mestranol or ethynodiol diacetate with mestranol). In contrast to an earlier report, no increase in the incidence of sister chromatid exchanges was observed in 52 women taking oral contraceptives as compared with 63 controls when results were adjusted for smoking[87].

No significant difference in the frequency of abnormal karyotypes or in sex ratio was seen in a study of spontaneous abortuses of women who had taken oral contraceptives; the contraceptives used were norgestrel, norethisterone acetate or medroxyprogesterone acetate in combination with ethinyloestradiol; or ethynodiol diacetate, megestrol acetate or lynoestrenol in combination with mestranol. Similarly, a large cohort study showed no increase in risk for chromosomal anomalies in live births and abortuses of oral contraceptive users[87].

High doses of one oral contraceptive (lynoestrenol and mestranol) administered to two strains of female mice induced dominant lethal mutations, whereas high doses of another (norethisterone and ethinyloestradiol) did not. In a later report using even higher doses of the oral contraceptive that induced dominant lethal mutations and another (norethisterone acetate and ethinyloestradiol), the same authors reported no increase in the incidence of dominant lethal, recessive lethal or visible mutations in mice. Combinations of progestins (norethynodrel and ethynodiol diacetate) and oestrogens (mestranol and ethinyloestradiol) did not induce sex-linked recessive lethal mutations in *Drosophila*[87].

References

[1]*IARC Monographs*, *21*, 103-129, 133-134, 1979

[2]Rooks, J.B., Ory, H.W., Ishak, K.G., Strauss, L.T., Greenspan, J.R. & Tyler, C.W., Jr (1977) The association between oral contraception and hepatocellular adenoma — a preliminary report. *Int. J. Gynaecol. Obstet.*, *15*, 143-144

[3]Edmondson, H.A., Henderson, B. & Benton, B. (1976) Liver-cell adenomas associated with use of oral contraceptives. *New Engl. J. Med.*, *294*, 470-472

[4]Henderson, B.E., Preston-Martin, S., Edmondson, H.A., Peters, R.L. & Pike, M.C. (1983) Hepatocellular carcinoma and oral contraceptives. *Br. J. Cancer*, *48*, 437-440

[5]Neuberger, J., Forman, D., Doll, R. & Williams, R. (1986) Oral contraceptives and hepatocellular carcinoma. *Br. med. J.*, *292*, 1355-1357

[6]Forman, D., Vincent, T.J. & Doll, R. (1986) Cancer of the liver and the use of oral contraceptives. *Br. med. J.*, *292*, 1357-1361

[7]Newhouse, M.L., Pearson, R.M., Fullerton, J.M., Boesen, E.A.M. & Shannon, H.S. (1977) A case control study of carcinoma of the ovary. *Br. J. prev. soc. Med.*, *31*, 148-153

[8]Casagrande, J.T., Pike, M.C., Ross, R.K., Louie, E.W., Roy, S. & Henderson, B.E. (1979) 'Incessant ovulation' and ovarian cancer. *Lancet*, *ii*, 170-173

[9]Willett, W.C., Bain, C., Hennekens, C.H., Rosner, B. & Speizer, F.E. (1981) Oral contraceptives and risk of ovarian cancer. *Cancer*, *48*, 1684-1687

[10]Hildreth, N.G., Kelsey, J.L., LiVolsi, V.A., Fischer, D.B., Holford, T.R., Mostow, E.D., Schwartz, P.E. & White, C. (1981) An epidemiologic study of epithelial carcinoma of the ovary. *Am. J. Epidemiol.*, *114*, 398-405

[11]Weiss, N.S., Lyon, J.L., Liff, J.M., Vollmer, W.M. & Daling, J.R. (1981) Incidence of ovarian cancer in relation to the use of oral contraceptives. *Int. J. Cancer*, *28*, 669-671

[12]Franceschi, S., La Vecchia, C., Helmrich, S.P., Mangioni, C. & Tognoni, G. (1982) Risk factors for epithelial ovarian cancer in Italy. *Am. J. Epidemiol.*, *115*, 714-719

[13]Cramer, D.W., Hutchison, G.B., Welch, W.R., Scully, R.E. & Knapp, R.C. (1982) Factors affecting the association of oral contraceptives and ovarian cancer. *New Engl. J. Med.*, *307*, 1047-1051

[14]Rosenberg, L., Shapiro, S., Slone, D., Kaufman, D.W., Helmrich, S.P., Miettinen, O.S., Stolley, P.D., Rosenshein, N.B., Schottenfeld, D. & Engle, R.L., Jr (1982) Epithelial ovarian cancer and combination oral contraceptives. *J. Am. med. Assoc.*, *247*, 3210-3212

[15]Centers for Disease Control Cancer and Steroid Hormone Study (1983) Oral contraceptive use and the risk of ovarian cancer. *J. Am. med. Assoc.*, *249*, 1596-1599

[16]La Vecchia, C., Decarli, A., Fasoli, M., Franceschi, S., Gentile, A., Negri, E., Parazzini, F. & Tognoni, G. (1986) Oral contraceptives and cancers of the breast and of the female genital tract. Interim results from a case-control study. *Br. J. Cancer*, *54*, 311-317

[17]Weiss, N.S. & Sayvetz, T.A. (1980) Incidence of endometrial cancer in relation to the use of oral contraceptives. *New Engl. J. Med.*, *302*, 551-554

[18]Kaufman, D.W., Shapiro, S., Slone, D., Rosenberg, L., Miettinen, O.S., Stolley, P.D., Knapp, R.C., Leavitt, T., Jr, Watring, W.G., Rosenshein, N.B., Lewis, J.L., Jr, Schottenfeld, D. & Engle, R.L., Jr (1980) Decreased risk of endometrial cancer among oral-contraceptive users. *New Engl. J. Med.*, *303*, 1045-1047

[19]Hulka, B.S., Chambless, L.E., Kaufman, D.G., Fowler, W.C., Jr & Greenberg, B.G. (1982) Protection against endometrial carcinoma by combination-product oral contraceptives. *J. Am. med. Assoc.*, *247*, 475-477

[20]Centers for Disease Control Cancer and Steroid Hormone Study (1983) Oral contraceptive use and the risk of endometrial cancer. *J. Am. med. Assoc.*, *249*, 1600-1604

[21]Kelsey, J.L., LiVolsi, V.A., Holford, T.R., Fischer, D.B., Mostow, E.D., Schwartz, P.E., O'Connor, T. & White, C. (1982) A case-control study of cancer of the endometrium. *Am. J. Epidemiol.*, *116*, 333-342

[22]Henderson, B.E., Casagrande, J.T., Pike, M.C., Mack, T., Rosario, I. & Duke, A. (1983) The epidemiology of endometrial cancer in young women. *Br. J. Cancer*, *47*, 749-756

[23]Thomas, D.B. (1972) Relationship of oral contraceptives to cervical carcinogenesis. *Obstet. Gynecol.*, *40*, 508-518

[24]Ory, H.W., Conger, S.B., Naib, Z., Tyler, C.W., Jr & Hatcher, R.A. (1977) *Preliminary analysis of oral contraceptive use and risk for developing premalignant lesions of the uterine cervix.* In: Garattini, S. & Berendes, H.W., eds, *Pharmacology of Steroid Contraceptive Drugs*, New York, Raven Press, pp. 211-218

[25]Fasal, E., Simmons, M.E. & Kampert, J.B. (1981) Factors associated with high and low risk of cervical neoplasia. *J. natl Cancer Inst.*, *66*, 631-636

[26]Clarke, E.A., Hatcher, J., McKeown-Eyssen, G.E. & Lickrish, G.M. (1985) Cervical dysplasia: association with sexual behavior, smoking, and oral contraceptive use? *Am. J. Obstet. Gynecol.*, *151*, 612-616

[27]Vessey, M.P., McPherson, K., Lawless, M. & Yeates, D. (1983) Neoplasia of the cervix uteri and contraception: a possible adverse effect of the pill. *Lancet*, *ii*, 930-934

[28]Andolsek, L., Kovacic, J., Kozuh, M. & Litt, B. (1983) Influence of oral contraceptives on the incidence of premalignant and malignant lesions of the cervix. *Contraception*, *28*, 505-519

[29]WHO Collaborative Study of Neoplasia and Steroid Contraceptives (1985) Invasive cervical cancer and combined oral contraceptives. *Br. med. J.*, *290*, 961-965

[30]Brinton, L.A., Huggins, G.R., Lehman, H.F., Mallin, K., Savitz, D.A., Trapido, E., Rosenthal, J. & Hoover, R. (1986) Long-term use of oral contraceptives and risk of invasive cervical cancer. *Int. J. Cancer*, *38*, 339-344

[31]Kay, C.R. (1983) Oral contraceptives and cancer. *Lancet*, *ii*, 1018

[32]Henderson, B.E., Powell, D., Rosario, I., Keys, C., Hanisch, R., Young, M., Casagrande, J., Gerkins, V. & Pike, M.C. (1974) An epidemiologic study of breast cancer. *J. natl Cancer Inst.*, *53*, 609-614

[33]Ravnihar, B., Seigel, D.G. & Lindtner, J. (1979) An epidemiologic study of breast cancer and benign breast neoplasias in relation to the oral contraceptive and estrogen use. *Eur. J. Cancer*, *15*, 395-405

[34]Pike, M.C., Henderson, B.E., Casagrande, J.T., Rosario, I. & Gray, G.E. (1981) Oral contraceptive use and early abortion as risk factors for breast cancer in young women. *Br. J. Cancer*, *43*, 72-76

35Kelsey, J.L., Fischer, D.B., Holford, T.R., LiVolsi, V.A., Mostow, E.D., Goldenberg, I.S. & White, C. (1981) Exogenous estrogens and other factors in the epidemiology of breast cancer. *J. natl Cancer Inst.*, *67*, 327-333

36Brinton, L.A., Hoover, R., Szklo, M. & Fraumeni, J.F., Jr (1982) Oral contraceptives and breast cancer. *Int. J. Epidemiol.*, *11*, 316-322

37Harris, N.V., Weiss, N.S., Francis, A.M. & Polissar, L. (1982) Breast cancer in relation to patterns of oral contraceptive use. *Am. J. Epidemiol.*, *116*, 643-651

38Vessey, M., Baron, J., Doll, R., McPherson, K. & Yeates, D. (1983) Oral contraceptives and breast cancer: final report of an epidemiological study. *Br. J. Cancer*, *47*, 455-462

39Hennekens, C.H., Speizer, F.E., Lipnick, R.J., Rosner, B., Bain, C., Belanger, C., Stampfer, M.J., Willett, W. & Peto, R. (1984) A case-control study of oral contraceptive use and breast cancer. *J. natl Cancer Inst.*, *72*, 39-42

40Rosenberg, L., Miller, D.R., Kaufman, D.W., Helmrich, S.P., Stolley, P.D., Schottenfeld, D. & Shapiro, S. (1984) Breast cancer and oral contraceptive use. *Am. J. Epidemiol.*, *119*, 167-176

41Talamini, R., La Vecchia, C., Franceschi, S., Colombo, F., Decarli, A., Grattoni, E., Grigoletto, E. & Tognoni, G. (1985) Reproductive and hormonal factors and breast cancer in a northern Italian population. *Int. J. Epidemiol.*, *14*, 70-74

42The Cancer and Steroid Hormone Study of the Centers for Disease Control and the National Institute of Child Health and Human Development (1986) Oral-contraceptive use and the risk of breast cancer. *New Engl. J. Med.*, *315*, 405-411

43Paul, C., Skegg, D.C.G., Spears, G.F.S. & Kaldor, J.M. (1986) Oral contraceptives and breast cancer: a national study. *Br. med. J.*, *293*, 723-726

44Vessey, M.P., McPherson, K. & Doll, R. (1981) Breast cancer and oral contraceptives: findings in Oxford-Family Planning Association contraceptive study. *Br. med. J.*, *282*, 2093-2094

45Trapido, E.J. (1981) A prospective cohort study of oral contraceptives and breast cancer. *J. natl Cancer Inst.*, *67*, 1011-1015

46Royal College of General Practitioners (1981) Breast cancer and oral contraceptives: findings in Royal College of General Practitioners' study. *Br. med. J.*, *282*, 2089-2093

47Lipnick, R.J., Buring, J.E., Hennekens, C.H., Rosner, B., Willett, W., Bain, C., Stampfer, M.J., Colditz, G.A., Peto, R. & Speizer, F.E. (1986) Oral contraceptives and breast cancer. A prospective cohort study. *J. Am. med. Assoc.*, *255*, 58-61

48Meirik, O., Adami, H.-O., Christoffersen, T., Lund, E., Bergström, R. & Bergsjö, P. (1986) Oral contraceptive use and breast cancer in young women. A joint national case-control study in Sweden and Norway. *Lancet*, *ii*, 650-654

49Vessey, M.P., McPherson, K., Yeates, D. & Doll, R. (1982) Oral contraceptive use and abortion before first term pregnancy in relation to breast cancer risk. *Br. J. Cancer*, *45*, 327-331

50Stadel, B.V., Webster, L.A., Rubin, G.L., Schlesselman, J.J. & Wingo, P.A. (1985) Oral contraceptives and breast cancer in young women. *Lancet*, *ii*, 970-973

51McPherson, K., Neil, A., Vessey, M.P. & Doll, R. (1983) Oral contraceptives and breast cancer. *Lancet*, *ii*, 1414-1415

52Paffenbarger, R.S., Jr, Kampert, J.B. & Chang, H.-G. (1980) Characteristics that predict risk of breast cancer before and after the menopause. *Am. J. Epidemiol.*, *112*, 258-268

[53]Pike, M.C., Krailo, M.D., Henderson, B.E., Duke, A. & Roy, S. (1983) Breast cancer in young women and use of oral contraceptives: possible modifying effect of formulation and age at use. *Lancet, ii*, 926-930

[54]Olsson, H., Olsson, M.L., Möller, T.R., Ranstam, J. & Holm, P. (1985) Oral contraceptive use and breast cancer in young women in Sweden. *Lancet, i*, 748-749

[55]Adam, S.A., Sheaves, J.K., Wright, N.H., Mosser, G., Harris, R.W. & Vessey, M.P. (1981) A case-control study of the possible association between oral contraceptives and malignant melanoma. *Br. J. Cancer, 44*, 45-50

[56]Bain, C., Hennekens, C.H., Speizer, F.E., Rosner, B., Willett, W. & Belanger, C. (1982) Oral contraceptive use and malignant melanoma. *J. natl Cancer Inst., 68*, 537-539

[57]Holly, E.A., Weiss, N.S. & Liff, J.M. (1983) Cutaneous melanoma in relation to exogenous hormones and reproductive factors. *J. natl Cancer Inst., 70*, 827-831

[58]Helmrich, S.P., Rosenberg, L., Kaufman, D.W., Miller, D.R., Schottenfeld, D., Stolley, P.D. & Shapiro, S. (1984) Lack of an elevated risk of malignant melanoma in relation to oral contraceptive use. *J. natl Cancer Inst., 72*, 617-620

[59]Beral, V., Evans, S., Shaw, H. & Milton, G. (1984) Oral contraceptive use and malignant melanoma in Australia. *Br. J. Cancer, 50*, 681-685

[60]Holman, C.D.J., Armstrong, B.K. & Heenan, P.J. (1984) Cutaneous malignant melanoma in women: exogenous sex hormones and reproductive factors. *Br. J. Cancer, 50*, 673-780

[61]Gallagher, R.P., Elwood, J.M., Hill, G.B., Coldman, A.J., Threlfall, W.J. & Spinelli, J.J. (1985) Reproductive factors, oral contraceptives and risk of malignant melanoma: Western Canada melanoma study. *Br. J. Cancer, 52*, 901-907

[62]Kay, C.R. (1981) Malignant melanoma and oral contraceptives. *Br. J. Cancer, 44*, 479

[63]Ramcharan, S., Pellegrin, F.A., Ray, R. & Hsu, J.-P. (1981) *The Walnut Creek Contraceptive Drug Study. A Prospective Study of the Side Effects of Oral Contraceptives (NIH Publ. No. 81-564)*, Bethesda, MD, National Institutes of Health, pp. 49, 53-55

[64]Wingrave, S.J., Kay, C.R. & Vessey, M.P. (1980) Oral contraceptives and pituitary adenomas. *Br. med. J., i*, 685-686

[65]Shy, K.K., McTiernan, A.M., Daling, J.R. & Weiss, N.S. (1983) Oral contraceptive use and the occurrence of pituitary prolactinoma. *J. Am. med. Assoc., 249*, 2204-2207

[66]Berkowitz, R.S., Marean, A.R., Goldstein, D.P. & Bernstein, M.R. (1980) Oral contraceptives and post-molar trophoblastic tumours. *Lancet, ii*, 752

[67]Potter, J.D. & McMichael, A.J. (1983) Large bowel cancer in women in relation to reproductive and hormonal factors: a case-control study. *J. natl Cancer Inst., 71*, 703-709

[68]Weiss, N.S., Daling, J.R. & Chow, W.H. (1981) Incidence of cancer of the large bowel in women in relation to reproductive and hormonal factors. *J. natl Cancer Inst., 67*, 57-60

[69]Brinton, L.A., Vessey, M.P., Flavel, R. & Yeates, D. (1981) Risk factors for benign breast disease. *Am. J. Epidemiol., 113*, 203-214

[70]Pastides, H., Kelsey, J.L., LiVolsi, V.A., Holford, T.R., Fischer, D.B. & Goldenberg, I.S. (1983) Oral contraceptive use and fibrocystic breast disease with special reference to its histopathology. *J. natl Cancer Inst., 71*, 5-9

[71]Hsieh, C.-C., Crosson, A.W., Walker, A.M., Trapido, E.J. & MacMahon, B. (1984) Oral contraceptive use and fibrocystic breast disease of different histologic classifications. *J. natl Cancer Inst., 72*, 285-290

[72]Hislop, T.G. & Threlfall, W.J. (1984) Oral contraceptives and benign breast disease. *Am. J. Epidemiol.*, *120*, 273-280

[73]Berkowitz, G.S., Kelsey, J.L., LiVolsi, V.A., Holford, T.R., Merino, M.J., Ort, S., O'Connor, T.Z., Goldenberg, I.S. & White, C. (1984) Oral contraceptive use and fibrocystic breast disease among pre-and postmenopausal women. *Am. J. Epidemiol.*, *120*, 87-96

[74]Ross, R.K., Pike, M.C., Vessey, M.P., Bull, D., Yeates, D. & Casagrande, J.T. (1986) Risk factors for uterine fibroids: reduced risk associated with oral contraceptives. *Br. med. J.*, *293*, 359-362

[75]*IARC Monographs*, *21*, 233-255, 257-278, 365-375, 1979

[76]*IARC Monographs*, *21*, 233-255, 257-278, 387-395, 1979

[77]*IARC Monographs*, *21*, 233-255, 407-415, 1979

[78]*IARC Monographs*, *21*, 257-278, 431-439, 1979

[79]*IARC Monographs*, *21*, 233-255, 257-278, 441-460, 1979

[80]El Etreby, M.F. & Neumann, F. (1980) *Influence of sex steroids and steroid antagonists on hormone-dependent tumors in experimental animals*. In: Iacobelli, S., King, R.J.B., Lindner, H.R. & Lippman, M.E., eds, *Hormones and Cancer*, New York, Raven Press, pp. 321-336

[81]Higashi, S., Tomita, T., Mizumoto, R. & Nakakuki, K. (1980) Development of hepatoma in rats following oral administration of synthetic oestrogen and progesterone. *Gann*, *71*, 576-577

[82]Fitzgerald, J., de la Iglesia, F. & Goldenthal, E.I. (1982) Ten-year oral toxicity study with norlestin in rhesus monkeys. *J. Toxicol. environ. Health*, *10*, 879-896

[83]*IARC Monographs*, *21*, 233-255, 461-477, 1979

[84]*IARC Monographs*, *21*, 257-278, 479-490, 1979

[85]*IARC Monographs*, *21*, 279-326, 491-515, 1979

[86]Kwapien, R.P., Giles, R.C., Gell, R.G. & Casey, H.W. (1980) Malignant mammary tumors in beagle dogs dosed with investigational oral contraceptive steroids. *J. natl Cancer Inst.*, *65*, 137-144

[87]*IARC Monographs*, *Suppl. 6*, 444, 1987

OESTROGEN-PROGESTIN REPLACEMENT THERAPY (Group 3)

A. Evidence for carcinogenicity to humans (*inadequate*)

Progestins, when administered for at least ten days per 28-day oestrogen replacement therapy cycle, prevent adenomatous hyperplasia, a precursor of endometrial carcinoma, and cause regression of pre-existing adenomatous hyperplasia in some patients[1]. When administered alone, progestins are effective in the treatment of carcinoma *in situ* of the endometrium[2] and of more advanced disease[3,4].

Progestins increase the conversion of oestradiol-17β to oestrone, a biologically less active oestrogen[5], and they reduce the concentration of oestrogen receptors[6]. Maximal mitotic activity in the endometrium occurs during the follicular phase of the cycle; luteal-phase progesterone effectively stops mitotic activity and causes differentiation of endo-metrial cells to a secretory state[7].

Support for a protective effect of progestins against endometrial cancer risk is obtained from the results of studies of the effects of oral contraceptives on endometrial cancer risk (see p. 298). Case-control studies have consistently shown that, whereas ingestion of sequential oral contraceptives containing an oestrogen alone throughout most of the menstrual cycle increases risk, ingestion of combined oral contraceptives, in which each pill contains an oestrogen and a progestin, substantially decreases risk.

The effect of progestins on the breast is markedly different from that on the endometrium. Endometrial cancer risk is considerably reduced with combined oral contraceptives (see p. 298), but there is no evidence of a reduced risk of breast cancer, even after long periods of combined oral contraceptive use[8]. Maximal mitotic activity in breast tissue occurs during the luteal phase of the normal menstrual cycle in the face of maximal progesterone levels[9]. These results concerning the effects of combined oral contraceptives suggest strongly that progestins do not have an antioestrogen, anticancer effect on the breast. A number of studies[10-12] have addressed the relationship between oestrogen-progestin replacement therapy and cancer, but in each instance either the small size of the study or apparently inadequate study design or data analysis prevent conclusions from being drawn.

B. Other relevant data

No data were available to the Working Group.

References

[1]Gambrell, R.D., Jr (1982) Clinical use of progestins in the menopausal patient. Dosage and duration. *J. reprod. Med.*, *27*, 531-538

[2]Kohorn, E.I. (1976) Gestagens and endometrial carcinoma. *Gynecol. Oncol.*, *4*, 398-411

[3]Thornton, J.G., Brown, L.A., Wells, M. & Scott, J.S. (1985) Primary treatment of endometrial cancer with progestogen alone. *Lancet, ii*, 207-208

[4]Mackillop, W.J. & Pringle, J.F. (1985) Stage III endometrial carcinoma: a review of 90 cases. *Cancer, 56*, 2519-2523

[5]Tseng, L. & Gurpide, E. (1975) Induction of human endometrial estradiol dehydrogenase by progestins. *Endocrinology*, *97*, 825-833

[6]Hsueh, A.J.W., Peck, E.J., Jr & Clark, J.H. (1975) Progesterone antagonism of the oestrogen receptor and oestrogen-induced uterine growth. *Nature, 254*, 337-339

[7]Novak, E.R. & Woodruff, J.D. (1979) *Novak's Gynecologic and Obstetric Pathology with Clinical and Endocrine Relations*, Philadelphia, PA, W.B. Saunders, pp. 171-184

[8]Kelsey, J.L. (1979) A review of the epidemiology of human breast cancer. *Epidemiol. Rev., 1*, 74-109

[9]Anderson, T.J., Ferguson, D.J.P. & Raab, G.M. (1982) Cell turnover in the 'resting' human breast: influence of parity, contraceptive pill, age and laterality. *Br. J. Cancer, 46*, 376-382

[10]Gambrell, R.D., Jr, Massey, F.M., Castaneda, T.A., Ugenas, A.J. & Ricci, C.A. (1979) Reduced incidence of endometrial cancer among postmenopausal women treated with progestogens. *J. Am. Geriatr. Soc., 27*, 389-394

[11]Nachtigall, L.E., Nachtigall, R.H., Nachtigall, R.D. & Beckman, E.M. (1979) Estrogen replacement therapy. II. A prospective study in the relationship to carcinoma and cardiovascular and metabolic problems. *Obstet. Gynecol.*, *54*, 74-79

[12]Gambrell, R.D., Jr, Maier, R.C. & Sanders, B.I. (1983) Decreased incidence of breast cancer in postmenopausal estrogen-progestogen users. *Obstet. Gynecol.*, *62*, 435-443

PHENACETIN (Group 2A) and
ANALGESIC MIXTURES CONTAINING PHENACETIN (Group 1)

A. Evidence for carcinogenicity to humans (*limited* for phenacetin; *sufficient* for analgesic mixtures containing phenacetin)

There have been many case reports of renal pelvic and other urothelial tumours in patients who had used large amounts of phenacetin-containing analgesics[1-13]. Case-control studies have been consistent in showing a positive association between cancer of the renal pelvis and cancer of the bladder and use of phenacetin-containing analgesics, with relative risks varying from 2.4 to over 6; these associations have not been explained by confounding with other causes of urothelial cancer, and, where looked for, a positive dose-response relationship has been evident[14-19]. In one study[14], use of nonphenacetin-containing analgesics appeared to increase the risk of cancer of the renal pelvis to the same extent as did phenacetin-containing analgesics. This result was not obtained in other studies[15,17,18].

B. Evidence for carcinogenicity to animals (*sufficient* for phenacetin; *limited* for analgesic mixtures containing phenacetin)

Phenacetin given orally induced benign and malignant tumours of the urinary tract in mice[20] and rats[1,21] and of the nasal cavity in rats[1]. When given in combination with aspirin and caffeine to rats or mice, no significant association was found with the incidence of tumours[1]. In rats, phenacetin alone or in combination with phenazone slightly increased the incidences of renal-cell and renal-pelvic tumours; rats treated with phenacetin, phenazone and caffeine in combination developed hepatomas[22]. Also in rats, phenacetin enhanced the incidence of urinary bladder tumours induced by N-nitrosobutyl-N-(4-hydroxybutyl)-amine[1], and prevented the induction of hepatocellular carcinomas by 2-acetylamino-fluorene[23].

C. Other relevant data

No data were available on the genetic and related effects of phenacetin in humans.

The results of studies on the induction of chromosomal aberrations, sister chromatid exchanges and micronuclei in rodents treated with phenacetin *in vivo* were equivocal. Phenacetin induced chromosomal aberrations in Chinese hamster cells *in vitro* but not DNA strand breaks in rat hepatocytes. It did not induce sex-linked recessive lethal mutations in *Drosophila*. Phenacetin was mutagenic to bacteria when tested in the presence of a metabolic system derived from hamster but not mouse or rat liver. The urine from phenacetin-treated Chinese hamsters, but not that from rats, was mutagenic to bacteria[24].

References

[1]*IARC Monographs, 24*, 135-161, 1980

[2]Christensen, T.E. & Ladefoged, J. (1979) Carcinomata in the urinary tract in patients with contracted kidneys and massive abuse of analgesics (phenacetin) (Dan.). *Ugeskr. Laeg., 141*, 3522-3524

[3]Gonwa, T.A., Corbett, W.T., Schey, H.M. & Buckalew, V.M., Jr (1980) Analgesic-associated nephropathy and transitional cell carcinoma of the urinary tract. *Ann. intern. Med., 93*, 249-252

[4]Mihatsch, M.J., Manz, T., Knüsli, C., Hofer, H.O., Rist, M., Guetg, R., Rutishauser, G. & Zollinger, H.U. (1980) Phenacetin abuse. III. Malignant urinary tract tumours with phenacetin abuse in Basel, 1963-1977 (Ger.). *Schweiz. med. Wochenschr., 110*, 255-264

[5]Orell, S.R., Nanra, R.S. & Ferguson, N.W. (1979) Renal pelvic carcinoma in the Hunter Valley. *Med. J. Aust., 524*, 555-557

[6]Blohmé, I. & Johansson, S. (1981) Renal pelvic neoplasms and atypical urothelium in patients with end-stage analgesic nephropathy. *Kidney int., 20*, 671-675

[7]Syré, G. & Matejka, M. (1981) Phenacetin abuse and renal pelvis carcinomas (Ger.). *Wien. klin. Wochenschr., 93*, 420-423

[8]Porpáczy, P. & Schramek, P. (1981) Analgesic nephropathy and phenacetin-induced transitional cell carcinoma — analysis of 300 patients with long-term consumption of phenacetin-containing drugs. *Eur. Urol., 7*, 349-354

[9]Mihatsch, M.J., Brunner, F.P., Korteweg, E., Rist, M., Dalquen, P. & Thiel, G. (1982) Phenacetin abuse. VII. Tumours of the urinary tract in haemodialysis and kidney transplant patients (Ger.). *Schweiz. med. Wochenschr., 112*, 1468-1472

[10]Novák, J. & Žídek, I. (1983) Phenacetin as a carcinogen for the renal pelvis (Czech.). *Čas. Lék. čes., 122*, 1149-1152

[11]Mihatsch, M.J. & Knüsli, C. (1982) Phenacetin abuse and malignant tumors. An autopsy study covering 25 years (1953-1977). *Klin. Wochenschr., 60*, 1339-1349

[12]Marek, J. & Hradec, E. (1985) Chronic sclerosing ureteritis and nephrogenic adenoma of the ureter in analgesic abuse. *Pathol. Res. Pract., 180*, 569-573

[13]Kliment, J. (1979) Renal pelvis tumours and abuse of analgesics (Czech.). *Bratisl. lék. Listy, 72*, 641-764

[14]McCredie, M., Ford, J.M., Taylor, J.S. & Stewart, J.H. (1982) Analgesics and cancer of the renal pelvis in New South Wales. *Cancer, 49*, 2617-2625

[15]McCredie, M., Stewart, J.H., Ford, J.M. & MacLennan, R.A. (1983) Phenacetin-containing analgesics and cancer of the bladder or renal pelvis in women. *Br. J. Urol., 55*, 220-224

[16]McCredie, M., Stewart, J.H. & Ford, J.M. (1983) Analgesics and tobacco as risk factors for cancer of the ureter and renal pelvis. *J. Urol., 130*, 28-30

[17]McLaughlin, J.K., Mandel, J.S., Blot, W.J., Schuman, L.M., Mehl, E.S. & Fraumeni, J.F., Jr (1984) A population-based case-control study of renal cell carcinoma. *J. natl Cancer Inst., 72*, 275-284

[18]Piper, J.M., Tonascia, J. & Matanoski, G.M. (1985) Heavy phenacetin use and bladder cancer in women aged 20 to 49 years. *New Engl. J. Med., 313*, 292-295

[19]Piper, J.M., Matanoski, G.M. & Tonascia, J. (1986) Bladder cancer in young women. *Am. J. Epidemiol.*, *123*, 1033-1042

[20]Nakanishi, K., Kurata, Y., Oshima, M., Fukushima, S. & Ito, N. (1982) Carcinogenicity of phenacetin: long-term feeding study in B6C3F$_1$ mice. *Int. J. Cancer*, *29*, 439-444

[21]Muradyan, R.Y. (1986) Experimental studies of phenacetin carcinogenicity (Russ.). *Vopr. Onkol.*, *32*, 63-70

[22]Johansson, S.L. (1981) Carcinogenicity of analgesics: long-term treatment of Sprague-Dawley rats with phenacetin, phenazone, caffeine and paracetamol (acetamidophen). *Int. J. Cancer*, *27*, 521-529

[23]Yamamoto, R.S., Frankel, H.H. & Weisburger, E.K. (1979) Effect of phenacetin and *N*-alkyl-acetanilides on *N*-2-fluorenylacetamide hepatocarcinogenesis. *Cancer Lett.*, *8*, 183-188

[24]*IARC Monographs*, *Suppl. 6*, 448-450, 1987

PHENAZOPYRIDINE HYDROCHLORIDE (Group 2B)

A. Evidence for carcinogenicity to humans (*inadequate*)

In one limited epidemiological study, no significant excess of any cancer was observed among 2214 patients who received phenazopyridine hydrochloride and were followed for a minimum of three years[1].

B. Evidence for carcinogenicity to animals (*sufficient*)

Oral administration of phenazopyridine hydrochloride increased the incidence of hepatocellular adenomas and carcinomas in female mice and induced tumours of the colon and rectum in rats[1].

C. Other relevant data

No data were available on the genetic and related effects of phenazopyridine hydrochloride in humans. It did not induce sex-linked recessive lethal mutations in *Drosophila* and was not mutagenic to bacteria[2].

References

[1]*IARC Monographs*, *24*, 175-184, 1980

[2]*IARC Monographs*, *Suppl. 6*, 451-452, 1987

PHENELZINE SULPHATE (Group 3)

A. Evidence for carcinogenicity to humans (*inadequate*)

A liver angiosarcoma was reported in one person who had taken phenelzine sulphate for six years preceding tumour diagnosis[1].

B. Evidence for carcinogenicity to animals (*limited*)

When phenelzine sulphate was administered to mice in drinking-water for life, incidences of lung and blood-vessel tumours were significantly increased in female but not in male animals[1].

C. Other relevant data

No data were available on the genetic and related effects of phenelzine sulphate in humans. It did not induce DNA strand breaks in mice treated *in vivo*. In bacteria, it was mutagenic and induced DNA damage[2].

References

[1]*IARC Monographs*, *24*, 175-184, 1980
[2]*IARC Monographs*, *Suppl. 6*, 453-454, 1987

PHENOBARBITAL (Group 2B)

A. Evidence for carcinogenicity to humans (*inadequate*)

Phenobarbital has been associated with increased frequencies of several cancers[1]. Excesses of brain tumours have been reported in studies of epileptics, most of whom were treated with phenobarbital, often in combination with other drugs[2,3]. The role of anticonvulsant therapy in the origin of these brain tumours is not clear, however, since the tumours may have been the precipitating cause or secondary to the cause of the epilepsy. In the largest study[2,4], there was an almost 12-fold excess of brain tumours in the first ten years of follow-up (45 observed, 3.8 expected), but this decreased with duration of follow-up to 1.3 (2 observed, 1.5 expected) 30 or more years following admission. A case-control study involving 84 children with brain tumours[5] showed a two-fold increase in the incidence of these tumours associated with prenatal or childhood exposure to barbiturates (mostly phenobarbital[6]). In a study of 11 169 matched case-control pairs of childhood cancers and controls, epilepsy was reported by 39 mothers of cases and 22 mothers of controls (20 and 12, respectively, having used phenobarbital). The number of brain tumours among the 39 cancers was not reported[7].

Lung cancer was reported in excess in 5834 members of a prepaid health plan prescribed phenobarbital during 1969-1973 and followed to 1976. The standardized mortality ratio (SMR) was 1.5 [95% confidence interval, 1.1-1.9]. Excesses were also found in users of pentobarbital sodium and secobarbital sodium. When users of the three drugs were considered together, the excess of lung cancer was found in both men and women, appeared to be accounted for only partly by cigarette smoking and persisted when cases diagnosed during the first two years of follow-up were excluded. There was no apparent relation with duration of use[8]. Small increases in lung cancer incidence were also observed in two cohort studies of epileptics[3,4], 'largely ascribable to tobacco' in one study[4], although the effects of smoking were not studied. In the larger of the two[4], the SMR was 1.3 [1.0-1.6]; in the other[3], it was 1.4 (0.9-2.1).

Liver cancer occurred in excess in the larger cohort study of epileptics[4] (SMR, 3.8 [2.7-4.9]). However, ten of the 13 observed cancers occurred in individuals exposed to thorotrast. Histology was available for nine of these: two were reported to be haemangiosarcomas, four, cholangiocarcinomas, one, a hepatocellular carcinoma, and two, adenocarcinomas[2]. In the other cohort study with data available[3], no primary liver tumour was observed although 0.6 cases of cancer of the liver and gall-bladder were expected.

B. Evidence for carcinogenicity to animals (*sufficient*)

Phenobarbital produced benign and malignant hepatocellular tumours in mice and hepatocellular tumours in rats after its oral administration[1,9,10]. Experiments with mice and rats in which phenobarbital was studied for its promoting activity included comparison groups given phenobarbital alone. Oral administration of phenobarbital enhanced the incidences of liver tumours induced in mice by *N*-nitrosodimethylamine[11] or *N*-ethyl-*N*-nitrosourea[12] and of benign and malignant liver tumours induced in rats by 2-acetylaminofluorene[13-16], *N*-nitrosodiethylamine[17,18], 2-methyl-*N*,*N*-dimethyl-4-aminoazobenzene[19], benzo[*a*]pyrene[20], cycasin[21], *N*-hydroxy-*N*-formyl- or -acetylaminobiphenyl[22], *N*-nitroso-*N*-(4-hydroxybutyl)butylamine[16] or *N*-nitrosomorpholine[23]. In rats, oral administration of phenobarbital in combination with DDT resulted in a high incidence of liver tumours[24]. Phenobarbital enhanced the development of thyroid tumours[25,26] and of liver foci[26] induced in rats by *N*-nitrosodi(2-hydroxypropyl)amine and enhanced the incidences of liver foci, thyroid adenocarcinomas and forestomach carcinomas induced in rats by *N*-methyl-*N*-nitrosourea[27].

C. Other relevant data

No data were available on the genetic and related effects of phenobarbital in humans.

Neither phenobarbital nor its sodium salt induced sister chromatid exchanges, chromosomal aberrations, micronuclei or sperm abnormalities in mice treated *in vivo*. Phenobarbital induced chromosomal aberrations and mutation but not sister chromatid exchanges in cultured human cells. Both positive and negative results were obtained for transformation in rodent cells *in vitro*. Phenobarbital enhanced transformation of virus-infected rat embryo cells initiated with 3-methylcholanthrene in a two-stage transformation assay. It induced sister chromatid exchanges and chromosomal aberrations in cultured Chinese hamster cells, but not in cultured rat liver cells; micronuclei and aneuploidy were not induced in Chinese hamster cells. Phenobarbital induced mutation in Chinese hamster cells, but conflicting or negative results were obtained in other rodent cells. Phenobarbital and its sodium salt did not induce DNA strand breaks, and phenobarbital did not induce unscheduled DNA synthesis, in cultured rodent cells. Phenobarbital inhibited intercellular communication in human hepatoma cells and both phenobarbital and its sodium salt did so in rodent systems. Phenobarbital induced neither somatic mutation nor recombination in *Drosophila*; the sodium salt did not induce sex-linked recessive lethal mutations.

Phenobarbital induced aneuploidy but not mutation or gene conversion in fungi. Conflicting results were obtained concerning the mutagenicity of these compounds in bacteria[28].

References

[1]*IARC Monographs*, 13, 157-181, 1977

[2]Clemmesen, J. & Hjalgrim-Jensen, S. (1978) Is phenobarbital carcinogenic? A follow-up of 8078 epileptics. *Ecotoxicol. environ. Saf.*, 1, 457-470

[3]White, S.J., McLean, A.E.M. & Howland, C. (1979) Anticonvulsant drugs and cancer. A cohort study in patients with severe epilepsy. *Lancet*, ii, 458-461

[4]Clemmesen, J. & Hjalgrim-Jensen, S. (1981) Does phenobarbital cause intracranial tumors? A follow-up through 35 years. *Ecotoxicol. environ. Saf.*, 5, 255-260

[5]Gold, E., Gordis, L., Tonascia, J. & Szklo, M. (1978) Increased risk of brain tumors in children exposed to barbiturates. *J. natl Cancer Inst.*, 61, 1031-1034

[6]Gold, E.B., Gordis, L., Tonascia, J.A. & Szklo, M. (1979) Brain tumors in children exposed to barbiturates. *J. natl Cancer Inst.*, 63, 3-4

[7]Sanders, B.M. & Draper, G.J. (1979) Childhood cancer and drugs in pregnancy. *Br. med. J.*, i, 717-718

[8]Friedman, G.D. (1981) Barbiturates and lung cancer in humans. *J. natl Cancer Inst.*, 67, 291-295

[9]Feldman, D., Swarm, R.L. & Becker, J. (1981) Ultrastructural study of rat liver and liver neoplasms after long-term treatment with phenobarbital. *Cancer Res.*, 41, 2151-2162

[10]Ward, J.M. (1983) Increased susceptibility of livers of aged F344/NCr rats to the effects of phenobarbital on the incidence, morphology, and histochemistry of hepatocellular foci and neoplasms. *J. natl Cancer Inst.*, 71, 815-823

[11]Uchida, E. & Hirono, I. (1979) Effect of phenobarbital on induction of liver and lung tumors by dimethylnitrosamine in newborn mice. *Gann*, 70, 639-644

[12]Pereira, M.A., Knutsen, G.L. & Herren-Freund, S.L. (1985) Effect of subsequent treatment of chloroform or phenobarbital on the incidence of liver and lung tumors initiated by ethyl-nitrosourea in 15 day old mice. *Carcinogenesis*, 6, 203-207

[13]Watanabe, K. & Williams, G.M. (1978) Enhancement of rat hepatocellular-altered foci by the liver tumor promoter phenobarbital: evidence that foci are precursors of neoplasms and that the promoter acts on carcinogenic-induced lesions. *J. natl Cancer Inst.*, 61, 1311-1314

[14]Peraino, C., Staffeldt, E.F., Haugen, D.A., Lombard, L.S., Stevens, F.J. & Fry, R.J.M. (1980) Effects of varying the dietary concentration of phenobarbital on its enhancement of 2-acetylaminofluorene-induced hepatic tumorigenesis. *Cancer Res.*, 40, 3268-3273

[15]Takano, T., Tatematsu, M., Hasegawa, R., Imaida, K. & Ito, N. (1980) Dose-response relationship for the promoting effect of phenobarbital on the induction of liver hyperplastic nodules in rats exposed to 2-fluorenylacetamide and carbon tetrachloride. *Gann*, 71, 580-581

[16]Nakanishi, K., Fukushima, S., Hagiwara, A., Tamano, S. & Ito, N. (1982) Organ-specific promoting effects of phenobarbital sodium and sodium saccharin in the induction of liver and urinary bladder tumors in male F344 rats. *J. natl Cancer Inst.*, 68, 497-500

[17]Farwell, D.C., Nolan, C.E. & Herbst, E.J. (1978) Liver ornithine decarboxylase during pheno-barbital promotion of nitrosamine carcinogenesis. *Cancer Lett.*, 5, 139-144

[18]Nishizumi, M. (1979) Effect of phenobarbital, dichlorodiphenyltrichloroethane, and poly-chlorinated biphenyls on diethylnitrosamine-induced hepatocarcinogenesis. *Gann, 70*, 835-837

[19]Kitagawa, T., Pitot, H.C., Miller, E.C. & Miller, J.A. (1979) Promotion by dietary phenobarbital of hepatocarcinogenesis by 2-methyl-*N,N*-dimethyl-4-aminoazobenzene in the rat. *Cancer Res., 39*, 112-115

[20]Kitagawa, T., Hirakawa, T., Ishikawa, T., Nemoto, N. & Takayama, S. (1980) Induction of hepatocellular carcinoma in rat liver by initial treatment with benzo[*a*]pyrene after partial hepatectomy and promotion by phenobarbital. *Toxicol. Lett., 6*, 167-171

[21]Uchida, E. & Hirono, I. (1981) Effect of phenobarbital on the development of neoplastic lesions in the liver of cycasin-treated rats. *J. Cancer Res. clin. Oncol., 100*, 231-238

[22]Shirai, T., Lee, M.-S., Wang, C.Y. & King, C.M. (1981) Effects of partial hepatectomy and dietary phenobarbital on liver and mammary tumorigenesis by two *N*-hydroxy-*N*-acylaminobiphenyls in female CD rats. *Cancer Res., 41*, 2450-2456

[23]Moore, M.A., Hacker, H.-J., Kunz, H.W. & Bannasch, P. (1983) Enhancement of NNM-induced carcinogenesis in the rat liver by phenobarbital: a combined morphological and enzyme histochemical approach. *Carcinogenesis, 4*, 473-479

[24]Barbieri, O., Rossi, L., Cabral, J.R.P. & Santi, L. (1983) Carcinogenic effects induced in Wistar rats by combined treatment with technical-grade dichlorodiphenyltrichloroethane and sodium phenobarbital. *Cancer Lett., 20*, 223-229

[25]Hiasa, Y., Kitahori, Y., Ohshima, M., Fujita, T., Yuasa, T., Konishi, N. & Miyashiro, A. (1982) Promoting effects of phenobarbital and barbital on development of thyroid tumors in rats treated with *N*-bis(2-hydroxypropyl)nitrosamine. *Carcinogenesis, 3*, 1187-1190

[26]Moore, M.A., Thamavit, W., Tsuda, H. & Ito, N. (1986) The influence of subsequent dehydro-epiandrosterone, diaminopropane, phenobarbital, butylated hydroxyanisole and butylated hydroxytoluene treatment on the development of preneoplastic and neoplastic lesions in the rat initiated with di-hydroxy-di-*N*-propyl nitrosamine. *Cancer Lett., 30*, 153-160

[27]Tsuda, H., Sakata, T., Shirai, T., Kurata, Y., Tamano, S. & Ito, N. (1984) Modification of *N*-methyl-*N*-nitrosourea initiated carcinogenesis in the rat by subsequent treatment with antioxidants, phenobarbital and ethinyl estradiol. *Cancer Lett., 24*, 19-27

[28]*IARC Monographs, Suppl. 6*, 455-458, 1987

PHENYLBUTAZONE (Group 3)

A. Evidence for carcinogenicity to humans (*inadequate*)

Cases of leukaemia have been reported in patients following phenylbutazone therapy[1,2], but their significance cannot be evaluated, given the widespread use of phenylbutazone[1]. No significant excess of leukaemia or other malignancy was observed during 1969-1976 among 3660 members of a prepaid health plan prescribed phenylbutazone during 1969-1973[3]. In a case-control study of 409 patients with leukaemia or lymphoma and a subset of 127 patients with myelocytic leukaemia, who were compared with equal numbers of hospital controls and with a second control series of members of a prepaid health plan, prior use of phenylbutazone was more frequent in cases than in members of the health plan (relative risk, 1.26; 95% confidence interval, 0.86-1.86). This appeared to be explained by an association of musculo-skeletal disease with these cancers. There was no clear association between the amount or duration of phenylbutazone therapy and risk of leukaemia[4]. In a cohort study of 489 patients with rheumatoid arthritis, followed for an average of 12.2 years, seven patients developed non-Hodgkin's lymphoma compared to 0.29 expected from regional rates (relative risk, 24.1 [20.4-27.9]), two developed Hodgkin's disease, one, a chronic lymphatic leukaemia and one, an acute myeloid leukaemia. A study of hospital charts indicated that 60% of those with malignancies had received phenylbutazone compared to 3% of the whole cohort; however, the author considered it likely that far more than 3% of the whole cohort had received phenylbutazone. Those patients with malignancies had also received other drugs: 40% had received gold, 20%, steroids and 10%, chloroquine, but none had received cytotoxic agents or radiotherapy. Further, 30% were believed not to have received any of these agents (including phenylbutazone)[5]. Lymphoproliferative malignancies have been recognized as a complication of other immune disorders, and it is possible that phenyl-butazone therapy did not play a causal role in this study.

B. Evidence for carcinogenicity to animals

No data were available to the Working Group.

C. Other relevant data

In one study of patients given high doses of phenylbutazone, no chromosomal aber-ration was found in bone-marrow cells[6].

Phenylbutazone did not induce dominant lethality, micronuclei or chromosomal anom-alies in bone-marrow cells of mice treated *in vivo*. It induced chromosomal aberrations in cultured Chinese hamster fibroblasts, but did not induce sister chromatid exchanges or chromosomal aberrations in cultured human cells. Phenylbutazone was not mutagenic to bacteria[6].

References

[1]*IARC Monographs*, *13*, 183-199, 1977

[2]Mitarnun, W. & Peerabool, R. (1983) Blood dyscrasia evolving into acute lymphoblastic leukemia following ingestion of phenylbutazone, indomethacin, dexamethasone and prednisolone. *J. med. Assoc. Thailand*, *66*, 649-654

[3]Friedman, G.D. & Ury, H.K. (1980) Initial screening for carcinogenicity of commonly used drugs. *J. natl Cancer Inst.*, *65*, 723-733

[4]Friedman, G.D. (1982) Phenylbutazone, musculoskeletal disease, and leukemia. *J. chron. Dis.*, *35*, 233-243

[5]Symmons, D.P.M. (1985) Neoplasms of the immune system in rheumatoid arthritis. *Am. J. Med.*, *78* (*Suppl. 1A*), 22-28

[6]*IARC Monographs*, *Suppl. 6*, 459-460, 1987

N-PHENYL-2-NAPHTHYLAMINE (Group 3)

A. Evidence for carcinogenicity to humans (*inadequate*)

No excess of bladder tumours was found among men in a rubber processing factory with known exposure to *N*-phenyl-2-naphthylamine (which contained small amounts of 2-naphthylamine [see p. 261]); however, a study of rubber workers who were not exposed to 2-naphthylamine did show an increased incidence of bladder tumours. In the latter study, the men were exposed to several compounds, which probably included *N*-phenyl-2-naphthylamine[1].

B. Evidence for carcinogenicity to animals (*limited*)

N-Phenyl-2-naphthylamine was tested for carcinogenicity by oral administration in mice, rats, hamsters and dogs. No carcinogenicity was reported in most experiments[1-4]. In one experiment, the total tumour incidence and the incidence of hepatocellular tumours were increased in male mice of one strain[1]. In another experiment, two rare kidney tumours were seen in female mice[2]. Subcutaneous administration to mice increased the total tumour incidence[1] and the incidences of lung[5] and liver neoplasms[1]. Repeated subcutaneous injection after previous unilateral nephrectomy in mice resulted in a significant increase in the total tumour incidence and in the incidences of haemangiosarcomas of the kidney and of carcinomas of the lung[6,7]. Following exposure of mice by inhalation in one study, lung carcinomas were reported[8].

C. Other relevant data

There is some evidence from one study of 19 human volunteers that up to 0.03% of a single 10-mg dose of *N*-phenyl-2-naphthylamine is converted to 2-naphthylamine. Similarly, the urine of workers exposed to *N*-phenyl-2-naphthylamine was found to contain 2-naphthylamine, indicating that *N*-phenyl-2-naphthylamine is dephenylated in the human body[1]. No data were available on the genetic effects of *N*-phenyl-2-naphthylamine in humans. It was reported not to be mutagenic to bacteria[9].

References

[1]*IARC Monographs*, *16*, 325-341, 1978

[2]National Toxicology Program (1987) *Technical Report on the Toxicology and Carcinogenesis Studies of N-Phenyl-2-naphthylamine (CAS No. 135-88-6) in F344/N Rats and B6C3F₁ Mice (Feed Studies)* (*Tech. Rep. No. 333; NIH Publ. No. 87-2589*), Research Triangle Park, NC

[3]Ketkar, M.B. & Mohr, U. (1982) The chronic effects of magenta, paramagenta and phenyl-β-naphthylamine in rats after intragastric administration. *Cancer Lett.*, *16*, 203-206

[4]Green, U., Holste, J. & Spikermann, A.R. (1979) A comparative study of the chronic effects of magenta, paramagenta and phenyl-β-naphthylamine in Syrian golden hamsters. *J. Cancer Res. clin. Oncol.*, *95*, 51-55

[5]Wang, H., Dzeng, R. & Wang, D. (1982) The carcinogenicity of *N*-phenyl-2-naphthylamine in ICR mice (Chin.). *Acta biol. exp. sin.*, *15*, 199-207

[6]Wang, D., Zeng, R. & Wang, H. (1983) A comparative study on carcinogenic activity of PBNA and PANA in unilaterally nephrectomized TA-1 mice (Chin.). *Acta sci. circumstantiae*, *3*, 262-266

[7]Wang, H., Wang, D. & Dzeng, R. (1984) Carcinogenicity of N-phenyl-1-naphthylamine and N-phenyl-2-naphthylamine in mice. *Cancer Res.*, *44*, 3098-3100

[8]You, X. & Yao, Y. (1981) Experimental study of inhalation carcinogenesis of N-phenyl-2-naphthylamine aerosol on mice (Chin.). *Acta biol. exp. sin.*, *14*, 139-143

[9]*IARC Monographs, Suppl. 6*, 461-462, 1987

PHENYTOIN (Group 2B)

A. Evidence for carcinogenicity to humans (*limited*)

Cases of cancer, mainly neuroblastoma, were reported in ten children under the age of four years who had been diagnosed as having an unusual constellation of congenital abnormalities (fetal hydantoin syndrome) thought to be induced by prenatal exposure to phenytoin or who had just received prenatal exposure to phenytoin[1-9]. Although the number of patients is small, the concordance of rare events suggests that phenytoin may be a transplacental carcinogen in humans. There is also one report of malignant mesenchymoma in an 18-year-old patient with phenytoin-associated malformations[10]. In a large case-control study[11] of 11 169 pairs of childhood cancer cases (about 8% of which would have been neuroblastomas[12]) and matched controls, epilepsy was reported among the mothers of 39 cancer cases compared with 22 controls (relative risk [RR], 1.77 [95% confidence interval, 1.02-3.10]). Review of available antenatal records indicated that 37% of case mothers had used phenytoin during pregnancy (RR, 1.57 [0.56-4.48]) and 67% had used phenobarbital (RR, 1.67 [0.78-3.62]).

There have been a number of case reports of lymphomas among individuals receiving phenytoin[1,13-21] with or without other antiepileptic drugs. No significant excess of lymphoma, however, was reported in two follow-up studies of epilepsy patients: the observed and expected numbers of lymphoma-leukaemia were 23 and 23.7 in the larger survey[22], and 6 and 4.7 in the smaller survey[23]. An excess of brain and other neurological tumours during 1969-1976 (8 observed, 0.5 expected) was reported among 954 people prescribed phenytoin during 1969-1973[24]. The excess is similar to that reported among epileptics [see summary of data on phenobarbital, p. 313] and may reflect the underlying disease rather than use of the drug *per se*. There was also no appreciable excess of phenytoin use in cases of Hodgkin's disease in a small case-control study[25].

B. Evidence for carcinogenicity to animals (*limited*)

Phenytoin and its sodium salt have been tested for carcinogenicity in mice by oral and intraperitoneal administration, producing lymphomas and leukaemias[1,26,27]. The effects of oral administration varied with the strain of mouse: no effect was observed in the resistant C3Hf strain; in the C57BL strain, thymic lymphomas were produced in 12% of treated mice, starting at about eight months of age, as compared with 4% in control mice starting at about

18 months of age; 25% of SJL/J mice had thymic lymphomas early in the study, but late in the study the majority of both treated and control SJL/J mice had extrathymic tumours[26]. The experiments were complicated by the use of a liquid diet. Studies by oral administration in rats were considered to be inadequate[1].

C. Other relevant data

Conflicting results have been obtained concerning the induction of sister chromatid exchanges in patients treated with phenytoin; no increase in the incidence of chromosomal aberrations was found[28].

Phenytoin induced sperm abnormalities and micronuclei but not dominant lethal mutations in mice treated *in vivo*; it did not induce chromosomal aberrations in bone-marrow cells of rats. It did not induce chromosomal aberrations in cultured human lymphocytes. It enhanced virus-induced transformation of Syrian hamster embryo cells and was a weak inhibitor of intercellular communication in Chinese hamster V79 cells. Phenytoin induced prophage but was not mutagenic to bacteria[28].

References

[1] *IARC Monographs, 13*, 201-225, 1977

[2] Seeler, R.A., Israel, J.N., Royal, J.E., Kaye, C.I., Rao, S. & Abulaban, M. (1979) Ganglioneuroblastoma and fetal hydantoin-alcohol syndromes. *Pediatrics, 63*, 524-527

[3] Allen, R.W., Jr, Ogden, B., Bentley, F.L. & Jung, A.L. (1980) Fetal hydantoin syndrome, neuroblastoma and hemorrhagic disease in a neonate. *J. Am. med. Assoc., 244*, 1464-1465

[4] Ehrenbard, L.T. & Chaganti, R.S.K. (1981) Cancer in the fetal hydantoin syndrome. *Lancet, ii*, 97

[5] Taylor, W.F., Myers, M. & Taylor, W.R. (1980) Extrarenal Wilms' tumour in an infant exposed to intrauterine phenytoin. *Lancet, ii*, 481-482

[6] Jimenez, J.F., Brown, R.E., Seibert, R.W., Seiberg, J.J. & Char, F. (1981) Melanotic neuroectodermal tumor of infancy and fetal hydantoin syndrome. *Am. J. pediatr. Hematol./Oncol., 3*, 9-15

[7] Ramilo, J. & Harris, V.J. (1979) Neuroblastoma in a child with the hydantoin and fetal alcohol syndrome. The radiographic features. *Br. J. Radiol., 52*, 993-995

[8] Bostrom, B. & Nesbit, M.E., Jr (1983) Hodgkin disease in a child with fetal alcohol-hydantoin syndrome. *J. Pediatr., 103*, 760-762

[9] Lipson, A. & Bale, P. (1985) Ependymoblastoma associated with prenatal exposure to diphenylhydantoin and methylphenobarbitone. *Cancer, 55*, 1859-1862

[10] Blattner, W.A., Henson, D.E., Young, R.C. & Fraumeni, J.F., Jr (1977) Malignant mesenchymoma and birth defects. Prenatal exposure to phenytoin. *J. Am. med. Assoc., 238*, 334-335

[11] Sanders, B.M. & Draper, G.J. (1979) Childhood cancer and drugs in pregnancy. *Br. med. J., i*, 717-718

[12] Bithell, J.F. & Stewart, A.M. (1975) Pre-natal irradiation and childhood malignancy: a review of British data from the Oxford survey. *Br. J. Cancer, 31*, 271-287

[13] Isobe, T., Horimatsu, T., Fujita, T., Miyazaki, K. & Sugiyama, T. (1980) Adult T-cell lymphoma following diphenylhydantoin therapy. *Acta haematol. jpn., 43*, 711-714

[14]Creixenti, J.B., Porta, F.S., Xarau, S.N., Marin, E.S. & San Miguel, J.G. (1980) Hodgkin's disease following treatment with hydantoins. Report of a case and review of the literature (Sp.). *Med. clin. (Barcelona)*, *75*, 24-26

[15]Aymard, J.P., Lederlin, P., Witz, F., Colomb, J.N., Faure, G., Guerci, O. & Herbeuval, R. (1981) Multiple myeloma after phenytoin therapy. *Scand. J. Haematol.*, *26*, 330-332

[16]Gabryś, K., Medraś, E., Kowalski, P. & Gola, A. (1983) Malignant lymphoma in the course of antiepileptic therapy (Pol.). *Polsk. Tyg. Lek.*, *38*, 505-507

[17]Guerin, J.M., Tibourtine, O., Segrestaa, J.M., Nemeth, J. & Wassef, M. (1983) Hodgkin's disease in an epileptic treated with hydantoins (Fr.). *Presse méd.*, *12*, 1491

[18]Gyte, G.M.L., Richmond, J.E., Williams, J.R.B. & Atwood, J.L. (1985) Hairy cell leukaemia occurring during phenytoin (diphenylhydantoin) treatment. *Scand. J. Haematol.*, *35*, 358-362

[19]Pereira, A., Cervantes, F. & Rozman, C. (1985) Folic acid deficiency with macrocytic anaemia and non-Hodgkin's lymphoma associated with prolonged diphenylhydantoin therapy (Sp.). *Med. Clin. (Barcelona)*, *85*, 503-505

[20]Rubinstein, N., Weinrauch, L. & Matzner, Y. (1985) Generalized pruritis as a presenting symptom of phenytoin-induced Hodgkin's disease. *Int. J. Dermatol.*, *24*, 54-55

[21]Rubinstein, I., Langevitz, P. & Shibi, G. (1985) Isolated malignant lymphoma of the jejunum and long-term diphenylhydantoin therapy. *Oncology*, *42*, 104-106

[22]Clemmesen, J. & Hjalgrim-Jensen, S. (1981) Does phenobarbital cause intracranial tumors? A follow-up through 35 years. *Ecotoxicol. environ. Saf.*, *5*, 255-260

[23]White, S.J., McLean, A.E.M. & Howland, C. (1979) Anticonvulsant drugs and cancer. A cohort study in patients with severe epilepsy. *Lancet*, *ii*, 458-461

[24]Friedman, G.D. & Ury, H.K. (1980) Initial screening for carcinogenicity of commonly used drugs. *J. natl Cancer Inst.*, *65*, 723-733

[25]Kirchhoff, L.V., Evans, A.S., McClelland, K.E., Carvalho, R.P.S. & Pannuti, C.S. (1980) A case-control study of Hodgkin's disease in Brazil. I. Epidemiologic aspects. *Am. J. Epidemiol.*, *112*, 595-608

[26]Krueger, G.R.F. & Bedoya, V.A. (1978) Hydantoin-induced lymphadenopathies and lymphomas: experimental studies in mice. *Recent Results Cancer Res.*, *64*, 265-270

[27]Bedoya, V. & Krueger, G.R.F. (1978) Ultrastructural studies on hydantoin induced lymphomas in mice. *Z. Krebsforsch.*, *91*, 195-204

[28]*IARC Monographs, Suppl. 6*, 463-465, 1987

POLYBROMINATED BIPHENYLS (Group 2B)

A. Evidence for carcinogenicity to humans (*inadequate*)

The mortality has been studied of a cohort of over 3500 male workers with potential exposure to several brominated compounds, including polybrominated biphenyls, who were employed between 1935 and 1976 at chemical plants. Due to a lack of quantitative data, potential exposures of workers to polybrominated biphenyls were categorized as 'routine' and 'nonroutine'. Of the 91 workers potentially exposed on a 'routine' basis, none died during the study period; among the 237 'nonroutinely' exposed, two deaths were observed, with 6.4 expected, one of which was due to cancer of the large intestine[1].

B. Evidence for carcinogenicity to animals (*sufficient*)

The carcinogenicity of a commercial preparation of polybrominated biphenyls (FireMaster FF-1, various lots), composed primarily of hexabromobiphenyl with smaller amounts of penta- and heptabrominated isomers, was tested by oral administration in mice and rats. In mice, it produced malignant liver tumours. In five studies in rats, it produced benign and malignant hepatic tumours, including cholangiocarcinomas, depending on the exposure conditions. Oral administration of polybrominated biphenyls enhanced the incidence of liver nodules induced by *N*-nitrosodiethylamine[2], but cutaneous application did not increase the incidence of skin tumours induced by 2-acetylaminofluorene[1].

C. Other relevant data

No data were available on the genetic and related effects of polybrominated biphenyls in humans.

Polybrominated biphenyls did not induce chromosomal aberrations in bone-marrow cells of rats or mice nor in rat spermatogonia and did not induce micronuclei in mice treated *in vivo*. They did not induce mutation in human or rodent cells *in vitro* or unscheduled DNA synthesis in rodent hepatocytes *in vitro*. Polybrominated biphenyls were not mutagenic to bacteria *in vitro* or in a host-mediated assay[3].

2,4,5,2′,4′,5′-Hexabromobiphenyl, 2,3,4,5,2′,4′,5′-heptabromobiphenyl and 2,3,4,5,2′,3′,4′,5′-octabromobiphenyl inhibited intercellular communication in Chinese hamster V79 cells; other congeners tested were only weakly active or were inactive[3].

References

[1] *IARC Monographs, 41*, 261-292, 1986

[2] Jensen, R.K. & Sleight, S.D. (1986) Sequential study on the synergistic effects of 2,2′,4,4′,5,5′-hexabromobiphenyl and 3,3′,4,4′,5,5′-hexabromobiphenyl on hepatic tumour promotion. *Carcinogenesis, 7*, 1771-1774

[3] *IARC Monographs, Suppl. 6*, 466-468, 1987

POLYCHLORINATED BIPHENYLS (Group 2A)

A. Evidence for carcinogenicity to humans (*limited*)

Information on the possible carcinogenic risk of human exposure to polychlorinated biphenyls (PCBs) comes from studies of occupational populations and of populations exposed to the compounds accidentally. PCB mixtures may be contaminated with polychlorinated dibenzofurans and polychlorinated dibenzodioxins (see, e.g., p. 350).

A slight increase in the incidence of cancer, particularly melanoma of the skin, was reported in a small group of men exposed to Aroclor 1254, a mixture of PCBs[1]. In a study of over 2500 US workers exposed to a similar mixture of PCBs during the manufacture of electrical capacitors, five deaths due to cancer of the liver and biliary passages were observed, whereas 1.9 would have been expected. This increase was sustained mainly by female workers in one of the two plants in the study (four of the five deaths), and all five workers had first been employed before the early 1950s[2,3]. Another study of workers in a capacitor plant was conducted in Italy. Exposure in the early years of production (until 1964) was to PCB mixtures containing 54% chlorine (mainly Aroclor 1254 and Pyralene 1476), which were later replaced by mixtures containing 42% chlorine (mainly Pyralene 3010 and 3011). Early results showed a significant excess of all cancers among male workers, which was due mainly to cancers of the digestive system and of the lymphatic and haematopoietic tissues. Among female workers, a slight increase in mortality from cancer of the lymphatic and haematopoietic tissues was reported[4]. The study was later enlarged and extended to include 2100 workers and to cover the period 1946-1982. Both male and female workers exhibited significantly increased cancer mortality in comparison with rates for the local population (14 observed, 7.6 expected; and 12 and 5.3, respectively, for men and women). Among male workers, cancers of the gastrointestinal tract (two stomach, two pancreas, one liver and one biliary passages) taken together were significantly increased (6 observed, 2.2 expected). Female workers showed a significant increase in deaths from haematological neoplasms (4 observed, 1.1 expected)[5]. In Sweden, among 142 male workers employed between 1965 and 1978 in a capacitor manufacturing plant when PCB mixtures containing up to 42% chlorine had been used, no significant excess of cancer deaths was noted. Cancer incidence was also examined: the number of cases observed corresponded well to that expected. One individual in a subgroup with higher exposure developed two relatively rare tumours, both of which occurred ten years after the start of exposure: a slow-growing mesenchymal tumour (desmoid) and a malignant lymphoma[6].

After contamination of cooking oil with a mixture of PCBs (Kanechlor 400) in Japan in 1968, a large population was intoxicated ('Yusho' disease). An early report on mortality from 1963-1983 showed a significantly increased risk of all cancers, and an almost five-fold significantly elevated risk of primary liver cancer. The edible rice oil had also been contaminated by polychlorinated quaterphenyls and polychlorinated dibenzofurans. Dose-response relationships were not clarified[7]. A further comprehensive study of 887 male 'Yusho' patients showed statistically significantly increased mortality from all malignancies (33 observed, 15.5 expected), from liver cancer (9 observed, 1.6 expected) and from lung cancer (8 observed, 2.5 expected). Use of local rather than national rates in calculating expected number of deaths decreased the observed:expected ratio for liver cancer from 5.6 to 3.9, which was still statistically significant. A closer look at the geographical distribution of liver cancer cases did not allow exclusion of factors other than PCB poisoning as a possible explanation for this finding. For the 874 female patients examined, none of the noted observed:expected ratios was significant[8]. In a series of ten autopsies of 'Yusho' patients, two adenocarcinomas of the liver were found, with no indication of a direct association with exposure to PCBs[9]. Ultrasonic and tumour marker examination of two series of 79 and 125 patients with 'Yusho' disease in 1983 and 1984, respectively, did not reveal any case of hepatic-cell carcinoma[10]. Two studies of the PCB content of fat tissues and cancer occurrence were available. An association was suggested between PCB concentrations in subcutaneous abdominal adipose tissue and the occurrence of cancers of the stomach, colon, pancreas, ovaries and prostate[11]. No indication emerged of a relationship between PCB content in extractable breast fat tissue and the occurrence of breast cancer[12].

The available studies suggest an association between cancer and exposure to PCBs. The increased risk from hepatobiliary cancer emerged consistently in different studies. Since, however, the numbers were small, dose-response relationships could not be evaluated, and the role of compounds other than PCBs could not be excluded, the evidence was considered to be limited.

B. Evidence for carcinogenicity to animals (*sufficient*)

Certain PCBs (particularly with greater than 50% chlorination) produced benign and malignant liver neoplasms in mice and rats after their oral administration[1,13,14]. Oral administration of Aroclor 1254 to rats yielded hepatocellular adenomas and carcinomas as well as intestinal metaplasia and a low, statistically nonsignificant incidence of stomach adenocarcinomas[15]. PCBs were inadequately tested in mice for induction of skin tumours[16,17]. In several studies, oral or intraperitoneal administration of PCBs enhanced the incidences of preneoplastic lesions[18-20] and of neoplasms[21,22] of the liver induced in rats by *N*-nitrosodiethylamine or 2-acetylaminofluorene. In one study, intragastric administration of PCBs to mice increased the incidence of lung tumours induced by intraperitoneal administration of *N*-nitrosodimethylamine[23].

C. Other relevant data

No data were available on the genetic and related effects of PCBs in humans.

Dominant lethal effects were not induced in rats administered PCBs orally, but were produced in rats nursed by females that had received PCBs orally. PCBs did not induce chromosomal aberrations in bone-marrow cells or spermatagonia of rats treated *in vivo*; micronuclei were not induced in bone-marrow cells of mice in one study, while equivocal results were obtained in a second study in which the PCBs were administered in corn oil. They did not transform Syrian hamster embryo cells *in vitro*. PCBs induced DNA strand breaks and unscheduled DNA synthesis in rat hepatocytes *in vitro*. Neither chromosomal breakage nor aneuploidy was induced in *Drosophila*. PCB mixtures did not induce SOS repair and were not mutagenic to bacteria[24].

2,2',5,5'-Tetrachlorobiphenyl induced DNA strand breaks in mouse cells *in vitro*. 2,4,5,2',4',5'-Hexachlorobiphenyl but not 3,4,5,3',4',5'-hexachlorobiphenyl inhibited intercellular communication in Chinese hamster V79 cells. Purified 2,4,2',4'-, 2,5,2',5'- and

3,4,3',4'-tetrachloro- and 2,4,6,2',4',6'-hexachlorobiphenyl were not mutagenic to bacteria[24].

References

[1]*IARC Monographs, 18*, 43-103, 1978

[2]Brown, D.P. & Jones, M. (1981) Mortality and industrial hygiene study of workers exposed to polychlorinated biphenyls. *Arch. environ. Health, 36*, 120-129

[3]Brown, D.P. (1987) Mortality of workers exposed to polychlorinated biphenyls. An update. *Arch. environ. Health* (in press)

[4]Bertazzi, P.A., Zocchetti, C., Guercilena, S., Della Foglia, M., Pesatori, A. & Riboldi, L. (1982) *Mortality study of male and female workers exposed to PCB's.* In: *Proceedings of the International Symposium on Prevention of Occupational Cancer, Helsinki, 1981*, Geneva, International Labour Office, pp. 242-248

[5]Bertazzi, P.A., Riboldi, L., Pesatori, A., Radice, L. & Zocchetti, C. (1987) Cancer mortality of capacitor manufacturing workers. *Am. J. ind. Med., 11*, 165-176

[6]Gustavsson, P., Hogstedt, C. & Rappe, C. (1986) Short-term mortality and cancer incidence in capacitor manufacturing workers exposed to polychlorinated biphenyls (PCBs). *Am. J. ind. Med., 10*, 341-344

[7]Umeda, G. (1984) *Studies on long-term effects of PCBs on human body: mortality from primary liver cancer and prevalence of ischemic heart disease* (Abstract No. 19.8). In: Eustace, I.E., ed., *Proceedings of the XXI International Congress on Occupational Health, Dublin, 1984*, p. 166

[8]Kuratsune, M., Nakamura, Y., Ikeda, M. & Hirohata, T. (1986) *Analysis of deaths seen among patients with Yusho* (Abstract FL17). In: *Dioxin 86. Proceedings of the VI International Symposium on Chlorinated Dioxins and Related Compounds, Fukuoka, Japan, 1986*, p. 179

[9]Kikuchi, M. (1984) Autopsy of patients with Yusho. *Am. J. ind. Med., 5*, 19-30

[10]Okumura, M. & Sakaguchi, S. (1985) Hepatic cell carcinoma and the patients with Yusho (Jpn.). *Fukuoka Igaku Zasshi, 76*, 229-232

[11]Unger, M., Olsen, J. & Clausen, J. (1982) Organochlorine compounds in the adipose tissue of deceased persons with and without cancer: a statistical survey of some potential confounders. *Environ. Res., 29*, 371-376

[12]Unger, M., Kiaer, H., Blichert-Toft, M., Olsen, J. & Clausen, J. (1984) Organochlorine compounds in human breast fat from deceased persons with and without breast cancer and in a biopsy material from newly diagnosed patients undergoing breast surgery. *Environ. Res., 34*, 24-28

[13]Norback, D.H. & Weltman, R.H. (1985) Polychlorinated biphenyl induction of hepatocellular carcinoma in the Sprague-Dawley rat. *Environ. Health Perspect., 60*, 97-105

[14]Schaeffer, E., Greim, H. & Goessner, W. (1984) Pathology of chronic polychlorinated biphenyl (PCB) feeding in rats. *Toxicol. appl. Pharmacol., 75*, 278-288

[15]Ward, J.M. (1985) Proliferative lesions of the glandular stomach and liver in F344 rats fed diets containing Aroclor 1254. *Environ. Health Perspect., 40*, 89-95

[16]DiGiovanni, J., Viaje, A., Berry, D.L., Slaga, T.J. & Juchau, M.R. (1977) Tumor-initiating ability of 2,3,7,8-tetrachlorodibenzo-*p*-dioxin (TCDD) and Aroclor 1254 in the two-stage system of mouse skin carcinogenesis. *Bull. environ. Contam. Toxicol., 18*, 552-557

[17]Hori, M., Fujita, K., Yamashiro, K., Toriyama, F., Hirose, R., Shukuwa, T., Toyoshima, H. & Yoshida, H. (1985) Methylcholanthrene induced mouse skin cancer. *Fukuoka Igaku Zasshi, 76*, 208-214

[18]Pereira, M.A., Herren, S.L., Britt, A.L. & Khoury, M.M. (1982) Promotion by polychlorinated biphenyls of enzyme-altered foci in rat liver. *Cancer Lett., 15*, 185-190

[19]Buchmann, A., Kunz, W., Wolf, C.R., Oesch, F. & Robertson, L.W. (1986) Polychlorinated biphenyls, classified as either phenobarbital- or 3-methylcholanthrene-type inducers of cytochrome *P*-450, are both hepatic tumor promoters in diethylnitrosamine-initiated rats. *Cancer Lett., 32*, 243-253

[20]Tatematsu, M., Nakanishi, K., Murasaki, G., Miyata, Y., Hirose, M. & Ito, N. (1979) Enhancing effect of inducers of liver microsomal enzymes on induction of hyperplastic liver nodules by *N*-2-fluorenylacetamine in rats. *J. natl Cancer Inst., 63*, 1411-1416

[21]Nishizumi, M. (1979) Effect of phenobarbital, dichlorodiphenyltrichloroethane, and polychlorinated biphenyls on diethylnitrosamine-induced hepatocarcinogenesis. *Gann, 70*, 835-837

[22]Preston, B.D., Van Miller, J.P., Moore, R.W. & Allen, J.R. (1981) Promoting effects of polychlorinated biphenyls (Aroclor 1254) and polychlorinated dibenzofuran-free Aroclor 1254 on diethylnitrosamine-induced tumorigenesis in the rat. *J. natl Cancer Inst., 66*, 509-515

[23]Anderson, L.M., Ward, J.M., Fox, S.D., Isaaq, H.J. & Riggs, C.W. (1986) Effects of a single dose of polychlorinated biphenyls to infant mice on *N*-nitrosodimethylamine-initiated lung and liver tumors. *Int. J. Cancer, 38*, 109-116

[24]*IARC Monographs, Suppl. 6*, 469-471, 1987

PREDNISONE (Group 3)

A. Evidence for carcinogenicity to humans (*inadequate*)

Many case reports of cancer include a mention of previous treatment with prednisone, as would be expected by chance alone in view of the very wide use of this drug in many different disorders. Prednisone is a common drug, prescribed for long periods in the treatment of many chronic conditions[1]. Patients treated with prednisone for rheumatoid arthritis appear to have, if anything, a lower than expected cancer risk. Over an average follow-up period of 12 years, 11% of 153 deaths that occurred in patients who had received prednisone were due to malignancies, compared to 20% of 74 deaths among patients who had not received prednisone[2]. The strong link between combination therapy for Hodgkin's disease and subsequent second malignancies (see summary of data on MOPP and other chemotherapy including alkylating agents, p. 254) is much more plausibly explained on the basis of concurrent administration of clearly carcinogenic agents than of prednisone.

A study of cancers that appeared within four years after documented use of common drugs showed that prednisone was among the 53 (of 95) drugs associated positively with cancer at least once. However, the excess consisted of 12 cases of lung cancer (31 observed, 19 expected), known to be largely related to cigarette smoking (which was not measured) and known to occur after a latent period much longer than the interval under observation.

Of more interest is the absence of those neoplasms, such as acute nonlymphocytic leukaemia and non-Hodgkin's lymphoma, which have been linked to chemotherapy and immuno-suppression[3].

Thus, the evidence for a carcinogenic action of prednisone was not compelling. The evidence did not, however 'suggest lack of carcinogenicity', because there is no well-designed analytical study of prednisone alone.

B. Evidence for carcinogenicity to animals (*inadequate*)

Prednisone was tested for carcinogenicity in mice and rats by intraperitoneal adminis-tration. A significant increase in the total number of tumours was reported in female rats, but the study suffered from limitations in both design and reporting[1].

C. Other relevant data

No data were available on the genetic and related effects of prednisone in humans. It did not induce chromosomal aberrations in bone-marrow cells of rats treated *in vivo*. It was not mutagenic to bacteria[4].

References

[1]*IARC Monographs*, 26, 293-309, 1981

[2]Fries, J.F., Bloch, D., Spitz, P. & Mitchell, D.M. (1985) Cancer in rheumatoid arthritis: a prospective long-term study of mortality. *Am. J. Med.*, 78 (*Suppl. 1A*), 56-59

[3]Friedman, G.D. & Ury, H.K. (1980) Initial screening for carcinogenicity of commonly used drugs. *J. natl Cancer Inst.*, 65, 723-733

[4]*IARC Monographs*, Suppl. 6, 472-473, 1987

PROCARBAZINE HYDROCHLORIDE (Group 2A)

A. Evidence for carcinogenicity to humans (*inadequate*)

No epidemiological study of procarbazine as a single agent was available to the Working Group. In various combinations with other chemotherapeutic agents, given for Hodgkin's disease, procarbazine use has repeatedly been shown to lead to the appearance of acute nonlymphocytic leukaemia. These combinations usually also include nitrogen mustard (see p. 269), an alkylating agent which is also a potent animal carcinogen, and these many observations do not permit conclusions about the independent effect of either drug[1].

B. Evidence for carcinogenicity to animals (*sufficient*)

Procarbazine hydrochloride administered by repeated intraperitoneal injections produced malignant tumours of the nervous system and haematopoietic system in mice and rats of each sex and adenocarcinomas of the mammary gland in rats only[1]. Repeated intravenous injections induced malignant tumours in different organs of rats[1]. Oral administration produced pulmonary tumours and leukaemias in mice[1,2] and mammary tumours in rats[1,3]. Leukaemias, haemangioendothelial sarcomas and osteogenic sarcomas were induced in rhesus, cynomolgus and African green monkeys of each sex by intraperitoneal, subcutaneous, intravenous or oral administration of procarbazine hydrochloride[1,4].

C. Other relevant data

Procarbazine generates an alkylating species[1].

No data were available on the genetic and related effects of procarbazine hydrochloride in humans.

Procarbazine gave positive results for germinal mutation in the mouse specific-locus test and caused mutation in the mouse spot test. It induced micronuclei and structural chromosomal aberrations in mice treated *in vivo*, but conflicting results were obtained in tests for dominant lethal mutations and negative results in the heritable-translocation test. It induced sister chromatid exchanges in mice and Chinese hamsters and caused DNA damage in rodents treated *in vivo*. Procarbazine did not transform Syrian hamster embryo cells. It induced mutation but not sister chromatid exchanges in rodent cells *in vitro*. It induced aneuploidy, dominant lethal mutations, sex-linked recessive lethal mutations and somatic mutation and recombination in *Drosophila*, but did not cause heritable translocations. It induced mutation, gene conversion and mitotic recombination in fungi. Conflicting results were obtained for mutation in bacteria, both *in vitro* and in host-mediated assays; it induced DNA damage in bacteria[5].

References

[1]*IARC Monographs*, 26, 311-339, 1981

[2]Bacci, M., Cavaliere, A. & Fratini, D. (1982) Lung carcinogenesis by procarbazine chlorate in BALB/c mice. *Carcinogenesis*, 3, 71-73

[3]Bacci, M., Cavaliere, A. & Amorosi, A. (1984) Procarbazine hydrochlorate carcinogenesis in Osborne-Mendel rats. *Oncology*, 41, 106-108

[4]Adamson, R.H. & Sieber, S.M. (1982) *Studies on the oncogenicity of procarbazine and other compounds in nonhuman primates.* In: Rosenberg, S. & Kaplan, H., eds, *Malignant Lymphomas: Etiology, Immunology, Pathology, Treatment* (*Bristol-Myers Cancer Symposia Series Vol. 3*), Orlando, FL, Academic Press, pp. 239-257

[5]*IARC Monographs*, Suppl. 6, 474-478, 1987

PROPYLENE OXIDE (Group 2A)

A. Evidence for carcinogenicity to humans (*inadequate*)

In a cohort study of 602 workers, some of whom were exposed to propylene oxide, as well as to ethylene oxide (see p. 205) and a mixture of other chemicals (including benzene [see p. 120] and ethylene chlorohydrin), there was no statistically significant excess of cancer deaths. The study is uninformative in relation to the carcinogenicity of propylene oxide[1].

B. Evidence for carcinogenicity to animals (*sufficient*)

Propylene oxide was tested by oral gavage in rats and produced local tumours, mainly squamous-cell carcinomas and papillomas of the forestomach[1]. When tested by inhalation in mice and in rats, it produced haemangiomas and haemangiosarcomas of the nasal submucosa in mice and an increased incidence of papillary adenomas of the nasal turbinates in rats[1,2]. In one experiment by inhalation in male rats, an increased incidence of adrenal pheochromocytomas and of peritoneal mesotheliomas was observed[1]. Propylene oxide was also tested by subcutaneous administration in mice, inducing local sarcomas, mainly fibrosarcomas[1].

C. Other relevant data

Propylene oxide is structurally related to ethylene oxide.

No data were available on the genetic effects of propylene oxide in humans. Haemoglobin alkylation was observed in exposed workers[3].

Propylene oxide induced micronuclei in mice but did not cause dominant lethal mutations in mice or rats exposed *in vivo*. It induced chromosomal aberrations in human cells *in vitro* and DNA strand breaks, mutation, sister chromatid exchanges and chromosomal aberrations in rodent cells *in vitro*. It induced sex-linked recessive lethal mutations in *Drosophila*, mutation in fungi and bacteria and DNA damage in bacteria[3].

References

[1]*IARC Monographs*, *36*, 227-243, 1985

[2]Renne, R.A., Giddens, W.E., Boorman, G.A., Kovatch, R., Haseman, J.E. & Clarke, W.J. (1986) Nasal cavity neoplasia in F344/N rats and (C57BL/6 × C3H)F$_1$ mice inhaling propylene oxide for up to two years. *J. natl Cancer Inst.*, *77*, 573-582

[3]*IARC Monographs*, *Suppl. 6*, 482-484, 1987

PROPYLTHIOURACIL (Group 2B)

A. Evidence for carcinogenicity to humans (*inadequate*)

In one survey of 331 hyperthyroid patients treated with antithyroid drugs, including propylthiouracil, and later with thyroidectomy, four thyroid cancers (an excess of unspecified proportion) were diagnosed more than one year after the beginning of drug therapy[1]. There has been one case report of acute myeloblastic leukaemia following propylthiouracil treatment[2].

B. Evidence for carcinogenicity to animals (*sufficient*)

Propylthiouracil produced thyroid tumours in mice, rats, hamsters and guinea-pigs and pituitary adenomas in mice after its oral administration[3]. When administered orally to rats with N-methyl-N-nitrosourea given intravenously[4] or N-nitrosobis(2-hydroxypropyl)-amine intraperitoneally[5], it induced malignant thyroid tumours.

C. Other relevant data

No adequate data were available to the Working Group.

References

[1]Dobyns, B.M., Sheline, G.E., Workman, J.B., Tompkins, E.A., McConahey, W.M. & Becker, D.V. (1974) Malignant and benign neoplasms of the thyroid in patients treated for hyperthyroidism: a report of the cooperative thyrotoxicosis therapy follow-up study. *J. clin. Endocrinol. Metab.*, *38*, 976-998

[2]Aksoy, M., Erdem, S., Tezel, H. & Tezel, T. (1974) Acute myeloblastic leukaemia after propylthiouracil. *Lancet*, *i*, 928-929

[3]*IARC Monographs*, *7*, 67-76, 1974

[4]Milmore, J.E., Chandrasekaran, V. & Weisburger, J.H. (1982) Effects of hypothyroidism on development of nitrosomethylurea-induced tumors of the mammary gland, thyroid gland, and other tissues. *Proc. Soc. exp. Biol. Med.*, *169*, 487-493

[5]Kitahori, Y., Hiasa, Y., Konishi, N., Enoki, N., Shimoyama, T. & Miyashiro, A. (1984) Effect of propylthiouracil on the thyroid tumorigenesis induced by N-bis(2-hydroxypropyl)nitrosamine in rats. *Carcinogenesis*, *5*, 657-660

RESERPINE (Group 3)

A. Evidence for carcinogenicity to humans (*inadequate*)

Sixteen case-control and three cohort studies on the relationship between reserpine and breast cancer were available to the Working Group[1-6]. Between and within studies, estimates of relative risk for different degrees of reserpine use varied from 0.6 to over 3. Many of the positive findings were not coherent with one another; and the studies considered to be most satisfactory methodologically showed little or no evidence of increased risk. However, a recent, large case-control study of breast screening participants showed that, although use of rauwolfia (reserpine) was not significantly associated with an overall increase in risk (odds ratio, 1.2; 95% confidence interval, 0.9-1.8), users for ten years or more had a risk ratio of 4.5 [2.3-11.6][7]. A study of prolactin levels in 15 women who had taken reserpine for five years or longer showed only 50% greater elevation of levels than in 15 women taking non-reserpine-containing medications and in 15 women taking no hypertensive medication. Elevated prolactin levels have been postulated as the mechanism for increased breast cancer risk following reserpine use, and the authors postulated that the increase in prolactin observed would probably cause only small increases in breast cancer risk[8].

B. Evidence for carcinogenicity to animals (*limited*)

Reserpine was tested for carcinogenicity in three experiments in mice by oral administration; in two experiments, it induced malignant mammary tumours in females, and in one experiment it induced carcinomas of the seminal vesicles in males[1,9]. It was tested in four experiments in rats by oral administration; in two, it increased the incidence of phaeochromocytomas[1,9]. An increase in tumour incidence was observed after repeated subcutaneous injections to mice and rats[9].

When reserpine was administered orally either prior to and concurrently with or following treatment with 3-methylcholanthrene, it had a protective effect against the induction of mammary tumours in rats[10]. Concurrent subcutaneous administration of reserpine reduced mammary tumour multiplicity and increased the percentage of well-differentiated tumours induced in rats by *N*-methyl-*N*-nitrosourea given intravenously[11]; its intravenous administration decreased skin tumour growth in 3-methylcholanthrene-treated mice[12].

C. Other relevant data

No data were available on the genetic and related effects of reserpine in humans.

Reserpine did not induce dominant lethal mutations in mice *in vivo*. In human cells *in vitro*, it did not induce chromosomal aberrations or sister chromatid exchanges. It did not induce chromosomal aberrations in cultured rodent cells or unscheduled DNA synthesis in rat hepatocytes. Reserpine was not mutagenic to bacteria[13].

References

[1]*IARC Monographs*, 24, 211-241, 1980

[2]Labarthe, D.R. & O'Fallon, W.M. (1980) Reserpine and breast cancer. A community-based longitudinal study of 2000 hypertensive women. *J. Am. med. Assoc.*, 243, 2304-2310

[3]Kewitz, H., Jesdinksy, H.-J., Kreutz, G. & Schulz, R. (1980) Reserpine and breast cancer. *Arch. int. Pharmacodynam. Ther., Suppl.*, 22-24

[4]Danielson, D.A., Jick, H., Hunter, J.R., Stergachis, A. & Madsen, S. (1982) Nonestrogenic drugs and breast cancer. *Am. J. Epidemiol.*, 116, 329-332

[5]Curb, J.D., Hardy, R.J., Labarthe, D.R., Borhani, N.O. & Taylor, J.O. (1982) Reserpine and breast cancer in the hypertension detection and follow-up program. *Hypertension*, 4, 307-311

[6]Horwitz, R.I. & Feinstein, A.R. (1985) Exclusion bias and the false relationship of reserpine and breast cancer. *Arch. intern. Med.*, 145, 1873-1875

[7]Stanford, J.L., Martin, E.J., Brinton, L.A. & Hoover, R.N. (1986) Rauwolfia use and breast cancer: a case-control study. *J. natl Cancer Inst.*, 76, 817-822

[8]Ross, R.K., Paganini-Hill, A., Krailo, M.D., Gerkins, V.R., Henderson, B.E. & Pike, M.C. (1984) Effects of reserpine on prolactin levels and incidence of breast cancer in postmenopausal women. *Cancer Res., 44*, 3106-3108

[9]Muradyan, R.Y. (1986) A study of possible carcinogenicity of reserpine (Russ.). *Vopr. Onkol., 32*, 76-81

[10]Gerard, S.S., Gardner, B., Patti, J., Husain, V., Shouten, J. & Alfonso, A.E. (1980) Effects of triiodothyronine and reserpine on induction and growth of mammary tumors in rats by 3-methylcholanthrene. *J. surg. Oncol., 14*, 213-218

[11]Verdeal, K., Ertürk, E. & Rose, D.P. (1983) Effects of reserpine administration on rat mammary tumors and uterine disease induced by *N*-nitrosomethylurea. *Eur. J. Cancer clin. Oncol., 19*, 825-834

[12]Lupulescu, A. (1983) Reserpine and carcinogenesis: inhibition of carcinoma formation in mice. *J. natl Cancer Inst., 71*, 1077-1083

[13]*IARC Monographs, Suppl. 6*, 485-487, 1987

THE RUBBER INDUSTRY (Group 1)

A. Evidence for carcinogenicity to humans (*sufficient*)

A large number of studies have been conducted on rubber industries in Canada, China, Finland, Norway, Sweden, Switzerland, the UK and the USA[1-19]. Workers employed in the industry before 1950 have a high risk of bladder cancer, probably associated with exposure to aromatic amines. Leukaemias have been associated with exposure to solvents and with employment in back processing, tyre curing, synthetic rubber production and vulcanization. Excess occurrence of lymphomas has been noted among workers exposed to solvents in such departments as footwear and in tyre plants[20]. Other cancers, including those of the lung, renal tract, stomach, pancreas, oesophagus, liver, skin, colon, larynx and brain, have been reported as occurring in excess in workers in various product areas and departments, but no consistent excess of any of these cancers is seen across the various studies.

B. Evidence for carcinogenicity to animals (*inadequate*)

In one inadequately reported experiment, three groups of rats were kept either in the compounding room or in the mixing or mastication area of a Banbury mill at a tyre factory. Increased incidences of respiratory and digestive carcinomas were found in rats maintained for two years at the latter two locations when compared with control rats maintained in the institute laboratory[17].

C. Other relevant data

No increase in the incidence of chromosomal aberrations was observed among 55 rubber workers as compared to 35 control subjects, with the exception of a small group of nonsmokers involved in weighing rubber chemicals. Increased frequencies of sister chromatid exchanges were observed both in smoking and nonsmoking weighers and in mixers who smoked, compared with unexposed controls; the frequency of sister chromatid exchanges in vulcanizers was not statistically significantly increased. Negative results for chromosomal aberrations and sister chromatid exchanges were also obtained in another study of vulcanizers[21].

Urine samples from 55 workers in two rubber factories and from 35 controls were analysed for mutagenicity in bacteria in the presence of an exogenous metabolic system. Mutagenic activity was observed in the urine of workers involved in weighing and mixing rubber components and in the urine of some vulcanizers. Similar results were reported in an extension of this study. No increase in bacterial mutagenicity was observed in urine samples from 72 tyre builders in a rubber factory and from 23 controls[21].

References

[1]*IARC Monographs, 28,* 1982

[2]Delzell, E. & Monson, R.R. (1981) Mortality among rubber workers. IV. General mortality patterns. *J. occup. Med., 23,* 850-856

[3]Delzell, E. & Monson, R.R. (1982) Mortality among rubber workers. V. Processing workers. *J. occup. Med., 24,* 539-545

[4]Delzell, E. & Monson, R.R. (1982) Mortality among rubber workers. VI. Men with potential exposure to acrylonitrile. *J. occup. Med., 24,* 767-769

[5]Delzell, E. & Monson, R.R. (1984) Mortality among rubber workers. VIII. Industrial products workers. *Am. J. ind. Med., 6,* 273-279

[6]Delzell, E. & Monson, R.R. (1985) Mortality among rubber workers. IX. Curing workers. *Am. J. ind. Med., 8,* 537-544

[7]Delzell, E. & Monson, R.R. (1985) Mortality among rubber workers. X. Reclaim workers. *Am. J. ind. Med., 7,* 307-313

[8]Delzell, E., Andjelkovich, D. & Tyroler, H.A. (1982) A case-control study of employment experience and lung cancer among rubber workers. *Am. J. ind. Med., 3,* 393-404

[9]Holmberg, B., Westerholm, P., Maasing, R., Kestrup, L., Gumaelius, K., Holmlund, L. & Englund, A. (1983) Retrospective cohort study of two plants in the Swedish rubber industry. *Scand. J. Work Environ. Health, 9 (Suppl. 2),* 59-68

[10]Holmes, T.M., Buffler, P.A., Holguin, A.H. & Hsi, B.P. (1986) A mortality study of employees at a synthetic rubber manufacturing plant. *Am. J. ind. Med., 9,* 355-362

[11]Kilpikari, I. (1982) Mortality among male rubber workers in Finland. *Arch. environ. Health, 37,* 295-299

[12]Kilpikari, I., Pukkala, E., Lehtonen, M. & Hakama, M. (1982) Cancer incidence among Finnish rubber workers. *Int. Arch. occup. environ. Health, 51,* 65-71

[13]Meinhardt, T.J., Lemen, R.A., Crandall, M.S. & Young, R.J. (1982) Environmental epidemiologic investigation of the styrene-butadiene rubber industry. *Scand. J. Work Environ. Health, 8,* 250-259

[14]Norell, S., Ahlbom, A., Lipping, H. & Österblom, L. (1983) Oesophageal cancer and vulcanisation work. *Lancet, i,* 462-463

[15]Norseth, T., Andersen, A. & Giltvedt, J. (1983) Cancer incidence in the rubber industry in Norway. *Scand. J. Work Environ. Health*, *9* (*Suppl. 2*), 69-71

[16]Wilcosky, T.C., Checkoway, H., Marshall, E.G. & Tyroler, H.A. (1984) Cancer mortality and solvent exposures in the rubber industry. *Am. ind. Hyg. Assoc. J.*, *45*, 809-811

[17]Wang, H.-W., You, X.-J., Qu, Y.-H., Wang, W.-F., Wang, D., Long, Y.-M. & Ni, J.A. (1984) Investigation of cancer epidemiology and study of carcinogenic agents in the Shanghai rubber industry. *Cancer Res.*, *44*, 3101-3105

[18]Arp, E.W., Jr, Wolf, P.H. & Checkoway, H. (1983) Lymphocytic leukemia and exposures to benzene and other solvents in the rubber industry. *J. occup. Med.*, *25*, 598-602

[19]Gustavsson, P., Hogstedt, C. & Holmberg, B. (1986) Mortality and incidence of cancer among Swedish rubber workers. *Scand. J. Work Environ. Health*, *12*, 538-544

[20]Veys, C. (1982) *The rubber industry: reflections on health risks.* In: Gardner, A.W., ed., *Current Approaches to Occupational Health*, Vol. 2, Bristol, Wright PSG, pp. 1-29

[21]*IARC Monographs*, *Suppl. 6*, 488, 1987

SACCHARIN (Group 2B)

A. Evidence for carcinogenicity to humans (*inadequate*)

The evidence that the risk of cancer is increased among users of artificial sweeteners is inconsistent[1]. Since the positive report of Howe *et al.*[2], reports have become available on seven case-control studies and on one population study of bladder cancer.

The largest was a population-based study in ten areas of the USA, with 3010 bladder cancer cases and 5783 controls. The relative risk for bladder cancer associated with use of artificial sweeteners was 1.0 (95% confidence interval, 0.9-1.1) among men and 1.1 (0.9-1.3) among women. Significant trends of increasing risk with increasing average daily consumption were found in certain subgroups examined *a priori* on the basis of the results of animal experiments; these subgroups were female nonsmokers and male heavy smokers[3]. Subsequent, independent re-analysis of the same data by a different statistical technique (multiple logistic regression) confirmed the original findings overall but cast doubt on the significance of the findings in the two subgroups because of inconsistent dose-response trends, especially among the male heavy smokers[4]. In response, the original investigators noted that the inconsistency derived from the development of risk scores which, in their opinion, were not correctly derived, as two relevant variables had been omitted[5]. In a subsequent report on data from one of the areas participating in this study, the use of hospital and population controls was compared. A higher proportion of hospital controls was found to have used artificial sweeteners than population controls[6]. This had been postulated earlier[2] as a possible reason for the negative findings of a hospital-based case-control study[7]. Bias resulting from use of prevalent rather than incident cases[8] has been suggested as a possible reason for the negative findings of another hospital-based case-control study[9].

Three other case-control studies have also shown increased risks among subgroups. In one, conducted simultaneously in Japan, the UK and the USA, the relative risks among women in the US component of the study associated with 'any' use of diet drinks and of sugar substitutes were 1.6 and 1.5, respectively, and 2.6 and 2.1, respectively, for nonsmokers[10]. In the other two areas, however, a history of the use of sugar substitutes, primarily saccharin, was not associated with an elevated bladder cancer risk[11]. In a second study, conducted in West Yorkshire, UK, elevated risks were found for saccharin takers who were nonsmokers. In men, the relative risk was 2.2 (95% confidence interval, 1.3-3.8); that in women was 1.6 (0.8-3.2)[12]. In a third study, conducted in a rural district of Denmark, a relative risk of 2.5 (1.0-6.6) was reported for saccharin consumption in men and women combined. This risk was not reduced after controlling for tobacco use and industrial work[13].

Two studies in Denmark[14,15], one in the USA[16] and a further case-control study in Canada[17], however, gave negative results. In one of the Danish studies, incidence of bladder cancer at ages 20-34 among people born 1941-1945 (when use of saccharin was high in Denmark) was compared with that among those born 1931-1940. The risk for men was 1.0 (0.7-1.6) and that for women, 0.3 (0.1-1.0). This study indirectly assessed intrauterine exposure to saccharin[14]. The other two studies were population-based case-control studies of bladder cancer. In Denmark, the relative risk for people of each sex combined was 0.8 (0.6-1.1)[15]. In a study in the USA of bladder cancer in women aged 20-49, the odds ratio for regular use of artificially sweetened beverages, table-top sweetener or both was 1.1 (0.7-1.7)[16]. In Canada, the odds ratio for use of saccharin was 1.0 (0.9-1.2) in men and 1.0 (0.8-1.2) in women[17]. The increased risks seen in subgroups in other studies were not replicated in either study.

In the USA, in a study of 1862 patients hospitalized for cancer and of 10 874 control patients, a greater proportion of artificial sweetener users was found only among women with cancer of the stomach. Little information was available on urinary-tract cancer. No overall association was found between artificial sweetener use and cancer[18].

B. Evidence for carcinogenicity to animals (*sufficient*)

Saccharin (unspecified or commercial) has been tested for carcinogenicity by oral administration to mice, rats and hamsters. In mice, saccharin produced no difference in tumour incidence between treated and control animals in one single- and in one multi-generation study. Two further studies by oral administration in mice and three in rats were considered to be inadequate for evaluation. A study in hamsters by oral administration and one study in mice by skin application could not be evaluated. A study in mice by bladder insertion provided evidence for the induction of bladder carcinomas[1]. Oral administration to mice produced thyroid tumours[19].

Sodium saccharin has been tested for carcinogenicity by oral administration to mice, rats and monkeys. One study in mice was inadequate for evaluation[1]. One single-generation study in rats showed an increased incidence of bladder tumours in males; two further studies showed a few bladder tumours; another study showed no difference in tumour incidence between treated and control animals; and two others were inadequate for evaluation[1]. In four two-generation studies in rats, sodium saccharin produced a statistically significant increase in the incidence of bladder tumours in F_1 males fed either 5% or 7.5% sodium saccharin[1,20]. In a further two-generation study of rats, a dose-related increase in the incidences of benign, malignant and/or combined bladder neoplasms was observed in males treated with doses ranging from 4-7.5% in the diet, while no tumorigenic effect was observed with 1%[21,22]. Transplacental exposure of rats to sodium saccharin and to saccharin (commercial) did not produce any treatment-related neoplasm[21,23]. Sodium saccharin has also been tested in mice by bladder insertion: it increased the incidence of bladder carcinomas. Experiments in which it was tested by oral administration to monkeys and by intraperitoneal administration to mice were considered to be inadequate for evaluation[1].

The combination of sodium saccharin with sodium cyclamate in a ratio of 1:10 has been tested by oral administration in a multigeneration experiment in mice and in single experiments in rats. In one study in rats, transitional-cell carcinomas in the bladder were produced in male animals given the highest dose; in two further studies in rats and in the study in mice, there was no difference in tumour incidence between treated and control animals[1,24]. Another study in rats was inadequate for evaluation[1].

Pretreatment with a single instillation into the bladder of a low dose of N-methyl-N-nitrosourea or feeding of N-[4-(5-nitro-2-furyl)-2-thiazolyl]formamide and subsequent oral administration of sodium saccharin for long periods increased the incidence of bladder neoplasms in rats over that induced by the nitrosourea or the amide alone[1]. Simultaneous administration of N-nitroso-N-(4-hydroxybutyl)butylamine and sodium saccharin significantly enhanced the induction of bladder papillomas over that seen after treatment with the nitrosamine alone[25]. Commercial saccharin preparations enhanced lung tumour induction in mice when given before or during intraperitoneal administration of urethane[26]. In rats, oral administration of sodium saccharin significantly increased the incidence of bladder neoplasms induced by ulceration of bladder mucosa[27,28]. Other studies of simultaneous or consecutive treatment with saccharin and known carcinogens were inadequate for evaluation[1].

ortho-Toluenesulphonamide was tested for carcinogenicity by oral administration in rats in a two-generation study: no increase in bladder tumour incidence was noted in animals of either generation. In one of two single-generation studies in rats, benign and malignant bladder tumours were found[1].

C. Other relevant data

No data were available on the genetic and related effects of saccharin, sodium saccharin or ortho-toluenesulphonamide in humans[29].

It should be noted that many studies do not differentiate between saccharin ('insoluble' form) and sodium saccharin. Additionally, when it is reported that 'saccharin' (presumably sodium saccharin) causes a positive response, primarily in assays for chromosomal effects, the effect is seen only with very high concentrations, at which simple salts also give responses[29].

Treatment of mice with saccharin did not induce micronuclei or chromosomal aberrations in bone-marrow cells or spermatocytes; conflicting results were obtained for the induction of dominant lethal mutations. A commercial preparation (of unknown purity) caused somatic mutations in the mouse spot test. Injection of radioactive saccharin into rats revealed no DNA binding in the liver or bladder, nor did treatment of rats result in DNA damage in bladder tissue. Saccharin did not induce sister chromatid exchanges in cultured human lymphocytes. Negative results were obtained in assays for transformation in cultured rodent cells, but saccharin enhanced transformation of virus-infected rat embryo cells and of C3H 10T1/2 mouse embryo cells initiated with 3-methylcholanthrene in two-state transformation assays. Results obtained with rodent cell systems were inconclusive with regard to inhibition of intercellular communication. It caused DNA strand breaks in rat hepatocytes but no chromosomal aberration in Chinese hamster cells. Saccharin induced aneuploidy but not recombination or gene conversion in yeast. It was not mutagenic and did not induce prophage in bacteria[29].

Treatment of mice with sodium saccharin did not induce micronuclei, somatic mutations (in the spot test) or sperm abnormalities. Treatment of Chinese hamsters did not induce chromosomal aberrations in bone-marrow cells or spermatogonia but induced sister chromatid exchanges in bone-marrow cells. Treatment of mice with commercial sodium saccharin resulted in the induction of dominant lethal mutations, but treatment with a preparation 'purified' by undefined criteria did not. Sodium saccharin induced chromosomal aberrations and sister chromatid exchanges in cultured human lymphocytes and induced sister chromatid exchanges and chromosomal aberrations in cultured Chinese hamster cells but no mutation in mouse lymphoma cells. It did not induce transformation of BALB/c 3T3 cells. Contradictory results have been reported concerning the ability of sodium saccharin to induce sex-linked recessive lethal mutations in *Drosophila*, and it did not cause a significant increase in heritable translocations. Sodium saccharin induced mutation, gene conversion and recombination in yeast, but was not mutagenic to bacteria[29].

ortho-Toluenesulphonamide did not induce micronuclei or somatic mutation (in the spot test) in mice treated *in vivo*. Contradictory results have been obtained for the induction of sex-linked recessive lethal mutations in *Drosophila*. It was not mutagenic to bacteria[29].

References

[1] *IARC Monographs*, *22*, 55-109, 171-185, 1980

[2] Howe, G.R., Burch, J.D., Miller, A.B., Cook, G.M., Estève, J., Morrison, B., Gordon, P., Chambers, L.W., Fodor, G. & Winsor, G.M. (1980) Tobacco use, occupation, coffee, various nutrients and bladder cancer. *J. natl Cancer Inst.*, *64*, 701-713

[3] Hoover, R.M. & Strasser, P.H. (1980) Artificial sweeteners and human bladder cancer. Preliminary results. *Lancet*, *i*, 837-840

[4] Walker, A.M., Dreyer, N.A., Friedlander, E., Loughlin, J., Rothman, K.J. & Kohn, H.I. (1982) An independent analysis of the National Cancer Institute study on non-nutritive sweeteners and bladder cancer. *Am. J. public. Health*, *72*, 376-381

[5]Hoover, R. & Hartge, P. (1982) Non-nutritive sweeteners and bladder cancer. *Am. J. public Health,* *72*, 382-383

[6]Silverman, D.T., Hoover, R.N. & Swanson, G.M. (1983) Artificial sweeteners and lower urinary tract cancer: hospital vs. population controls. *Am. J. Epidemiol., 117*, 326-334

[7]Wynder, E.L. & Stellman, S.D. (1980) Artificial sweetener use and bladder cancer: a case-control study. *Science, 207*, 1214-1216

[8]Goldsmith, D.F. (1982) Calculation of potential bias in the odds ratio illustrated by a study of saccharin use and bladder cancer. *Environ. Res., 27*, 298-306

[9]Kessler, I.I. & Clark, J.P. (1978) Saccharin, cyclamate, and human bladder cancer. No evidence of an association. *J. Am. med. Assoc., 240*, 349-355

[10]Morrison, A.S. & Buring, J.E. (1980) Artificial sweeteners and cancer of the lower urinary tract. *New Engl. J. Med., 302*, 537-541

[11]Morrison, A.S., Verhoek, W.G., Leck, I., Aoki, K., Ohno, Y. & Obata, K. (1982) Artificial sweeteners and bladder cancer in Manchester, UK, and Nagoya, Japan. *Br. J. Cancer, 45*, 332-336

[12]Cartwright, R.A., Adib, R., Glashan, R. & Gray, B.K. (1981) The epidemiology of bladder cancer in West Yorkshire. A preliminary report on non-occupational aetiologies. *Carcinogenesis, 2*, 343-347

[13]Mommsen, S., Aagaard, J. & Sell, A. (1983) An epidemiological study of bladder cancer in a predominantly rural district. *Scand. J. Urol. Nephrol., 17*, 307-312

[14]Jensen, O.M. & Kamby, C. (1982) Intra-uterine exposure to saccharin and risk of bladder cancer in man. *Int. J. Cancer, 29*, 507-509

[15]Møller-Jensen, O., Knudsen, J.B., Sørensen, B.L. & Clemmesen, J. (1983) Artificial sweeteners and absence of bladder cancer risk in Copenhagen. *Int. J. Cancer, 32*, 577-582

[16]Piper, J.M., Matanoski, G.M. & Tonascia, J. (1986) Bladder cancer in young women. *Am. J. Epidemiol., 123*, 1033-1042

[17]Risch, H.A., Burch, J.D., Miller, A.B., Hill, G.B., Steele, R. & Howe, G.R. (1987) Dietary factors and the incidence of cancer of the urinary bladder. *Am. J. Epidemiol.* (in press)

[18]Morrison, A.S. (1979) Use of artificial sweeteners by cancer patients. *J. natl Cancer Inst., 62*, 1397-1399

[19]Prasad, O. & Rai, G. (1986) Induction of papillary adenocarcinoma of thyroid in albino mice by saccharin feeding. *Indian J. exp. Biol., 24*, 197-199

[20]Taylor, J.M., Weinberger, M.A. & Friedman, L. (1980) Chronic toxicity and carcinogenicity to the urinary bladder of sodium saccharin in the in utero-exposed rat. *Toxicol. appl. Pharmacol., 54*, 57-75

[21]Schoenig, G.P., Goldenthal, E.I., Geil, R.G., Frith, C.H., Richter, W.R. & Carlborg, F.W. (1985) Evaluation of the dose response and in utero exposure to saccharin in the rat. *Food chem. Toxicol., 23*, 475-490

[22]Squire, R.A. (1985) Histopathological evaluation of rat urinary bladders from the IRDC two-generation bioassay of sodium saccharin. *Food chem. Toxicol., 23*, 491-497

[23]Schmähl, D. & Habs, M. (1980) Absence of a carcinogenic response to cyclamate and saccharin in Sprague-Dawley rats after transplacental application. *Arzneimittelforschung, 30*, 1905-1906

[24]Schmähl, D. & Habs, M. (1984) Investigations on the carcinogenicity of the artificial sweeteners sodium cyclamate and sodium saccharin in rats in a two-generation experiment. *Arzneimittelforschung, 34,* 604-606

[25]Nakanishi, K., Hirose, M., Ogiso, T., Hasegawa, R., Arai, M. & Ito, N. (1980) Effects of sodium saccharin and caffeine on the urinary bladder of rats treated with *N*-butyl-*N*-(4-hydroxybutyl)-nitrosamine. *Gann, 71,* 490-500

[26]Theiss, J.C., Arnold, L.J. & Shimkin, M.B. (1980) Effect of commercial saccharin preparations on urethan-induced lung tumorigenesis in strain A mice. *Cancer Res., 40,* 4322-4324

[27]Cohen, S.M., Murasaki, G., Fukushima, S. & Greenfield, R.E. (1982) Effect of regenerative hyperplasia on the urinary bladder: carcinogenicity of sodium saccharin and *N*-[4-(5-nitro-2-furyl)-2-thiazolyl]formamide. *Cancer Res., 42,* 65-71

[28]Hasegawa, R., Greenfield, R.E., Murasaki, G., Suzuki, T. & Cohen, S.M. (1985) Initiation of urinary bladder carcinogenesis in rats by freeze ulceration with sodium saccharin promotion. *Cancer Res., 45,* 1469-1473

[29]*IARC Monographs, Suppl. 6,* 488-493, 520-522, 1987

SHALE-OILS (Group 1)

A. Evidence for carcinogenicity to humans (*sufficient*)

The association between shale-oils and skin cancers, particularly of the scrotum, was demonstrated by analyses of 65 cases of skin cancer, including 31 of the scrotum, from the Scottish shale-oil industry. In the UK, over 2000 cases of skin cancer ('mule-spinners' cancer') were recorded among cotton-textile workers and others exposed to lubricating oils (many of which are believed to have been shale-derived). The occupational etiology of these cases is supported by occupational mortality statistics for the UK and by an occupational comparison with fatal cases of penile cancer. In contrast, one study showed very few scrotal cancers among US cotton-textile workers employed in mills where shale-derived lubricants were not used. A cohort study of shale-oil workers in western USA showed statistically significant excesses of all cancers and of colon cancer, although data on duration and time since first exposure were not available. A cohort study of shale-oil workers in Estonia showed a significant excess of skin cancer but not of cancers at other sites[1]. A follow-up of 6064 men who had worked in the Scottish oil-shale industry between 1950 and 1962 showed a significant excess of skin cancer[2]. A case-control study of lung cancer in the shale area showed no association with work in the shale industry[2].

Two basal- and two squamous-cell carcinomas were found among 325 workers employed at an oil-shale demonstration facility during 1948-1969 in Utah, USA. The incidence was about that expected[3].

B. Evidence for carcinogenicity to animals (*sufficient*)

Inhalation of either raw oil shale or spent oil shale produced lung tumours in rats. Application of an extract of spent oil shale produced skin tumours in mice[1].

Skin application of crude oils from both low- and high-temperature retorting induced skin tumours in mice and rabbits; the high-temperature retorted oils had greater carcinogenic activity. A low-temperature crude oil produced lung tumours in mice after intratracheal instillation[1].

Various fractions of shale-oils were carcinogenic when applied to the skin of mice and rabbits[1].

Shale-oil distillates, residues, blends and commercial products of the oil-shale industry were tested in mice by skin application, producing skin tumours. Distillation fractions from less highly refined shale-oils were more carcinogenic than the more highly refined products[1].

C. Other relevant data

No data were available on the genetic and related effects of shale-oils in humans.

All shale-derived materials assayed in tests for genetic and related effects came from sources in the USA and were therefore all produced by low-temperature processes[4].

Chromosomal aberrations were induced in bone-marrow cells of rats following administration by gavage of a suspension of raw oil-shale. In-vitro tests of extracts of raw oil-shale in cultured rodent cells, yeast and bacteria gave negative results[4].

Preparations of spent oil-shale yielded negative results in an assay for chromosomal aberrations *in vivo* and in mutation assays with eukaryotic cells *in vitro*; contradictory results were obtained in bacterial mutation assays[4].

Preparations of shale-derived crude oils from various sources and retort processes gave both positive and negative results in assays for chromosomal effects in rodents *in vivo*. Two crude shale-oil preparations induced sister chromatid exchanges in cultured human lymphocytes; three others did not induce mitotic gene conversion in yeast. Shale-derived crude oils were mutagenic to cultured rodent cells, yeast and bacteria following metabolic or photoinduced activation[4].

As compared with the corresponding crude shale-oils, preparations of hydrotreated oils showed less activity or gave negative results in various short-term tests[4].

Oil-shale retort process-waters induced chromosomal aberrations, but not sister chromatid exchanges, in cells of mice treated *in vivo*, chromosomal aberrations in cultured rodent cells and mutation and DNA damage in cultured rodent cells and bacteria following metabolic activation or photoactivation[4].

Extracts of oil-shale ash were not mutagenic to fungi but were mutagenic to bacteria in the absence of a metabolic system[4].

References

[1]*IARC Monographs*, 35, 161-217, 243-247, 1985

[2]Miller, B.G., Cowie, H.A., Middleton, W.G. & Seaton, A. (1986) Epidemiologic studies of Scottish oil shale workers. III. Causes of death. *Am. J. ind. Med.*, 9, 433-446

[3]Rom, W.N., Krueger, G., Zone, J., Attfield, M.D., Costello, J., Burkart, J. & Turner, E.R. (1985) Morbidity survey of US oil shale workers employed during 1948-1969. *Arch. environ. Health*, *40*, 58-62

[4]*IARC Monographs, Suppl. 6*, 494, 1987

SILICA:
CRYSTALLINE SILICA (Group 2A)
AMORPHOUS SILICA (Group 3)

A. Evidence for carcinogenicity to humans (*limited* for crystalline silica; *inadequate* for amorphous silica)

A number of studies have shown that persons diagnosed as having silicosis after occupational exposure to dust containing crystalline silica have an increased risk for dying from lung cancer[1,2]. This increase has been seen among miners, quarry workers, foundry workers, ceramic workers, granite workers and stone cutters.

Workers in the granite industry have shown increased risks for lung cancer in some studies; the excesses were of the order of 10-30% and were not usually statistically significant[1]. An extended follow-up of Finnish granite workers showed 22 lung cancer cases, with 17.1 expected. When allowing for a latency of 15 years, 21 cases were observed, whereas nine were expected ($p < 0.01$; Poisson distribution). Smoking habits were similar to those of the active Finnish male population, and exposures to radon and asbestos were considered unlikely to have occurred[3]. A recent joint Nordic register linkage study, combining lung cancer mortality and incidence data from the cancer registries with census-based records on previous occupation of 20-64-year-old males, showed an elevated risk of lung cancer among stone cutters in Finland and Denmark, but not in Sweden or Norway. Excess risk was also seen for Finnish males in excavation work, whereas no such risk was evident in the other countries[4].

Three epidemiological studies of workers in the ceramics, glass and refractory brick industries, using different designs, have shown a roughly two-fold increase in mortality from lung cancer. Only one case-referent study took smoking into account[1]. The Nordic register study also found an excess of lung cancer for Danish glass-workers, but workers in the ceramics industry did not have an elevated risk in any of the countries[4]. A US cohort study of pottery workers exposed to silica and talc showed a nonsignificant standardized mortality ratio of 137 for workers exposed to high levels of silica dust with no talc exposure[5].

Several studies of metal miners have shown mortality rates from lung cancer some 20-50% higher than expected[1]. In the Nordic register study[4], relative risks from 1.0 (Norwegian metal miners) to 5.0 (Finnish nonferrous ore miners) were seen. The largest group was Swedish iron ore miners; their relative risk was 3.2 (95% confidence interval, 2.9-3.5), based on 124 observed cases. However, in repeated cohort studies of workers in a gold mine, no excess lung cancer risk was seen[1,6]. The contribution of radon has not in general been assessed.

Coal miners appear not to be at increased risk of lung cancer[1].

Studies of foundry workers (see p. 224) have consistently shown moderate increases in mortality from lung cancer[1,7]. The Nordic register study also showed lung cancer risk to be elevated for foundry workers in all Nordic countries[4]. However, several contaminants other than silica dust occur in the foundry environment, including polycyclic aromatic hydrocarbons.

Epidemiological studies of both exposed populations and silicotics give indications of the carcinogenicity of a working environment contaminated with crystalline silica, particularly in combination with other exposures. In most industries studied, such an effect cannot be separated from those of other concomitant carcinogenic exposures, but in the granite and stone industry the exposure to silica is fairly pure. Few studies provide data on smoking. It is not clear whether the mechanisms of a possible carcinogenic effect of crystalline silica requires a fibrotic process.

No adequate epidemiological study or case report was available to evaluate the carcinogenicity of amorphous silica to humans.

B. Evidence for carcinogenicity to animals (*sufficient* for crystalline silica; *inadequate* for amorphous silica)

Various forms and preparations of crystalline silica produced adenocarcinomas and squamous-cell carcinomas of the lung in rats after inhalation or repeated intratracheal instillation. Thoracic and abdominal malignant lymphomas developed in rats after single intrapleural and intraperitoneal injections of suspensions of several types of quartz. Malignant lymphomas developed after intrapleural injection of cristobalite and tridymite. No tumorigenic response was observed in hamsters after repeated intratracheal instillation of quartz dusts or in a mouse-lung adenoma assay with one sample of quartz[1].

Tests of different preparations of amorphous silica administered by various routes to mice and rats either gave negative results or were inadequate. In two limited tests (one by intraperitoneal injection and one by inhalation) in mice, increased incidences of lymphosarcomas in the abdominal cavity and of lung tumours, respectively, were observed[1].

C. Other relevant data

No data were available on the genetic and related effects of silica in humans.

Quartz did not induce micronuclei in mice treated *in vivo*. In Syrian hamster embryo cells *in vitro*, it induced cell transformation and micronuclei; it did not induce sister chromatid exchanges in Chinese hamster cells. Quartz did not inhibit intercellular communication in Chinese hamster cells *in vitro*. Silica was not mutagenic to bacteria[8].

References

[1]*IARC Monographs*, *42*, 39-143, 1987

[2]Zambon, P., Simonato, L., Mastrangelo, G., Winkelmann, R., Saia, B. & Crepet, M. (1987) Mortality of workers compensated for silicosis during the period 1959-1963 in the Veneto region of Italy. *Scand. J. Work Environ. Health*, *13*, 118-123

[3]Koskela, R.-S., Klockars, M., Järvinen, E., Kolari, P.J. & Rossi, A. (1987) Cancer mortality of granite workers. *Scand. J. Work Environ. Health*, *13*, 26-31

[4]Lynge, E., Kurppa, K., Kristofersen, L., Malker, H. & Sauli, H. (1986) Silica dust and lung cancer: results from the Nordic occupational mortality and cancer incidence registers. *J. natl Cancer Inst.*, *77*, 883-889

[5]Thomas, T.L. & Stewart, P.A. (1987) Mortality from lung cancer and respiratory disease among pottery workers exposed to silica and talc. *Am. J. Epidemiol.*, *125*, 35-43

[6]Hessel, P.A., Sluis-Cremer, G.K. & Hnizdo, E. (1986) Case-control study of silicosis, silica exposure, and lung cancer in white South African gold miners. *Am. J. ind. Med.*, *10*, 57-62

[7]*IARC Monographs*, *34*, 133-190, 1984

[8]*IARC Monographs*, *Suppl. 6*, 494-496, 1987

SOOTS (Group 1)

A. Evidence for carcinogenicity to humans (*sufficient*)

The carcinogenicity of soot is demonstrated by numerous case reports, dating back over 200 years, of skin cancer, particularly of the scrotum, among chimney-sweeps. More recent cohort studies of mortality among chimney-sweeps in Sweden and Denmark have shown a significantly increased risk of lung cancer. Supporting evidence for an association with lung cancer was provided by two earlier epidemiological studies in the German Democratic Republic and the UK. The potentially confounding and interactive effects of smoking could not be evaluated; however, cigarette smoking is not believed to have seriously biased these estimates. In addition to lung cancer, statistically significant excess mortality from oesophageal cancer, primary liver cancer and leukaemia was found among chimney-sweeps in one study[1].

B. Evidence for carcinogenicity to animals (*inadequate* for soots; *sufficient* for soot extracts)

Coal soot was tested in two experiments in mice by whole-body exposure, but the studies were inadequate for evaluation. Coal-soot extracts applied to the skin of mice produced skin tumours in two studies. A wood-soot extract applied to the skin of mice was inadequately tested. In limited studies, subcutaneous implants of wood soot in female rats produced a few local sarcomas; similar implants in the scrotal sac of rats did not. An extract of fuel-oil soot was inadequately tested by application to the skin of mice. Extracts of soot from the combustion of oil shale produced skin tumours in mice after dermal application and lung tumours in rats after intratracheal instillation. Extracts of soot from the combustion of a heating oil produced from shale-oil produced skin tumours in mice in two experiments when applied to the skin[1].

C. Other relevant data

No data were available on the genetic and related effects of soots in humans.

Extracts of soot samples from domestic sources were mutagenic to *Salmonella typhimurium* both in the presence and absence of an exogenous metabolic system. Extracts of experimentally-derived soots were mutagenic in forward mutation assays in *S. typhimurium* and in cultured human lymphoblasts in the presence of an exogenous metabolic system. Extracts of particulate emissions from wood combustion were shown to induce sister chromatid exchanges in Chinese hamster ovary cells, transformation of Syrian hamster embryo cells and mutation in *S. typhimurium*. An experimentally-derived, intact particulate soot and an extract of this material were mutagenic in a human lymphoblastoid cell line[2].

References

[1]*IARC Monographs*, *35*, 219-246, 1985

[2]*IARC Monographs*, *Suppl. 6*, 497, 1987

SPIRONOLACTONE (Group 3)

A. Evidence for carcinogenicity to humans (*inadequate*)

Cases of breast cancer have been reported in women who had used spironolactone. Four analytical studies, however, showed no consistent evidence of an association[1].

B. Evidence for carcinogenicity to animals (*limited*)

Spironolactone was tested for carcinogenicity by oral administration in two experiments in rats. Increased incidences of thyroid and testicular tumours were reported in one experiment but not in another experiment of longer duration with lower doses[1].

C. Other relevant data

No data were available to the Working Group.

Reference

[1]*IARC Monographs*, *24*, 259-273, 1980

STYRENE (Group 2B)

A. Evidence for carcinogenicity to humans (*inadequate*)

Three studies have suggested an association between leukaemia and lymphomas and exposure to styrene. In a mortality analysis of 2904 US workers exposed to low or moderate levels of styrene (not exceeding 100 ppm [420 mg/m³]), six cases of leukaemia (3.4 expected; standardized mortality ratio [SMR], 176) and seven cases of lymphoma (5.3 expected; SMR, 132) were observed. When the incidence was analysed, seven cases of lymphatic leukaemia (1.6 expected), four cases of all other leukaemias (2.9 expected) and four cases of multiple myeloma (1.6 expected) were found. However, six of the leukaemia cases occurred in a group with concomitant exposure to colourants; moreover, a subset of the cohort had also been exposed to benzene in the past[1].

In a cohort study of 622 men exposed for at least one year in the production, polymerization and processing of styrene in the UK, three deaths from non-Hodgkin's lymphoma were found (0.6 expected; $P_u = 0.02$, upper tail). Two of them occurred in the age group 15-44 years (0.3 expected; $P_u = 0.032$). A cancer incidence study of the same group revealed a further case of lymphatic leukaemia (0.2 expected), and three cases of laryngeal cancer (0.5 expected; $p = 0.041$). Two of the men were under 45 years of age (0.1 expected). The men with lymphoma and leukaemia had had potential exposure to other agents, i.e., acrylonitrile (see p. 79), benzene (see p. 120), ethylene oxide (see p. 205) and dyestuffs, but styrene was the main agent to which they were exposed[2].

A slight excess of cancers of the lymphatic and haematopoietic tissues (SMR, 155; not significant) was found in a US cohort of 1662 men employed for at least six months in styrene-butadiene rubber production. A subset of workers employed in the early 1940s had an SMR of 212 (9 observed, 4.3 expected; $p < 0.05$); for leukaemias alone, the SMR was 278 (5 observed, 1.8 expected; $p < 0.05$). In another plant where exposure to styrene had been about twice as high, no such excess was seen. The mean levels of exposure to styrene had, according to measurements carried out at the end of follow-up, been approximately 1-2 ppm (4.2-8.4 mg/m³); however, this level was probably not representative of that during the whole period. Concomitant exposure to 1,3-butadiene (see p. 136) and to low levels of benzene renders it difficult to single out styrene or any other agent as the causative factor[3].

A UK cohort study of 7949 men and women employed during 1947-1984 in eight companies manufacturing glass-reinforced plastics involving high exposure to styrene showed no excess mortality from cancer (181 observed, 223.7 expected). There was a deficit of deaths from lymphoid and haematopoietic cancer (6 observed, 14.9 expected). Only one death from lymphoma and none from leukaemia was found among 3494 workers with the highest exposure. An additional eight cases of lymphoma and leukaemia occurred in workers still alive or who had died from other causes. A small excess of lung cancer (89 observed, 80.1 expected) was not statistically significant. Analysis by level of exposure gave some indication of a dose-response relationship, but there was no clear relationship with time since first exposure. Concomitant exposure to asbestos could not explain the findings.

Smoking habits were not controlled for, but a low mortality from respiratory and cardiovascular diseases suggests that smoking rates were not excessively high[4].

Two cohort studies showed no excess of lymphoma or leukaemia, or of any other cancer. Both studies had low statistical power because the cohorts had a young age structure and there had been short follow-up since the commencement of exposure; they will provide useful information only when updated[5,6].

Two other studies are uninformative because of diluting errors in design and analysis[7,8]. There is an anecdotal report of three deaths from leukaemia and two from lymphoma among a group of workers exposed to styrene, benzene and butadiene, but the study population was ill-defined[9].

In a case-referent study, designed to investigate a possible connection between background radiation and acute myeloid leukaemia, three cases out of 59 (rate ratio, 18.9; 95% confidence interval, 1.9-357) and one referent out of 354 reported past exposure to styrene[10].

B. Evidence for carcinogenicity to animals (*limited*)

Styrene has been tested for carcinogenicity by oral administration to dams and to offspring of two strains of mice and of one strain of rats. In mice, it increased the incidence of lung tumours in male and female offspring of one strain after administration of a high dose. In rats, no statistically significant increase in tumour incidence was observed[9]. In experiments by oral administration to mice and rats, an increased incidence of lung tumours was observed only in male mice[11]. In an inadequately reported study in rats, exposure to styrene by inhalation or ingestion was associated with a small, nonstatistically significant increase in the incidence of brain tumours[12]. A further study in rats by oral administration using a small number of animals gave equivocal results[13].

There is *sufficient evidence* for the carcinogenicity in experimental animals of styrene oxide, a metabolite of styrene *in vivo*[14].

C. Other relevant data

Styrene is metabolized in humans and mammals to styrene oxide. In humans exposed to styrene, chromosomal aberrations and micronuclei were induced in peripheral lymphocytes; a slight increase in the incidence of sister chromatid exchanges was noted in one study, while no increase was reported in several others[15].

In animals treated *in vivo*, styrene induced micronuclei, sister chromatid exchanges and DNA strand breaks; however, conflicting results were obtained for chromosomal aberrations. Styrene bound covalently to DNA in mice *in vivo*. In human lymphocytes *in vitro*, styrene induced chromosomal aberrations, micronuclei and sister chromatid exchanges. In Chinese hamster cells *in vitro*, it induced chromosomal aberrations, sister chromatid exchanges (the latter only when epoxide hydratase was inhibited) and mutation, and, in rat hepatocytes, DNA strand breaks. It induced sex-linked recessive lethal mutations but not sex-chromosome loss or nondisjunction in *Drosophila*. Styrene induced mutation and mitotic recombination in yeast and chromosomal aberrations in plants. It was mutagenic to bacteria when the test protocol was adjusted for the volatility of styrene or the metabolic system was depleted of epoxide hydratase[15].

References

[1]Ott, M.G., Kolesar, R.C., Scharnweber, H.C., Schneider, E.J. & Venable, J.R. (1980) A mortality survey of employees engaged in the development or manufacture of styrene-based products. *J. occup. Med.*, *22*, 445-460

[2]Hodgson, J.T. & Jones, R.D. (1985) Mortality of styrene production, polymerization and processing workers at a site in northwest England. *Scand. J. Work Environ. Health*, *11*, 347-352

[3]Meinhardt, T.J., Lemen, R.A., Crandall, M.S. & Young, R.J. (1982) Environmental epidemiologic investigation of the styrene-butadiene rubber industry. Mortality patterns with discussion of the hematopoietic and lymphatic malignancies. *Scand. J. Work Environ. Health*, *8*, 250-259

[4]Coggon, D., Osmond, C., Pannett, B., Simmonds, S., Winter, P.D. & Acheson, E.D. (1987) Mortality of workers exposed to styrene in the manufacture of glass-reinforced plastics. *Scand. J. Work Environ. Health*, *13*, 94-99

[5]Härkönen, H., Tola, S., Korkala, M.L. & Hernberg, S. (1984) Congenital malformations, mortality and styrene exposure. *Ann. Acad. Med. (Singapore)*, *13*, 404-407

[6]Okun, A.H., Beaumont, J.J., Meinhardt, T.J. & Crandall, M.S. (1985) Mortality patterns among styrene-exposed boatbuilders. *Am. J. ind. Med.*, *8*, 193-205

[7]Nicholson, W.J., Selikoff, I.J. & Seidman, H. (1978) Mortality experience of styrene-polystyrene polymerization workers. Initial findings. *Scand. J. Work Environ. Health, 4 (Suppl. 2)*, 247-252

[8]Frentzel-Beyme, R., Thiess, A.M. & Wieland, R. (1978) Survey of mortality among employees engaged in the manufacture of styrene and polystyrene at the BASF Ludwigshafen works. *Scand. J. Work Environ. Health, 4 (Suppl. 2)*, 231-239

[9]*IARC Monographs*, *19*, 231-274, 1979

[10]Flodin, U., Fredriksson, M., Axelson, O., Persson, B. & Hardell, L. (1986) Background radiation, electrical work, and some other exposures associated with acute myeloid leukemia in a case-referent study. *Arch. environ. Health*, *41*, 77-84

[11]National Cancer Institute (1979) *Bioassay of Styrene for Possible Carcinogenicity (Tech. Rep. Ser. No. 185; DHEW Publ. No. (NIH) 79-1741)*, Washington DC, US Government Printing Office

[12]Maltoni, C., Ciliberti, A. & Carretti, P. (1982) Experimental contributions in identifying brain potential carcinogens in the petrochemical industry. *Ann. N.Y. Acad. Sci.*, *381*, 216-249

[13]Radeva, M. & Krástev, L. (1982) Studies on the effect of monomer styrene on albino rats during long-term per oral administration (Russ.). *Knig. Zdraveopaz*, *25*, 464-468

[14]*IARC Monographs*, *36*, 245-263, 1985

[15]*IARC Monographs*, *Suppl. 6*, 497-501, 1987

SULFAFURAZOLE (SULPHISOXAZOLE) (Group 3)

A. Evidence for carcinogenicity to humans (*inadequate*)

No significant association with cancer at any site was observed during 1969-1976 among 11 659 members of a prepaid health plan prescribed sulfafurazole during 1969-1973[1].

B. Evidence for carcinogenicity to animals (*inadequate*)

Sulfafurazole was tested for carcinogenicity in mice and rats by oral administration; no increase in tumour incidence was observed[2].

C. Other relevant data

No data were available to the Working Group.

References

[1]Friedman, G.D. & Ury, H.K. (1980) Initial screening for carcinogenicity of commonly used drugs. *J. natl Cancer Inst.*, *65*, 723-733

[2]*IARC Monographs*, *24*, 275-285, 1980

SULFAMETHOXAZOLE (Group 3)

A. Evidence for carcinogenicity to humans (*inadequate*)

Although no increase in the incidence of cancers at all sites combined was noted during 1969-1976 among 1709 members of a prepaid health plan prescribed sulfamethoxazole during 1969-1973, significant increases in the incidences of nasopharyngeal carcinoma (3 observed, 0.1 expected; relative risk, 30.0 [95% confidence interval, 23.7-36.3]) and of cancer of the cervix after a two-year lag period (7 observed, 2.2 expected; relative risk, 3.2 [1.8-4.5]) were observed. However, a significant deficit of colon cancer was also seen (none observed, 4.7 expected)[1].

B. Evidence for carcinogenicity to animals (*limited*)

Sulfamethoxazole produced thyroid tumours in rats following its oral administration; no information on other tumour types was reported[2].

C. Other relevant data

In a single study, sulfamethoxazole did not induce chromosomal aberrations in human lymphocytes *in vivo* or *in vitro*. It was not mutagenic to bacteria[3].

References

[1]Friedman, G.D. & Ury, H.K. (1980) Initial screening for carcinogenicity of commonly used drugs. *J. natl Cancer Inst.*, *65*, 723-733

[2]*IARC Monographs*, *24*, 285-295, 1980

[3]*IARC Monographs*, *Suppl. 6*, 502-503, 1987

TALC NOT CONTAINING ASBESTIFORM FIBRES (Group 3) and TALC CONTAINING ASBESTIFORM FIBRES (Group 1)

A. Evidence for carcinogenicity to humans (*inadequate* for talc not containing asbestiform fibres; *sufficient* for talc containing asbestiform fibres)

Evaluation of the effects of talc is confused by the fact that talc deposits may be contaminated with various other minerals, including carbonates, quartz (see p. 341), serpentines and amphiboles (asbestiform [see p. 106] and nonasbestiform)[1].

Case studies have suggested an association between mesothelioma and exposure to talc containing asbestiform fibres[1].

A proportionate mortality study of miners and millers of talc containing asbestiform tremolite has shown an excess of lung cancer and one case of mesothelioma. Another cohort study of workers mining and milling talc containing tremolite, anthophyllite and serpentine minerals revealed significant excess mortality from lung cancer and from nonmalignant respiratory disease. Mortality from lung cancer increased with latency[1].

Several mortality studies have assessed cancer risk among miners and millers of talc that was reported to contain no more than trace amounts of asbestos. A cohort mortality study of talc miners and millers showed an excess of lung cancer among underground miners but not among millers; a contributory etiological role of radon daughters to the lung cancer risk in miners could not be excluded. The three other studies published suffered from methodological limitations and could not be interpreted[1].

A cohort study of pottery workers exposed to silica and talc showed an excess risk of lung cancer (standardized mortality ratio [SMR], 143; 52 observed, 36.3 expected). Among those exposed to high levels of silica, an SMR of 254 (21 observed, 8.3 expected; $p < 0.05$) occurred among those with exposure to nonfibrous talc in contrast to an SMR of 137 (18 observed, 13.2 expected; $p > 0.05$) among those without talc exposure. Mortality from lung cancer increased with duration of exposure to talc (SMR, 364 for those with $\geqslant 15$ years of exposure), but not with duration of exposure to silica[2].

A case-control study has suggested an approximate doubling in relative risk for ovarian cancer among women with perineal use of talc, but the possibility of recall bias cannot be ruled out[1].

B. Evidence for carcinogenicity to animals (*inadequate* for talc not containing asbestiform fibres and for talc containing asbestiform fibres)

Talc of different grades was tested for carcinogenicity in mice, rats and hamsters by various routes of administration, including intraperitoneal, intrathoracic and intrapleural routes. Most of these studies were inadequate. No tumour was induced in rats following either a single intrapleural administration or four intraperitoneal injections of talc, or following administration of talc in the diet. No local tumour developed in mice following a single subcutaneous injection of talc[1].

C. Other relevant data

No data were available on the genetic and related effects of talc in humans.

Talc did not induce dominant lethal mutations or chromosomal aberrations in bone-marrow cells of rats treated *in vivo*, or chromosomal aberrations in human cells *in vitro*. Talc was not mutagenic to yeast or to bacteria in a host-mediated assay[3].

References

[1] *IARC Monographs*, *42*, 185-224, 1987

[2] Thomas, T.L. & Stewart, P.A. (1987) Mortality from lung cancer and respiratory disease among pottery workers exposed to silica and talc. *Am. J. Epidemiol.*, *125*, 35-43

[3] *IARC Monographs*, *Suppl. 6*, 504-505, 1987

2,3,7,8-TETRACHLORODIBENZO-*para*-DIOXIN (TCDD) (Group 2B)

A. Evidence for carcinogenicity to humans (*inadequate*)

The epidemiological studies and case reports considered with regard to producers and users of 2,4,5-trichlorophenol and 2,4,5-trichlorophenoxyacetic acid (2,4,5-T) (see also summaries on chlorophenols and chlorophenoxy herbicides, pp. 154 and 156) also relate to TCDD exposure, since those products may contain TCDD as an impurity. Only studies of particular relevance to TCDD exposure are considered here.

Aggregation of six relatively small cohorts[1-6] shows 37 deaths from cancer, with 33.3 expected, among 956 men likely to have been exposed to TCDD during the manufacture or use of 2,4,5-trichlorophenol and/or 2,4,5-T. The total number of deaths was 135, with 157.3 expected. Two of the deaths were from Hodgkin's lymphoma and two from soft-tissue sarcoma. Five more cases of soft-tissue sarcoma have been reported in men with potential exposure to TCDD during the manufacture of 2,4,5-trichlorophenol or 2,4,5-T[7-9]. A histological review and a reassessment of the exposure in seven of the cases in these various reports indicated that only five were actually soft-tissue sarcomas, and that only two of the cases had had definite exposure to 2,4,5-trichlorophenol or 2,4,5-T; the population background for these two cases was assumed to be fewer than 1000 workers[10].

Three other small cohorts with potential exposure to TCDD have been studied. In one, there were two non-Hodgkin's lymphomas, with 0.3 expected, in 158 individuals with chloracne[11], whereas another, similar group of 79 individuals with chloracne had no cancer[12]. In the third group of 55 individuals with chloracne, there were two lung cancers[13]. A cohort study of 2189 men involved in the manufacture of 2,4,5-trichlorophenol and 2,4,5-T showed no excess of deaths from all cancers (61 observed, 63.5 expected; standardized mortality ratio [SMR], 96), but five non-Hodgkin's lymphomas were seen (SMR, 238; 95% confidence interval, 77-556), although there was no dose-response relationship with TCDD exposure[14]. In the USA, 14 cases of soft-tissue sarcoma among the employees of a large chemical company showed no association with potential TCDD exposure in reference to nine controls per case from the same company[15].

In Seveso, Italy, 15 cases of soft-tissue sarcoma were observed in polluted and 44 cases in unpolluted areas, resulting in rates of 5.7 and 3.2 per 100 000 inhabitants, respectively. However, the rate in the polluted area was high even before the accident, possibly reflecting earlier emissions[16]. Three cases of soft-tissue sarcoma have been reported in Viet Nam veterans who had been in contact with TCDD-containing defoliants[17].

In view of these findings and with regard to chlorophenoxy herbicides, it may be noted that some excesses of soft-tissue sarcoma, nasal cancer and non-Hodgkin's lymphoma, respectively, have been observed in two cohort and one case-control studies, in which no substantial TCDD exposure was likely to have occurred[18-20]. No association between soft-tissue sarcoma and military service in Viet Nam could be demonstrated in the published studies in this respect, despite potential exposure to the heavily TCDD-contaminated chlorophenoxy herbicides that were used[21,22].

B. Evidence for carcinogenicity to animals (*sufficient*)

TCDD was tested in several studies in mice and rats by oral administration and in mice by skin application, but no evaluation of its carcinogenicity could be made[23]. In subsequent, more complete reports and in other studies in mice, oral administration of TCDD alone or, in one study, in combination with 2,4,5-trichlorophenoxyethanol increased the incidence of liver tumours[24-26] and, in one study, produced thyroid tumours in female mice[26]. In rats, oral administration of TCDD increased the incidences of a variety of tumours, including hepatocellular carcinomas, squamous-cell carcinomas of the lung and tumours of the hard palate/nasal turbinates, tongue and thyroid[26-29]. Application of TCDD to the skin of mice was associated with an increased incidence of fibrosarcomas in the integument in females[30].

Intraperitoneal administration of TCDD to infant mice induced thymic lymphomas and liver tumours. Oral administration of TCDD to infant mice increased the incidence of liver tumours[31].

In female rats, TCDD given subcutaneously enhanced the incidences of foci of altered hepatocytes and of hepatocellular carcinomas induced by *N*-nitrosodiethylamine[32]. TCDD did not increase skin carcinogenesis when applied to the skin of mice before administration of polycyclic aromatic hydrocarbons[33,34] or after administration of 7,12-dimethylbenz[*a*]-anthracene[35], but it enhanced the incidence of subcutaneous tumours induced by 3-methyl-cholanthrene[36].

C. Other relevant data

Conflicting results have been reported from studies of chromosomal aberrations in peripheral blood lymphocytes of individuals exposed to TCDD occupationally or as a result of industrial accidents. No convincing evidence for the induction of chromosomal aberrations was obtained in a study of abortuses of women accidentally exposed to TCDD[37].

TCDD did not induce dominant lethal mutations, chromosomal aberrations, micronuclei or sister chromatid exchanges in rodents treated *in vivo*. It did not induce transformation of mouse C3H 10T1/2 cells *in vitro* but did enhance transformation induced by *N*-methyl-*N'*-nitro-*N*-nitrosoguanidine. In another study using the same cell type, it did not inhibit intercellular communication. It was mutagenic to mouse lymphoma cells but did not induce unscheduled DNA synthesis in rat hepatocytes *in vitro*. TCDD was not mutagenic to bacteria[37].

References

[1]Axelson, O., Sundell, L., Andersson, K., Edling, C., Hogstedt, C. & Kling, H. (1980) Herbicide exposure and tumor mortality. An updated epidemiologic investigation on Swedish railroad workers. *Scand. J. Work Environ. Health, 6*, 73-79

[2]Cook, R.R., Townsend, J.C., Ott, M.G. & Silverstein, L.G. (1980) Mortality experience of employees exposed to 2,3,7,8-tetrachlorodibenzo-*p*-dioxin (TCDD). *J. occup. Med., 22*, 530-532

[3]Hogstedt, C. & Westerlund, B. (1980) Cohort studies of cause of death of forest workers with and without exposure to phenoxy acid preparations (Swed.). *Läkartidningen, 77*, 1828-1831

[4]Ott, M.G., Holder, B.B. & Olson, R.D. (1980) A mortality analysis of employees engaged in the manufacture of 2,4,5-trichlorophenoxyacetic acid. *J. occup. Med., 22*, 47-50

[5]Thiess, A.M., Frentzel-Beyme, R. & Link, R. (1982) Mortality study of persons exposed to dioxin in a trichlorophenol-process accident that occurred in the BASF AG on November 17, 1953. *Am. J. ind. Med., 3*, 179-189

[6]Zack, J.A. & Suskind, R.R. (1980) The mortality experience of workers exposed to tetrachloro-dibenzodioxin in a trichlorophenol process accident. *J. occup. Med., 22*, 11-14

[7]Cook, R.R. (1981) Dioxin, chloracne, and soft-tissue sarcoma. *Lancet, i*, 618-619

[8]Moses, M. & Selikoff, I.J. (1981) Soft tissue sarcomas, phenoxy herbicides, and chlorinated phenols. *Lancet, i*, 1370

[9]Johnson, F.E., Kugler, M.A. & Brown, S.M. (1981) Soft tissue sarcomas and chlorinated phenols. *Lancet, ii*, 40

[10]Fingerhut, M.A., Halperin, W.E., Honchar, P.A., Smith, A.B., Groth, D.H. & Russell, W.O. (1984) An evaluation of reports of dioxin exposure and soft tissue sarcoma pathology among chemical workers in the United States. *Scand. J. Work Environ. Health, 10*, 299-303

[11]Bishop, C.M. & Jones, A.H. (1981) Non-Hodgkin's lymphoma of the scalp in workers exposed to dioxins. *Lancet, ii*, 369

[12]May, G. (1982) Tetrachlorodibenzodioxin: a survey of subjects ten years after exposure. *Br. J. ind. Med., 39*, 128-135

[13]Pazderova-Vejlupková, J., Némcova, M., Pícková, J., Jirásek, L. & Lukáš, E. (1981) The development and prognosis of chronic intoxication by tetrachlorodibenzo-*p*-dioxin in men. *Arch. environ. Health, 36*, 5-11

[14]Cook, R.R., Bond, G.G., Olson, R.A., Ott, M.G. & Gondek, M.R. (1986) Evaluation of the mortality experience of workers exposed to the chlorinated dioxins. *Chemosphere, 15*, 1769-1776

[15]Sobel, W., Bond, G.G., Skowronski, B.J., Brownson, P.J. & Cook, R.R. (1986) Soft-tissue sarcoma: case-control study. *J. occup. Med., 28*, 804, 806, 808

[16]Puntoni, R., Merlo, F., Fini, A., Meazza, L. & Santi, L. (1986) Soft tissue sarcomas in Seveso. *Lancet, ii*, 525

[17]Sarma, P.R. & Jacobs, J. (1982) Thoracic soft-tissue sarcoma in Vietnam veterans exposed to Agent Orange. *New Engl. J. Med., 306*, 1109

[18]Lynge, E. (1985) A follow-up study of cancer incidence among workers in manufacture of phenoxy herbicides in Denmark. *Br. J. Cancer, 52*, 259-270

[19]Coggon, D., Pannett, B., Winter, P.D., Acheson, E.D. & Bonsall, J. (1986) Mortality of workers exposed to 2 methyl-4 chlorophenoxyacetic acid. *Scand. J. Work Environ. Health, 12*, 448-454

[20]Riihimäki, V., Asp, S. Pukkala, E. & Hernberg, S. (1983) Mortality and cancer morbidity among chlorinated phenoxyacid applicators in Finland. *Chemosphere, 12*, 779-784

[21]Greenwald, P., Kovasznay, B., Collins, D.N. & Therriault, G. (1984) Sarcomas of soft tissues after Vietnam service. *J. natl Cancer Inst., 73*, 1107-1109

[22]Kang, H.K., Weatherbee, L., Breslin, P.P., Lee, Y. & Shepard, B.M. (1986) Soft tissue sarcomas and military service in Vietnam: a case comparison group analysis of hospital patients. *J. occup. Med., 28*, 1215-1218

[23]*IARC Monographs, 15*, 41-102, 1977

[24]Tóth, K., Sugár, J., Somfai-Relle, S. & Bence, J. (1978) Carcinogenic bioassay of the herbicide, 2,4,5-trichlorophenoxyethanol (TCPE) with different 2,3,7,8-tetrachlorodibenzo-*p*-dioxin (dioxin) content in Swiss mice. *Progr. Biochem. Pharmacol., 14*, 82-93

[25]Tóth, K., Somfai-Relle, S., Sugár, J. & Bence, J. (1979) Carcinogenicity testing of herbicide 2,4,5-trichlorophenoxyethanol containing dioxin and of pure dioxin in Swiss mice. *Nature, 278*, 548-549

[26]National Toxicology Program (1982) *Carcinogenesis Bioassay of 2,3,7,8-Tetrachlorodibenzo-p-dioxin (CAS No. 1746-01-6) in Osborne-Mendel Rats and B6C3F$_1$ Mice (Gavage Study) (Tech. Rep. Ser. No. 209; NIH Publ. No. 82-1765*), Bethesda, MD

[27]Van Miller, J.P., Lalich, J.J. & Allen, J.R. (1977) Increased incidence of neoplasms in rats exposed to low levels of 2,3,7,8-tetrachlorodibenzo-*p*-dioxin. *Chemosphere, 6*, 537-544

[28]Kociba, R.J., Keyes, D.G., Beyer, J.E., Carreon, R.M., Wade, C.E., Dittenber, D.A., Kalnins, R.P., Frauson, L.E., Park, C.N., Barnard, S.D., Hummel, R.A. & Humiston, C.G. (1978) Results of a two-year chronic toxicity and oncogenicity study of 2,3,7,8-tetrachlorodibenzo-*p*-dioxin in rats. *Toxicol. appl. Pharmacol., 46*, 279-303

[29]Kociba, R.J., Keyes, D.G., Beyer, J.E. & Carreon, R.M. (1979) *Toxicologic studies of 2,3,7,8-tetrachlorobenzo-p-dioxin (TCDD) in rats.* In: Deichmann, W.B., ed., *Toxicology and Occupational Medicine*, New York, Elsevier/North-Holland, pp. 281-287

[30]National Toxicology Program (1982) *Carcinogenesis Bioassay of 2,3,7,8-Tetrachlorodibenzo-p-dioxin (CAS No. 1746-01-6) in Swiss-Webster Mice (Dermal Study) (Tech. Rep. Ser. No. 201; NIH Publ. No. 82-1757*), Bethesda, MD

[31] Della Porta, G., Dragani, T.A. & Sozzi, G. (1987) Carcinogenic effects of infantile and long-term 2,3,7,8-tetrachlorodibenzo-*p*-dioxin treatment in the mouse. *Tumori* (in press)

[32] Pitot, H.C., Goldsworthy, T., Campbell, H.A. & Poland, A. (1980) Quantitative evaluation of the promotion by 2,3,7,8-tetrachlorodibenzo-*p*-dioxin of hepatocarcinogenesis from diethylnitrosamine. *Cancer Res., 40*, 3616-3620

[33] DiGiovanni, J., Berry, D.L., Gleason, G.L., Kishore, G.S. & Slaga, T.J. (1980) Time-dependent inhibition by 2,3,7,8-tetrachlorodibenzo-*p*-dioxin of skin tumorigenesis with polycyclic hydrocarbons. *Cancer Res., 40*, 1580-1587

[34] DiGiovanni, J., Decina, P.C. & Diamond, L. (1983) Tumor initiating activity of 9- and 10-fluoro-7,12-dimethylbenz[*a*]anthracene (DMBA) and the effect of 2,3,7,8-tetrachlorodibenzo-*p*-dioxin on tumor initiation by monofluoro derivatives of DMBA in SENCAR mice. *Carcinogenesis, 4*, 1045-1049

[35] Berry, D.L., DiGiovanni, J., Juchau, M.R., Bracken, W.M., Gleason, G.L. & Slaga, T.J. (1978) Lack of tumor-promoting ability of certain environmental chemicals in a two-stage mouse skin tumorigenesis assay. *Res. Commun. chem. Pathol. Pharmacol., 20*, 101-108

[36] Kouri, R.E., Rude, T.H., Joglekar, R., Dansette, P.M., Jerina, D.M., Atlas, S.A., Owens, I.S. & Nebert, D.W. (1978) 2,3,7,8-Tetrachlorodibenzo-*p*-dioxin as cocarcinogen causing 3-methylcholanthrene-initiated subcutaneous tumors in mice genetically 'nonresponsive' at *Ah* locus. *Cancer Res., 38*, 2777-2783

[37] *IARC Monographs, Suppl. 6*, 508-510, 1987

1,1,2,2-TETRACHLOROETHANE (Group 3)

A. Evidence for carcinogenicity to humans (*inadequate*)

The only epidemiological study available evaluated the mortality experience of Second World War army personnel engaged in treating clothing as a defence against gas warfare. In one treatment process, tetrachloroethane was the solvent used for the impregnate. Of the 3859 persons assigned to this process, 1099 whites and 124 blacks had had job duties with probably exposure to the solvent. Among these persons, no statistically significant excess mortality from cancer occurred. Slight excesses were reported for leukaemia (standardized mortality ratio [SMR], 272; based on four deaths) and cancer of the genital organs (SMR, 158; based on three deaths)[1].

B. Evidence for carcinogenicity to animals (*limited*)

1,1,2,2-Tetrachloroethane was tested for carcinogenicity in one experiment in mice and in one in rats by oral administration. In male and female mice, it produced hepatocellular carcinomas. No significant increase in the incidence of tumours was observed in rats of either sex. The compound was inadequately tested in one experiment in mice by intraperitoneal injection[2].

C. Other relevant data

No data were available on the genetic and related effects of 1,1,2,2-tetrachloroethane in humans.

1,1,2,2-Tetrachloroethane did not transform BALB/c 3T3 cells and did not induce sex-linked recessive lethal mutations in *Drosophila*. It induced recombination, gene conversion and mutation in *Saccharomyces cerevisiae* under conditions in which endogenous levels of cytochrome P450 were enhanced. It was not mutagenic to bacteria but caused DNA damage[3].

References

[1]Norman, J.E., Jr, Robinette, C.D. & Fraumeni, J.F., Jr (1981) The mortality experience of army World War II chemical processing companies. *J. occup. Med.*, *23*, 818-822

[2]*IARC Monographs*, *20*, 477-489, 1979

[3]*IARC Monographs*, *Suppl. 6*, 511-513, 1987

TETRACHLOROETHYLENE (Group 2B)

A. Evidence for carcinogenicity to humans (*inadequate*)

Tetrachloroethylene has been studied by observing laundry and dry-cleaning workers, who may also have been exposed to other solvents, especially trichloroethylene (see p. 364), but also petroleum solvents. In several cohort and proportionate mortality studies, excesses have been reported of lymphosarcomas[1], leukaemias[2] and cancers of the skin[1,2], colon[3], lung[2,4] and urogenital tract[1-5], although in one study no excess of urogenital cancer was seen among persons exposed mainly to tetrachloroethylene[5]. Some excess of lymphomas and of cancers of the larynx and bladder was seen in a large cohort of dry cleaners[6]. A familial cluster of chronic lymphocytic leukaemia has also been related to dry-cleaning[7]. A large case-control study of bladder cancer did not show any clear association with dry-cleaning[8]. In other case-control studies, dry-cleaning appeared to be a risk factor for pancreatic cancer[9] and for liver cancer[10]. Some excess of liver cancer was also seen in one of the proportionate mortality studies[2]. In two case-control studies of liver cancer[11,12], an increased risk with occupational exposure to organic solvents (in one of the studies in women only[12]) was observed; in the first study, one case and no control had had exposure to tetrachloroethylene; in the second, one of six female cases was in dry-cleaning workers. Even if there is some consistency in several studies with regard to an association between lymphatic malignancies and urogenital cancers, taken together, and exposure to tetrachloroethylene, this broad grouping and the small numbers involved do not permit any definite conclusion to be drawn about any causal connection.

B. Evidence for carcinogenicity to animals (*sufficient*)

Tetrachloroethylene was tested for carcinogenicity in mice and rats by oral administration and by inhalation. In mice, it produced hepatocellular carcinomas in animals of each sex by each route of administration[13,14]. One experiment in rats by oral administration was considered to be inadequate[13]. Exposure of rats by inhalation produced an increased incidence of leukaemias[14]; the other experiment by inhalation was inadequate[13]. Tetrachloroethylene was also tested inadequately by intraperitoneal injection in mice[13].

C. Other relevant data

In one study, tetrachloroethylene did not induce chromosomal aberrations or sister chromatid exchanges in lymphocytes from persons occupationally exposed to low concentrations[15].

Tetrachloroethylene induced DNA strand breaks in liver and kidney cells of mice treated *in vivo*. It induced transformation of rat embryo cells but not of BALB/c 3T3 cells; it did not induce unscheduled DNA synthesis in rat hepatocytes. It induced sex-linked recessive lethal mutations in *Drosophila*. Tetrachloroethylene induced gene conversion and mitotic recombination in yeast in one study under conditions in which endogenous levels of cytochrome P450 were enhanced. It was mutagenic to plants but not to yeast *in vitro* or in a host-mediated assay or to bacteria[15].

References

[1]Katz, R.M. & Jowett, D. (1981) Female laundry and dry cleaning workers in Wisconsin: a mortality analysis. *Am. J. public Health, 71*, 305-307

[2]Blair, A., Decouflé, P. & Grauman, D. (1979) Causes of death among laundry and dry cleaning workers. *Am. J. public Health, 69*, 508-511

[3]Kaplan, S.D. (1980) *Dry Cleaners Workers Exposed to Perchloroethylene. A Retrospective Cohort Mortality Study (PB 81-231367)*, Springfield, VA, National Technical Information Service

[4]Duh, R.W. & Asal, N.R. (1984) Mortality among laundry and dry cleaning workers in Oklahoma. *Am. J. public Health, 74*, 1278-1280

[5]Brown, D.P. & Kaplan, S.D. (1987) Retrospective cohort mortality study of dry cleaner workers using perchloroethylene. *J. occup. Med., 29*, 535-541

[6]Blair, A., Tolbert, P., Thomas, D. & Grauman, D. (1986) Mortality among dry cleaners. *Med. Lav., 77*, 82-83

[7]Blattner, W.A., Strober, W., Muchmore, A.V., Blaese, R.M., Broder, S. & Fraumeni, J.F., Jr (1976) Familial chronic lymphocytic leukemia. Immunologic and cellular characterization. *Ann. intern. Med., 84*, 554-557

[8]Smith, E.M., Miller, E.R., Woolson, R.F. & Brown, C.K. (1985) Bladder cancer risk among laundry workers, dry cleaners, and others in chemically-related occupations. *J. occup. Med., 27*, 295-297

[9]Lin, R.S. & Kessler, I.I. (1981) A multifactorial model for pancreatic cancer in man. Epidemiologic evidence. *J. Am. med. Assoc., 245*, 147-152

[10]Stemhagen, A., Slade, J., Altman, R. & Bill, J. (1983) Occupational risk factors and liver cancer. A retrospective case-control study of primary liver cancer in New Jersey. *Am. J. Epidemiol., 117*, 443-454

[11]Hardell, L., Bengtsson, N.O., Jonsson, U., Eriksson, S. & Larsson, L.G. (1984) Aetiological aspects of primary liver cancer with special regard to alcohol, organic solvents and acute intermittent porphyria — an epidemiological investigation. *Br. J. Cancer, 50*, 389-397

[12]Hernberg, S., Korkala, M.-L., Asikainen, U. & Riala, R. (1984) Primary liver cancer and exposure to solvents. *Int. Arch. occup. environ. Health, 54*, 147-153

[13]*IARC Monographs, 20*, 491-514, 1979

[14]National Toxicology Program (1986) *Toxicology and Carcinogenesis Studies of Tetrachloroethylene (Perchloroethylene) (CAS No. 127-18-4) in F344/N Rats and B6C3F₁ Mice (Inhalation Studies) (Tech. Rep. Ser. No. 311; NIH Publ. No. 86-2567)*, Research Triangle Park, NC

[15]*IARC Monographs, Suppl. 6*, 514-516, 1987

TOBACCO PRODUCTS, SMOKELESS (Group 1)

A. Evidence for carcinogenicity to humans (*sufficient*)

In North America and western Europe, case reports indicate an association between tobacco chewing and oral cancer at the site where the quid was placed habitually. In those case-control studies in which an association between tobacco chewing and cancer of the oral cavity, pharynx and larynx has been observed, confounding by tobacco smoking or alcohol consumption could not be excluded. A slight increase in the incidence of oesophageal cancer related to tobacco chewing has been seen in four case-control studies[1].

Case reports indicate an association between oral use of snuff and oral cancer. Four case-control studies imply a causal association between snuff use and oral, and possibly pharyngeal, cancer. That oral use of snuff increases the risk of nasal-sinus cancer was suggested in one case-control study[1].

Three case series also show a high relative frequency of smokeless-tobacco use (chewing tobacco or oral snuff, unspecified) among oral cancer patients. Four case-control studies have shown an association between smokeless-tobacco use and the risk of oral cancer. Two cohort mortality studies provide evidence of a positive association with oesophageal cancer, and one suggests an increased risk for oral and pharyngeal cancer[1].

Two large case-control studies from Pakistan and India reported substantial increases in the risk for oral cancer related to tobacco-lime (*khaini*) chewing[1]. In addition, evidence is available from various studies in which cancer risks were studied in relation to unspecified habits of betel-tobacco-lime chewing[2].

Case series have indicated an association between use of *shammah* and *nass* and oral cancer. Oral cancer was found to develop at the site at which *nass* was placed habitually. Two case-control studies showed substantial increases in the risk of oral cancer associated with *nass* use and one with *naswar* use; however, in these studies positive confounding by smoking and other factors could not be excluded. Oral cancer in users of *mishri* and *gudakhu* was studied in a prevalence survey; no case was found[1]. A study of 64 patients with squamous-cell carcinoma of the head and neck in Saudi Arabia showed that 81% were *alshammah* users and 34% were *alqat* users, but only 14% were cigarette smokers; none used alcohol to excess[3].

No association has been seen between nasal use of snuff and oral cancer. In two case-control studies an association between snuff inhaling and nasal-sinus cancer has been reported. One case-control study reported snuff inhaling to be more common among patients with cancers of the oesophagus, hypopharynx or oropharynx than among controls[1].

B. Evidence for carcinogenicity to animals (*inadequate*)

Various chewing tobaccos and unburnt cigarette tobaccos and their extracts were tested for carcinogenicity by oral administration in mice, by topical application to the oral mucosa of mice, rats and hamsters, and by subcutaneous administration, skin application, inhalation, intravesicular implantation and intravaginal application to mice. All of these studies suffered from certain deficiencies[1].

In a two-stage mouse-skin assay, applications of tobacco extract followed by treatment with croton oil induced papillomas and squamous-cell carcinomas of the skin. In further two-stage mouse-skin assays, application of tobacco extracts following initiation by 7,12-dimethylbenz[*a*]anthracene resulted in papillomas[1].

A commercial Swedish snuff was tested for carcinogenicity in rats by topical administration in a surgically-created oral canal, alone or in combination with herpes simplex type 1 infection. Two squamous-cell carcinomas of the oral cavity were observed in the group receiving both treatments, but this result was not statistically significant[1]. A commercial North American snuff was tested in rats by the same route. One squamous-cell carcinoma and two papillomas of the oral cavity were found, but this result was not statistically significant[4].

An aqueous extract of a commercial North American snuff was also tested by topical application to the oral mucosa in rats, alone or enriched with the tobacco-specific nitrosamines, N'-nitrosonornicotine and 4-(nitrosomethylamino)-1-(3-pyridyl)-1-butanone. Some papillomas of the oral cavity were observed in rats treated with the enriched snuff extract, but this result was not statistically significant[4].

Snuff was tested by oral administration in hamsters, alone and in combination with calcium hydroxide, but the data were insufficient for evaluation. Several studies in hamsters in which snuff was administered as single or repeated applications into the cheek pouch or fed in the diet yielded insufficient data for evaluation. Subcutaneous injection of ethanol extracts of snuff to rats did not produce an increase in tumour incidence[1].

Nass was tested for carcinogenicity in hamsters by administration into the cheek pouch or by skin application. No tumour was found at the site of application. Although *nass* administration was associated with an apparent excess of liver tumours in various groups receiving cheek-pouch administration, which may be indicative of carcinogenicity, deficiencies in reporting do not allow an evaluation to be made[1].

C. Other relevant data

An increased incidence of micronuclei was observed in exfoliated epithelial cells from chewers of *khaini* and *nass*. Saliva collected from chewers of Indian tobacco induced chromosomal aberrations in Chinese hamster ovary cells *in vitro*[5].

Ethanol extracts of Indian chewing tobacco induced micronuclei in bone-marrow cells of Swiss mice treated *in vivo* and were mutagenic to Chinese hamster V79 cells *in vitro*, both in the presence and absence of an exogenous metabolic system, and to *Salmonella typhimurium*. Both ethanol and ethyl acetate extracts of Sri Lankan chewing tobacco induced transformation of Syrian hamster embryo cells. Ethyl acetate extracts induced sister chromatid exchanges in cultured human cells, but not mutation in Chinese hamster V79 cells when tested in the absence of an exogenous metabolic system[5].

Aqueous extracts of *nass* and *khaini* induced chromosomal aberrations in Chinese hamster ovary cells. Powdered tobacco fed to larvae of *Drosophila* did not induce sex-linked recessive lethal mutations, autosomal translocations or sex-chromosome loss[5].

Chloroform extracts of *shammah* induced transformation in mouse C3H 10T1/2 cells. The same extracts also induced aberrant colonies and gene conversion in yeast and were mutagenic to *S. typhimurium*, both in the presence and absence of an exogenous metabolic system[5].

Extracts of North American oral snuff (at pH 3.0) and extracts of North American chewing tobacco treated with sodium nitrite under acidic conditions were mutagenic to *S. typhimurium* in the presence and absence of a metabolic system. Organic solvent extracts of snuff induced a dose-related increase in the frequency of sister chromatid exchanges in human peripheral lymphocytes *in vitro* in the absence of a metabolic system[5].

References

[1]*IARC Monographs, 37*, 37-136, 1985

[2]*IARC Monographs, 37*, 141-209, 1985

[3]Ibrahim, E.M., Satti, M.B., Al Idrissi, H.Y., Higazi, M.M., Magbool, G.M. & Al Quorain, A. (1986) Oral cancer in Saudi Arabia: the role of alqat and alshammah. *Cancer Detect. Prev., 9*, 215-218

[4]Hecht, S.S., Rivenson, A., Braley, J., DiBello, J., Adams, J.D. & Hoffmann, D. (1986) Induction of oral cavity tumors in F344 rats by tobacco-specific nitrosamines and snuff. *Cancer Res., 46*, 4162-4166

[5]*IARC Monographs, Suppl. 6*, 519, 1987

TOBACCO SMOKE (Group 1)

A. Evidence for carcinogenicity to humans (*sufficient*)

Cigarette smoking has been shown to cause lung cancer, bladder cancer, cancer of the renal pelvis (and possibly renal adenocarcinoma), cancer of the lip, and oropharyngeal, hypopharyngeal, laryngeal, oesophageal and pancreatic cancers. In some studies, increased risks of cancers of the stomach, liver and cervix have been noted, but the data were inadequate to decide whether the association is causal or not. The risk for lung cancer due to cigarette smoking is substantially increased in conjunction with exposure to radon daughters or asbestos (see p. 106). An increase in the incidence of lung cancer also results from smoking other forms of tobacco, i.e., pipe, cigars and *bidis*. Pipe and cigar smoking probably increase the risk of bladder cancer, but at lower levels than that caused by cigarette smoking. They also increase the risks of oral, oropharyngeal, hypopharyngeal, laryngeal and oesophageal cancers to approximately the same extent as cigarette smoking, and, as with cigarette smoking, the risk is substantially augmented in conjunction with high-dose exposure to alcohol[1].

Tobacco smoke affects not only people who smoke but also those who are exposed to the combustion products of other people's tobacco (passive smokers). The most numerous observations hitherto available concern lung cancer, and the results of most of the 13 main epidemiological studies[2] carried out so far are compatible with either an increased risk from passive smoking or an absence of risk. However, the aggregate evidence from these studies, taken together with knowledge of the nature of sidestream and mainstream smoke, of the materials absorbed during passive smoking and of the quantitative relationships between dose and effect that are commonly observed after exposure to carcinogens, leads to the conclusion that passive smoking does carry some risk for lung cancer.

B. Evidence for carcinogenicity to animals (*sufficient*)

Cigarette smoke has been tested for carcinogenicity by inhalation in mice, rats, hamsters and dogs. Exposure of hamsters and rats to whole smoke produced malignant respiratory-tract tumours[1]. In mice, inhalation of whole tobacco smoke resulted in a slightly increased incidence of alveologenic lung tumours, but this was not statistically significant in some of the studies[1,3]. An increased incidence of lung tumours has also been reported in dogs exposed to cigarette smoke, but the data were insufficient for evaluation. More tumours of the respiratory tract occurred in rodents exposed to both cigarette smoke and 7,12-dimethyl-benz[a]anthracene than to either one alone; the same is true for concomitant exposure to benzo[a]pyrene or radon daughters[1].

Cigarette-smoke condensate induced benign and malignant skin tumours in mice and rabbits after application to the skin. Following its topical administration to oral mucosa, it resulted in an increased incidence of lung tumours and tumours of other organs, primarily lymphomas, in one strain of mice. In rats, cigarette-smoke condensate produced lung cancer after intrapulmonary injection. In two-stage mouse-skin assays, a single topical administration of cigarette-smoke condensate induced changes resulting in benign and malignant skin tumours after additional application of croton oil. Skin tumours were also produced when cigarette-smoke condensate was applied chronically subsequent to a single treatment with other agents, such as 7,12-dimethylbenz[a]anthracene[1].

C. Other relevant data

Structural chromosomal aberrations, sister chromatid exchanges and micronuclei have been observed in peripheral blood lymphocytes of tobacco smokers. Although in some studies there was no increase in the incidence of sister chromatid exchanges, in several others a dose-response relationship was reported between the amount and duration of cigarette smoking and the frequency of sister chromatid exchange. Long-term heavy smokers generally also had higher frequencies of chromosomal aberrations in peripheral blood lymphocytes. In a large study, a significant dose-response relationship was found between the frequency of structural chromosomal aberrations and the estimated daily uptake of condensate. In a single study, it was reported that DNA adducts associated with cigarette smoke were detected in the bronchus of one smoker and in the larynx of another, but not in the bronchus of a nonsmoker. In another study, one of several DNA adducts detected in 16/17 placentas from smokers and 3/14 placentas from nonsmokers was claimed to be related to maternal smoking. Antigenicity against polycyclic aromatic hydrocarbon-DNA adducts has been demonstrated in peripheral lymphocytes and lung samples from cigarette smokers, although the occurrence of these adducts could not be correlated with cigarette smoking[4].

Extracts of urine from smokers induced chromosomal aberrations in Chinese hamster ovary cells and were mutagenic to bacteria in the presence of an exogenous metabolic system. Passive exposure to tobacco smoke has also been reported to increase urinary mutagenicity. In studies of amniotic fluid samples from smoking and nonsmoking mothers, more mutagenicity to *Salmonella typhimurium* was reported in samples taken at term from heavy smokers as compared to nonsmokers, but not in samples taken at 16 weeks by amniocentesis. One study of the mutagenicity of cervical mucus from smoking and non-smoking women was difficult to interpret due to inadequate reporting[4].

Tobacco smoke inhibited DNA repair capacity in mice and increased the frequency of sister chromatid exchanges in bone-marrow cells of mice exposed *in vivo* and in human lymphocytes *in vitro*; it also induced single-strand breaks in cultured human cells. It induced sex-linked recessive lethal mutations in *Drosophila* and mitotic recombination, gene conversion and mutation in yeast. The urine of rats and baboons exposed to cigarette smoke was mutagenic to bacteria[4].

Tobacco smoke and extracts of particulate matter collected on filters in rooms containing cigarette smoke were mutagenic to bacteria. The extracts also induced sister chromatid exchanges in cultured Chinese hamster ovary cells[4].

Tobacco condensates induced mutation, sister chromatid exchanges and transformation in rodent cells in culture, sex-linked recessive lethal mutations in *Drosophila* and mutation and gene conversion in fungi. Tobacco-smoke condensate inhibited intercellular communication of Chinese hamster V79 cells. All tobacco-smoke condensates tested were mutagenic to bacteria[4].

References

[1]*IARC Monographs*, 38, 1986

[2]Wald, N.J., Nanchahal, K., Thompson, S.G. & Cuckle, H.S. (1986) Does breathing other people's tobacco smoke cause lung cancer? *Br. med. J.*, 293, 1217-1222

[3]Henry, C.J. & Kouri, R.E. (1986) Chronic inhalation studies in mice. II. Effects of long-term exposure to 2R1 cigarette smoke on (C57BL/Cum × C3H/AnfCum)F₁ mice. *J. natl Cancer Inst.*, 77, 203-212

[4]*IARC Monographs, Suppl. 6*, 519-520, 1987

ortho-TOLUIDINE (Group 2B)

A. Evidence for carcinogenicity to humans (*inadequate*)

There are numerous studies of dyestuffs workers, dating back to the classical cohort studies in 1954. Although an excess of bladder tumours has often been found in workers exposed to varying combinations of dyestuffs and dyestuff intermediates, no population of workers exposed to *ortho*-toluidine alone has been described[1]. Occasional cases of bladder tumours have been reported in workers classified as being exposed primarily to *ortho*-toluidine, but either insufficient data or insufficient follow-up time have prevented a clear association being made with the exposure. An excess of bladder tumours was noted in workers exposed to toluene, *ortho*-nitrotoluene, *ortho*-toluidine and 4,4′-methylene bis(2-methylaniline) (see p. 248) during the manufacture of new fuchsin ('new' magenta, see p. 238) and safranine T[1,2].

B. Evidence for carcinogenicity to animals (*sufficient*)

ortho-Toluidine hydrochloride was tested for carcinogenicity in mice and rats by oral administration, producing neoplasms at various sites in both species; in particular, vascular tumours were induced, including tumours of the spleen and other abdominal haemangiosarcomas[1,3]. Following subcutaneous injection in a limited study in hamsters, no treatment-related neoplasm was observed[4]. Experiments in rabbits and guinea-pigs by subcutaneous administration were inadequate for evaluation[1].

C. Other relevant data

No data were available on the genetic and related effects of *ortho*-toluidine in humans.

ortho-Toluidine did not induce micronuclei in mice treated *in vivo*; equivocal results were obtained for sister chromatid exchanges in Chinese hamsters. It induced sister chromatid exchanges, mutation and unscheduled DNA synthesis in human cells *in vitro*. It induced transformation, aneuploidy and chromosomal aberrations in cultured rodent cells; conflicting results were obtained for sister chromatid exchanges, mutation and DNA damage. *ortho*-Toluidine caused somatic mutation in *Drosophila*. Conflicting results were obtained for mutagenicity to yeast; it induced aneuploidy, but not mitotic recombination. *ortho*-Toluidine was mutagenic to bacteria when larger amounts of an exogenous metabolic system were used than in the standard assay[5].

References

[1]*IARC Monographs*, 27, 155-175, 1982

[2]Rubino, G.F., Scansetti, G., Piolatto, G. & Pira, E. (1982) The carcinogenic effect of aromatic amines: an epidemiological study of the role of *o*-toluidine and 4,4'-methylene bis(2-methyl-aniline) in inducing bladder cancer in man. *Environ. Res.*, 27, 241-254

[3]Hecht, S.S., El-Bayoumy, K., Rivenson, A. & Fiala, E. (1982) Comparative carcinogenicity of *o*-toluidine hydrochloride and *o*-nitrosotoluene in F-344 rats. *Cancer Lett.*, 16, 103-108

[4]Hecht, S.S., El-Bayoumy, K., Rivenson, A. & Fiala, E.S. (1983) Bioassay for carcinogenicity of 3,2'-dimethyl-4-nitrosobiphenyl, *o*-nitrosotoluene, nitrosobenzene and the corresponding amines in Syrian golden hamsters. *Cancer Lett.*, 20, 349-354

[5]*IARC Monographs, Suppl. 6*, 523-527, 1987

TREOSULPHAN (Group 1)

A. Evidence for carcinogenicity to humans (*sufficient*)

In one epidemiological study of 553 patients with ovarian cancer treated only with treosulphan and followed for nine years (over 1700 person-years) after treatment, 13 patients developed acute nonlymphocytic leukaemia, mostly within five years after the start of chemotherapy; the expected number of cases among the patients was less than 0.1, giving a relative risk in excess of 100. There was a significant correlation between cumulative dose of treosulphan and risk of leukaemia[1,2].

B. Evidence for carcinogenicity to animals

No data were available to the Working Group.

C. Other relevant data

Treosulphan is a bifunctional alkylating agent. No data were available on the genetic and related effects of this compound in humans. It induced chromosomal aberrations in plant cells[3].

References

[1]*IARC Monographs*, 26, 341-349, 1981

[2]Pedersen-Bjergaard, J., Ersbøll, J., Sørensen, H.M., Keiding, N., Larsen, S.O., Philip, P., Larsen, M.S., Schultz, H. & Nissen, N.I. (1985) Risk of acute nonlymphocytic leukemia and preleukemia in patients treated with cyclophosphamide for non-Hodgkin's lymphomas. Comparison with results obtained in patients treated for Hodgkin's disease and ovarian carcinoma with other alkylating agents. *Ann. intern. Med.*, 103, 195-200

[3]*IARC Monographs, Suppl. 6*, 528-529, 1987

TRICHLOROETHYLENE (Group 3)

A. Evidence for carcinogenicity to humans (*inadequate*)

Three cohort studies have been reported, two of which showed no excess of cancer[1,2]; the third[3], in an extended and updated version[4], showed slightly increased incidences of cancer of the bladder (3 observed, 0.8 expected) and prostate (4 observed, 2.4 expected) and of lymphoma (2 observed, 0.3 expected). Two case-control studies of lymphoma have been reported: one on Hodgkin's lymphoma, in which three of 25 cases and none of 50 controls had had exposure to trichloroethylene[5], and the other on Hodgkin's and non-Hodgkin's lymphomas combined in which seven of 169 cases and three of 338 controls had been exposed[6]. Four studies of liver cancer have indicated no clear association with exposure to trichloroethylene[7-10]. A few more cases than controls were exposed in two of the studies, especially when the two studies were analysed together[7,9]. In a proportionate mortality study of polishers and platers with potential exposure to trichloroethylene, but also to chromates (see p. 165) and nickel (see p. 264), there were excesses of oesophageal and primary liver cancers. There were also slight excesses of cancers of the buccal cavity and pharynx, pancreas and larynx and of lymphoma (Hodgkin's and non-Hodgkin's lymphomas combined, 13 observed, 9.3 expected)[11].

Exposure to trichloroethylene may occur to some extent in laundry and dry-cleaning work, although exposure to tetrachloroethylene (see p. 355) probably predominates. Decaffeinated coffee, which is often extracted with trichloroethylene, appeared to be a risk factor for pancreatic cancer in one study, as did dry-cleaning[12].

The inconsistent relationship between liver cancer and dry-cleaning is considered in the summary on tetrachloroethylene. Even if there is some consistency among several studies with regard to an association between lymphatic malignancies and exposure to trichloroethylene, the small numbers involved do not permit any definite conclusion to be drawn about a causal association.

B. Evidence for carcinogenicity to animals (*limited*)

Trichloroethylene was tested for carcinogenicity by oral administration in mice in one experiment and in rats in two experiments. In mice, it produced hepatocellular carcinomas and lung tumours in both males and females. One study in rats was considered to be inadequate, and the other showed equivocal evidence of carcinogenicity[3]. Inhalation studies with trichloroethylene have been conducted in mice, rats and hamsters[13,14]. In one study in female mice, it caused lung tumours[13], but it gave negative results in the other study in mice and in rats and hamsters. Administration by skin painting and by subcutaneous injection to mice also gave negative results[15]. In inhalation experiments using two strains of mice, trichloroethylene increased the incidences of liver tumours in males of one strain and in males and females of the other strain, and of lung tumours in males of one strain and in females of the other. In rats, a low incidence of adenocarcinomas of the renal tubules was observed following exposure to trichloroethylene by inhalation[16]. In mice, oral administration of trichloroethylene containing epichlorohydrin (see p. 202) as a stabilizer induced forestomach carcinomas but no liver or lung carcinoma[17]. Pure trichloroethylene was tested by oral administration in mice and rats. Hepatocellular carcinomas were induced in male and female mice; none were induced in female rats, and the experiment in male rats was considered inadequate[18]. A study by oral administration was conducted in four strains of rats, but it was inadequate because of toxicity and poor survival[19].

C. Other relevant data

Oral administration of trichloroethylene to mice induced hepatic peroxisome proliferation; however, no such effect was observed in rats[20].

No adequate data were available on the genetic and related effects of trichloroethylene in humans.

Many commercial preparations of trichloroethylene contain stabilizers which are known to be mutagenic. As a rule, the purities of the preparations tested are not given. Trichloroethylene induced micronuclei, somatic mutation (in the spot test), sperm anomalies and DNA strand breaks in the kidney and liver, but not lung, of mice treated *in vivo*; it did not induce dominant lethal mutations. It induced sister chromatid exchanges and unscheduled DNA synthesis in human lymphocytes *in vitro*. It induced transformation of mouse and rat cells but not of Syrian hamster cells; it did not induce sister chromatid exchanges in Chinese hamster cells *in vitro* or unscheduled DNA synthesis in rat hepatocytes. It was mutagenic to plant cells and induced mutation, gene conversion and mitotic recombination in *Saccharomyces cerevisiae* both *in vivo* and in host-mediated assays, but mutation was not induced in *Schizosaccharomyces pombe in vitro* or in a host-mediated assay. It was mutagenic to bacteria when tested as a gas but not when tested as a liquid, except in one study using a mouse-liver metabolic system[21].

References

[1]Tola, S., Vilhunen, R., Järvinen, E. & Korkala, M.-L. (1980) A cohort study on workers exposed to trichloroethylene. *J. occup. Med.*, *22*, 737-740

[2]Shindell, S. & Ulrich, S. (1985) A cohort study of employees of a manufacturing plant using trichloroethylene. *J. occup. Med.*, *27*, 577-579

[3]*IARC Monographs*, *20*, 545-572, 1979

[4]Axelson, O. (1985) *Halogenated alkanes and alkenes and cancer: epidemiological aspects.* In: Fishbein, L. & O'Neill, I.K., eds, *Environmental Carcinogens. Selected Methods of Analysis*, Vol. 7, *Some Volatile Halogenated Hydrocarbons (IARC Scientific Publications No. 68)*, Lyon, International Agency for Research on Cancer, pp. 5-20

[5]Olsson, H. & Brandt, L. (1980) Occupational exposure to organic solvents and Hodgkin's disease in men. A case-referent study. *Scand. J. Work Environ. Health*, *6*, 302-305

[6]Hardell, L., Eriksson, M., Lenner, P. & Lundgren, E. (1981) Malignant lymphoma and exposure to chemicals, especially organic solvents, chlorophenols and phenoxy acids: a case-control study. *Br. J. Cancer*, *43*, 169-176

[7]Hardell, L., Bengtsson, N.O., Jonsson, U., Eriksson, S. & Larsson, L.G. (1984) Aetiological aspects of primary liver cancer with special regard to alcohol, organic solvents and acute intermittent porphyria — an epidemiological investigation. *Br. J. Cancer*, *50*, 389-397

[8]Novotná, E., David, A. & Málek, B. (1979) An epidemiological study on hepatic tumour incidence in subjects working with trichloroethylene. I. Negative result of retrospective investigations in subjects with primary liver carcinoma (Pol.). *Pracov. Lék., 31*, 121-123

[9]Hernberg, S., Korkala, M.-L., Asikainen, U. & Riala, R. (1984) Primary liver cancer and exposure to solvents. *Int. Arch. occup. environ. Health, 54*, 147-153

[10]Paddle, G.M. (1983) Incidence of liver cancer and trichloroethylene manufacture: joint study by industry and a cancer registry. *Br. med. J., 286*, 846

[11]Blair, A. (1980) Mortality among workers in the metal polishing and plating industry, 1951-1969. *J. occup. Med., 22*, 158-162

[12]Lin, R.S. & Kessler, I.I. (1981) A multifactorial model for pancreatic cancer in man. Epidemiologic evidence. *J. Am. med. Assoc., 245*, 147-152

[13]Fukuda, K., Takemoto, K. & Tsuruta, H. (1983) Inhalation carcinogenicity of trichloroethylene in mice and rats. *Ind. Health, 21*, 243-254

[14]Henschler, D., Romen, W., Elsässer, H.M., Reichert, D., Eder, E. & Radwan, Z. (1980) Carcinogenicity study of trichloroethylene by longterm inhalation in three animal species. *Arch. Toxicol., 43*, 237-248

[15]Van Duuren, B.L., Kline, S.A., Melchionne, S. & Seidman, I. (1983) Chemical structure and carcinogenicity relationships of some chloroalkene oxides and their parent olefins. *Cancer Res., 43*, 159-162

[16]Maltoni, C., Lefemine, G. & Cotti, G. (1986) *Archives of Research on Industrial Carcinogenesis, Vol. V, Experimental Research on Trichloroethylene Carcinogenesis*, Princeton, Princeton Scientific Publishing Co.

[17]Henschler, D., Elsässer, H.M., Romen, W. & Eder, E. (1984) Carcinogenicity study of trichloroethylene, with and without epoxide stabilizers, in mice. *J. Cancer Res. clin. Oncol., 107*, 149-156

[18]National Toxicology Program (1982) *Carcinogenesis Bioassay of Trichloroethylene (CAS No. 79-01-6) in F344/N Rats and B6C3F₁/N Mice (Gavage Studies)* (*Tech. Rep. Ser. No. 243; NIH Publ. No. 82-1799*), Research Triangle Park, NC

[19]National Toxicology Program (1986) *Toxicology and Carcinogenesis Studies of Trichloroethylene (CAS No. 79-01-6) in Four Strains of Rats (ACI, August, Marshall, Osborne-Mendel) (Gavage Studies)* (*Tech. Rep. Ser. No. 273; NIH Publ. No. 86-2529*), Research Triangle Park, NC

[20]Elcombe, C.R., Rose, M.S. & Pratt, I.S. (1985) Biochemical, histological and ultrastructural changes in rat and mouse liver following the administration of trichloroethylene: possible relevance of species differences in hepatocarcinogenicity. *Toxicol. appl. Pharmacol., 79*, 365-376

[21]*IARC Monographs, Suppl. 6*, 530-532, 1987

4,5′,8-TRIMETHYLPSORALEN (Group 3)

A. Evidence for carcinogenicity to humans (*inadequate*)

Malignant melanoma was diagnosed in a 30-year-old male shortly after commencement of treatment with 4,5′,8-trimethylpsoralen for vitiligo. No skin cancer was observed during two to 14 months of follow-up in 57 patients with psoriasis treated for one to 23 months with 4,5′,8-trimethylpsoralen[1].

B. Evidence for carcinogenicity to animals (*inadequate*)

No skin tumour was observed in mice given thrice-weekly skin applications of 4,5′,8-trimethylpsoralen followed by low doses of ultraviolet A irradiation for nine months[1,2].

C. Other relevant data

No data were available on the genetic and related effects of 4,5′,8-trimethylpsoralen in humans.

In combination with ultraviolet A radiation, 4,5′,8-trimethylpsoralen bound covalently to DNA in guinea-pig skin *in vivo*. It induced sister chromatid exchanges and unscheduled DNA synthesis in human cells *in vitro*, and DNA cross-links in human and rodent cells *in vitro*. It induced mutation in yeast and DNA damage in bacteria. Results on the induction of mutation in bacteria were inconclusive[3].

In the absence of ultraviolet A radiation, 4,5′,8-trimethylpsoralen did not induce sister chromatid exchanges in human lymphocytes *in vitro*; results for induction of unscheduled DNA synthesis were equivocal. Mutagenicity studies in bacteria were inconclusive[3].

References

[1]*IARC Monographs*, *40*, 357-371, 1986

[2]Hannuksela, M., Stenbäck, F. & Lahti, A. (1986) The carcinogenic properties of topical PUVA. A lifelong study in mice. *Arch. dermatol. Res.*, *278*, 347-351

[3]*IARC Monographs*, *Suppl. 6*, 541-544, 1987

TRIS(AZIRIDINYL)-*para*-BENZOQUINONE (TRIAZIQUONE) (Group 3)

A. Evidence for carcinogenicity to humans (*inadequate*)

No epidemiological study of triaziquone as a single agent was available to the Working Group. Occasional case reports of exposure to triaziquone, especially in the presence of concurrent therapy with other putative carcinogens, such as ionizing radiation, alkylating agents and other potent oncotherapeutic drugs, do not constitute evidence of carcinogenesis[1].

B. Evidence for carcinogenicity to animals (*limited*)

Triaziquone produced a small number of different types of malignant tumours in rats after repeated intravenous injections or after repeated intravenous injections followed by repeated intraperitoneal injections[1].

C. Other relevant data

Triaziquone is an alkylating agent[2]. No data were available on its genetic and related effects in humans.

Triaziquone induced dominant lethal mutations, heritable translocations, chromosomal aberrations and micronuclei in bone-marrow cells of mice and chromosomal aberrations in oocytes of mice and hamsters treated *in vivo*. In human cells *in vitro*, it induced chromosomal aberrations and sister chromatid exchanges. In Chinese hamster cells *in vitro*, triaziquone induced chromosomal aberrations, micronuclei and sister chromatid exchanges; it induced unscheduled DNA synthesis in mouse testicular cells. It induced aneuploidy, chromosomal aberrations and sex-linked recessive lethal mutations in *Drosophila*, mutation in plant cells, gene conversion in yeast and mutation and DNA damage in bacteria[2].

References

[1]*IARC Monographs*, 9, 67-73, 1975
[2]*IARC Monographs*, *Suppl. 6*, 545-548, 1987

TRIS(1-AZIRIDINYL)PHOSPHINE SULPHIDE (THIOTEPA) (Group 2A)

A. Evidence for carcinogenicity to humans (*inadequate*)

Occasional case reports of exposure to Thiotepa, especially in the presence of concurrent therapy with other putative carcinogens, such as ionizing radiation, alkylating agents and other potent oncotherapeutic drugs, do not constitute evidence of carcinogenesis[1].

No increased risk of second malignancies was found among 470 patients with colorectal cancer randomized to low-dose (four doses of 0.2 mg/kg bw) adjuvant therapy with Thiotepa, followed for 3102 person-years (30 second noncolorectal malignancies observed, 31.4 expected)[1]. No increased risk of second malignancies was found among 90 patients with breast cancer randomized to adjuvant therapy with Thiotepa for one year (0.8 mg/kg bw in divided doses followed by 0.2 mg/kg bw weekly maintenance); after an average follow-up of approximately five years, five nonskin, nonbreast cancers had occurred in 5819 person-years among 90 treated subjects compared with six in 4746 person-years among the 77 nonexposed patients[2].

B. Evidence for carcinogenicity to animals (*sufficient*)

Thiotepa was tested for carcinogenicity in mice by intraperitoneal injection and in rats by intraperitoneal and intravenous injection, producing a variety of malignant tumours[3,4,5].

C. Other relevant data

Thiotepa is an alkylating agent. An increased frequency of chromosomal aberrations was observed in one study of cancer patients receiving therapeutic doses of this compound[6].

Thiotepa induced dominant lethal mutations, chromosomal aberrations, micronuclei and sister chromatid exchanges in rodents treated *in vivo*. It induced sister chromatid exchanges and chromosomal aberrations in human and rodent cells *in vitro* and transformation of C3H 10T1/2 mouse cells. It was mutagenic to Chinese hamster cells *in vitro* and to mouse lymphoma cells in a host-mediated assay. Thiotepa induced sex-linked recessive lethal mutations in *Drosophila*, caused sister chromatid exchanges and chromosomal aberrations in plant cells and was mutagenic to fungi and to bacteria *in vitro* and in host-mediated assays[6].

References

[1]Boice, J.D., Greene, M.H., Keehn, R.J., Higgins, G.A. & Fraumeni, J.F., Jr (1980) Late effects of low-dose adjuvant chemotherapy in colorectal cancer. *J. natl Cancer Inst.*, *64*, 501-511

[2]Kardinal, C.G. & Donegan, W.L. (1980) Second cancers after prolonged adjuvant Thiotepa for operable carcinoma of the breast. *Cancer*, *45*, 2042-2046

[3]*IARC Monographs*, *9*, 85-94, 1975

[4]National Cancer Institute (1978) *Bioassay of Thio-tepa for Possible Carcinogenicity (Tech. Rep. Ser. No. 58; DHEW Publ. No. (NIH) 78-1308)*, Washington DC, US Government Printing Office

[5]Schmähl, D. (1975) *Experimental investigations with anti-cancer drugs for carcinogenicity with special reference to immunodepression*. In: Grundmann, E. & Gross, R., eds, *The Ambivalence of Cytostatic Therapy*, New York, Springer, pp. 18-28

[6]*IARC Monographs*, *Suppl. 6*, 549-553, 1987

TRIS(2,3-DIBROMOPROPYL) PHOSPHATE (Group 2A)

A. Evidence for carcinogenicity to humans (*inadequate*)

In a cohort mortality study in the USA of workers with multiple exposures, exposure to tris(2,3-dibromopropyl) phosphate was considered. A group of 628 male workers was classified as exposed either on a 'routine' or 'nonroutine' basis; 36 deaths occurred in this group (35 expected), seven of which were due to cancer compared to 6.6 that would have been expected[1].

B. Evidence for carcinogenicity to animals (*sufficient*)

Tris(2,3-dibromopropyl) phosphate was tested for carcinogenicity in mice and rats by oral administration. In mice, it produced tumours of the forestomach and lung in animals of each sex, benign and malignant liver tumours in females and benign and malignant tumours of the kidney in males[2]. In rats, it produced benign and malignant tumours of the kidney in males[2,3] and benign kidney tumours in females[2]. In a study of limited duration in male rats, benign colon tumours were reported[3]. After skin application to female mice, it produced tumours of the skin, lung, forestomach and oral cavity[2].

C. Other relevant data

No data were available on the genetic and related effects of tris(2,3-dibromopropyl) phosphate in humans.

Tris(2,3-dibromopropyl) phosphate induced micronuclei in bone-marrow cells and sperm abnormalities in mice treated *in vivo*. It induced sister chromatid exchanges and DNA damage in human cells *in vitro*. It transformed Syrian hamster embryo and mouse C3H 10T1/2 cells and induced chromosomal aberrations, sister chromatid exchanges and mutation in cultured rodent cells. It induced heritable translocations in *Drosophila* and DNA damage and mutation in bacteria[4].

References

[1]Wong, O., Brocker, W., Davis, H.V. & Nagle, G.S. (1984) Mortality of workers potentially exposed to organic and inorganic brominated chemicals, DBCP, Tris, PBB, and DDT. *Br. J. ind. Med.*, *41*, 15-24

[2]*IARC Monographs, 20*, 575-588, 1979

[3]Reznik, G., Reznik-Schüller, H.M., Rice, J.M. & Hague, B.F., Jr (1981) Pathogenesis of toxic and neoplastic renal lesions induced by the flame retardant tris(2,3-dibromopropyl)phosphate in F344 rats, and development of colonic adenomas after prolonged oral administration. *Lab. Invest.*, *44*, 74-83

[4]*IARC Monographs, Suppl. 6*, 554-557, 1987

URACIL MUSTARD (Group 2B)

A. Evidence for carcinogenicity to humans (*inadequate*)

No epidemiological study of uracil mustard as a single agent was available to the Working Group. Occasional case reports of treatment with uracil mustard, especially in the presence of concurrent therapy with other putative carcinogens, such as ionizing radiation, alkylating agents and other potent oncotherapeutic drugs, do not constitute evidence of carcinogenesis[1-5].

B. Evidence for carcinogenicity to animals (*sufficient*)

Intraperitoneal administration of uracil mustard to mice of three strains induced lung adenomas and adenocarcinomas in a dose-dependent incidence; in one of the strains, liver, ovarian and lymphatic tumours were also observed. In rats, intraperitoneal administration induced peritoneal sarcomas and lymphomas and tumours in the pancreas, ovary and mammary gland[6].

C. Other relevant data

Uracil mustard is an alkylating agent[7]. No data were available on its genetic and related effects in humans.

Uracil mustard did not induce dominant lethal mutations in mice in one study using low doses. It induced mutation in mouse lymphoma cells *in vitro*, aneuploidy and sex-linked recessive lethal mutations in *Drosophila* and mitotic recombination in yeast. It caused DNA damage and was mutagenic in bacteria[7].

References

[1]Reimer, R.R., Hoover, R., Fraumeni, J.F., Jr & Young, R.C. (1977) Acute leukemia after alkylating-agent therapy of ovarian cancer. *New Engl. J. Med.*, *297*, 177-181

[2]Zarrabi, M.H. & Rosner, F. (1979) Acute myeloblastic leukemia following treatment for non-hematopoietic cancers. Report of 19 cases and review of the literature. *Am. J. Hematol.*, *7*, 357-367

[3]McKenna, R.W., Parkin, J.L., Foucar, K. & Brunning, R.D. (1981) Ultrastructural characteristics of therapy-related acute nonlymphocytic leukemia: evidence for a panmyelosis. *Cancer*, *48*, 725-737

[4]Rosner, F. (1976) Acute leukemia as a delayed consequence of cancer chemotherapy. *Cancer*, *37*, 1033-1036

[5]Zarrabi, M.H. (1980) Association of non-Hodgkin's lymphoma (NHL) and second neoplasms. *Semin. Oncol.*, *7*, 340-351

[6]*IARC Monographs*, *9*, 235-241, 1975

[7]*IARC Monographs*, *Suppl. 6*, 558-560, 1987

VINBLASTINE SULPHATE (Group 3)

A. Evidence for carcinogenicity to humans (*inadequate*)

No epidemiological study of vinblastine sulphate as a single agent was available to the Working Group. Occasional case reports of exposure to vinblastine sulphate, especially in the presence of concurrent therapy with other putative carcinogens, such as ionizing radiation, alkylating agents and other potent oncotherapeutic drugs, do not constitute evidence of carcinogenesis[1].

In a large systematic follow-up of patients with Hodgkin's disease treated with an intensive chemotherapeutic combination including vinblastine (plus adriamycin [see p. 81], bleomycins [see p. 134] and dacarbazine [see p. 184]) but no alkylating agent, preliminary evidence suggested no excess of acute nonlymphocytic leukaemia in the first decade after therapy[2,3].

B. Evidence for carcinogenicity to animals (*inadequate*)

No evidence of carcinogenicity was found after intraperitoneal administration of vinblastine sulphate to mice and rats or after its intravenous administration to rats, but it has not been adequately tested at high doses[1].

C. Other relevant data

No data were available on the genetic and related effects of vinblastine sulphate in humans.

Vinblastine sulphate weakly induced micronuclei in a single study using low doses, but it did not induce dominant lethal mutations in mice treated *in vivo*. It induced chromosomal aberrations but not mutation in Chinese hamster cells *in vitro* and was not mutagenic to bacteria[4].

References

[1]*IARC Monographs*, 26, 349-363, 1981

[2]Santoro, A., Viviani, S., Villarreal, C.J.R., Bonfante, V., Delfino, A., Valagussa, P. & Bonadonna, G. (1986) Salvage chemotherapy in Hodgkin's disease irradiation failures: superiority of doxorubicin containing regimens over MOPP. *Cancer Treat. Rep.*, 70, 343-348

[3]Valagussa, P., Santoro, A., Fossati Bellani, F., Franchi, F., Banfi, A. & Bonadonna, G. (1982) Absence of treatment-induced second neoplasms after ABVD in Hodgkin's disease. *Blood*, 59, 488-494

[4]*IARC Monographs, Suppl. 6*, 561-562, 1987

VINCRISTINE SULPHATE (Group 3)

A. Evidence for carcinogenicity to humans (*inadequate*)

No epidemiological study of vincristine sulphate as a single agent was available to the Working Group. Intensive combination chemotherapy with regimens including vincristine has been shown to result in increased risks for acute nonlymphocytic leukaemia (ANLL). (See also the summary of data on MOPP and other combined chemotherapy including alkylating agents, p. 254.) Such combinations usually include procarbazine (see p. 327) together with an alkylating agent such as nitrogen mustard (see p. 269), both of which are potent animal carcinogens, suggesting more plausible explanations for the association between combination chemotherapy and ANLL. In the presence of concurrent therapy with other putative carcinogens, including ionizing radiation and other potent drugs, occasional case reports of exposure to vincristine sulphate do not constitute evidence of carcinogenesis[1].

B. Evidence for carcinogenicity to animals (*inadequate*)

In limited studies in mice and rats, no evidence of carcinogenicity was found after intraperitoneal administration of vincristine sulphate[1].

C. Other relevant data

No data were available on the genetic and related effects of vincristine sulphate in humans.

Vincristine sulphate induced micronuclei in bone-marrow cells of mice and hamsters treated *in vivo*. Conflicting results were obtained for induction of sister chromatid exchanges in human lymphocytes *in vitro*. It induced aneuploidy in and transformation of Syrian hamster embryo cells, but it did not transform mouse C3H 10T1/2 cells. It did not induce chromosomal aberrations, sister chromatid exchanges or unscheduled DNA synthesis in rodent cells *in vitro*. It induced mutation in mouse lymphoma cells but not in other rodent cells. It did not induce sex-linked recessive lethal mutations in *Drosophila* and was not mutagenic to bacteria[2].

References

[1]*IARC Monographs*, 26, 365-384, 1981

[2]*IARC Monographs, Suppl. 6*, 563-565, 1987

VINYL CHLORIDE (Group 1)

A. Evidence for carcinogenicity to humans (*sufficient*)

Vinyl chloride has been associated with tumours of the liver, brain, lung and haematolymphopoietic system[1]. A large number of epidemiological studies[2-12] and case reports[13-25] have substantiated the causal association between vinyl chloride and angiosarcoma of the liver. Several studies also confirm that exposure to vinyl chloride causes other forms of cancer, i.e., hepatocellular carcinoma[13,19,23,26], brain tumours[11,27], lung tumours[12,28-30] and malignancies of the lymphatic and haematopoietic system[11,29,31]. Exposure to polyvinyl chloride dust was associated with an increased incidence of lung tumours in one study; the authors suggested that trapped vinyl chloride monomer was responsible[30]. Melanoma occurred in excess in one study[12] but has not been mentioned in others. Slightly elevated risks for gastric[29] and gastrointestinal cancer (other than liver cancer)[32] were indicated in some studies, but these were not confirmed in others.

B. Evidence for carcinogenicity to animals (*sufficient*)

Vinyl chloride administered orally or by inhalation to mice, rats and hamsters produced tumours in the mammary gland, lung, Zymbal gland and skin and angiosarcomas of the liver[1]. Similar findings were made in more recent studies[33-39]. In one, a combination of oral administration of ethanol and inhalation of vinyl chloride resulted in more liver tumours (including angiosarcomas) than after treatment with vinyl chloride alone[40].

C. Other relevant data

Chromosomal aberrations were induced in peripheral blood lymphocytes of workers exposed to vinyl chloride at levels of 5-500 ppm (13-1300 mg/m[3]). Two studies reported negative results for sister chromatid exchanges in exposed workers, while in another study a weakly positive response was found[41].

Vinyl chloride induced chromosomal aberrations, sister chromatid exchanges and micronuclei in rodents exposed *in vivo* but did not induce mutation in the mouse spot test or dominant lethal mutations in rats or mice. It alkylated DNA in several tissues of mice and rats exposed *in vivo*. Vinyl chloride induced sister chromatid exchanges in human lymphocytes *in vitro*. It induced mutation in Chinese hamster cells and unscheduled DNA synthesis in rat hepatocytes *in vitro* and induced transformation of BALB/c 3T3 cells and virus-infected Syrian hamster cells. It induced sex-linked recessive lethal mutations, but not aneuploidy, heritable translocations or dominant lethal mutations in *Drosophila*. It was mutagenic to plants and to *Schizosaccharomyces pombe* but not to other fungi; it induced gene conversion in yeast. It caused DNA damage and mutation in bacteria. Vinyl chloride bound covalently to isolated DNA in the presence of a metabolic system[41].

References

[1]*IARC Monographs*, *19*, 377-438, 1979

[2]Baxter, P.J., Anthony, P.P., MacSween, R.N.M. & Scheuer, P.J. (1977) Angiosarcoma of the liver in Great Britain 1963-73. *Br. med. J.*, *ii*, 919-921

[3]Brady, J., Liberatore, F., Harper, P., Greenwald, P., Burnett, W., Davies, J.N.P., Bishop, M., Polan, A. & Viana, N. (1977) Angiosarcoma of the liver: an epidemiologic survey. *J. natl Cancer Inst.*, *59*, 1383-1385

[4]Baxter, P.J., Anthony, P.P., MacSween, R.N.M. & Scheuer, P.J. (1980) Angiosarcoma of the liver: annual occurrence and aetiology in Great Britain. *Br. J. ind. Med.*, *37*, 213-221

[5]Baxter, P.J. (1981) The British hepatic angiosarcoma register. *Environ. Health Perspect.*, *41*, 115-116

[6]Falk, H., Herbert, J., Crowley, S., Ishak, K.G., Thomas, L.B., Popper, H. & Caldwell, G.G. (1981) Epidemiology of hepatic angiosarcoma in the United States, 1964-1974. *Environ. Health Perspect.*, *41*, 107-113

[7]Thériault, G. & Allard, P. (1981) Cancer mortality of a group of Canadian workers exposed to vinyl chloride monomer. *J. occup. Med.*, *23*, 671-676

[8]Vianna, N.J., Brady, J.A. & Cardamone, A.T. (1981) Epidemiology of angiosarcoma of liver in New York State. *N.Y. State J. Med.*, *6*, 895-899

[9]Weber, H., Reinl, W. & Greiser, E. (1981) German investigations on morbidity and mortality of workers exposed to vinyl chloride. *Environ. Health Perspect.*, *41*, 95-99

[10]Forman, D., Bennett, B., Stafford, J. & Doll, R. (1985) Exposure to vinyl chloride and angiosarcoma of the liver: a report of the register of cases. *Br. J. ind. Med.*, *42*, 750-753

[11]von Greiser, E., Reinl, W. & Weber, H. (1982) Vinyl chloride exposure and mortality of German chemical workers in comparison to mortality of non-exposed chemical workers and PVC workers (Ger.). *Zbl. Arbeitsmed.*, *32*, 44-62

[12]Heldaas, S.S., Langård, S.L. & Andersen, A. (1984) Incidence of cancer among vinyl chloride and polyvinyl chloride workers. *Br. J. ind. Med.*, *41*, 25-30

[13]Gokel, J.M., Liebezeit, E. & Eder, M. (1976) Hemangiosarcoma and hepatocellular carcinoma of the liver following vinyl chloride exposure. A report of two cases. *Virchows Arch. Pathol. Anat. Histol.*, *372*, 195-203

[14]Bonneton, G., Champetier, J., Fournet, J., Guidicelli, H., Legrand, J., Dupré, A., Hostein, M., Marty, F. & Pahn, M. (1977) Angiosarcoma of the liver and portal fibrosis in vinyl chloride workers. Two cases (Fr.). *Nouv. Presse méd.*, *6*, 735-742

[15]Puech, A.-M., Fournet, A., Laulhere, L., Faure, J., Cau, G. & Mallion, J.-M. (1977) Study of hepatic lesions seen in 5 subjects exposed to vinyl chloride, including 3 cases of angiosarcoma of the liver (Fr.). *Arch. Mal. prof.*, *38*, 787-795

[16]Réty, J., Lambert, R. & Pialat, J. (1981) Medical surveillance of persons exposed to occupational toxic compounds with late or carcinogenic effects. The 11th French case of angiosarcoma of the liver in a PVC worker (Fr.). *Arch. Mal. prof.*, *42*, 405-406

[17]Pialat, J., Pasquier, B., Pahn, M. & Kopp, N. (1979) Hepatic lesions caused by vinyl chloride monomer. Study of eight clinicopathological cases (Fr.). *Arch. Anat. Cytol. pathol.*, *27*, 361-375

[18]Ghandur-Mnaymneh, L. & Gonzalez, M.S. (1981) Angiosarcoma of the penis with hepatic angiomas in a patient with low vinyl chloride exposure. *Cancer*, *47*, 1318-1324

[19]Koischwitz, D., Lelbach, W.K., Lackner, K. & Hermanutz, D. (1981) Angiosarcoma of the liver and hepatocellular carcinomas induced by vinyl chloride (Ger.). *Fortschr. Röntgenstr.*, *134*, 283-290

[20]Vianna, N.J, Brady, J. & Harper, P. (1981) Angiosarcoma of the liver: a signal lesion of vinyl chloride exposure. *Environ. Health Perspect.*, *41*, 207-210

[21]Chiappino, G., Bertazzi, P.A., Baroni, M. & Masini, T. (1982) Hepatic angiosarcoma from vinyl chloride. Report of a new Italian case. *Med. Lav.*, *6*, 555-563

[22]Jones, D.B. & Smith, P.M. (1982) Progression of vinyl chloride induced hepatic fibrosis to angiosarcoma of the liver. *Br. J. ind. Med.*, *39*, 306-307

[23]Evans, D.M.D., Williams, W.J. & Kung, I.T.M. (1983) Angiosarcoma and hepatocellular carcinoma in vinyl chloride workers. *Histopathology*, *7*, 377-388

[24]Maltoni, C., Clini, C., Vicini, F. & Masina, A. (1984) Two cases of liver angiosarcoma among polyvinyl chloride (PVC) extruders of an Italian factory producing PVC bags and other containers. *Am. J. ind. Med.*, *5*, 297-302

[25]Louagie, Y.A., Gianello, P., Kestens, P.J., Bonbled, F. & Haot, J.G. (1984) Vinyl chloride induced hepatic angiosarcoma. *Br. J. Surg.*, *71*, 322-323

[26]Langbein, G., Permanetter, W. & Dietz, A. (1983) Hepatocellular carcinoma after vinyl chloride exposure (Ger.). *Dtsch. med. Wochenschr.*, *108*, 741-745

[27]Cooper, W.C. (1981) Epidemiologic study of vinyl chloride workers: mortality through December 31, 1972. *Environ. Health Perspect.*, *41*, 101-106

[28]Buffler, P.A., Wood, S., Eifler, C., Suarez, L. & Kilian, D.J. (1979) Mortality experience of workers in a vinyl chloride monomer production plant. *J. occup. Med.*, *21*, 195-203

[29]Fedotova, I.V. (1983) The incidence of malignant tumours among workers engaged in the manufacture of vinyl chloride and polyvinyl chloride (Russ.). *Gig. Tr. prof. Zabol.*, *4*, 30-32

[30]Waxweiler, R.J., Smith, A.H., Falk, H. & Tyroler, H.A. (1981) Excess lung cancer risk in a synthetic chemicals plant. *Environ. Health Perspect.*, *41*, 159-165

[31]Filatova, V.S., Antonyuzhenko, V.A., Smulevich, V.B., Fedotova, I.V., Kryzhanovskaya, N.A., Bochkareva, T.V., Goryacheva, L.A. & Bulbulyan, M.A. (1982) Blastomogenic hazard of vinyl chloride (clinico-hygienic and epidemiologic study) (Russ.). *Gig. Tr. prof. Zabol.*, *1*, 28-31

[32]Molina, G., Holmberg, B., Elofsson, S., Holmlund, L., Moosing, R. & Westerholm, P. (1981) Mortality and cancer rates among workers in the Swedish PVC processing industry. *Environ. Health Perspect.*, *41*, 145-151

[33]Hong, C.B., Winston, J.M., Thornburg, L.P., Lee, C.C. & Woods, J.S. (1981) Follow-up study on the carcinogenicity of vinyl chloride and vinylidene chloride in rats and mice: tumor incidence and mortality subsequent to exposure. *J. Toxicol. environ. Health*, *7*, 909-924

[34]Feron, V.J., Hendriksen, C.F.M., Speek, A.J., Til, H.P. & Spit, B.J. (1981) Lifespan oral toxicity study of vinyl chloride in rats. *Food Cosmet. Toxicol.*, *19*, 317-333

[35]Hehir, R.M., McNamara, B.P., McLaughlin, J., Jr, Willigan, D.A., Bierbower, G. & Hardisty, J.F. (1981) Cancer induction following single and multiple exposures to a constant amount of vinyl chloride monomer. *Environ. Health Perspect.*, *41*, 63-72

[36]Maltoni, C., Lefemine, G., Ciliberti, A., Cotti, G. & Carretti, D. (1981) Carcinogenicity bioassays of vinyl chloride monomer: a model of risk assessment on an experimental basis. *Environ. Health Perspect.*, *41*, 3-29

[37]Drew, R.T., Boorman, G.A., Haseman, J.K., McConnell, E.E., Busey, W.M. & Moore, J.A. (1983) The effect of age and exposure duration on cancer induction by a known carcinogen in rats, mice and hamsters. *Toxicol. appl. Pharmacol.*, *68*, 120-130

[38]Suzuki, Y. (1983) Neoplastic effect of vinyl chloride in mouse lung — lower doses and short-term exposure. *Environ. Res.*, *32*, 91-103

[39]Groth, D.H., Coate, W.B., Ulland, B.M. & Hornung, R.W. (1981) Effects of aging on the induction of angiosarcoma. *Environ. Health Perspect.*, *41*, 53-57

[40]Radike, M.J., Stemmer, K.L. & Bingham, E. (1981) Effect of ethanol on vinyl chloride carcinogenesis. *Environ. Health Perspect.*, *44*, 59-62

[41]*IARC Monographs*, Suppl. *6*, 566-569, 1987

VINYLIDENE CHLORIDE (Group 3)

A. Evidence for carcinogenicity to humans (*inadequate*)

In one epidemiological study of 138 US workers exposed to vinylidene chloride, no excess of cancer was found, but follow-up was incomplete, and nearly 40% of the workers had less than 15 years' latency since first exposure[1]. In a study in the Federal Republic of Germany of 629 workers exposed to vinylidene chloride, seven deaths from cancer (five bronchial carcinomas) were reported; this number was not in excess of the expected value. Two cases of bronchial carcinoma were found in workers, both of whom were 37 years old, whereas 0.07 were expected for persons aged 35-39 years[1,2]. The limitations of these two studies do not permit assessment of the carcinogenicity of the agent to humans. No specific association was found between exposure to vinylidene chloride and the excess of lung cancer noted previously in a US synthetic chemicals plant[1].

B. Evidence for carcinogenicity to animals (*limited*)

Vinylidene chloride was tested for carcinogenicity in mice and rats by oral adminis-tration and by inhalation, in mice by subcutaneous administration and by topical application, and in hamsters by inhalation. Studies in mice and rats by oral administration gave negative results. In inhalation studies, no treatment-related neoplasm was observed in rats or hamsters. In mice, a treatment-related increase in the incidence of kidney adenocarcinomas was observed in male mice, as were increases in the incidences of mammary carcinomas in females and of pulmonary adenomas in male and female mice. In skin-painting studies in female mice, vinylidene chloride showed activity as an initiator, but, in a study of repeated skin application, no skin tumour occurred. No tumour at the injection site was seen in mice given repeated subcutaneous administrations[1].

C. Other relevant data

No data were available on the genetic and related effects of vinylidene chloride in humans.

Vinylidene chloride did not induce dominant lethal mutations in mice or rats and did not induce chromosomal aberrations in bone-marrow cells of rats treated *in vivo*; however, it induced unscheduled DNA synthesis in treated mice. It did not induce chromosomal aberrations or mutation in Chinese hamster cells *in vitro* but did induce unscheduled DNA synthesis in rat hepatocytes. Vinylidene chloride was mutagenic to plant cells and induced mutation and gene conversion in yeast. It was mutagenic to bacteria[3].

References

[1]*IARC Monographs*, *39*, 195-226, 1986

[2]Theiss, A.M., Frentzel-Beyme, R. & Penning, E. (1979) *Mortality study of vinylidene chloride exposed persons.* In: Heir, C. & Kilian, D.J., eds, *Proceedings of the 5th Medichem Congress, San Francisco CA, September 1977*, San Francisco, CA, University of California at San Franciso, pp. 270-278

[3]*IARC Monographs*, *Suppl. 6*, 570-572, 1987

WOLLASTONITE (Group 3)

A. Evidence for carcinogenicity to humans (*inadequate*)

In a small cohort mortality study of 192 male and 46 female workers exposed to wollastonite who were followed from first employment during the period 1923-1980, 79 deaths had occurred by the end of 1980, with 96 expected. Death was due to cancer in ten men (15.6 expected) and two women (3.0 expected). Four lung cancer cases (5.0 expected) were found among the men and none among the women. A rare malignant mesenchymal tumour of the retroperitoneum was reported in one woman[1]. The limited power of this study does not allow any conclusion as to the carcinogenicity of wollastonite.

B. Evidence for carcinogenicity to animals (*limited*)

In one experiment in rats, a significant increase in the incidence of pleural sarcomas was observed after intrapleural implantation of wollastonite fibres >4 μm in length and <0.5 μm in diameter[1].

C. Other relevant data

No data were available to the Working Group.

Reference

[1]*IARC Monographs*, 42, 145-158, 1987

WOOD INDUSTRIES: CARPENTRY AND JOINERY (Group 2B)

Evidence for carcinogenicity to humans (*limited*)

The epidemiological data available suggest that there may be a carcinogenic risk connected with employment as a carpenter or joiner, although some of the studies produced negative results[1].

The connection between nasal cancer other than adenocarcinoma and exposure to wood dust among carpenters and joiners, found in some studies, if true, cannot be ascribed to any specific exposure. Carpenters and joiners usually work with impregnated wood, use a variety of types of wood and are exposed to many chemicals used in carpentry[1].

Several studies raise the possibility of an increased risk of Hodgkin's disease. A number of studies suggest an association between work as a joiner and nasal adenocarcinoma, but it is possible that the workers involved may have worked in the furniture industry[1].

There is also some evidence of an association between nasal carcinomas other than adenocarcinoma and work as a carpenter. In a case-control study based on an analysis of occupational data in the hospital records of 121 men seen for nasal cancer in British Columbia, Canada, between 1939 and 1977, a relative risk of 2.5 (adjusted for smoking and ethnic origin) was associated with exposure to wood. There was an increased risk for most histological types of epithelial tumour, except for transitional tumours. Of the 28 wood workers with nasal cancer, 16 had worked in the forestry industry, seven had been carpenters, four had been construction workers and one had been a cabinet-maker[2].

A case-control study on nasal and sinonasal cancer in Denmark, Finland and Sweden found a connection with exposure to spruce, pine and birch dust and the cancers studied, especially epidermoid and anaplastic carcinomas. There were 13 cases with exposure only to these types of wood *versus* four controls (relative risk, 3.2; 95% confidence interval, 1.1-9.4). Of the cases, five were in construction carpenters and one in a cabinet-maker with no exposure to hardwood; there were two construction carpenters among the controls[3].

In a Norwegian study of 70 cases of nasal carcinoma, three cases of squamous-cell carcinoma had had exposure to pine and spruce dust in joinery and carpentry *versus* 1.5 expected on the basis of the occupational distribution in Norway according to the 1946 census[4]. In France, carpenters were not found to have an increased risk of nasal cancer, but no quantitative data were given[5]. A case-control study of nasal cancer from North Carolina and Virginia, USA, showed a nonsignificant relative risk of 1.6 for carpentry[6].

In a national study of nasal cancer in England and Wales in 1963-1967, the occupations of 925 men were studied, using postal questionnaires and data from hospital and death records. Among wood workers, the standard incidence ratios (SIRs) for cabinet- and chairmakers, machinists and 'other' wood workers were 966, 616 and 293, respectively. For carpenters and joiners, the SIR was 149[7]. Another case-control study[8] showed no significantly increased risk for 'woodworkers and carpenters' residing in certain areas of London, selected for the study because of high incidences of nasal and bladder cancer.

A Swedish register-linkage study gave a two-fold excess of adenocarcinoma, based on five cases, among carpenters and joiners but no overall excess of nasal cancer in this group[9].

A cohort study comparing the experience of 10 322 men employed in wood-working industries with that of 406 798 non-wood workers showed no excess for all cancers combined. In the subcohort of carpenters and joiners, 36 cases of stomach cancer were found, yielding a standardized mortality ratio (SMR) of 170 ($p < 0.01$). There were 101 deaths from lung cancer, resulting in a SMR of 120 ($p < 0.05$). Nonsignificantly elevated SMRs were found for cancers of the liver, biliary ducts and gall-bladder (11 cases; SMR, 121), nonmelanocytic skin cancer (4 cases; SMR, 333) and melanoma (5 cases; SMR, 161). There were two cases of nasal cancer (SMR, 333; nonsignificant)[10].

A proportionate mortality study showed an elevated risk for death from all cancers (proportionate mortality ratio [PMR], 112; $p < 0.01$), stomach cancer (PMR, 128; $p < 0.01$) and non-Hodgkin's lymphoma (PMR, 139; $p < 0.05$) among woodworkers (including carpenters, cabinet-makers and furniture workers, lumber graders and scalers, sawyers in sawmills and woodworkers not classified elsewhere). In this mixed category, there was no death from sinonasal cancer[11].

A Dutch case-control study[12] of 116 male patients with primary sinonasal malignancies of epithelial origin showed an increased risk of adenocarcinoma for those employed in joinery and carpentry work in factories (odds ratio, 16.3; 90% confidence interval, 2.8-85.3). This work included production of doors and window frames; hence, exposure to oak dust was likely.

References

[1]*IARC Monographs*, 25, 139-156, 1981

[2]Elwood, J.M. (1981) Wood exposure and smoking: association with cancer of the nasal cavity and paranasal sinuses in British Columbia. *Can. med. Assoc. J.*, *124*, 1573-1577

[3]Hernberg, S., Westerholm, P., Schultz-Larsen, K., Degerth, R., Kuosma, E., Englund, A., Engzell, U., Sand Hansen, H. & Mutanen, P. (1983) Nasal and sinonasal cancer. Connection with occupational exposures in Denmark, Finland and Sweden. *Scand. J. Work Environ. Health*, *9*, 315-326

[4]Voss, R., Stenersen, T., Oppedal, B.R. & Boysen, M. (1985) Sinonasal cancer and exposure to softwood. *Acta otolaryngol.*, *99*, 172-178

[5]Duclos, J.-C., Dubreuil, C., Contassot, J.C., Guinchard, R. & Arnould, G. (1979) Nasal ethmoid adenocarcinomas in woodworkers. Clinical and forensic aspects (Fr.). *Arch. Mal. prof.*, *40*, 909-917

[6]Brinton, L.A., Blot, W.J., Becker, J.A., Winn, D.M., Browder, J.P., Farmer, J.C., Jr & Fraumeni, J.F., Jr (1984) A case-control study of cancers of the nasal cavity and paranasal sinuses. *Am. J. Epidemiol.*, *119*, 896-906

[7]Acheson, E.D., Cowdell, R.H. & Rang, E.H. (1981) Nasal cancer in England and Wales: an occupational survey. *Br. J. ind. Med.*, *38*, 218-224

[8]Baxter, P.J. & McDowall, M.E. (1986) Occupation and cancer in London: an investigation into nasal and bladder cancer using the Cancer Atlas. *Br. J. ind. Med.*, *43*, 44-49

[9]Malker, H.S.R., McLaughlin, J.K., Blot, W.J., Weiner, J.A., Malker, B.K., Ericsson J.L.E. & Stone, B.J. (1986) Nasal cancer and occupation in Sweden, 1961-1979. *Am. J. ind. Med.*, *9*, 477-485

[10]Stellman, S.D. & Garfinkel, L. (1984) Cancer mortality among woodworkers. *Am. J. ind. Med.*, *5*, 343-357

[11]Gallagher, R.P., Threlfall, W.J., Band, P.R. & Spinelli, J.J. (1985) Cancer mortality experience of woodworkers, loggers, fishermen, farmers, and miners in British Columbia. *Natl Cancer Inst. Monogr.*, *69*, 163-167

[12]Hayes, R.B., Gerin, M., Raatgever, J.W. & de Bruyn, A. (1986) Wood-related occupations, wood dust exposure, and sinonasal cancer. *Am. J. Epidemiol.*, *124*, 569-577

FURNITURE AND CABINET-MAKING (Group 1)

A. Evidence for carcinogenicity to humans (*sufficient*)

Employment in the furniture-making industry has been associated with nasal adeno-carcinoma; an increased risk for other nasal cancers has also been suggested[1]. Subsequent case reports[2-11] and epidemiological studies[12-18] have clearly corroborated an increased risk of nasal adenocarcinoma among workers in the furniture and cabinet-making industry.

A study was made of the incidence of and mortality from cancer in 5371 men employed in the Buckinghamshire, UK, furniture industry and followed for an average of 19 years since commencing work. The incidence of nasal adenocarcinoma was about 100 times that expected from the local population. For cancer of the bronchus, the standard registration ratio was 82 (95% confidence interval, 61-107), based on 53 cases, and the SMR (corrected for the Oxford region) was 79 (59-105). However, a significant trend of increasing SMR with increasing dustiness of work was found. A trend of increasing SMR for bronchial cancer with increasing duration of work (not significant) was also found. A sample of the work-force alive in 1969 contained a lower percentage of current smokers than the general population, and there were slightly fewer smokers among the men in the dustiest jobs than in the less dusty jobs[12]. However, an update of the same study at the end of 1982 found no significant increase in mortality nor any trend towards increasing mortality with increased dustiness of work for cancer at any site apart from the nasal cavity[16].

A Swedish pilot case-control study found an odds ratio of 4.1 (1.6-10.6) for respiratory cancer other than nasal cancer in relation to wood work. This ratio was based on six exposed cases, four of which were in furniture workers (odds ratio, 6.0)[19]. In another Swedish study, 8141 furniture workers were followed for 19 years. Nasal adenocarcinoma was 63.4 times more common than expected, but no increased risk was found for laryngeal cancer, lung cancer or sinonasal cancer other than adenocarcinoma[17].

A cohort study of the Danish carpenters' and cabinet-makers' union[20] gives SMRs for lung cancer of 96 (68-114) in men aged 20-64 and 110 (92-127) in men aged 65-84.

Mortality from multiple myeloma among furniture workers was investigated in a US case-control study of 301 male cases and 858 controls who had died from other causes. Employment in the furniture industry was associated with a nonsignificant excess risk (odds ratio, 1.3) of multiple myeloma. The risk was somewhat higher for those who had died before age 65 (odds ratio, 1.7) and for those born before 1905 (odds ratio, 1.5), and was significantly elevated for those born before 1905 and who had died before age 65 (odds ratio, 5.4; based on five cases; $p < 0.05$)[21].

A proportionate mortality study showed an elevated risk for death from all cancers (PMR, 112; $p < 0.01$), stomach cancer (PMR, 128; $p < 0.01$) and non-Hodgkin's lymphoma (PMR, 139; $p < 0.05$) among woodworkers (including carpenters, cabinet-makers and furniture workers, lumber graders and scalers, sawyers in sawmills and woodworkers not classified elsewhere). In this mixed category, there was no death from sinonasal cancer[22].

Epidemiological data reported here and previously[1] thus provide sufficient evidence that nasal adenocarcinomas have been caused by employment in the furniture-making industry. The excess risk occurs (mainly) among those exposed to wood dust.

According to Acheson et al.[13], the fact that woodworking machinists (who saw timber) and cabinet- and chain makers (who shape, finish, sand and assemble furniture) experience similar risks makes it unlikely that the tumours are due to a chemical agent applied to the wood at a particular stage of the process, but that they are more probably due to a substance in wood itself. Beech and oak, especially, have been incriminated, but the possibility that other hardwoods are carcinogenic cannot be ruled out. The carcinogenic substances in hardwood are, however, unknown.

B. Evidence for carcinogenicity to animals (inadequate)

Among hamsters exposed by inhalation to fine particles of beech wood dust, one animal out of 22 had a nasal tumour. In these limited studies, inhalation of wood dust did not increase the incidence of nasal or respiratory-tract tumours induced by N-nitroso-diethylamine[23,24].

C. Other relevant data

A fraction of a methanol extract of beech-wood dust was mutagenic to *Salmonella typhimurium* in the presence of an exogenous metabolic system[25].

References

[1]*IARC Monographs*, *25*, 99-138, 1981

[2]Duclos, J.-C., Dubreuil, C., Contassot, J.C., Guinchard, R. & Arnould, G. (1979) Nasal ethmoid adenocarcinomas in woodworkers. Clinical and forensic aspects (Fr.). *Arch. Mal. prof.*, *40*, 909-917

[3]Cecchi, F., Buiatti, E., Kriebel, D., Nastasi, L. & Santucci, M. (1980) Adenocarcinoma of the nose and paranasal sinuses in shoemakers and woodworkers in the province of Florence, Italy (1963-77). *Br. J. ind. Med.*, *37*, 222-225

[4]Merler, E., Carnevale, F., D' Andrea, F., Macaccaro, G., Pisa, R., Capitanio, A., Cavazzani, M., Gentile, A. & Fantoni, G. (1981) Neoplasm of the nasal cavities and the paranasal sinuses and occupational exposure to wood dust (Ital.). *Med. Lav.*, *72*, 87-95

[5]Marandas, P., Schwaab, G. & Cachin, Y. (1980) Wood workers and ethmoid tumours (Fr.). *Ouest méd.*, *33*, 1149-1153

[6]Cabal, C. & Teyssier, J.-M. (1981) Ethmoid tumours in wood workers (Fr.). *Arch. Mal. prof.*, *42*, 303-305

[7]Duclos, J.C., Dubreuil, C., Guinchard, R. & Arnould, G. (1981) Ethmoid nasal adenocarcinomas in wood workers (Fr.). *Arch. Mal. prof.*, *42*, 292-294

[8]Marandas, P., Schwaab, G., Lecointre, F., Pene, F. & Vandenbrouck, C. (1981) Ethmoid tumours. Role of wood work and clinical aspects (Fr.). *Arch. Mal. prof.*, *42*, 294-300

[9]Klintenberg, C., Olofsson, J., Hellquist, H. & Sökjer, H. (1984) Adenocarcinoma of the ethmoid sinuses. A review of 28 cases with special reference to wood dust exposure. *Cancer*, *54*, 482-488

[10]von Thürauf, J. & Hartung, M. (1984) Adenocarcinoma of the nose and paranasal sinuses in people employed in the wood industry in the Federal Republic of Germany (Ger.). *Zbl. Arbeitsmed.*, *34*, 8-15

[11]Wolf, J., Hartung, M., Schaller, K.H., Kochem, W. & Valentin, H. (1986) Occurrence of adenocarcinoma of the nasal and paranasal sinuses in woodworkers (Ger.). *Arbeitsmed. Sozialmed. Präventivmed.*, *7*, 3-22

[12]Rang, E.H. & Acheson, E.D. (1981) Cancer in furniture workers. *Int. J. Epidemiol.*, *10*, 253-261

[13]Acheson, E.D., Winter, P.D., Hadfield, E. & Macbeth, R.G. (1982) Is nasal adenocarcinoma in the Buckinghamshire furniture industry declining? *Nature*, *299*, 263-265

[14]Battista, G., Cavallucci, F., Comba, P., Quercia, A., Vindigni, C. & Sartorelli, E. (1983) A case-referent study on nasal cancer and exposure to wood dust in the province of Sienna, Italy. *Scand. J. Work Environ. Health*, *9*, 25-29

[15]Hernberg, S., Westerholm, P., Schultz-Larsen, K., Degerth, R., Kuosma, E., Englund, A., Engzell, U., Sand Hansen, H. & Mutanen, P. (1983) Nasal and sinonasal cancer. Connection with occupational exposures in Denmark, Finland and Sweden. *Scand. J. Work Environ. Health*, *9*, 315-326

[16]Acheson, E.D., Pippard, E.C. & Winter, P.D. (1984) Mortality of English furniture makers. *Scand. J. Work Environ. Health*, *10*, 211-217

[17]Gerhardsson, M.R., Norell, S.E., Kiviranta, H.J. & Ahlbom, A. (1985) Respiratory cancers in furniture workers. *Br. J. ind. Med.*, *42*, 403-405

[18]Malker, H.S.R., McLaughlin, J.K., Blot, W.J., Weiner, J.A., Malker, B.K., Ericsson, J.L.E. & Stone, B.J. (1986) Nasal cancer and occupation in Sweden, 1961-1979. *Am. J. ind. Med.*, *9*, 477-485

[19]Esping, B. & Axelson, O. (1980) A pilot study on respiratory and digestive tract cancer among woodworkers. *Scand. J. Work Environ. Health, 6*, 201-205

[20]Olsen, J. & Sabroe, S. (1979) A follow-up study of non-retired and retired members of the Danish Carpenter/Cabinet Makers' Trade Union. *Int. J. Epidemiol., 8*, 375-382

[21]Tollerud, D.J., Brinton, L.A., Stone, B.J., Tobacman, J.K. & Blattner, W.A. (1985) Mortality from multiple myeloma among North Carolina furniture workers. *J. natl Cancer Inst., 74*, 799-801

[22]Gallagher, R.P., Threlfall, W.J., Band, P.R. & Spinelli, J.J. (1985) Cancer mortality experience of woodworkers, loggers, fishermen, farmers, and miners in British Columbia. *Natl Cancer Inst. Monogr., 69*, 163-167

[23]Wilhelmsson, B., Lundh, B., Drettner, B. & Stenkvist, B. (1985) Effects of wood dust exposure and diethylnitrosamine. A pilot study in Syrian golden hamsters. *Acta otolaryngol., 99*, 160-171

[24]Drettner, B., Wilhelmsson, B. & Lundh, B. (1985) Experimental studies on carcinogenesis in the nasal mucosa. *Acta otolaryngol., 99*, 205-207

[25]*IARC Monographs, Suppl. 6*, 573, 1987

LUMBER AND SAWMILL INDUSTRIES (INCLUDING LOGGING) (Group 3)

Evidence for carcinogenicity to humans (*inadequate*)

Information on the occurrence of cancer in lumber and sawmill workers is limited. The available epidemiological data come primarily from surveys of statements of occupation on death certificates. Nasal tumours, malignant lymphomas and leukaemias and soft-tissue sarcomas have been linked with work in the lumber and sawmill industries, but the results are not consistent[1].

In a case-control study based on an analysis of occupational data in the hospital records of 121 men seen for nasal cancer in British Columbia, Canada, between 1939 and 1977, a relative risk of 2.5 (adjusted for smoking and ethnic origin) was found to be associated with exposure to wood. There was increased risk for most histological types of epithelial tumour, except for transitional tumours. Of the 28 wood workers with nasal cancer, 16 had worked in the forestry industry, seven had been carpenters, four had been construction workers and one had been a cabinet-maker[2].

In a case-control study based on 167 cases of nasal or sinonasal cancer and 167 controls from Denmark, Finland and Sweden, exposure mainly to softwood dust (pine and spruce, but also some birch) was associated with epidermoid and anaplastic carcinomas, but not with adenocarcinomas. There were 13 cases with exposure only to softwood *versus* four controls (odds ratio, 3.3; 95% confidence interval, 1.1-9.4). Of these, four cases (all with epidermoid carcinoma) and two controls had been sawmill workers. Only two of the four cases had had potential exposure to chlorophenols (see p. 154)[3].

In a Norwegian study based on 70 cases of various forms of sinonasal cancer (4 observed, 0.4 expected in saw- and planingmill workers; 3 observed, 1.8 expected in forestry workers), three cases of non-Hodgkin's lymphoma were associated with employment in saw- and planingmill firms. The comparison was made between the number of cases observed in different occupations and the expected number of cases according to the 1946 census data of workers in these occupations[4].

A case-control study of Hodgkin's disease[5], using death certificates from North Carolina, USA, counties with a 'significant proportion' of the population employed in the furniture industry and in lumbering, showed an excess risk only among occupational groups with exposure to wood or paper. Carpenters and lumberers had a relative risk of 4.2 for Hodgkin's disease (95% confidence interval, 1.4-12.5). In Oregon, USA, a case-control study on leukaemia (ICD-9 codes 204-208)[6] showed a three-fold increase in risk for patients who had worked for ten years or more in the sawmill industry ($p = 0.017$), based on nine exposed cases.

In a proportionate mortality study of the causes of death of 375 union-affiliated Swedish lumberjacks who had died between 1968 and 1977, there were fewer deaths from cancer than expected (PMR, 88; 69-111). A marked deficiency of deaths from lung cancer (SMR, 33) and excesses of deaths from kidney cancer (SMR, 193; 92-407) and from cancers of the lymphatic and haematopoietic systems (SMR, 191; 105-349) were found. No information was given about the histology of these two groups of tumours. The mortality experience of Swedish males during that period was used as the standard for comparison[7].

A cohort study comparing the mortality experience of 10 322 men employed in wood-working industries with that of 406 798 non-wood workers showed no excess risk for all cancers combined. In the subcohort of lumber and sawmill workers, there was no statistically significant increase in the incidence of cancer at any site. No case of nasal cancer was reported[8].

A nested case-control study[9], based on an average of 25 years' follow-up of 3805 men working in the Finnish particle-board, plywood, sawmill or formaldehyde glue industries between 1944 and 1965, showed no clear connection between respiratory cancer incidence and most of the exposures studied, although some odds ratios were statistically significantly increased. For example, exposure to pesticides (in wood dust) and phenol was associated with elevated odds ratios, which became more marked among workers with more than ten years' exposure to pesticides. The raised odds ratios for exposure to phenol were partly explained by smoking and exposure to pesticides. Because of the mixed exposure, no single pesticide could be linked with respiratory cancer. Exposure to terpenes and other products of coniferous wood was also significantly associated with respiratory cancer when the duration of exposure exceeded five years. None of the odds ratios for exposure to wood dust and chlorophenols was statistically significant.

A proportionate mortality study showed an elevated risk for death from all cancers (PMR, 112; $p < 0.01$), stomach cancer (PMR, 128; $p < 0.01$) and non-Hodgkin's lymphoma (PMR, 139; $p < 0.05$) among woodworkers (including carpenters, cabinet-makers and furniture workers, lumber graders and scalers, sawyers in sawmills and woodworkers not classified elsewhere). In this mixed category, there was no death from sinonasal cancer[10].

The epidemiological data reported here and previously[1] are not sufficient to make a definite assessment of the carcinogenic risks of employment in the lumber and sawmill industries. It should also be noted that these two industries differ greatly with regard to exposures other than wood dust. Some studies suggest that the incidences of nasal cancers, lung cancer and Hodgkin's and non-Hodgkin's lymphoma may be increased. The patterns are not consistent, the results are based on few cases, and, in some studies, work in furniture manufacture has not been excluded sufficiently well. The hypothesis of a link with Hodgkin's disease is not adequately supported. Soft-tissue sarcomas and histiocytic lymphomas have been reported following exposure to chlorophenols and phenoxyacetic acid herbicides (see pp. 154 and 156), but the risk to sawmill and lumber workers was not quantified directly. Stomach cancer incidence was slightly elevated in these occupational groups in six mortality series; however, this might be related to nonoccupational factors.

References

[1] *IARC Monographs*, *25*, 49-97, 1981

[2] Elwood, J.M. (1981) Wood exposure and smoking: association with cancer of the nasal cavity and paranasal sinuses in British Columbia. *Can. med. Assoc. J.*, *15*, 1573-1577

[3] Hernberg, S., Westerholm, P., Schultz-Larsen, K., Degerth, R., Kuosma, E., Englund, A., Engzell, U., Sand Hansen, H. & Mutanen, P. (1983) Nasal and sinonasal cancer. Connection with occupational exposures in Denmark, Finland and Sweden. *Scand. J. Work Environ. Health*, *9*, 315-326

[4] Voss, R., Stenersen, T., Oppedal, B.R. & Boysen, M. (1985) Sinonasal cancer and exposure to softwood. *Acta otolaryngol.*, *99*, 172-178

[5] Greene, M.H., Brinton, L.A., Fraumeni, J.F. & D'Amico, R. (1978) Familial and sporadic Hodgkin's disease associated with occupational wood exposure. *Lancet*, *ii*, 626-627

[6] Burkart, J.A. (1982) Leukemia in hospital patients with occupational exposure to the sawmill industry. *West J. Med.*, *137*, 440-441

[7] Edling, C. & Granstam, S. (1980) Causes of death among lumberjacks — a pilot study. *J. occup. Med.*, *22*, 403-406

[8] Stellman, S. & Garfinkel, L. (1984) Cancer mortality among woodworkers. *Am. J. ind. Med.*, *5*, 343-357

[9] Kauppinen, T.P., Partanen, T.J., Nurminen, M.M., Nickels, J.I., Hernberg, S.G., Hakulinen, T.R., Pukkala, E.I. & Savonen, E.T. (1986) Respiratory cancers and chemical exposures in the wood industry: a nested case-control study. *Br. J. ind. Med.*, *43*, 84-90

[10] Gallagher, R.P., Threlfall, W.J., Band, P.R. & Spinelli, J.J. (1985) Cancer mortality experience of woodworkers, loggers, fishermen, farmers, and miners in British Columbia. *Natl Cancer Inst. Monogr.*, *69*, 163-167

PULP AND PAPER MANUFACTURE (Group 3)

A. Evidence for carcinogenicity to humans (*inadequate*)

Excess incidences of oral and pharyngeal and/or laryngeal cancers were reported in two studies designed to generate hypotheses. These cancer forms have not been evaluated in independent studies[1].

Some studies, based on a few cases, suggest that an increased risk of lymphoproliferative neoplasms, particularly Hodgkin's disease, may be linked to employment in the pulp and paper industries[1-3].

In a prospective cohort study of viscose workers exposed to carbon disulphide, 343 pulp and paper workers served as the reference group. During 15 years of follow-up, nine pulp and paper workers had died of lung cancer, compared with four viscose workers (rate ratio, 2.2; [95% confidence interval, 0.7-6.7]). The pulp and paper workers smoked slightly less than the viscose workers[4]. When national rates were used as the reference, the SMR was 154 (70-292). However, a US proportionate mortality study[3] comprising 2113 deaths revealed no excess of lung cancer among pulp and paper workers.

A US cohort study of 3572 pulp and paper mill workers employed for at least one year between 1945 and 1955 and followed until 1977 showed statistically nonsignificant excesses of lymphosarcoma and reticulosarcoma (10 cases; SMR, 169; 92-287) and of stomach cancer (17 cases; SMR, 123; 78-185). There was no excess of lung cancer. The excess of lymphosarcoma and reticulosarcoma was present only for men who had worked in sulphate mills (6 observed; SMR, 207; 90-408), whereas the excess of stomach cancer occurred in sulphite mills (11 observed; SMR, 149; 83-246)[5].

Excesses of cancers at miscellaneous sites have been mentioned in some studies on pulp and paper workers[1,3,6-8]. The findings may be due to chance, because the cases were generally few and the patterns inconsistent.

A case-control study of the paternal occupations of 692 children who had died of cancer in Massachusetts, USA, showed that paternal employment as a pulp or paper mill worker was associated with tumours of the brain and other parts of the nervous system (six cases observed; relative risk, 2.8); however, as many comparisons were made, this may well be a chance finding[9].

B. Other relevant data

Workers employed for two to 30 years in a paper factory and exposed intermittently to high levels of formaldehyde (see p. 211) for short periods showed a significant increase in the incidence of structural chromosomal aberrations associated with mean exposure to formaldehyde; however, no increase in the incidence of sister chromatid exchanges was observed as compared with controls. An increase in the incidence of chromosomal and chromatid-type aberrations was reported among seven workers involved in boiling pulp and handling sulphuric acid in a sulphite factory, as compared to six workers exposed to chlorine during the bleaching of pulp, six workers exposed to dust in a paper mill and 15 control subjects; but the results remain uncertain due to methodological problems[10].

References

[1]*IARC Monographs, 25*, 157-197, 1981

[2]Greene, M.H., Brinton, L.A., Fraumeni, J.F. & D'Amico, R. (1978) Familial and sporadic Hodgkin's disease associated with occupational wood exposure. *Lancet, ii*, 626-627

[3]Milham, S., Jr & Demers, R.Y. (1984) Mortality among pulp and paper workers. *J. occup. Med.*, *26*, 844-846

[4]Nurminen, M. & Hernberg, S. (1984) Cancer mortality among carbon disulfide-exposed workers. *J. occup. Med.*, *26*, 341

[5]Robinson, C.F., Waxweiler, R.J. & Fowler, D.P. (1986) Mortality among production workers in pulp and paper mills. *Scand. J. Work Environ. Health*, *12*, 552-560

[6]Okubo, T. & Tsuchiya, K. (1974) An epidemiological study on the cancer mortality in various industries in Japan (Jpn.). *Jpn. J. ind. Health*, *16*, 438-452

[7]Malker, H.S.R., McLaughlin, J.K., Malker, B.K., Stone, B.J., Weiner, J.A., Erickson, J.L.E. & Blot, W.J. (1986) Biliary tract cancer and occupation in Sweden. *Br. J. ind. Med.*, *43*, 257-262

[8]Malker, H.S.R., McLaughlin, J.K., Malker, B.K., Stone, B.J., Weiner, J.A., Erickson, J.L.E. & Blot, W.J. (1985) Occupational risks for pleural mesothelioma in Sweden, 1961-79. *J. natl Cancer Inst.*, *74*, 61-66

[9]Kwa, S.-L. & Fine, L.J. (1980) The association between parental occupation and childhood malignancy. *J. occup. Med.*, *22*, 792-794

[10]*IARC Monographs, Suppl. 6*, 573, 1987

ADDITIONAL SUMMARIES AND EVALUATIONS OF EVIDENCE FOR CARCINOGENICITY IN EXPERIMENTAL ANIMALS, AND SUMMARIES OF OTHER RELEVANT DATA, FOR SELECTED AGENTS FOR WHICH THERE ARE NO DATA ON CARCINOGENICITY IN HUMANS

The Working Group also examined the available experimental data on chemicals evaluated by previous Working Groups as being *sufficient evidence* of carcinogenicity to experimental animals, but for which there are no data on humans. The Working Group confirmed the evaluation of *sufficient evidence* of carcinogenicity for these chemicals, except in one case (gyromitrin), for which the evidence for carcinogenicity, on the basis of the present criteria, was considered to be *limited*. A new summary of the data on this chemical was prepared (see p. 391).

The Working Group also reviewed the data on certain chemicals for which there are no data in humans but for which the evidence of carcinogenicity in experimental animals had previously been evaluated as being *limited*. Taking into account new data, the evidence for four chemicals (acetamide, *para*-aminoazobenzene, griseofulvin and sodium *ortho*-phenyl-phenate was re-evaluated as representing *sufficient evidence* of carcinogenicity in experimental animals, and new summaries were prepared for these chemicals (see below and pp. 390, 391 and 392). Thus, there are now 123 agents for which no human data are available but for which there is *sufficient evidence* of carcinogenicity in experimental animals.

In addition, the Working Group re-evaluated the available experimental data as given in the *Monographs* on 11 chemicals previously evaluated by IARC working groups as representing *no evidence* of carcinogenicity to experimental animals. On the basis of the present criteria for *evidence suggesting lack of carcinogenicity* in experimental animals, as given in the Preamble, the evidence for two chemicals (caprolactam and methyl parathion) was re-evaluated as meeting the criteria for placement in this category. For the data on the remaining nine chemicals, an evaluation of *inadequate evidence* was adopted. Summaries of the available data on the two chemicals evaluated as representing *evidence suggesting lack of carcinogenicity* were prepared (see pp. 390 and 392).

ACETAMIDE

Evidence for carcinogenicity to animals (*sufficient*)

Acetamide produced benign and malignant liver tumours in rats following its oral administration[1-3]. In male mice, an increased incidence of malignant lymphomas was also observed[3].

References

[1]*IARC Monographs*, 7, 197-202, 1974

[2]Flaks, B., Trevan, M.T. & Flaks, A. (1983) An electron microscope study of hepatocellular changes in the rat during chronic treatment with acetamide. Parenchyma, foci and neoplasms. *Carcinogenesis*, 4, 1117-1125

[3]Fleischman, R.W., Baker, J.R., Hagopian, M., Wade, G.G., Hayden, D.W., Smith, E.R., Weisburger, J.H. & Weisburger, E.K. (1980) Carcinogenesis bioassay of acetamide, hexanamide, adipamide, urea and p-tolylurea in mice and rats. *J. environ. Pathol. Toxicol.*, 3, 149-170

para-AMINOAZOBENZENE

Evidence for carcinogenicity to animals (*sufficient*)

para-Aminoazobenzene produced liver tumours in rats following its oral administration and produced epidermal tumours in rats after application to the skin[1]. In mice, hepatomas were found in 50-100% of males after one or four intraperitoneal injections of *para*-aminoazobenzene, compared to 3% in controls and in females. In two other strains of mice, 93% and 46% of males had hepatomas at 11 months of age after a single intraperitoneal injection of the compound[2]. When pregnant and newborn male and female mice were administered high doses of *para*-aminoazobenzene by subcutaneous injection, there was a borderline increase in the incidences of tumours of the liver and of the haematopoietic and lymphoid tissues in mice treated transplacentally and a statistically significant increase in the incidence of these tumours in neonates[3].

References

[1]*IARC Monographs*, 8, 53-60, 1975

[2]Delclos, K.B., Tarpley, W.G., Miller, E.C. & Miller, J.A. (1984) 4-Aminoazobenzene and *N,N*-dimethyl-4-aminoazobenzene as equipotent hepatic carcinogens in male C57BL/6×C3H/HeF$_1$ mice and characterization of *N*-(deoxyguanosin-8-yl)-4-aminoazobenzene as the major persistent hepatic DNA-bound dye in these mice. *Cancer Res.*, 44, 2540-2550

[3]Fujii, K. (1983) Induction of tumors in transplacental or neonatal mice administered 3'-methyl-4-dimethylaminoazobenzene or 4-aminoazobenzene. *Cancer Lett.*, 17, 321-325

CAPROLACTAM

A. Evidence for carcinogenicity to animals (*evidence suggesting lack of carcinogenicity*)

Caprolactam was tested adequately by oral administration in the diet of mice and rats. There was no increase in tumour incidence over that in controls[1].

B. Other relevant data

Caprolactam gave negative results in a wide range of in-vitro short-term tests: it did not induce DNA damage, DNA repair, point mutation, sister chromatid exchange, micronuclei, aneuploidy or polyploidy in cultured mammalian cells, recombination or aneuploidy in fungi or mutation in *Salmonella typhimurium* in the presence or absence of an exogenous metabolic system. Results of borderline positivity were obtained in tests for morphological transformation in cultured mammalian cells and for gene conversion in yeast. Caprolactam induced somatic-cell mutations in *Drosophila melanogaster*. There is some evidence that it induces chromosomal aberrations in cultured human cells and point mutations in yeast[1].

Reference

[1]*IARC Monographs, 39*, 247-276, 1986

GRISEOFULVIN

Evidence for carcinogenicity to animals (*sufficient*)

Griseofulvin induced liver tumours following its oral administration to adult mice[1-3] or its subcutaneous administration to infant male mice[1]. When given orally to rats and hamsters, it produced a significant increase in the incidence of thyroid tumours in rats but had no carcinogenic effect in hamsters[2].

References

[1]*IARC Monographs, 10*, 153-161, 1976

[2]Rustia, M. & Shubik, P. (1978) Thyroid tumours in rats and hepatomas in mice after griseofulvin treatment. *Br. J. Cancer, 38*, 237-249

[3]Chlumská, A.A. & Janoušek, V. (1981) Hepatomas after long-term administration of griseofulvin (Czech.). *Cesk. Patol., 17*, 83-87

GYROMITRIN

Evidence for carcinogenicity to animals (*limited*)

In one study, gyromitrin was administered by intragastric intubation to mice, producing increased incidences of tumours of the forestomach, clitoral gland and lung in females and of tumours of the preputial gland in males[1].

Reference

[1]*IARC Monographs, 31*, 163-170, 1983

METHYL PARATHION

A. Evidence for carcinogenicity to animals (*evidence suggesting lack of carcinogenicity*)

Methyl parathion was tested adequately by oral administration in the diet of mice and rats. There was no increase in tumour incidence over that in controls[1].

B. Other relevant data

The incidences of chromosomal aberrations and of dominant lethal mutations were not increased in mice treated *in vivo* with methyl parathion. In mammalian cells, sister chromatid exchange and presumed gene mutations were induced, but neither chromosomal aberration nor unscheduled DNA synthesis was elicited. Methyl parathion was weakly or nonmutagenic in *Drosophila melanogaster* and in bacterial systems, but it was mutagenic in yeasts[1].

Reference

[1]*IARC Monographs*, *30*, 131-152, 1983

SODIUM *ortho*-PHENYLPHENATE

Evidence for carcinogenicity to animals (*sufficient*)

Sodium *ortho*-phenylphenate produced urinary bladder carcinomas in rats following its oral administration[1-3]. It increased the incidences of haemangiosarcomas of the liver and of hepatocellular carcinomas in male mice after its oral administration[4]. When given in the diet to rats, it enhanced the incidence of bladder cancer induced by oral administration of N-nitroso-N-(4-hydroxybutyl)-N-butylamine[5].

References

[1]*IARC Monographs*, *30*, 329-344, 1983

[2]Fujii, T. & Hiraga, K. (1985) Carcinogenicity testing of sodium *ortho*-phenylphenate in F344 rats (Jpn.). *J. Saitama med. School*, *12*, 277-287

[3]Fujii, T., Mikuriya, H., Kamiya, N. & Hiraga, K. (1986) Enhancing effect of thiabendazole on urinary bladder carcinogenesis induced by sodium *o*-phenylphenate in F344 rats. *Food chem. Toxicol.*, *24*, 207-211

[4]Hagiwara, A., Shibata, M., Hirose, M., Fukushima, S. & Ito, N. (1984) Long-term toxicity and carcinogenicity study of sodium *o*-phenylphenate in B6C3F$_1$ mice. *Food chem. Toxicol.*, *22*, 809-814

[5]Fukushima, S., Kurata, Y., Shibata, M., Ikawa, E. & Ito, N. (1983) Promoting effect of sodium *o*-phenylphenate and *o*-phenylphenol on two-stage urinary bladder carcinogenesis in rats. *Gann*, *74*, 625-632

APPENDIX 1.
SUMMARY OF DATA ON GENETIC AND RELATED EFFECTS

Appendix 1. Summary of data on genetic and related effects

Agent	Nonmammalian systems													Mammalian systems																									
	Proka-ryotes		Lower eukaryotes				Plants			Insects			In vitro														In vivo											
													Animal cells								Human cells						Animals							Humans				
	D	G	D	R	G	A	D	G	C	R	G	C	D	G	S	M	C	A	T	I	D	G	S	M	C	A	D	G	S	M	C	DL	A	D	S	M	C	A
Acetaldehyde	+	+											+*	+	+	+*	+*				+*	+	+	+					+		+*							
Acrolein	+	+	*										+	+	+*	+*	?		*		+*	+		+	+						+*							
Acrylonitrile	+*	+	*	+		+*	+*	+*		-			+	+	+	+	+				+	+*	*	+*	+		+			+*	-*				*		-	
Actinomycin D	-*	-	-*	?	+*				-*				+	+	+	+	+	-		*	+*	+*		+			+	+		+*	+	-*		+*	*		+*	*
Adriamycin	+	+	-*	+*	+*	+*		+*	+	+*			+	+*	+	+*	+	+	+*	+*	+*	+*	*	+	+*	*	+*	+		+	+	*	+*	+*	+	+	+	
Aflatoxin B	+	+		+	+*	+					+*		+	+	+	+*	+	+	+*	+*	+*	+	+	+			+*	+			+							
Aflatoxin B1	+	+	-*	+*	-*	+*					+*		+	+	+*	+*	+*	+*	+	+*	+*	+	+*	+	+	-	+*	+*	-		+			+*		+	?	
Aflatoxin B2	-	+		+*	+*					+*			+	+	+*	+*	+		+	+	+	+*		+	+*			+			+							
Aflatoxin G1	+	+	*	+*		+*					+		+	+	-*	+*	+			*	+	+*		+		?		+			+							
Aflatoxin G2	-	?							+				-	-	-*		+*				?	+		-*			+*	-			+*							
Aflatoxin M1	-	+	-*	+*	+								+	+	+	+					+*			-*			?				+							
Aldrin	-*	-		+*									+	+*	+*	+					?	-	-	?			+*	+			+							
4-Aminobiphenyl	+*	-	-*	-*	+*	+						?		-		+*					+	+*					+	-											
Amitrole	-	+			?							-	+*	+	+	+*					?	-					+				+				+				
Aniline	-*	+	-*	+*	+*							*	+*	+	+*	+*	+*	+	*	*	+*	-*		?	-		+*	+*	+*	+*	+	*		-	?	+	?	+
Arsenic, trivalent	+		+*	+*	+*	+*					*		+	+	+	+*	+*	+	+		*	?	-	+*	+*	+	+*	+*	+	+*	+*	*	+	+	*	-	+	
Arsenic, pentavalent	+		*	+*	-*						*		+	+	?	+*	+	+	+			?	-	+	+	+	+*	+	?	+*	*		+	+*	+	+	+	
Asbestos	-		+										+*	+*	+*	+*	+				+*	?		+	*		*	+*		+		*						
Attapulgite	-											?		-							+*				-			+	?										
Auramine	+	+	+		+	+				+	+		+*	+*	+	+*	+				+			-	+			+			+							
Azathioprine	+	+	+*		*			*	+	+*	+*	*	+*	-*	+*	+*	+*	+*	+*	+*	+	+	*	-*	+	+	*	+*	+*	+		+*	+	+	*	+*	+*	*
Benzal chloride	+	+	+										+	+		+	+				*	+	-	+*	+		-			*	+				+*		+	*
Benzene	+*		+*		+*	+*				*	+		+	+	+*	+	+	+	+		*	+	+	+	+		*	+	+	+	+	-*		+	-	+*	+	+
Benzidine	+*	+	+	+*			+	+					+*	+*	+	+*	+				?	-		-			+	?			+							
Benzotrichloride	+*	+	+*	+*	+*						+*	*	+		+	-					+*	*	?		+*	?	+*	+*	+*	+		*		+	*+		*	
Benzoyl chloride	+*	+									+*		+	+	+*	+*	+		*		+*	?		+*			+			+								
Benzyl chloride	+										+*		+	+	+	+	+				+*	+																
Beryllium and beryllium compounds	+	?	-*	+	+	-				?			+	+*	+*	+	+				+*	+*					+									*+		
N,N-Bis(2-chloroethyl)-2-naphthyl-amine (Chlornaphazine)	+		+		+						+		+		+*	+*	+			*	+*						+								?			
Bischloroethyl nitrosourea (BCNU)	+	+	+*		+						+*		+	+	+*	+*	+				+*	+		*			+*	+							?	*+		
Bis(chloromethyl)ether	+	+	+		+								+	+	+	+	+				+*	+					+*	+							*+	+		
Bleomycins	+	+	+		+				+				+	+	+*	+	+				+	+*		+*	+		+		+*	*	?				+*	?	?	*
1,3-Butadiene	+	+											+		*	+	+				+	+*		*+	+		*		+*	+*	*+				*	*+	+*	+
1,4-Butanediol dimethanesulphonate (Myleran)	+	+				-			+		+*		+	+	+	+	+				+	+	+	+	+		*+		+	+	+	+*		+		+	+*	

Agent	Prokaryotes		Lower eukaryotes				Plants			Insects				Animal cells (in vitro)							Human cells								Animals (in vivo)								Humans					
	D	G	D	R	G	A	D	G	C	R	G	C	A	D	G	S	M	C	A	T	I	D	G	S	M	C	A	T	I	D	G	S	M	C	DL	A	A	D	S	M	C	A
Cadmium and cadmium compounds	−*	−*	−	+*	*								−	+	?	−		−	+	+	+	+	−	*		+								−	−	?		+*		*	+?	?
Carbon tetrachloride	+	−	+*	+	+*								−	+	?		*	+		+		?	+	+	−	+*	+					*	+*	*	−			+			?	?
Chlorambucil	+	+	+*	+*	+*	*	+		+*		+*	+		+	+	−*	+	+	*			+	+	+*	*		+					*	+*	*	?						+?	+?
Chloramphenicol	−*	−	+*	+	*	*		+*			−*		−	−	−	+*	+*	+*	−	+		−		+*	−	+					+	+*	+*	−		−					+?
Chlordane	*	*	+*	+*	+*	*	+*	+*					−	+	?	+		+		+		?	+*	+										*	*		+				
Chlormadinone acetate	+	+	*	+*	+*									+	?							?	−			?								+							
Chlorodifluoromethane	+	+	+*	+*	+*									+	−					−												−	+	−							
1-(2-Chloroethyl)-3-cyclohexyl-1-nitrosourea (CCNU)	+*	+*	+*	+*	+*	+																							+												
Chloroform	−	−	+*	+*	+*									−			+	*		+													−	+*	−	−						
Chloromethyl methyl ether	+*	+*																+		*														+*	+*	+?						
(4-Chloro-2-methylphenoxy)acetic acid (MCPA)	−	−	+*	+*	+*	*	*	+*		+*	+*		*	*	*	*		*	*	+	*	*	*	+*	+		+					*	+	+	−							
Chloroprene	+*	+*			+							?		+	?			+		*			?	?											?	?	?					
Cholesterol	−	−												+	+	+				*			+	+		+																
Chromium [VI]	+	+	+*	+	*	*					+*	+	+	+	+*	−*	+*	+*	+*	+	*	+*	+*	+		+*	?			+	+*	+*	+*	*	?		*	−			+	+
Chromium [III]	+	+	+*	+	*						+*	+		+	?	+*		?	+	+	?	+	+	?		+	+			+		+	+*	+	?						?	?
Chrysoidine	+*	+*	+*	+*	+*									+				+*			*															*							
Cisplatin	+	+*	+*	+*	+*		+	+*		+	+*		+	+	+	+	*	+	+*	+	*	+	+	*		+		+	+	+			+	+	*		+					
Clofibrate	+		+	+	+						−		−	+	+				?			+	−			?							+	+	−			+	+			
Clomiphene citrate	−	*									?		−			*				*			+	+					+				+		−	*		+	?			
Conjugated oestrogens	+*	*	+*	+	+*						?		−	*	*	+	+	*	+	+	*	*	+	*		*	?			*	+*	+*	+	*	−		*	+		*	+	+
Cyclamate, calcium	−	−											+	+	?	−	−		+		+		?	−		−						+	−	−	−							
Cyclamate, sodium	−	−	+*	+*	+*					+*	?		−	−	?	+		*	+	+		+	?	+		*		−			+		−	−	?							
Cyclohexylamine	−	−	+	−							+		+	+	+	+		*	+	+	+	+	+			*							+	*	−							
Cyclophosphamide	−	+	+*	+*	+*	+		+		+	+*		+	+	+	+*	+	+*	+*	+	+	*	+*	+	*	+			+		+	+*	+*	*	?		+	+		*	+*	+
Cyclopropane	+	+									−		−	−	−					+					−		+															
Dacarbazine	+	+									?		−	+	+	+	*	?	?		+	−				+		?					?	*	?							
Dapsone	−	−									+*		−	+	?	+		*	+			?	−			*					+		+*	+*	?		*			*	?	−
DDT	−	−	+	+	+*	*		+*		+*	+*		+	+	?	+		*	+*	+		+	?	+		*			+				+	+*	+						?	
Diazepam	−	−									−		+	*	*	+		*	*	+		+	+			*							+	+*								
1,2-Dibromo-3-chloropropane	+	+	+*	+*	+*		+*	+*			+*		+*	+*	+*	+*		+*	+*	+		+*	+			+	?						+*	+*	?						?	
ortho-Dichlorobenzene	−	−	−	−	+*						+*		−	+	?	−		*		+		+	+			?							+	*	?			+			?	
para-Dichlorobenzene	+	+	−	−	+*						?			+	?							+								+				*	+							
3,3'-Dichlorobenzidine	+	+	+*	+	+*		+*			+*			+*	+		?		+*	+*		+	+*		?	+*	+*							+*	+*	+		+	+*			+*	
Dichloromethane	*	+	+*	+*	+*						−		+	+	−	?		+	+	+		−	−			−	−						+	+	+						?	−

Agent	Nonmammalian systems													Mammalian systems																																				
	Proka-ryotes		Lower eukaryotes				Plants			Insects				*In vitro*																					*In vivo*															
														Animal cells														Human cells						Animals									Humans					
	D	G	D	R	G	A	A	D	G	R	G	C	A	D	G	S	M	C	A	T	I	D	G	S	M	C	A	T	I	D	G	S	M	C	A	T	I	D	G	S	M	C	DL	A	D	A	S	M	C	A
2,4-Dichlorophenol	*													*																																				
2,4-Dichlorophenoxyacetic acid (2,4-D)																																																		
1,3-Dichloropropene		*																																																
Dicyclohexylamine																																																		
Dieldrin																																																		
Dienoestrol																																																		
Diethyl ether																																																		
Diethylstilboestrol																																																		
Diethyl sulphate																																																		
Dimethisterone																																																		
3,3'-Dimethoxybenzidine (ortho-Dianisidine)																																																		
Dimethylcarbamoyl chloride																																																		
Dimethyl sulphate																																																		
1,4-Dioxane																																																		
Direct Black 38																																																		
Direct Blue 6																																																		
Direct Brown 95																																																		
Divinyl ether																																																		
Enflurane																																																		
Epichlorohydrin																																																		
Erionite																																																		
Ethinyloestradiol																																																		
Ethylene dibromide																																																		
Ethylene oxide																																																		
Ethylene thiourea																																																		
Ethynodiol diacetate																																																		
Ferric oxide																																																		
Fluorides (inorganic) Sodium fluoride Sodium monofluorophosphate Sodium silicofluoride Stannous fluoride																																																		
5-Fluorouracil																																																		
Fluroxene																																																		
Formaldehyde																																																		
Halothane																																																		
Heptachlor																																																		
Hexachlorobenzene																																																		

Agent	Nonmammalian systems																Mammalian systems																								
	Prokaryotes		Lower eukaryotes				Plants			Insects				In vitro														In vivo												
														Animal cells								Human cells						Animals							Humans					
	D	G	D	R	G	A	D	G	C	R	G	C	A	D	G	S	M	C	A	T	I	D	G	S	M	C	A	I	D	G	S	M	C	DL	A	D	S	M	C	A
Hexachlorocyclohexanes																																								
Hexoestrol																																								
Hydralazine																																								
Hydrazine																																								
Isoflurane																																								
Isonicotinic acid hydrazide (Isoniazid)																																								
Lead and lead compounds																																								
Lead and inorganic lead compounds																																								
Tetraethyl- and tetramethyllead																																								
Magenta																																								
para-Magenta																																								
Magenta I																																								
Medroxyprogesterone acetate																																								
Megestrol acetate																																								
Melphalan																																								
6-Mercaptopurine																																								
Mestranol																																								
Methotrexate																																								
Methoxyflurane																																								
5-Methoxypsoralen +ultraviolet A radiation in the dark																																								
8-Methoxypsoralen (Methoxsalen) + ultraviolet A radiation in the dark																																								
Methyl bromide																																								
Methyl chloride																																								
4,4'-Methylene bis(2-chloroaniline) (MOCA)																																								
N-Methyl-N'-nitro-N-nitrosoguanidine																																								
Metronidazole																																								
Mustard gas (Sulphur mustard)																																								
1-Naphthylamine																																								
2-Naphthylamine																																								
1-Naphthylthiourea (ANTU)																																								
Nickel and nickel compounds																																								
Nitrogen mustard																																								
Nitrous oxide																																								
Norethisterone																																								
Norethynodrel																																								
Norgestrel																																								

Genetic and related effects: activity profile table.

	Nonmammalian systems													Mammalian systems																									
	Prokaryotes		Lower eukaryotes				Plants			Insects				In vitro															In vivo											
														Animal cells								Human cells								Animals						Humans				
Agent	D	G	D	R	G	A	D	G	C	R	G	C	A	D	G	S	M	C	A	T	I	D	G	S	M	C	A	T	I	D	G	S	M	C	DL	A	D	S	M	C	A
Ochratoxin A																																									
Oestradiol-17β																																									
Oestriol																																									
Oestrone																																									
Pentachlorophenol																																									
Phenacetin																																									
Phenazopyridine hydrochloride																																									
Phenelzine sulphate																																									
Phenobarbital																																									
Phenylbutazone																																									
N-Phenyl-2-naphthylamine																																									
Phenytoin																																									
Polybrominated biphenyls																																									
Polychlorinated biphenyls																																									
Prednisone																																									
Procarbazine hydrochloride																																									
Progesterone																																									
Propylene oxide																																									
Reserpine																																									
Saccharin, unspecified																																									
Saccharin, sodium																																									
Silica																																									
Styrene																																									
Sulfamethoxazole																																									
Talc																																									
Testosterone																																									
2,3,7,8-Tetrachlorodibenzo-para-dioxin (TCDD)																																									
1,1,2,2-Tetrachloroethane																																									
Tetrachloroethylene																																									
2,3,4,6-Tetrachlorophenol																																									
ortho-Toluenesulphonamide																																									
ortho-Toluidine																																									
Treosulphan																																									
Trichloroethylene																																									
2,4,5-Trichlorophenol																																									
2,4,6-Trichlorophenol																																									

Agent	Nonmammalian systems													Mammalian systems																									
	Prokaryotes		Lower eukaryotes				Plants			Insects				In vitro														In vivo											
														Animal cells							Human cells								Animals							Humans				
	D	G	D	R	G	A	D	G	C	R	G	C	A	D	G	S	M	C	A	T	I	D	G	S	M	C	A	T	D	G	S	M	C	DL	A	D	S	M	C	A
2,4,5-Trichlorophenoxyacetic acid (2,4,5-T)	–									?									–		+*														+*	?	?			
4,5',8-Trimethylpsoralen + ultraviolet A radiation in the dark	+			+	+*									+*		+					+*	+	?						+*				–* +*	–	+*				+*	
Tris(aziridinyl)para-benzoquinone (Triaziquone)	+*	+*					+*	+		+*	+*	+*		+*	+*	+	+*	+*	+			+	+	+	+	+			+	+ +*	+*	+	–* +*		+*				+	
Tris(1-aziridinyl)phosphine sulphide (Thiotepa)	+	+		+*						+*	+	+*		+*	+*	+*	+	+	?	+*		+*	+	+ +*	+	+	+	*	+ +*	+	?	+*	?	+			?		+	
Tris(2,3-dibromopropyl)phosphate	+* +	+		+*			+	+*		+*	+			+* +	+*	+*	–	+*	?			+*	+*	+*					+* +	+*			+*	+						
Uracil mustard	+*	+										+*	+*						+*	+*	+*	+*											+*	+*						
Vinblastine sulphate	–*																–*	.								–*				+*	+*	+*	+*	+*					+*	
Vincristine sulphate	–*																		+*					? +*							+?		+*				?			
Vinyl chloride	+	+	+*	+*	+*	+*	+	+*			+			+*	+*	–	.	+				?		? +*					+	+	+	+	+	–			?		+	
Vinylidene chloride	+	+		+*	+*		+*	+ +*			+			+*	+*			–				–			–* +*	–			+*	+	+*			–					+	

A, aneuploidy; C, chromosomal aberrations; D, DNA damage; DL, dominant lethal mutations; G, gene mutation; I, inhibition of intercellular communication; M, micronuclei; R, mitotic recombination and gene conversion; S, sister chromatid exchange; T, cell transformation

*Only one valid study was available to the Working Group.

SUPPLEMENTARY CORRIGENDA TO SUPPLEMENT 4

p. 47	A, last line	*replace footnote* 9 *by footnote* 3.
p. 53	A, lines 3-6	*replace* An increased risk of bladder cancer was reported to be associated with the manufacture of auramine in two further studies[3,4]. No information on exposure to auramine alone was available to the Working Group. *by* Data reported in two further studies[3,4] of workers involved in the manufacture of auramine were judged to show an increased risk of bladder cancer; however, workers had also been exposed to other chemicals, including β-naphthylamine. Data on exposure to auramine alone were considered inadequate for evaluation.
p. 56	B. Evidence of carcinogenicity to animals	*replace* (limited) *by* (inadequate)** *and add footnote:* **More recent data would provide an evaluation of *limited evidence* (*IARC Monographs*, *29*, 93-148, 1982)
p. 65	B, line 1	*add* to mice *after* administration
p. 122	A, line 2	*replace* 8.74 *by* 7.28 [data pooled by the Working Group]
	A, line 3	*delete* This difference is significant.
p. 149	A, line 7	*replace* extended[3-5] *by* extended[3,4]
p. 158	A, lines 9-11	*delete sentence starting* In a case-control study...
p. 160	Reference 4	*delete*
p. 262	last line	*replace* vinyl chloride *by* vinylidene chloride
p. 268		*replace* Indeno[1,2-*cd*]pyrene *by* Indeno[1,2,3-*cd*]pyrene

CUMULATIVE CROSS INDEX TO IARC MONOGRAPHS ON THE EVALUATION OF CARCINOGENIC RISKS TO HUMANS

The volume, page and year are given. References to corrigenda are given in parentheses.

A

A-α-C	*40*, 245 (1986)
	Suppl. 7, 56 (1987)
Acetaldehyde	*36*, 101 (1985) (*corr. 42*, 263)
	Suppl. 7, 77 (1987)
Acetaldehyde formylmethylhydrazone (*see* Gyromitrin)	
Acetamide	*7*, 197 (1974)
	Suppl. 7, 389 (1987)
Acetic acid, (4-chloro-2-methylphenoxy)- (*see* MCPA)	
Acridine orange	*16*, 145 (1978)
	Suppl. 7, 56 (1987)
Acriflavinium chloride	*13*, 31 (1977)
	Suppl. 7, 56 (1987)
Acrolein	*19*, 479 (1979)
	36, 133 (1985)
	Suppl. 7, 78 (1987)
Acrylamide	*39*, 41 (1986)
	Suppl. 7, 56 (1987)
Acrylic acid	*19*, 47 (1979)
	Suppl. 7, 56 (1987)
Acrylic fibres	*19*, 86 (1979)
	Suppl. 7, 56 (1987)
Acrylonitrile	*19*, 73 (1979)
	Suppl. 7, 79 (1987)
Acrylonitrile-butadiene-styrene copolymers	*19*, 9 (1979)
	Suppl. 7, 56 (1987)
Actinolite (*see* Asbestos)	
Actinomycins	*10*, 29 (1976) (*corr. 42*, 255)
	Suppl. 7, 80 (1987)
Adriamycin	*10*, 43 (1976)
	Suppl. 7, 81 (1987)

AF-2   *31*, 47 (1983)
                                                  Suppl. 7, 56 (1987)

Aflatoxins   *1*, 145 (1972) (*corr. 42*, 251)
                                                  10, 51 (1976)
                                                  Suppl. 7, 82 (1987)

Aflatoxin B₁ (*see* Aflatoxins)
Aflatoxin B₂ (*see* Aflatoxins)
Aflatoxin G₁ (*see* Aflatoxins)
Aflatoxin G₂ (*see* Aflatoxins)
Aflatoxin M₁ (*see* Aflatoxins)
Agaritine   *31*, 63 (1983)
                                                  Suppl. 7, 56 (1987)
Aldrin   *5*, 25 (1974)
                                                  Suppl. 7, 88 (1987)
Allyl chloride   *36*, 39 (1985)
                                                  Suppl. 7, 56 (1987)
Allyl isothiocyanate   *36*, 55 (1985)
                                                  Suppl. 7, 56 (1987)
Allyl isovalerate   *36*, 69 (1985)
                                                  Suppl. 7, 56 (1987)
Aluminium production   *34*, 37 (1984)
                                                  Suppl. 7, 89 (1987)
Amaranth   *8*, 41 (1975)
                                                  Suppl. 7, 56 (1987)
5-Aminoacenaphthene   *16*, 243 (1978)
                                                  Suppl. 7, 56 (1987)
2-Aminoanthraquinone   *27*, 191 (1982)
                                                  Suppl. 7, 56 (1987)
para-Aminoazobenzene   *8*, 53 (1975)
                                                  Suppl. 7, 390 (1987)
ortho-Aminoazotoluene   *8*, 61 (1975) (*corr. 42*, 254)
                                                  Suppl. 7, 56 (1987)
para-Aminobenzoic acid   *16*, 249 (1978)
                                                  Suppl. 7, 56 (1987)
4-Aminobiphenyl   *1*, 74 (1971) (*corr. 42*, 251)
                                                  Suppl. 7, 91 (1987)

2-Amino-3,4-dimethylimidazo[4,5-*f*]quinoline (*see* MeIQ)
2-Amino-3,8-dimethylimidazo[4,5-*f*]quinoxaline (*see* MeIQx)
3-Amino-1,4-dimethyl-5*H*-pyrido[4,3-*b*]indole (*see* Trp-P-1)
2-Aminodipyrido[1,2-*a*:3′,2′-*d*]imidazole (*see* Glu-P-2)
1-Amino-2-methylanthraquinone   *27*, 199 (1982)
                                                  Suppl. 7, 57 (1987)

2-Amino-3-methylimidazo[4,5-*f*]quinoline (*see* IQ)
2-Amino-6-methyldipyrido[1,2-*a*:3′,2′-*d*]-imidazole (*see* Glu-P-1)
2-Amino-3-methyl-9*H*-pyrido[2,3-*b*]indole (*see* MeA-α-C)
3-Amino-1-methyl-5*H*-pyrido[4,3-*b*]indole (*see* Trp-P-2)

Arsenic and arsenic compounds	*1*, 41 (1972)
	2, 48 (1973)
	23, 39 (1980)
	Suppl. 7, 100 (1987)
Arsenic pentoxide (*see* Arsenic and arsenic compounds)	
Arsenic sulphide (*see* Arsenic and arsenic compounds)	
Arsenic trioxide (*see* Arsenic and arsenic compounds)	
Arsine (*see* Arsenic and arsenic compounds)	
Asbestos	*2*, 17 (1973) (*corr. 42*, 252)
	14 (1977) (*corr. 42*, 256)
	Suppl. 7, 106 (1987)
Attapulgite	*42*, 159 (1987)
	Suppl. 7, 117 (1987)
Auramine (technical-grade)	*1*, 69 (1972) (*corr. 42*, 251)
	Suppl. 7, 118 (1987)
Auramine, manufacture of (*see also* Auramine, technical-grade)	*Suppl. 7*, 118 (1987)
Aurothioglucose	*13*, 39 (1977)
	Suppl. 7, 57 (1987)
5-Azacytidine	*26*, 37 (1981)
	Suppl. 7, 57 (1987)
Azaserine	*10*, 73 (1976) (*corr. 42*, 255)
	Suppl. 7, 57 (1987)
Azathioprine	*26*, 47 (1981)
	Suppl. 7, 119 (1987)
Aziridine	*9*, 37 (1975)
	Suppl. 7, 58 (1987)
2-(1-Aziridinyl)ethanol	*9*, 47 (1975)
	Suppl. 7, 58 (1987)
Aziridyl benzoquinone	*9*, 51 (1975)
	Suppl. 7, 58 (1987)
Azobenzene	*8*, 75 (1975)
	Suppl. 7, 58 (1987)

B

Barium chromate (*see* Chromium and chromium compounds)	
Basic chromic sulphate (*see* Chromium and chromium compounds)	
BCNU (*see* Bischloroethyl nitrosourea)	
Benz[*a*]acridine	*32*, 123 (1983)
	Suppl. 7, 58 (1987)
Benz[*c*]acridine	*3*, 241 (1973)
	32, 129 (1983)
	Suppl. 7, 58 (1987)
Benzal chloride (*see also* α-Chlorinated toluenes)	*29*, 65 (1982)
Benz[*a*]anthracene	*3*, 45 (1973)
	32, 135 (1983)
	Suppl. 7, 58 (1987)

Beryllium and beryllium compounds	*1*, 17 (1972)
	23, 143 (1980) (*corr. 42*, 260)
	Suppl. 7, 127 (1987)

Beryllium acetate (*see* Beryllium and beryllium compounds)

Beryllium acetate, basic (*see* Beryllium and beryllium compounds)

Beryllium-aluminium alloy (*see* Beryllium and beryllium compounds)

Beryllium carbonate (*see* Beryllium and beryllium compounds)

Beryllium chloride (*see* Beryllium and beryllium compounds)

Beryllium-copper alloy (*see* Beryllium and beryllium compounds)

Beryllium-copper-cobalt alloy (*see* Beryllium and beryllium compounds)

Beryllium fluoride (*see* Beryllium and beryllium compounds)

Beryllium hydroxide (*see* Beryllium and beryllium compounds)

Beryllium-nickel alloy (*see* Beryllium and beryllium compounds)

Beryllium oxide (*see* Beryllium and beryllium compounds)

Beryllium phosphate (*see* Beryllium and beryllium compounds)

Beryllium silicate (*see* Beryllium and beryllium compounds)

Beryllium sulphate (*see* Beryllium and beryllium compounds)

Beryl ore (*see* Beryllium and beryllium compounds)

Betel quid	*37*, 141 (1985)
	Suppl. 7, 128 (1987)

Betel-quid chewing (*see* Betel quid)

BHA (*see* Butylated hydroxyanisole)

BHT (*see* Butylated hydroxytoluene)

Bis(1-aziridinyl)morpholinophosphine sulphide	*9*, 55 (1975)
	Suppl. 7, 58 (1987)
Bis(2-chloroethyl)ether	*9*, 117 (1975)
	Suppl. 7, 58 (1987)
N, N-Bis(2-chloroethyl)-2-naphthylamine	*4*, 119 (1974) (*corr. 42*, 253)
	Suppl. 7, 130 (1987)
Bischloroethyl nitrosourea (*see also* Chloroethyl nitrosoureas)	*26*, 79 (1981)
	Suppl. 7, 150 (1987)
1,2-Bis(chloromethoxy)ethane	*15*, 31 (1977)
	Suppl. 7, 58 (1987)
1,4-Bis(chloromethoxymethyl)benzene	*15*, 37 (1977)
	Suppl. 7, 58 (1987)
Bis(chloromethyl)ether	*4*, 231 (1974) (*corr. 42*, 253)
	Suppl. 7, 131 (1987)
Bis(2-chloro-1-methylethyl)ether	*41*, 149 (1986)
	Suppl. 7, 59 (1987)
Bitumens	*35*, 39 (1985)
	Suppl. 7, 133 (1987)
Bleomycins	*26*, 97 (1981)
	Suppl. 7, 134 (1987)
Blue VRS	*16*, 163 (1978)
	Suppl. 7, 59 (1987)

Carbazole	*32*, 239 (1983)
	Suppl. 7, 59 (1987)
3-Carbethoxypsoralen	*40*, 317 (1986)
	Suppl. 7, 59 (1987)
Carbon blacks	*3*, 22 (1973)
	33, 35 (1984)
	Suppl. 7, 142 (1987)
Carbon tetrachloride	*1*, 53 (1972)
	20, 371 (1979)
	Suppl. 7, 143 (1987)
Carmoisine	*8*, 83 (1975)
	Suppl. 7, 59 (1987)
Carpentry and joinery	*25*, 139 (1981)
	Suppl. 7, 378 (1987)
Carrageenan	*10*, 181 (1976) (*corr. 42*, 255)
	31, 79 (1983)
	Suppl. 7, 59 (1987)
Catechol	*15*, 155 (1977)
	Suppl. 7, 59 (1987)
CCNU (*see* 1-(2-Chloroethyl)-3-cyclohexyl-1-nitrosourea)	
Chemotherapy, combined, including alkylating agents (*see* MOPP and other combined chemotherapy including alkylating agents)	
Chlorambucil	*9*, 125 (1975)
	26, 115 (1981)
	Suppl. 7, 144 (1987)
Chloramphenicol	*10*, 85 (1976)
	Suppl. 7, 145 (1987)
Chlordane (*see also* Chlordane/Heptachlor)	*20*, 45 (1979) (*corr. 42*, 258)
Chlordane/Heptachlor	*Suppl. 7*, 146 (1987)
Chlordecone	*20*, 67 (1979)
	Suppl. 7, 59 (1987)
Chlordimeform	*30*, 61 (1983)
	Suppl. 7, 59 (1987)
Chlorinated dibenzodioxins (other than TCDD)	*15*, 41 (1977)
	Suppl. 7, 59 (1987)
α-Chlorinated toluenes	*Suppl. 7*, 148 (1987)
Chlormadinone acetate (*see also* Progestins; Combined oral contraceptives)	*6*, 149 (1974)
	21, 365 (1979)
Chlornaphazine [*see* *N,N*-Bis(2-chloroethyl)-2-naphthylamine]	
Chlorobenzilate	*5*, 75 (1974)
	30, 73 (1983)
	Suppl. 7, 60 (1987)
Chlorodifluoromethane	*41*, 237 (1986)
	Suppl. 7, 149 (1987)
1-(2-Chloroethyl)-3-cyclohexyl-1-nitrosourea (*see also* Chloro-ethyl nitrosoureas)	*26*, 173 (1981) (*corr. 42*, 260)
	Suppl. 7, 150 (1987)

Chromium trioxide (*see* Chromium and chromium compounds)
Chrysene   *3*, 159 (1973)
                                                           32, 247 (1983)
                                                           Suppl. 7, 60 (1987)
Chrysoidine   *8*, 91 (1975)
                                                           Suppl. 7, 169 (1987)
Chrysotile (*see* Asbestos)
CI Disperse Yellow 3   *8*, 97 (1975)
                                                           Suppl. 7, 60 (1987)
Cinnamyl anthranilate   *16*, 287 (1978)
                                                           31, 133 (1983)
                                                           Suppl. 7, 60 (1987)
Cisplatin   *26*, 151 (1981)
                                                           Suppl. 7, 170 (1987)
Citrinin   *40*, 67 (1986)
                                                           Suppl. 7, 60 (1987)
Citrus Red No. 2   *8*, 101 (1975) (*corr. 42*, 254)
                                                           Suppl. 7, 60 (1987)
Clofibrate   *24*, 39 (1980)
                                                           Suppl. 7, 171 (1987)
Clomiphene citrate   *21*, 551 (1979)
                                                           Suppl. 7, 172 (1987)
Coal gasification   *34*, 65 (1984)
                                                           Suppl. 7, 173 (1987)
Coal-tar pitches (*see also* Coal-tars)   *Suppl. 7*, 174 (1987)
Coal-tars   *35*, 83 (1985)
                                                           Suppl. 7, 175 (1987)
Cobalt-chromium alloy (*see* Chromium and chromium
    compounds)
Coke production   *34*, 101 (1984)
                                                           Suppl. 7, 176 (1987)
Combined oral contraceptives (*see also* Oestrogens, progestins   *Suppl. 7*, 297 (1987)
    and combinations)
Conjugated oestrogens (*see also* Steroidal oestrogens)   *21*, 147 (1979)
Contraceptives, oral (*see* Combined oral contraceptives;
    Sequential oral contraceptives)
Copper 8-hydroxyquinoline   *15*, 103 (1977)
                                                           Suppl. 7, 61 (1987)
Coronene   *32*, 263 (1983)
                                                           Suppl. 7, 61 (1987)
Coumarin   *10*, 113 (1976)
                                                           Suppl. 7, 61 (1987)
Creosotes (*see also* Coal-tars)   *Suppl. 7*, 177 (1987)
meta-Cresidine   *27*, 91 (1982)
                                                           Suppl. 7, 61 (1987)
para-Cresidine   *27*, 92 (1982)
                                                           Suppl. 7, 61 (1987)

4,4'-Diaminodiphenyl ether   *16*, 301 (1978)
                                                         29, 203 (1982)
                                                         Suppl. 7, 61 (1987)
1,2-Diamino-4-nitrobenzene   *16*, 63 (1978)
                                                         Suppl. 7, 61 (1987)
1,4-Diamino-2-nitrobenzene   *16*, 73 (1978)
                                                         Suppl. 7, 61 (1987)

2,6-Diamino-3-(phenylazo)pyridine (*see* Phenazopyridine
    hydrochloride)
2,4-Diaminotoluene (*see also* Toluene diisocyanates)   *16*, 83 (1978)
                                                         Suppl. 7, 61 (1987)
2,5-Diaminotoluene (*see also* Toluene diisocyanates)   *16*, 97 (1978)
                                                         Suppl. 7, 61 (1987)

ortho-Dianisidine (*see* 3,3'-Dimethoxybenzidine)
Diazepam   *13*, 57 (1977)
                                                         Suppl. 7, 189 (1987)
Diazomethane   *7*, 223 (1974)
                                                         Suppl. 7, 61 (1987)
Dibenz[*a,h*]acridine   *3*, 247 (1973)
                                                         32, 277 (1983)
                                                         Suppl. 7, 61 (1987)
Dibenz[*a,j*]acridine   *3*, 254 (1973)
                                                         32, 283 (1983)
                                                         Suppl. 7, 61 (1987)
Dibenz[*a,c*]anthracene   *32*, 289 (1983) (*corr. 42*, 262)
                                                         Suppl. 7, 61 (1987)
Dibenz[*a,h*]anthracene   *3*, 178 (1973)
                                                         32, 299 (1983)
                                                         Suppl. 7, 61 (1987)
Dibenz[*a,j*]anthracene   *32*, 309 (1983)
                                                         Suppl. 7, 61 (1987)
7*H*-Dibenzo[*c,g*]carbazole   *3*, 260 (1973)
                                                         32, 315 (1983)
                                                         Suppl. 7, 61 (1987)

Dibenzodioxins, chlorinated (other than TCDD)
    [*see* Chlorinated dibenzodioxins (other than TCDD)]
Dibenzo[*a,e*]fluoranthene   *32*, 321 (1983)
                                                         Suppl. 7, 61 (1987)
Dibenzo[*h,rst*]pentaphene   *3*, 197 (1973)
                                                         Suppl. 7, 62 (1987)
Dibenzo[*a,e*]pyrene   *3*, 201 (1973)
                                                         32, 327 (1983)
                                                         Suppl. 7, 62 (1987)
Dibenzo[*a,h*]pyrene   *3*, 207 (1973)
                                                         32, 331 (1983)
                                                         Suppl. 7, 62 (1987)

Diepoxybutane   *11*, 115 (1976) (*corr. 42*, 255)
                                                       Suppl. 7, 62 (1987)

Diethyl ether (*see* Anaesthetics, volatile)

Di(2-ethylhexyl)adipate   *29*, 257 (1982)
                                                       Suppl. 7, 62 (1987)

Di(2-ethylhexyl)phthalate   *29*, 269 (1982) (*corr. 42*, 261)
                                                       Suppl. 7, 62 (1987)

1,2-Diethylhydrazine   *4*, 153 (1974)
                                                       Suppl. 7, 62 (1987)

Diethylstilboestrol   *6*, 55 (1974)
                                                       21, 172 (1979) (*corr. 42*, 259)
                                                       Suppl. 7, 273 (1987)

Diethylstilboestrol dipropionate (*see* Diethylstilboestrol)
Diethyl sulphate   *4*, 277 (1974)
                                                       Suppl. 7, 198 (1987)

Diglycidyl resorcinol ether   *11*, 125 (1976)
                                                       36, 181 (1985)
                                                       Suppl. 7, 62 (1987)

Dihydrosafrole   *1*, 170 (1972)
                                                       10, 233 (1976)
                                                       Suppl. 7, 62 (1987)

Dihydroxybenzenes (*see* Catechol; Hydroquinone; Resorcinol)
Dihydroxymethylfuratrizine   *24*, 77 (1980)
                                                       Suppl. 7, 62 (1987)

Dimethisterone (*see also* Progestins; Sequential oral   *6*, 167 (1974)
  contraceptives)   *21*, 377 (1979)

Dimethoxane   *15*, 177 (1977)
                                                       Suppl. 7, 62 (1987)

3,3'-Dimethoxybenzidine   *4*, 41 (1974)
                                                       Suppl. 7, 198 (1987)

3,3'-Dimethoxybenzidine-4,4'-diisocyanate   *39*, 279 (1986)
                                                       Suppl. 7, 62 (1987)

para-Dimethylaminoazobenzene   *8*, 125 (1975)
                                                       Suppl. 7, 62 (1987)

para-Dimethylaminoazobenzenediazo sodium sulphonate *8*, 147 (1975)
                                                       Suppl. 7, 62 (1987)

trans-2-[(Dimethylamino)methylimino]-5-[2-(5-nitro-2-furyl)-   *7*, 147 (1974) (*corr. 42*, 253)
  vinyl]-1,3,4-oxadiazole   *Suppl. 7*, 62 (1987)

4,4'-Dimethylangelicin plus ultraviolet radiation (*see also*
  Angelicin and some synthetic derivatives)   *Suppl. 7*, 57 (1987)

4,5'-Dimethylangelicin plus ultraviolet radiation (*see also*
  Angelicin and some synthetic derivatives)   *Suppl. 7*, 57 (1987)

Dimethylarsinic acid (*see* Arsenic and arsenic compounds)
3,3'-Dimethylbenzidine   *1*, 87 (1972)
                                                       Suppl. 7, 62 (1987)

Ethinyloestradiol (*see also* Steroidal oestrogens)	*6*, 77 (1974)
	21, 233 (1979)
Ethionamide	*13*, 83 (1977)
	Suppl. 7, 63 (1987)
Ethyl acrylate	*19*, 57 (1979)
	39, 81 (1986)
	Suppl. 7, 63 (1987)
Ethylene	*19*, 157 (1979)
	Suppl. 7, 63 (1987)
Ethylene dibromide	*15*, 195 (1977)
	Suppl. 7, 204 (1987)
Ethylene oxide	*11*, 157 (1976)
	36, 189 (1985) (*corr. 42*, 263)
	Suppl. 7, 205 (1987)
Ethylene sulphide	*11*, 257 (1976)
	Suppl. 7, 63 (1987)
Ethylene thiourea	*7*, 45 (1974)
	Suppl. 7, 207 (1987)
Ethyl methanesulphonate	*7*, 245 (1974)
	Suppl. 7, 63 (1987)
N-Ethyl-*N*-nitrosourea	*1*, 135 (1972)
	17, 191 (1978)
	Suppl. 7, 63 (1987)
Ethyl selenac (*see also* Selenium and selenium compounds)	*12*, 107 (1976)
	Suppl. 7, 63 (1987)
Ethyl tellurac	*12*, 115 (1976)
	Suppl. 7, 63 (1987)
Ethynodiol diacetate (*see also* Progestins; Combined oral contraceptives)	*6* 173 (1974)
	21, 387 (1979)
Eugenol	*36*, 75 (1985)
	Suppl. 7, 63 (1987)
Evans blue	*8*, 151 (1975)
	Suppl. 7, 63 (1987)

F

Fast Green FCF	*16*, 187 (1978)
	Suppl. 7, 63 (1987)
Ferbam	*12*, 121 (1976) (*corr. 42*, 256)
	Suppl. 7, 63 (1987)
Ferric oxide	*1*, 29 (1972)
	Suppl. 7, 216 (1987)
Ferrochromium (*see* Chromium and chromium compounds)	
Fluometuron	*30*, 245 (1983)
	Suppl. 7, 63 (1987)
Fluoranthene	*32*, 355 (1983)
	Suppl. 7, 63 (1987)

Haematite mining, underground, with exposure to radon   *1*, 29 (1972)
                                                                          Suppl. 7, 216 (1987)
Hair dyes, epidemiology of   *16*, 29 (1978)
                                                                          27, 307 (1982)

Halothane (*see* Anaesthetics, volatile)
α-HCH (*see* Hexachlorocyclohexanes)
β-HCH (*see* Hexachlorocyclohexanes)
γ-HCH (*see* Hexachlorocyclohexanes)
Heptachlor (*see also* Chlordane/ Heptachlor)   *5*, 173 (1974)
                                                                          20, 129 (1979)
Hexachlorobenzene   *20*, 155 (1979)
                                                                          Suppl. 7, 219 (1987)
Hexachlorobutadiene   *20*, 179 (1979)
                                                                          Suppl. 7, 64 (1987)
Hexachlorocyclohexanes   *5*, 47 (1974)
                                                                          20, 195 (1979) (*corr. 42*, 258)
                                                                          Suppl. 7, 220 (1987)

Hexachlorocyclohexane, technical-grade (*see* Hexachloro-
    cyclohexanes)
Hexachloroethane   *20*, 467 (1979)
                                                                          Suppl. 7, 64 (1987)
Hexachlorophene   *20*, 241 (1979)
                                                                          Suppl. 7, 64 (1987)
Hexamethylphosphoramide   *15*, 211 (1977)
                                                                          Suppl. 7, 64 (1987)
Hexoestrol (*see* Nonsteroidal oestrogens)
Hycanthone mesylate   *13*, 91 (1977)
                                                                          Suppl. 7, 64 (1987)
Hydralazine   *24*, 85 (1980)
                                                                          Suppl. 7, 222 (1987)
Hydrazine   *4*, 127 (1974)
                                                                          Suppl. 7, 223 (1987)
Hydrogen peroxide   *36*, 285 (1985)
                                                                          Suppl. 7, 64 (1987)
Hydroquinone   *15*, 155 (1977)
                                                                          Suppl. 7, 64 (1987)
4-Hydroxyazobenzene   *8*, 157 (1975)
                                                                          Suppl. 7, 64 (1987)
17α-Hydroxyprogesterone caproate (*see also* Progestins)   *21*, 399 (1979) (*corr. 42*, 259)
8-Hydroxyquinoline   *13*, 101 (1977)
                                                                          Suppl. 7, 64 (1987)
8-Hydroxysenkirkine   *10*, 265 (1976)
                                                                          Suppl. 7, 64 (1987)

L

Lasiocarpine

10, 281 (1976)
Suppl. 7, 65 (1987)

Lauroyl peroxide

36, 315 (1985)
Suppl. 7, 65 (1987)

Lead acetate (*see* Lead and lead compounds)
Lead and lead compounds

1, 40 (1972) (*corr. 42*, 251)
2, 52, 150 (1973)
12, 131 (1976)
23, 40, 208, 209, 325 (1980)
Suppl. 7, 230 (1987)

Lead arsenate (*see* Arsenic and arsenic compounds)
Lead carbonate (*see* Lead and lead compounds)
Lead chloride (*see* Lead and lead compounds)
Lead chromate (*see* Chromium and chromium compounds)
Lead chromate oxide (*see* Chromium and chromium compounds)
Lead naphthenate (*see* Lead and lead compounds)
Lead nitrate (*see* Lead and lead compounds)
Lead oxide (*see* Lead and lead compounds)
Lead phosphate (*see* Lead and lead compounds)
Lead subacetate (*see* Lead and lead compounds)
Lead tetroxide (*see* Lead and lead compounds)
Leather goods manufacture

25, 279 (1981)
Suppl. 7, 235 (1987)

Leather industries

25, 199 (1981)
Suppl. 7, 232 (1987)

Leather tanning and processing

25, 201 (1981)
Suppl. 7, 236 (1987)

Ledate (*see also* Lead and lead compounds)
Light Green SF

12, 131 (1976)
16, 209 (1978)
Suppl. 7, 65 (1987)

Lindane (*see* Hexachlorocyclohexanes)
The lumber and sawmill industries (including logging)

25, 49 (1981)
Suppl. 7, 383 (1987)

Luteoskyrin

10, 163 (1976)
Suppl. 7, 65 (1987)

Lynoestrenol (*see also* Progestins; Combined oral contraceptives)

21, 407 (1979)

M

Magenta

4, 57 (1974) (*corr. 42*, 252)
Suppl. 7, 238 (1987)

Magenta, manufacture of (*see also* Magenta)
Malathion

Suppl. 7, 238 (1987)
30, 103 (1983)
Suppl. 7, 65 (1987)

Maleic hydrazide

4, 173 (1974) (*corr. 42*, 253)
Suppl. 7, 65 (1987)

Methyl acrylate	*19*, 52 (1979)
	39, 99 (1986)
	Suppl. 7, 66 (1987)
5-Methylangelicin plus ultraviolet radiation (*see also* Angelicin and some synthetic derivatives)	*Suppl. 7*, 57 (1987)
2-Methylaziridine	*9*, 61 (1975)
	Suppl. 7, 66 (1987)
Methylazoxymethanol acetate	*1*, 164 (1972)
	10, 121 (1976)
	Suppl. 7, 66 (1987)
Methyl bromide	*41*, 187 (1986)
	Suppl. 7, 245 (1987)
Methyl carbamate	*12*, 151 (1976)
	Suppl. 7, 66 (1987)
Methyl-CCNU [*see* 1-(2-Chloroethyl)-3-(4-methyl-cyclohexyl)-1-nitrosourea]	
Methyl chloride	*41*, 161 (1986)
	Suppl. 7, 246 (1987)
1-, 2-, 3-, 4-, 5- and 6-Methylchrysenes	*32*, 379 (1983)
	Suppl. 7, 66 (1987)
N-Methyl-*N*,4-dinitrosoaniline	*1*, 141 (1972)
	Suppl. 7, 66 (1987)
4,4'-Methylene bis(2-chloroaniline)	*4*, 65 (1974) (*corr. 42*, 252)
	Suppl. 7, 246 (1987)
4,4'-Methylene bis(*N,N*-dimethyl)benzenamine	*27*, 119 (1982)
	Suppl. 7, 66 (1987)
4,4'-Methylene bis(2-methylaniline)	*4*, 73 (1974)
	Suppl. 7, 248 (1987)
4,4'-Methylenedianiline	*4*, 79 (1974) (*corr. 42*, 252)
	39, 347 (1986)
	Suppl. 7, 66 (1987)
4,4'-Methylenediphenyl diisocyanate	*19*, 314 (1979)
	Suppl. 7, 66 (1987)
2-Methylfluoranthene	*32*, 399 (1983)
	Suppl. 7, 66 (1987)
3-Methylfluoranthene	*32*, 399 (1983)
	Suppl. 7, 66 (1987)
Methyl iodide	*15*, 245 (1977)
	41, 213 (1986)
	Suppl. 7, 66 (1987)
Methyl methacrylate	*19*, 187 (1979)
	Suppl. 7, 66 (1987)
Methyl methanesulphonate	*7*, 253 (1974)
	Suppl. 7, 66 (1987)
2-Methyl-1-nitroanthraquinone	*27*, 205 (1982)
	Suppl. 7, 66 (1987)

5-(Morpholinomethyl)-3-[(5-nitrofurfurylidene)amino]-2- oxazolidinone	7, 161 (1974) *Suppl. 7*, 67 (1987)
Mustard gas	9. 181 (1975) (*corr. 42*, 254) *Suppl. 7*, 259 (1987)
Myleran (*see* 1,4-Butanediol dimethanesulphonate)	

N

Nafenopin	24, 125 (1980) *Suppl. 7*, 67 (1987)
1,5-Naphthalenediamine	27, 127 (1982) *Suppl. 7*, 67 (1987)
1,5-Naphthalene diisocyanate	19, 311 (1979) *Suppl. 7*, 67 (1987)
1-Naphthylamine	4, 87 (1974) (*corr. 42*, 253) *Suppl. 7*, 260 (1987)
2-Naphthylamine	4, 97 (1974) *Suppl. 7*, 261 (1987)
1-Naphthylthiourea	30, 347 (1983) *Suppl. 7*, 263 (1987)
Nickel acetate (*see* Nickel and nickel compounds)	
Nickel ammonium sulphate (*see* Nickel and nickel compounds)	
Nickel and nickel compounds	2, 126 (1973) (*corr. 42*, 252) 11, 75 (1976) *Suppl. 7*, 264 (1987)
Nickel carbonate (*see* Nickel and nickel compounds)	
Nickel carbonyl (*see* Nickel and nickel compounds)	
Nickel chloride (*see* Nickel and nickel compounds)	
Nickel-gallium alloy (*see* Nickel and nickel compounds)	
Nickel hydroxide (*see* Nickel and nickel compounds)	
Nickelocene (*see* Nickel and nickel compounds)	
Nickel oxide (*see* Nickel and nickel compounds)	
Nickel subsulphide (*see* Nickel and nickel compounds)	
Nickel sulphate (*see* Nickel and nickel compounds)	
Niridazole	13, 123 (1977) *Suppl. 7*, 67 (1987)
Nithiazide	31, 179 (1983) *Suppl. 7*, 67 (1987)
5-Nitroacenaphthene	16, 319 (1978) *Suppl. 7*, 67 (1987)
5-Nitro-*ortho*-anisidine	27, 133 (1982) *Suppl. 7*, 67 (1987)
9-Nitroanthracene	33, 179 (1984) *Suppl. 7*, 67 (1987)
6-Nitrobenzo[*a*]pyrene	33, 187 (1984) *Suppl. 7*, 67 (1987)
4-Nitrobiphenyl	4, 113 (1974) *Suppl. 7*, 67 (1987)

N-Nitrosoguvacine   37, 263 (1985)
                                                               Suppl. 7, 68 (1987)
N-Nitrosoguvacoline   37, 263 (1985)
                                                               Suppl. 7, 68 (1987)
N-Nitrosohydroxyproline   17, 304 (1978)
                                                               Suppl. 7, 68 (1987)
3-(N-Nitrosomethylamino)propionaldehyde   37, 263 (1985)
                                                               Suppl. 7, 68 (1987)
3-(N-Nitrosomethylamino)propionitrile   37, 263 (1985)
                                                               Suppl. 7, 68 (1987)
4-(N-Nitrosomethylamino)-4-(3-pyridyl)-1-butanal   37, 205 (1985)
                                                               Suppl. 7, 68 (1987)
4-(N-Nitrosomethylamino)-1-(3-pyridyl)-1-butanone   37, 209 (1985)
                                                               Suppl. 7,(1987)
N-Nitrosomethylethylamine   17, 221 (1978)
                                                               Suppl. 7, 68 (1987)
N-Nitroso-N-methylurea (see N-Methyl-N-nitrosourea)
N-Nitroso-N-methylurethane (see N-Methyl-N-nitrosourethane)
N-Nitrosomethylvinylamine   17, 257 (1978)
                                                               Suppl. 7, 68 (1987)
N-Nitrosomorpholine   17, 263 (1978)
                                                               Suppl. 7, 68 (1987)
N'-Nitrosonornicotine   17, 281 (1978)
                                                               37, 241 (1985)
                                                               Suppl. 7, 68 (1987)
N-Nitrosopiperidine   17, 287 (1978)
                                                               Suppl. 7, 68 (1987)
N-Nitrosoproline   17, 303 (1978)
                                                               Suppl. 7, 68 (1987)
N-Nitrosopyrrolidine   17, 313 (1978)
                                                               Suppl. 7, 68 (1987)
N-Nitrososarcosine   17, 327 (1978)
                                                               Suppl. 7, 68 (1987)
Nitrosoureas, chloroethyl (see Chloroethyl nitrosoureas)
Nitrous oxide (see Anaesthetics, volatile)
Nitrovin   31, 185 (1983)
                                                               Suppl. 7, 68 (1987)
NNA [see 4-(N-Nitrosomethylamino)-4-(3-pyridyl)-1-butanal]
NNK [see 4-(N-Nitrosomethylamino)-1-(3-pyridyl)-1-butanone]
Nonsteroidal oestrogens (see also Oestrogens, progestins   Suppl. 7, 272 (1987)
     and combinations)
Noresthisterone (see also Progestins; Combined oral   6, 179 (1974)
     contraceptives)   21, 441 (1979)
Norethynodrel (see also Progestins; Combined oral   6, 191 (1974)
     contraceptives)   21, 46 (1979) (corr. 42, 259)

Oxymetholone [*see also* Androgenic (anabolic) steroids]   *13*, 131 (1977)
Oxyphenbutazone   *13*, 185 (1977)
                                                             Suppl. 7, 69 (1987)

P

Panfuran S (*see also* Dihydroxymethylfuratrizine)   *24*, 77 (1980)
                                                             Suppl. 7, 69 (1987)

Paper manufacture (*see* Pulp and paper manufacture)
Parasorbic acid   *10*, 199 (1976) (*corr. 42*, 255)
                                                             Suppl. 7, 69 (1987)
Parathion   *30*, 153 (1983)
                                                             Suppl. 7, 69 (1987)
Patulin   *10*, 205 (1976)
                                                             40, 83 (1986)
                                                             Suppl. 7, 69 (1987)
Penicillic acid   *10*, 211 (1976)
                                                             Suppl. 7, 69 (1987)
Pentachloroethane   *41*, 99 (1986)
                                                             Suppl. 7, 69 (1987)

Pentachloronitrobenzene (*see* Quintozene)
Pentachlorophenol (*see also* Chlorophenols; Chlorophenols,   *20*, 203 (1979)
    occupational exposures to)
Perylene   *32*, 411 (1983)
                                                             Suppl. 7, 69 (1987)
Petasitenine   *31*, 207 (1983)
                                                             Suppl. 7, 69 (1987)

Petasites japonicus (*see* Pyrrolizidine alkaloids)
Phenacetin   *3*, 141 (1973)
                                                             24, 135 (1980)
                                                             Suppl. 7, 310 (1987)
Phenanthrene   *32*, 419 (1983)
                                                             Suppl. 7, 69 (1987)
Phenazopyridine hydrochloride   *8*, 117 (1975)
                                                             24, 163 (1980) (*corr. 42*, 260)
                                                             Suppl. 7, 312 (1987)
Phenelzine sulphate   *24*, 175 (1980)
                                                             Suppl. 7, 312 (1987)
Phenicarbazide   *12*, 177 (1976)
                                                             Suppl. 7, 70 (1987)
Phenobarbital   *13*, 157 (1977)
                                                             Suppl. 7, 313 (1987)

Phenoxyacetic acid herbicides (*see* Chlorophenoxy herbicides)
Phenoxybenzamine hydrochloride   *9*, 223 (1975)
                                                             24, 185 (1980)
                                                             Suppl. 7, 70 (1987)

Polyvinyl chloride	*7*, 306 (1974)
	19, 402 (1979)
	Suppl. 7, 70 (1987)
Polyvinyl pyrrolidone	*19*, 463 (1979)
	Suppl. 7, 70 (1987)
Ponceau MX	*8*, 189 (1975)
	Suppl. 7, 70 (1987)
Ponceau 3R	*8*, 199 (1975)
	Suppl. 7, 70 (1987)
Ponceau SX	*8*, 207 (1975)
	Suppl. 7, 70 (1987)
Potassium arsenate (*see* Arsenic and arsenic compounds)	
Potassium arsenite (*see* Arsenic and arsenic compounds)	
Potassium bis(2-hydroxyethyl)dithiocarbamate	*12*, 183 (1976)
	Suppl. 7, 70 (1987)
Potassium bromate	*40*, 207 (1986)
	Suppl. 7, 70 (1987)
Potassium chromate (*see* Chromium and chromium compounds)	
Potassium dichromate (*see* Chromium and chromium compounds)	
Prednisone	*26*, 293 (1981)
	Suppl. 7, 326 (1987)
Procarbazine hydrochloride	*26*, 311 (1981)
	Suppl. 7, 327 (1987)
Proflavine salts	*24*, 195 (1980)
	Suppl. 7, 70 (1987)
Progesterone (*see also* Progestins; Combined oral contraceptives	*6*, 135 (1974)
	21, 49 (1979) (*corr. 42*, 259)
Progestins (*see also* Oestrogens, progestins and combinations)	*Suppl. 7*, 289 (1987)
Pronetalol hydrochloride	*13*, 227 (1977) (*corr. 42*, 256)
	Suppl. 7, 70 (1987)
1,3-Propane sultone	*4*, 253 (1974) (*corr. 42*, 253)
	Suppl. 7, 70 (1987)
Propham	*12*, 189 (1976)
	Suppl. 7, 70 (1987)
β-Propiolactone	*4*, 259 (1974) (*corr. 42*, 253)
	Suppl. 7, 70 (1987)
n-Propyl carbamate	*12*, 201 (1976)
	Suppl. 7, 70 (1987)
Propylene	*19*, 213 (1979)
	Suppl. 7, 71 (1987)
Propylene oxide	*11*, 191 (1976)
	36, 227 (1985) (*corr. 42*, 263)
	Suppl. 7, 328 (1987)
Propylthiouracil	*7*, 67 (1974)
	Suppl. 7, 329 (1987)
Ptaquiloside (*see also* Bracken fern)	*40*, 55 (1986)
	Suppl. 7, 71 (1987)

Safrole   *1*, 169 (1972)
                                                                 10, 231 (1976)
                                                                 Suppl. 7, 71 (1987)

The sawmill industry (including logging) [*see* The lumber and
    sawmill industry (including logging)]
Scarlet Red   *8*, 217 (1975)
                                                                 Suppl. 7, 71 (1987)
Selenium and selenium compounds   *9*, 245 (1975) (*corr. 42*, 255)
                                                                 Suppl. 7, 71 (1987)

Selenium dioxide (*see* Selenium and selenium compounds)
Selenium oxide (*see* Selenium and selenium compounds)
Semicarbazide hydrochloride   *12*, 209 (1976) (*corr. 42*, 256)
                                                                 Suppl. 7, 71 (1987)

Senecio jacobaea L. (*see* Pyrrolizidine alkaloids)
Senecio longilobus (*see* Pyrrolizidine alkaloids)
Seneciphylline   *10*, 319, 335 (1976)
                                                                 Suppl. 7, 71 (1987)
Senkirkine   *10*, 327 (1976)
                                                                 31, 231 (1983)
                                                                 Suppl. 7, 71 (1987)
Sepiolite   *42*, 175 (1987)
                                                                 Suppl. 7, 71 (1987)
Sequential oral contraceptives (*see also* Oestrogens, progestins   *Suppl. 7*, 296 (1987)
    and combinations)
Shale-oils   *35*, 161 (1985)
                                                                 Suppl. 7, 339 (1987)
Shikimic acid (*see also* Bracken fern)   *40*, 55 (1986)
                                                                 Suppl. 7, 71 (1987)

Shoe manufacture and repair (*see* Boot and shoe manufacture
    and repair)
Silica (*see also* Amorphous silica; Crystalline silica)   *42*, 39 (1987)
Sodium arsenate (*see* Arsenic and arsenic compounds)
Sodium arsenite (*see* Arsenic and arsenic compounds)
Sodium cacodylate (*see* Arsenic and arsenic compounds)
Sodium chromate (*see* Chromium and chromium compounds)
Sodium cyclamate (*see* Cyclamates)
Sodium dichromate (*see* Chromium and chromium compounds)
Sodium diethyldithiocarbamate   *12*, 217 (1976)
                                                                 Suppl. 7, 71 (1987)

Sodium equilin sulphate (*see* Conjugated oestrogens)
Sodium fluoride (*see* Fluorides)
Sodium monofluorophosphate (*see* Fluorides)
Sodium oestrone sulphate (*see* Conjugated oestrogens)
Sodium *ortho*-phenylphenate (*see also ortho*-Phenylphenol)   *30*, 329 (1983)
                                                                 Suppl. 7, 392 (1987)

Sodium saccharin (*see* Saccharin)
Sodium selenate (*see* Selenium and selenium compounds)

Sulphisoxazole (*see* Sulfafurazole)
Sulphur mustard (*see* Mustard gas)
Sunset Yellow FCF   *8*, 257 (1975)
                                                        Suppl. 7, 72 (1987)
Symphytine   *31*, 239 (1983)
                                                        Suppl. 7, 72 (1987)

T

2,4,5-T (*see also* Chlorophenoxy herbicides; Chlorophenoxy   *15*, 273 (1977)
    herbicides, occupational exposures to)
Talc   *42*, 185 (1987)
                                                        Suppl. 7, 349 (1987)
Tannic acid   *10*, 253 (1976) (*corr. 42*, 255)
                                                        Suppl. 7, 72 (1987)
Tannins (*see also* Tannic acid)   *10*, 254 (1976)
                                                        Suppl. 7, 72 (1987)
TCDD (*see* 2,3,7,8-Tetrachlorodibenzo-*para*-dioxin)
TDE (*see* DDT)
Terpene polychlorinates   *5*, 219 (1974)
                                                        Suppl. 7, 72 (1987)
Testosterone [*see also* Androgenic (anabolic) steroids]   *6*, 209 (1974)
                                                        21, 519 (1979)
Testosterone oenanthate (*see* Testosterone)
Testosterone propionate (*see* Testosterone)
2,2',5,5'-Tetrachlorobenzidine   *27*, 141 (1982)
                                                        Suppl. 7, 72 (1987)
2,3,7,8-Tetrachlorodibenzo-*para*-dioxin   *15*, 41 (1977)
                                                        Suppl. 7, 350 (1987)
1,1,1,2-Tetrachloroethane   *41*, 87 (1986)
                                                        Suppl. 7, 72 (1987)
1,1,2,2-Tetrachloroethane   *20*, 477 (1979)
                                                        Suppl. 7, 354 (1987)
Tetrachloroethylene   *20*, 491 (1979)
                                                        Suppl. 7, 355 (1987)
2,3,4,6-Tetrachlorophenol (*see* Chlorophenols; Chlorophenols,
    occupational exposure to)
Tetrachlorvinphos   *30*, 197 (1983)
                                                        Suppl. 7, 72 (1987)
Tetraethyllead (*see* Lead and lead compounds)
Tetrafluoroethylene   *19*, 285 (1979)
                                                        Suppl. 7, 72 (1987)
Tetramethyllead (*see* Lead and lead compounds)
Thioacetamide   *7*, 77 (1974)
                                                        Suppl. 7, 72 (1987)

2,4,6-Trichlorophenols (*see also* Chlorophenols; Chlorophenols, occupational exposures to)   *20*, 349 (1979)

(2,4,5-Trichlorophenoxy)acetic acid (*see* 2,4,5-T)

Trichlorotriethylamine hydrochloride   *9*, 229 (1975)
    Suppl. 7, 73 (1987)

T_2-Trichothecene   *31*, 265 (1983)
    Suppl. 7, 73 (1987)

Triethylene glycol diglycidyl ether   *11*, 209 (1976)
    Suppl. 7, 73 (1987)

4,4',6-Trimethylangelicin plus ultraviolet radiation (*see also* Angelicin and some synthetic derivatives)   *Suppl. 7*, 57 (1987)

2,4,5-Trimethylaniline   *27*, 177 (1982)
    Suppl. 7, 73 (1987)

2,4,6-Trimethylaniline   *27*, 178 (1982)
    Suppl. 7, 73 (1987)

4,5',8-Trimethylpsoralen   *40*, 357 (1986)
    Suppl. 7, 366 (1987)

Triphenylene   *32*, 447 (1983)
    Suppl. 7, 73 (1987)

Tris(aziridinyl)-*para*-benzoquinone   *9*, 67 (1975)
    Suppl. 7, 367 (1987)

Tris(1-aziridinyl)phosphine oxide   *9*, 75 (1975)
    Suppl. 7, 73 (1987)

Tris(1-aziridinyl)phosphine sulphide   *9*, 85 (1975)
    Suppl. 7, 368 (1987)

2,4,6-Tris(1-aziridinyl)-*s*-triazine   *9*, 95 (1975)
    Suppl. 7, 73 (1987)

1,2,3-Tris(chloromethoxy)propane   *15*, 301 (1977)
    Suppl. 7, 73 (1987)

Tris(2,3-dibromopropyl) phosphate   *20*, 575 (1979)
    Suppl. 7, 369 (1987)

Tris(2-methyl-1-aziridinyl)phosphine oxide   *9*, 107 (1975)
    Suppl. 7, 73 (1987)

Trp-P-1   *31*, 247 (1983)
    Suppl. 7, 73 (1987)

Trp-P-2   *31*, 255 (1983)
    Suppl. 7, 73 (1987)

Trypan blue   *8*, 267 (1975)
    Suppl. 7, 73 (1987)

Tussilago farfara L. (*see* Pyrrolizidine alkaloids)

U

Underground haematite mining with exposure to radon   *1*, 29 (1972)
    Suppl. 7, 216 (1987)

Uracil mustard   *9*, 235 (1975)
    Suppl. 7, 370 (1987)

Y

Yellow AB   *8*, 279 (1975)
                                                               Suppl. 7, 74 (1987)
Yellow OB   *8*, 287 (1975)
                                                               Suppl. 7, 74 (1987)

Z

Zearalenone   *31*, 279 (1983)
                                                               Suppl. 7, 74 (1987)
Zectran   *12*, 237 (1976)
                                                               Suppl. 7, 74 (1987)

Zinc beryllium silicate (*see* Beryllium and beryllium compounds)
Zinc chromate (*see* Chromium and chromium compounds)
Zinc chromate hydroxide (*see* Chromium and chromium
    compounds)
Zinc potassium chromate (*see* Chromium and chromium
    compounds)
Zinc yellow (*see* Chromium and chromium compounds)
Zineb   *12*, 245 (1976)
                                                               Suppl. 7, 74 (1987)
Ziram   *12*, 259 (1976)
                                                               Suppl. 7, 74 (1987)

PUBLICATIONS OF THE INTERNATIONAL
AGENCY FOR RESEARCH ON CANCER
SCIENTIFIC PUBLICATIONS SERIES

(Available from Oxford University Press)
through local bookshops

Prices, valid for October 1987, are subject to change without notice

SCIENTIFIC PUBLICATIONS SERIES

No. 22 ENVIRONMENTAL CARCINOGENS:
SELECTED METHODS OF ANALYSIS
Editor-in-Chief H. Egan
VOLUME 2. METHODS FOR THE MEASUREMENT
OF VINYL CHLORIDE IN POLY(VINYL
CHLORIDE), AIR, WATER AND FOODSTUFFS
Edited by D.C.M. Squirrell & W. Thain
1978; 142 pages; out of print

No. 23 PATHOLOGY OF TUMOURS IN
LABORATORY ANIMALS. VOLUME II.
TUMOURS OF THE MOUSE
Editor-in-Chief V.S. Turusov
1979; 669 pages; £37.50

No. 24 ONCOGENESIS AND HERPESVIRUSES III
Edited by G. de-Thé, W. Henle & F. Rapp
1978; Part 1, 580 pages; Part 2, 522 pages; out of print

No. 25 CARCINOGENIC RISKS: STRATEGIES
FOR INTERVENTION
Edited by W. Davis & C. Rosenfeld
1979; 283 pages; out of print

No. 26 DIRECTORY OF ON-GOING RESEARCH
IN CANCER EPIDEMIOLOGY 1978
Edited by C.S. Muir & G. Wagner,
1978; 550 pages; out of print

No. 27 MOLECULAR AND CELLULAR ASPECTS
OF CARCINOGEN SCREENING TESTS
Edited by R. Montesano, H. Bartsch & L. Tomatis
1980; 371 pages; £22.50

No. 28 DIRECTORY OF ON-GOING RESEARCH
IN CANCER EPIDEMIOLOGY 1979
Edited by C.S. Muir & G. Wagner
1979; 672 pages; out of print

No. 29 ENVIRONMENTAL CARCINOGENS:
SELECTED METHODS OF ANALYSIS
Editor-in-Chief H. Egan
VOLUME 3. ANALYSIS OF POLYCYCLIC
AROMATIC HYDROCARBONS IN
ENVIRONMENTAL SAMPLES
Edited by M. Castegnaro, P. Bogovski, H. Kunte
& E.A. Walker
1979; 240 pages; out of print

No. 30 BIOLOGICAL EFFECTS OF MINERAL
FIBRES
Editor-in-Chief J.C. Wagner
1980; Volume 1, 494 pages; Volume 2, 513 pages;
£55.-

No. 31 N-NITROSO COMPOUNDS: ANALYSIS,
FORMATION AND OCCURRENCE
Edited by E.A. Walker, L. Griciute, M. Castegnaro
& M. Börzsönyi
1980; 841 pages; out of print

No. 32 STATISTICAL METHODS IN CANCER
RESEARCH. VOLUME 1. THE ANALYSIS OF
CASE-CONTROL STUDIES
By N.E. Breslow & N.E. Day
1980; 338 pages; £20.-

No. 33 HANDLING CHEMICAL CARCINOGENS IN
THE LABORATORY: PROBLEMS OF SAFETY
Edited by R. Montesano, H. Bartsch, E. Boyland,
G. Della Porta, L. Fishbein, R.A. Griesemer,
A.B. Swan & L. Tomatis
1979; 32 pages; out of print

No. 34 PATHOLOGY OF TUMOURS IN
LABORATORY ANIMALS. VOLUME III.
TUMOURS OF THE HAMSTER
Editor-in-Chief V.S. Turusov
1982; 461 pages; £32.50

No. 35 DIRECTORY OF ON-GOING RESEARCH
IN CANCER EPIDEMIOLOGY 1980
Edited by C.S. Muir & G. Wagner
1980; 660 pages; out of print

No. 36 CANCER MORTALITY BY OCCUPATION
AND SOCIAL CLASS 1851-1971
By W.P.D. Logan
1982; 253 pages; £22.50

No. 37 LABORATORY DECONTAMINATION
AND DESTRUCTION OF AFLATOXINS
B_1, B_2, G_1, G_2 IN LABORATORY WASTES
Edited by M. Castegnaro, D.C. Hunt, E.B. Sansone,
P.L. Schuller, M.G. Siriwardana, G.M. Telling,
H.P. Van Egmond & E.A. Walker
1980; 59 pages; £6.50

No. 38 DIRECTORY OF ON-GOING RESEARCH
IN CANCER EPIDEMIOLOGY 1981
Edited by C.S. Muir & G. Wagner
1981; 696 pages; out of print

No. 39 HOST FACTORS IN HUMAN
CARCINOGENESIS
Edited by H. Bartsch & B. Armstrong
1982; 583 pages; £37.50

No. 40 ENVIRONMENTAL CARCINOGENS:
SELECTED METHODS OF ANALYSIS
Edited-in-Chief H. Egan
VOLUME 4. SOME AROMATIC AMINES AND
AZO DYES IN THE GENERAL AND INDUSTRIAL
ENVIRONMENT
Edited by L. Fishbein, M. Castegnaro, I.K. O'Neill
& H. Bartsch
1981; 347 pages; £22.50

No. 41 N-NITROSO COMPOUNDS:
OCCURRENCE AND BIOLOGICAL EFFECTS
Edited by H. Bartsch, I.K. O'Neill, M. Castegnaro
& M. Okada
1982; 755 pages; £37.50

No. 42 CANCER INCIDENCE IN FIVE
CONTINENTS. VOLUME IV
Edited by J. Waterhouse, C. Muir,
K. Shanmugaratnam & J. Powell
1982; 811 pages; £37.50

No. 43 LABORATORY DECONTAMINATION
AND DESTRUCTION OF CARCINOGENS IN
LABORATORY WASTES: SOME N-NITROSAMINES
Edited by M. Castegnaro, G. Eisenbrand, G. Ellen,
L. Keefer, D. Klein, E.B. Sansone, D. Spincer,
G. Telling & K. Webb
1982; 73 pages; £7.50

No. 44 ENVIRONMENTAL CARCINOGENS:.
SELECTED METHODS OF ANALYSIS
Editor-in-Chief H. Egan
VOLUME 5. SOME MYCOTOXINS
Edited by L. Stoloff, M. Castegnaro, P. Scott,
I.K. O'Neill & H. Bartsch
1983; 455 pages; £22.50

No. 45 ENVIRONMENTAL CARCINOGENS:
SELECTED METHODS OF ANALYSIS
Editor-in-Chief H. Egan
VOLUME 6. N-NITROSO COMPOUNDS
Edited by R. Preussmann, I.K. O'Neill, G. Eisenbrand,
B. Spiegelhalder & H. Bartsch
1983; 508 pages; £22.50

No. 46 DIRECTORY OF ON-GOING RESEARCH
IN CANCER EPIDEMIOLOGY 1982
Edited by C.S. Muir & G. Wagner
1982; 722 pages; out of print

No. 47 CANCER INCIDENCE IN SINGAPORE
1968-1977
Edited by K. Shanmugaratnam, H.P. Lee & N.E. Day
1982; 171 pages; out of print

No. 48 CANCER INCIDENCE IN THE USSR
Second Revised Edition
Edited by N.P. Napalkov, G.F. Tserkovny,
V.M. Merabishvili, D.M. Parkin, M. Smans & C.S. Muir,
1983; 75 pages; £12.-

No. 49 LABORATORY DECONTAMINATION AND
DESTRUCTION OF CARCINOGENS IN
LABORATORY WASTES: SOME POLYCYCLIC
AROMATIC HYDROCARBONS
Edited by M. Castegnaro, G. Grimmer, O. Hutzinger,
W. Karcher, H. Kunte, M. Lafontaine, E.B. Sansone,
G. Telling & S.P. Tucker
1983; 81 pages; £9.-

No. 50 DIRECTORY OF ON-GOING RESEARCH
IN CANCER EPIDEMIOLOGY 1983
Edited by C.S. Muir & G. Wagner
1983; 740 pages; out of print

No. 51 MODULATORS OF EXPERIMENTAL
CARCINOGENESIS
Edited by V. Turusov & R. Montesano
1983; 307 pages; £22.50

No. 52 SECOND CANCER IN RELATION TO
RADIATION TREATMENT FOR CERVICAL
CANCER
Edited by N.E. Day & J.D. Boice, Jr
1984; 207 pages; £20.-

No. 53 NICKEL IN THE HUMAN ENVIRONMENT
Editor-in-Chief F.W. Sunderman, Jr
1984: 530 pages; £32.50

No. 54 LABORATORY DECONTAMINATION
AND DESTRUCTION OF CARCINOGENS IN
LABORATORY WASTES: SOME HYDRAZINES
Edited by M. Castegnaro, G. Ellen, M. Lafontaine,
H.C. van der Plas, E.B. Sansone & S.P. Tucker
1983; 87 pages; £9.-

No. 55 LABORATORY DECONTAMINATION
AND DESTRUCTION OF CARCINOGENS IN
LABORATORY WASTES: SOME N-NITROSAMIDES
Edited by M. Castegnaro, M. Benard,
L.W. van Broekhoven, D. Fine, R. Massey,
E.B. Sansone, P.L.R. Smith, B. Spiegelhalder,
A. Stacchini, G. Telling & J.J. Vallon
1984; 65 pages; £7.50

No. 56 MODELS, MECHANISMS AND ETIOLOGY
OF TUMOUR PROMOTION
Edited by M. Börszönyi, N.E. Day, K. Lapis
& H. Yamasaki
1984; 532 pages; £32.50

No. 57 N-NITROSO COMPOUNDS:
OCCURRENCE, BIOLOGICAL EFFECTS
AND RELEVANCE TO HUMAN CANCER
Edited by I.K. O'Neill, R.C. von Borstel, C.T. Miller,
J. Long & H. Bartsch
1984; 1011 pages; £80.-

No. 58 AGE-RELATED FACTORS IN
CARCINOGENESIS
Edited by A. Likhachev, V. Anisimov & R. Montesano
1985; 288 pages; £20.-

No. 59 MONITORING HUMAN EXPOSURE TO
CARCINOGENIC AND MUTAGENIC AGENTS
Edited by A. Berlin, M. Draper, K. Hemminki
& H. Vainio
1984; 457 pages; £27.50

No. 60 BURKITT'S LYMPHOMA: A HUMAN
CANCER MODEL
Edited by G. Lenoir, G. O'Conor & C.L.M. Olweny
1985; 484 pages; £22.50

No. 61 LABORATORY DECONTAMINATION
AND DESTRUCTION OF CARCINOGENS IN
LABORATORY WASTES: SOME HALOETHERS
Edited by M. Castegnaro, M. Alvarez, M. Iovu,
E.B. Sansone, G.M. Telling & D.T. Williams
1984; 53 pages; £7.50

No. 62 DIRECTORY OF ON-GOING RESEARCH
IN CANCER EPIDEMIOLOGY 1984
Edited by C.S. Muir & G. Wagner
1984; 728 pages; £26.-

No. 63 VIRUS-ASSOCIATED CANCERS IN AFRICA
Edited by A.O. Williams, G.T. O'Conor, G.B. de-Thé
& C.A. Johnson
1984; 774 pages; £22.-

No. 64 LABORATORY DECONTAMINATION
AND DESTRUCTION OF CARCINOGENS IN
LABORATORY WASTES: SOME AROMATIC
AMINES AND 4-NITROBIPHENYL
Edited by M. Castegnaro, J. Barek, J. Dennis,
G. Ellen M. Klibanov, M. Lafontaine, R. Mitchum,
P. Van Loosmalen, E.B. Sansone, L.A. Sternson
& M. Vahl
1985; 85 pages; £6.95

No. 65 INTERPRETATION OF NEGATIVE
EPIDEMIOLOGICAL EVIDENCE FOR
CARCINOGENICITY
Edited by N.J. Wald & R. Doll
1985; 232 pages; £20.-

No. 66 THE ROLE OF THE REGISTRY IN
CANCER CONTROL
Edited by D.M. Parkin, G. Wagner & C. Muir
1985; 152 pages; £10.-

No. 67 TRANSFORMATION ASSAY OF
ESTABLISHED CELL LINES: MECHANISMS
AND APPLICATION
Edited by T. Kakunaga & H. Yamasaki
1985; 225 pages; £20.-

No. 68 ENVIRONMENTAL CARCINOGENS:
SELECTED METHODS OF ANALYSIS
VOLUME 7. SOME VOLATILE HALOGENATED
HYDROCARBONS
Edited by L. Fishbein & I.K. O'Neill
1985; 479 pages; £20.-

No. 69 DIRECTORY OF ON-GOING RESEARCH
IN CANCER EPIDEMIOLOGY 1985
Edited by C.S. Muir & G. Wagner
1985; 756 pages; £22.

No. 70 THE ROLE OF CYCLIC NUCLEIC ACID
ADDUCTS IN CARCINOGENESIS AND
MUTAGENESIS
Edited by B. Singer & H. Bartsch
1986; 467 pages; £40.-

No. 71 ENVIRONMENTAL CARCINOGENS:
SELECTED METHODS OF ANALYSIS
VOLUME 8. SOME METALS: As, Be, Cd, Cr, Ni,
Pb, Se, Zn
Edited by I.K. O'Neill, P. Schuller & L. Fishbein
1986; 485 pages; £20.

No. 72 ATLAS OF CANCER IN SCOTLAND
1975-1980: INCIDENCE AND EPIDEMIOLOGICAL
PERSPECTIVE
Edited by I. Kemp, P. Boyle, M. Smans & C. Muir
1985; 282 pages; £35.-

No. 73 LABORATORY DECONTAMINATION
AND DESTRUCTION OF CARCINOGENS IN
LABORATORY WASTES: SOME
ANTINEOPLASTIC AGENTS
Edited by M. Castegnaro, J. Adams, M. Armour,
J. Barek, J. Benvenuto, C. Confalonieri, U. Goff,
S. Ludeman, D. Reed, E.B. Sansone & G. Telling
1985; 163 pages; £10.-

No. 74 TOBACCO: A MAJOR INTERNATIONAL
HEALTH HAZARD
Edited by D. Zaridze & R. Peto
1986; 324 pages; £20.-

No. 75 CANCER OCCURRENCE IN DEVELOPING
COUNTRIES
Edited by D.M. Parkin
1986; 339 pages; £20.-

No. 76 SCREENING FOR CANCER OF THE
UTERINE CERVIX
Edited by M. Hakama, A.B. Miller & N.E. Day
1986; 315 pages; £25.-

No. 77 HEXACHLOROBENZENE: PROCEEDINGS
OF AN INTERNATIONAL SYMPOSIUM
Edited by C.R. Morris & J.R.P. Cabral
1986; 668 pages; £50.-

No. 78 CARCINOGENICITY OF ALKYLATING
CYTOSTATIC DRUGS
Edited by D. Schmähl & J. M. Kaldor
1986; 338 pages; £25.-

No. 79 STATISTICAL METHODS IN CANCER
RESEARCH. VOLUME III. THE DESIGN AND
ANALYSIS OF LONG-TERM ANIMAL
EXPERIMENTS
By J.J. Gart, D. Krewski, P.N. Lee, R.E. Tarone
& J. Wahrendorf
1986; 219 pages; £20.-

No. 80 DIRECTORY OF ON-GOING RESEARCH
IN CANCER EPIDEMIOLOGY 1986
Edited by C.S. Muir & G. Wagner
1986; 805 pages; £22.-

No. 81 ENVIRONMENTAL CARCINOGENS:
METHODS OF ANALYSIS AND EXPOSURE
MEASUREMENT. VOLUME 9. PASSIVE
SMOKING
Edited by I.K. O'Neill, K.D. Brunnemann,
B. Dodet & D. Hoffmann
1987; 379 pages; £30.-

No. 82 STATISTICAL METHODS IN CANCER
RESEARCH. VOLUME II. THE DESIGN AND
ANALYSIS OF COHORT STUDIES
By N.E. Breslow & N.E. Day
1987; 404 pages; £30.-

No. 83 LONG-TERM AND SHORT-TERM
ASSAYS FOR CARCINOGENS: A CRITICAL
APPRAISAL
Edited by R. Montesano, H. Bartsch, H. Vainio,
J. Wilbourn & H. Yamasaki
1986; 575 pages; £32.50

No. 84 THE RELEVANCE OF N-NITROSO
COMPOUNDS TO HUMAN CANCER:
EXPOSURES AND MECHANISMS
Edited by H. Bartsch, I.K. O'Neill
& R. Schulte-Hermann
1987; 671 pages; £50.-

SCIENTIFIC PUBLICATIONS SERIES

IARC MONOGRAPHS ON THE EVALUATION OF THE CARCINOGENIC RISK OF CHEMICALS TO HUMANS

(English editions only)

(Available from booksellers through the network of WHO Sales Agents*)

Volume 1
Some inorganic substances, chlorinated hydrocarbons, aromatic amines, N-nitroso compounds, and natural products
1972; 184 pages; out of print

Volume 2
Some inorganic and organometallic compounds
1973; 181 pages; out of print

Volume 3
Certain polycyclic aromatic hydrocarbons and heterocyclic compounds
1973; 271 pages; out of print

Volume 4
Some aromatic amines, hydrazine and related substances, N-nitroso compounds and miscellaneous alkylating agents
1974; 286 pages;
Sw. fr. 18.-

Volume 5
Some organochlorine pesticides
1974; 241 pages; out of print

Volume 6
Sex hormones
1974; 243 pages;
out of print

Volume 7
Some anti-thyroid and related substances, nitrofurans and industrial chemicals
1974; 326 pages; out of print

Volume 8
Some aromatic azo compounds
1975; 357 pages; Sw.fr. 36.-

Volume 9
Some aziridines, N-, S- and O-mustards and selenium
1975; 268 pages; Sw. fr. 27.-

Volume 10
Some naturally occurring substances
1976; 353 pages; out of print

Volume 11
Cadmium, nickel, some epoxides, miscellaneous industrial chemicals and general considerations on volatile anaesthetics
1976; 306 pages; out of print

Volume 12
Some carbamates, thiocarbamates and carbazides
1976; 282 pages; Sw. fr. 34.-

Volume 13
Some miscellaneous pharmaceutical substances
1977; 255 pages; Sw. fr. 30.-

Volume 14
Asbestos
1977; 106 pages; out of print

Volume 15
Some fumigants, the herbicides 2,4-D and 2,4,5-T, chlorinated dibenzodioxins and miscellaneous industrial chemicals
1977; 354 pages; Sw. fr. 50.-

Volume 16
Some aromatic amines and related nitro compounds — hair dyes, colouring agents and miscellaneous industrial chemicals
1978; 400 pages; Sw. fr. 50.-

Volume 17
Some N-nitroso compounds
1978; 365 pages; Sw. fr. 50.

Volume 18
Polychlorinated biphenyls and polybrominated biphenyls
1978; 140 pages; Sw. fr. 20.-

Volume 19
Some monomers, plastics and synthetic elastomers, and acrolein
1979; 513 pages; Sw. fr. 60.-

Volume 20
Some halogenated hydrocarbons
1979; 609 pages; Sw. fr. 60.-

Volume 21
Sex hormones (II)
1979; 583 pages; Sw. fr. 60.-

Volume 22
Some non-nutritive sweetening agents
1980; 208 pages; Sw. fr. 25.-

Volume 23
Some metals and metallic compounds
1980; 438 pages; Sw. fr. 50.-

Volume 24
Some pharmaceutical drugs
1980; 337 pages; Sw. fr. 40.-

Volume 25
Wood, leather and some associated industries
1981; 412 pages; Sw. fr. 60.-

Volume 26
Some antineoplastic and immunosuppressive agents
1981; 411 pages; Sw. fr. 62.-

*A list of these Agents may be obtained by writing to the World Health Organization, Distribution and Sales Service, 1211 Geneva 27, Switzerland

IARC MONOGRAPHS SERIES

Volume 27
Some aromatic amines, anthraquinones and nitroso compounds, and inorganic fluorides used in drinking-water and dental preparations
1982; 341 pages; Sw. fr. 40.-

Volume 28
The rubber industry
1982; 486 pages; Sw. fr. 70.-

Volume 29
Some industrial chemicals and dyestuffs
1982; 416 pages; Sw. fr. 60.-

Volume 30
Miscellaneous pesticides
1983; 424 pages; Sw. fr. 60.-

Volume 31
Some food additives, feed additives and naturally occurring substances
1983; 14 pages; Sw. fr. 60.-

Volume 32
Polynuclear aromatic compounds, Part 1, Chemical, environmental and experimental data
1984; 477 pages; Sw. fr. 60.-

Volume 33
Polynuclear aromatic compounds, Part 2, Carbon blacks, mineral oils and some nitroarenes
1984; 245 pages; Sw. fr. 50.-

Volume 34
Polynuclear aromatic compounds, Part 3, Industrial exposures in aluminium production, coal gasification, coke production, and iron and steel founding
1984; 219 pages; Sw. fr. 48.-

Volume 35
Polynuclear aromatic compounds, Part 4, Bitumens, coal-tars and derived products, shale-oils and soots
1985; 271 pages; Sw. fr.70.-

Volume 36
Allyl compounds, aldehydes, epoxides and peroxides
1985; 369 pages; Sw. fr. 70.-

Volume 37
Tobacco habits other than smoking; betel-quid and areca-nut chewing; and some related nitrosamines
1985; 291 pages; Sw. fr. 70.-

Volume 38
Tobacco smoking
1986; 421 pages; Sw. fr. 75.-

Volume 39
Some chemicals used in plastics and elastomers
1986; 403 pages; Sw. fr. 60.-

Volume 40
Some naturally occurring and synthetic food components, furocoumarins and ultraviolet radiation
1986; 444 pages; Sw. fr. 65.-

Volume 41
Some halogenated hydrocarbons and pesticide exposures
1986; 434 pages; Sw. fr. 65.-

Volume 42
Silica and some silicates
1987; 289 pages; Sw. fr. 65.-

*Volume 43
Man-made mineral fibres and radon
(in press)

Volume 44
Alcohol and alcoholic beverages
(in preparation)

Supplement No. 1
Chemicals and industrial processes associated with cancer in humans (IARC Monographs, Volumes 1 to 20)
1979; 71 pages; out of print

Supplement No. 2
Long-term and short-term screening assays for carcinogens: a critical appraisal
1980; 426 pages; Sw. fr. 40.-

Supplement No. 3
Cross index of synonyms and trade names in Volumes 1 to 26
1982; 199 pages; Sw. fr. 60.-

Supplement No. 4
Chemicals, industrial processes and industries associated with cancer in humans (IARC Monographs, Volumes 1 to 29)
1982; 292 pages; Sw. fr. 60.-

Supplement No. 5
Cross index of synonyms and trade names in Volumes 1 to 36
1985; 259 pages; Sw. fr. 60.-

*Supplement No. 6
Genetic and related effects: An updating of selected IARC Monographs from Volumes 1-42
(in press)

*Supplement No. 7
Overall evaluations of carcinogenicity: An updating of IARC Monographs Volumes 1-42
1987; 440 pages; Sw. fr. 65

---

*From Volume 43 onwards, the series title has been changed to IARC MONOGRAPHS ON THE EVALUATION OF CARCINOGENIC RISKS TO HUMANS

INFORMATION BULLETINS ON THE SURVEY OF CHEMICALS BEING TESTED FOR CARCINOGENICITY

(Available from IARC and WHO Sales Agents)

No. 8 (1979)
Edited by M.-J. Ghess, H. Bartsch
& L. Tomatis
604 pages; Sw. fr. 40.-

No. 9 (1981)
Edited by M.-J. Ghess, J.D. Wilbourn,
H. Bartsch & L. Tomatis
294 pages; Sw. fr. 41.-

No. 10 (1982)
Edited by M.-J. Ghess, J.D. Wilbourn
& H. Bartsch
362 pages; Sw. fr. 42.-

No. 11 (1984)
Edited by M.-J. Ghess, J.D. Wilbourn,
H. Vainio & H. Bartsch
362 pages; Sw. fr. 50.-

No. 12 (1986)
Edited by M.-J. Ghess, J.D. Wilbourn,
A. Tossavainen & H. Vainio
385 pages; Sw. fr. 50.-

NON-SERIAL PUBLICATIONS

(Available from IARC)

ALCOOL ET CANCER
By A. Tuyns (in French only)
1978; 42 pages; Fr. fr. 35.-

CANCER MORBIDITY AND CAUSES OF
DEATH AMONG DANISH BREWERY
WORKERS
By O.M. Jensen
1980; 143 pages; Fr. fr. 75.-

DIRECTORY OF COMPUTER SYSTEMS
USED IN CANCER REGISTRIES
By H.R. Menck & D.M. Parkin
1986; 236 pages; Fr. fr. 50.-

**IARC Monographs are distributed
by the
World Health Organization,
Distribution and Sales Service,
1211 Geneva 27, Switzerland
and are available from booksellers
through the network of WHO Sales Agents.**

**A list of these Agents may be obtained
by writing to the above address.**